Active Commuting and Active Transportation

Active Commuting and Active Transportation

Editor

Adilson Marques

MDPI • Basel • Beijing • Wuhan • Barcelona • Belgrade • Manchester • Tokyo • Cluj • Tianjin

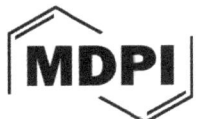

Editor
Adilson Marques
Universidade de Lisboa
Portugal

Editorial Office
MDPI
St. Alban-Anlage 66
4052 Basel, Switzerland

This is a reprint of articles from the Special Issue published online in the open access journal *International Journal of Environmental Research and Public Health* (ISSN 1660-4601) (available at: https://www.mdpi.com/journal/ijerph/special_issues/ACAT).

For citation purposes, cite each article independently as indicated on the article page online and as indicated below:

LastName, A.A.; LastName, B.B.; LastName, C.C. Article Title. *Journal Name* **Year**, *Volume Number*, Page Range.

ISBN 978-3-0365-6149-3 (Hbk)
ISBN 978-3-0365-6150-9 (PDF)

© 2022 by the authors. Articles in this book are Open Access and distributed under the Creative Commons Attribution (CC BY) license, which allows users to download, copy and build upon published articles, as long as the author and publisher are properly credited, which ensures maximum dissemination and a wider impact of our publications.

The book as a whole is distributed by MDPI under the terms and conditions of the Creative Commons license CC BY-NC-ND.

Contents

About the Editor ix

Adilson Marques, Miguel Peralta, Duarte Henriques-Neto, Diana Frasquilho, Élvio Rubio Gouveira and Diego Gomez-Baya
Active Commuting and Depression Symptoms in Adults: A Systematic Review
Reprinted from: *Int. J. Environ. Res. Public Health* **2020**, *17*, 1041, doi:10.3390/ijerph17031041 . . . **1**

Eun Jung Kim, Jiyeong Kim and Hyunjung Kim
Does Environmental Walkability Matter? The Role of Walkable Environment in Active Commuting
Reprinted from: *Int. J. Environ. Res. Public Health* **2020**, *17*, 1261, doi:10.3390/ijerph17041261 . . . **13**

Miguel Peralta, Duarte Henriques-Neto, Joana Bordado, Nuno Loureiro, Susana Diz and Adilson Marques
Active Commuting to School and Physical Activity Levels among 11 to 16 Year-Old Adolescents from 63 Low- and Middle-Income Countries
Reprinted from: *Int. J. Environ. Res. Public Health* **2020**, *17*, 1276, doi:10.3390/ijerph17041276 . . . **31**

João Costa, Manolis Adamakis, Wesley O'Brien and João Martins
A Scoping Review of Children and Adolescents' Active Travel in Ireland
Reprinted from: *Int. J. Environ. Res. Public Health* **2020**, *17*, 2016, doi:10.3390/ijerph17062016 . . . **39**

Eun Jung Kim, Jiyeong Kim and Hyunjung Kim
Neighborhood Walkability and Active Transportation: A Correlation Study in Leisure and Shopping Purposes
Reprinted from: *Int. J. Environ. Res. Public Health* **2020**, *17*, 2178, doi:10.3390/ijerph17072178 . . . **59**

Duarte Henriques-Neto, Miguel Peralta, Susana Garradas, Andreia Pelegrini, André Araújo Pinto, Pedro António Sánchez-Miguel and Adilson Marques
Active Commuting and Physical Fitness: A Systematic Review
Reprinted from: *Int. J. Environ. Res. Public Health* **2020**, *17*, 2721, doi:10.3390/ijerph17082721 . . . **75**

Adilson Marques, Duarte Henriques-Neto, Miguel Peralta, João Martins, Yolanda Demetriou, Dorothea M. I. Schönbach and Margarida Gaspar de Matos
Prevalence of Physical Activity among Adolescents from 105 Low, Middle, and High-Income Countries
Reprinted from: *Int. J. Environ. Res. Public Health* **2020**, *17*, 3145, doi:10.3390/ijerph17093145 . . . **91**

Senlai Zhu, Jie Ma, Tianpei Tang and Quan Shi
A Combined Modal and Route Choice Behavioral Complementarity Equilibrium Model with Users of Vehicles and Electric Bicycles
Reprinted from: *Int. J. Environ. Res. Public Health* **2020**, *17*, 3704, doi:10.3390/ijerph17103704 . . . **103**

Silvia A. González, Olga L. Sarmiento, Pablo D. Lemoine, Richard Larouche, Jose D. Meisel, Mark S. Tremblay, Melisa Naranjo, Stephanie T. Broyles, Mikael Fogelholm, Gustavo A. Holguin, Estelle V. Lambert and Peter T. Katzmarzyk
Active School Transport among Children from Canada, Colombia, Finland, South Africa, and the United States: A Tale of Two Journeys
Reprinted from: *Int. J. Environ. Res. Public Health* **2020**, *17*, 3847, doi:10.3390/ijerph17113847 . . . **121**

Xiaoyu Wang, Jinquan Gong and Chunan Wang
How Does Commute Time Affect Labor Supply in Urban China? Implications for Active Commuting
Reprinted from: *Int. J. Environ. Res. Public Health* **2020**, *17*, 4631, doi:10.3390/ijerph17134631 . . . **143**

Hedwig T. Stenner, Johanna Boyen, Markus Hein, Gudrun Protte, Momme Kück, Armin Finkel, Alexander A. Hanke and Uwe Tegtbur
Everyday Pedelec Use and Its Effect on Meeting Physical Activity Guidelines
Reprinted from: *Int. J. Environ. Res. Public Health* **2020**, *17*, 4807, doi:10.3390/ijerph17134807 . . . **161**

Silvia A. González, Salomé Aubert, Joel D. Barnes, Richard Larouche and Mark S. Tremblay
Profiles of Active Transportation among Children and Adolescents in the Global Matrix 3.0 Initiative: A 49-Country Comparison
Reprinted from: *Int. J. Environ. Res. Public Health* **2020**, *17*, 5997, doi:10.3390/ijerph17165997 . . . **171**

**Gerson Ferrari, André Oliveira Werneck, Danilo Rodrigues da Silva, Irina Kovalskys, Georgina Gómez, Attilio Rigotti, Lilia Yadira Cortés Sanabria, Martha Cecilia Yépez García, Rossina G. Pareja, Marianella Herrera-Cuenca, Ioná Zalcman Zimberg, Viviana Guajardo, Michael Pratt, Cristian Cofre Bolados, Emilio Jofré Saldía, Carlos Pires, Adilson Marques, Miguel Peralta, Eduardo Rossato de Victo, Mauro Fisberg
and on behalf of the ELANS Study Group**
Association between Perceived Neighborhood Built Environment and Walking and Cycling for Transport among Inhabitants from Latin America: The ELANS Study
Reprinted from: *Int. J. Environ. Res. Public Health* **2020**, *17*, 6858, doi:10.3390/ijerph17186858 . . . **201**

Dorothea M. I. Schönbach, Catherina Vondung, Lisan M. Hidding, Teatske M. Altenburg, Mai J. M. Chinapaw and Yolanda Demetriou
Gender Influence on Students, Parents, and Teachers' Perceptions of What Children and Adolescents in Germany Need to Cycle to School: A Concept Mapping Study
Reprinted from: *Int. J. Environ. Res. Public Health* **2020**, *17*, 6872, doi:10.3390/ijerph17186872 . . . **221**

Juan Guzmán Habinger, Javiera Lobos Chávez, Sandra Mahecha Matsudo, Irina Kovalskys, Georgina Gómez, Attilio Rigotti, Lilia Yadira Cortés Sanabria, Martha Cecilia Yépez García, Rossina G. Pareja, Marianella Herrera-Cuenca, Ioná Zalcman Zimberg, Viviana Guajardo, Michael Pratt, Cristian Cofre Bolados, Claudio Farías Valenzuela, Adilson Marques, Miguel Peralta, Ana Carolina B. Leme, Mauro Fisberg, André Oliveira Werneck, Danilo Rodrigues da Silva, Gerson Ferrari and on behalf of the ELANS Study Group
Active Transportation and Obesity Indicators in Adults from Latin America: ELANS Multi-Country Study
Reprinted from: *Int. J. Environ. Res. Public Health* **2020**, *17*, 6974, doi:10.3390/ijerph17196974 . . . **243**

Mabliny Thuany, João Carlos N. Melo, João Pedro B. Tavares, Filipe M. J. Santos, Ellen C. M. Silva, André O. Werneck, Sayuri Dantas, Gerson Ferrari, Thiago H. Sá and Danilo R. Silva
The Profile of Bicycle Users, Their Perceived Difficulty to Cycle, and the Most Frequent Trip Origins and Destinations in Aracaju, Brazil
Reprinted from: *Int. J. Environ. Res. Public Health* **2020**, *17*, 7983, doi:10.3390/ijerph17217983 . . . **255**

Dorota Kleszczewska, Joanna Mazur, Jens Bucksch, Anna Dzielska, Catherina Brindley and Agnieszka Michalska
Active Transport to School May Reduce Psychosomatic Symptoms in School-Aged Children: Data from Nine Countries
Reprinted from: *Int. J. Environ. Res. Public Health* **2020**, *17*, 8709, doi:10.3390/ijerph17238709 . . . **265**

Hamid Mostofi, Houshmand Masoumi and Hans-Liudger Dienel
The Association between the Regular Use of ICT Based Mobility Services and the Bicycle Mode Choice in Tehran and Cairo
Reprinted from: *Int. J. Environ. Res. Public Health* **2020**, *17*, 8767, doi:10.3390/ijerph17238767 . . . **277**

Yuanyuan Guo, Linchuan Yang, Wenke Huang and Yi Guo
Traffic Safety Perception, Attitude, and Feeder Mode Choice of Metro Commute: Evidence from Shenzhen
Reprinted from: *Int. J. Environ. Res. Public Health* **2020**, *17*, 9402, doi:10.3390/ijerph17249402 . . . **297**

Monika Teuber and Gorden Sudeck
Why Do Students Walk or Cycle for Transportation? Perceived Study Environment and Psychological Determinants as Predictors of Active Transportation by University Students
Reprinted from: *Int. J. Environ. Res. Public Health* **2021**, *18*, 1390, doi:10.3390/ijerph18041390 . . . **317**

Antonio Castillo-Paredes, Natalia Inostroza Jiménez, Maribel Parra-Saldías, Ximena Palma-Leal, José Luis Felipe, Itziar Págola Aldazabal, Ximena Díaz-Martínez and Fernando Rodríguez-Rodríguez
Environmental and Psychosocial Barriers Affect the Active Commuting to University in Chilean Students
Reprinted from: *Int. J. Environ. Res. Public Health* **2021**, *18*, 1818, doi:10.3390/ijerph18041818 . . . **343**

Ellen Haug, Otto Robert Frans Smith, Jens Bucksch, Catherina Brindley, Jan Pavelka, Zdenek Hamrik, Joanna Inchley, Chris Roberts, Frida Kathrine Sofie Mathisen and Dagmar Sigmundová
12-Year Trends in Active School Transport across Four European Countries—Findings from the Health Behaviour in School-Aged Children (HBSC) Study
Reprinted from: *Int. J. Environ. Res. Public Health* **2021**, *18*, 2118, doi:10.3390/ijerph18042118 . . . **357**

David Rojas-Rueda
Health Impacts of Urban Bicycling in Mexico
Reprinted from: *Int. J. Environ. Res. Public Health* **2021**, *18*, 2300, doi:10.3390/ijerph18052300 . . . **373**

Linda M. Nguyen and Lieze Mertens
Psychosocial and Social Environmental Factors as Moderators in the Relation between the Objective Environment and Older Adults' Active Transport
Reprinted from: *Int. J. Environ. Res. Public Health* **2021**, *18*, 2647, doi:10.3390/ijerph18052647 . . . **385**

About the Editor

Adilson Marques

Adilson Marques (PhD, MPH) is a professor at the University of Lisbon. His main research interest is the study of health promotion, physical activity, and mental health. He has published several international peer-reviewed original articles and has been an investigator in several research projects. He is a reviewer for several scientific journals in sports science and health promotion. He is a team member of the National Physical Activity Promotion Program at the Portuguese Ministry of Health.

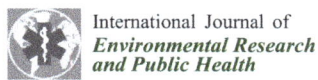 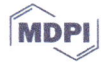

Article

Active Commuting and Depression Symptoms in Adults: A Systematic Review

Adilson Marques [1,2,3,*], Miguel Peralta [1,2], Duarte Henriques-Neto [1], Diana Frasquilho [4], Élvio Rubio Gouveira [5,6] and Diego Gomez-Baya [3,7]

1. CIPER, Faculdade de Motricidade Humana, Universidade de Lisboa, Estrada da Costa, 1499-002 Cruz Quebrada, Portugal; mperalta@fmh.ulisboa.pt (M.P.); duarteneto13@gmail.com (D.H.-N.)
2. ISAMB, Faculdade de Medicina, Universidade de Lisboa, 1649-028 Lisboa, Portugal
3. Escuela de Doctorado, University of Huelva, 21071 Huelva, Spain; diego.gomez@dpee.uhu.es
4. Champalimaud Clinical Center, Champalimaud Centre for the Unknown, Champalimaud Foundation, 1400-038 Lisbon, Portugal; diana.frasquilho@research.fchampalimaud.org
5. Departamento de Educação Física e Desporto, Universidade da Madeira, 9020-105 Funchal, Portugal; erubiog@staff.uma.pt
6. Interactive Technologies Institute, LARSyS, 9020-105 Funchal, Portugal
7. Department of Social, Developmental and Educational Psychology, University of Huelva, 21007 Huelva, Spain
* Correspondence: amarques@fmh.ulisboa.pt; Tel.: (+351)-214149100

Received: 8 January 2020; Accepted: 5 February 2020; Published: 6 February 2020

Abstract: Physical activity (PA) is suggested to have a protective effect against depression. One way of engaging in PA is through active commuting. This review summarises the literature regarding the relationship between active commuting and depression among adults and older adults. A systematic review of studies published up to December 2019, performed in accordance with the Preferred Reporting Items for Systematic Reviews and Meta-Analysis guidelines, was conducted using three databases (PubMed, Scopus, and Web of Science). A total of seven articles were identified as relevant. The results from these studies were inconsistent. Only two presented a significant relationship between active commuting and depression symptoms. In those two studies, switching to more active modes of travel and walking long distances were negatively related to the likelihood of developing new depressive symptoms. In the other five studies, no significant association between active travel or active commuting and depression was found. The relationship between active commuting and depression symptoms in adults is not clear. More studies on this topic are necessary in order to understand if active commuting can be used as a public health strategy to tackle mental health issues such as depression.

Keywords: active travel; walking; cycling; mental health

1. Introduction

Depression is a mental health problem that affects more than 300 million adults worldwide [1]. The prevalence of depression has been rising globally, and it was projected to be the second-largest cause for the burden of disease by 2020 [2]. Depression is already the greatest non-communicable disease contributing to the loss of health [1], due to its association with comorbidities [3], risk of suicide [4], and premature mortality [5]. Most cases of depression are treated using pharmacotherapy and psychotherapy [6,7]. However, both types of therapies are expensive and increase health costs for health care systems [8].

Physical activity (PA) is suggested to have a protective effect against depression and a positive effect on the treatment of depression in non-clinical and clinical populations, regardless of sex and age [9,10]. As non-pharmacology therapy, PA does not show drug side effects such as weight gain, insomnia, dry mouth, or withdrawal symptoms [11]. On the contrary, besides the positive benefits on depression, it is also associated with positive public health gains such as physical performance and cardiovascular improvements [11].

PA can be performed in several contexts, including sports activities, occupational context, leisure-time activities, domestic activities, and in active commuting. For some adults, walking or cycling while commuting to work or to other places seems to be important for enhancing their daily levels of PA [12,13], because is likely to be sustained when incorporated into people's daily routine [14]. As a result, active commuting has been related to health and wellbeing improvement [15,16] and associated with fewer transport-related carbon emissions [17]. Thus, it can be expected that commuting actively might also be related to depression symptoms. However, so far, there is no clear evidence of the relationship between active travel or active commuting and depression symptoms. Therefore, the purpose of this study was to review the literature regarding the relationship between PA in active commuting and depression among adults and older adults.

2. Materials and Methods

This systematic review was performed in accordance with the Preferred Reporting Items for Systematic Reviews and Meta-Analysis (PRISMA) guidelines [18].

2.1. Inclusion Criteria

Articles that presented a relationship between active travel and active commuting and depression symptoms published in peer-reviewed journals up to December 2019 were eligible for inclusion. Eligibility criteria included the following: (1) cross-sectional, prospective, and cohort studies (study design criterion); (2) outcomes included depression or depressive symptoms (outcome measure criterion); (3) active travel or active commuting (relationship criterion); (4) adults and older adults (participants criterion); (5) articles published in English, Portuguese, or Spanish (language criterion); and (6) articles that did not meet the inclusion criteria or did not include findings related to the inclusion criteria were excluded (exclusion criteria).

2.2. Search Strategy

Studies published up to December 2019 were identified by searching in electronic databases. The search was undertaken in the PubMed, Scopus, and Web of Science databases. Articles that assessed the relationship between active travel or active commuting and depression were included in this review. The search was performed using the following combination of terms: travel* OR transport* OR commute* OR cycle OR cycling OR bicycle* OR bike* OR walk* OR/AND depress* OR mental health OR psychological health OR anxiety OR psychological function*. Search terms were defined previously and used in each database to identify articles for review. Two reviewers (A.M. and M.P.) independently screened titles and abstracts to identify studies that met the inclusion criteria. Duplicate articles were removed. Relevant articles were retrieved for a full read. Two authors (A.M. and M.P.) reviewed the full text of potential studies, and decisions to include or exclude studies in the review were made by consensus. Disagreements were solved by consensus and, when necessary, a third reviewer served as a judge (D.H.-N. or D.F.).

2.3. Data Extraction and Harmonisation

Based on PRISMA [18], a data extraction form was developed. The following information was extracted from each article: authors' name and year of publication; study design; country; sample characteristics (number of participants, sex, and age); the instrument for assessing depression symptoms; the instrument for assessing active travel or active commuting; main results; and study quality. The extraction was performed by one author (A.M.), and coding was verified by two authors (M.P. and D.H.-N.).

2.4. Study Quality and Risk of Bias

Study methodological quality was assessed using a checklist criteria from the Quality Assessment Tool for Quantitative Studies [19]. The checklist comprises 19 items, assessing eight methodological domains: selection bias, study design, confounders, blinding, data collection methods, withdrawals and dropouts, intervention integrity, and analyses. Each section is classified as strong, moderate, and with weak methodological quality. Then, a global rating is determined based on the scores of each component. Two researchers rated the articles (M.P. and D.F.) in each domain and the studies' overall quality. Discrepancies were resolved by consensus.

2.5. Synthesis of Results

This review analysed the relationship between active travel or active commuting and depression. The details for each study, including design, participant characteristics and sample size, measures, main results, and study quality, are presented in a consistent manner.

3. Results

3.1. Search Results

Figure 1 presents the flow citation through the systematic review process. The systematic search yielded 3938 publications. After excluding the duplicates (*n* = 2246), the title and abstract of 1692 articles were screened. After eliminating 1606 articles at the title and abstract level, 86 articles remained and were subsequently read. From the 86 articles, 35 were eliminated for having a different outcome, 40 were eliminated because they were not focused on active travel or active commuting, three were eliminated for not being empirical studies, and one was deleted because it was written in Mandarin. Thus, seven articles were identified as relevant.

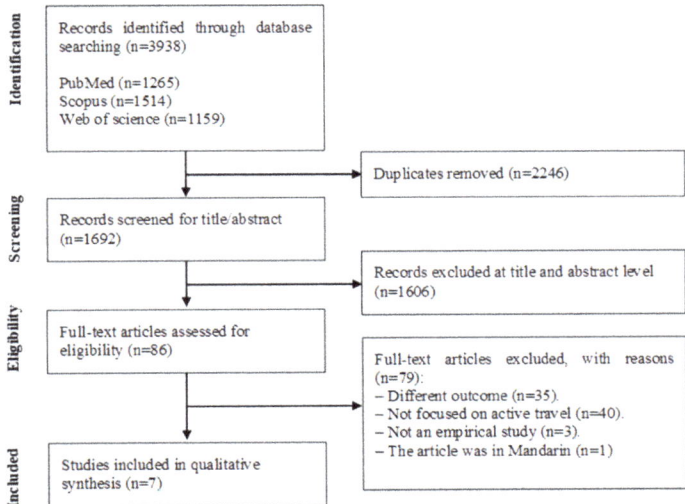

Figure 1. Flow diagram of study selection.

3.2. Study Characteristics

Table 1 presents the studies' characteristics. From the seven articles, five had prospective designs and two had cross-sectional designs. In total, all studies combined included 47,300 adults aged over 18 years. Geographically, two were performed in the United States; two in Japan; one in Canada; one in the United Kingdom; and one in several Latin American countries (Argentina, Bolivia, Brazil,

Colombia, Ecuador, México, Panamá, Peru, Uruguay, and Venezuela). The Center for Epidemiologic Studies Depression Scale (CES-D) was the most used scale to assess depression symptoms (in five articles). In most articles, the walking distance was self-reported and included leisure time and active commuting. The seven studies were considered of moderate quality.

The older study included in the systematic review was published in 2010, and it examined the effect of walking on incident depressive symptoms in Japanese-American older men with and without chronic disease [20]. The authors used a cohort of men from Hawaii born between 1900 and 1919. Several rounds of examinations were performed; the seventh (which was used in the study) was in 1999–2000. The CES-D 11 scale was used to screen for depressive symptoms, and walking activity was self-reported. It was found that older men, without chronic diseases, in the intermediate (odds ratio (OR) = 0.52, 95% confidence interval (CI): 0.32–0.83) and highest (OR = 0.61, 95% CI: 0.39–0.97) walking groups had significantly lower odds of developing eight-year incident depressive symptoms.

Posteriorly, using a one-year follow-up longitudinal survey, Kai et al. [21] examined the prospective association of walking to work with depressive symptoms among 634 Japanese workers. Depression symptoms were screened by the CES-D scale, and walking activity was self-reported. The authors reported that baseline mean walking to work time was 29.2 ± 18.0 min per day. Walking to work tertiles were calculated; mean values of the low, medium, and high walking to work time tertiles were 13.8 ± 7.0, 29.6 ± 1.9, and 49.7 ± 16.1, respectively. No significant association was found between the depressive symptoms and tertiles of walking to work duration.

In an effort to determine whether walking or depressive symptoms were the stronger predictor of each other, Julien et al. [22] examined the longitudinal associations between walking and depressive symptoms in a population-based sample of 498 Canadian urban-dwelling older adults. Four repeated measures over a five-year period were performed. The geriatric depression scale was used to assess depressive symptoms, and walking was self-reported. Although depressive symptoms predicted walking frequency, walking frequency did not predict depressive symptoms at subsequent time points.

Later, a cross-sectional study based on the National Survey of American Life investigated the odds of having depressive symptoms accordingly to walking frequency in 2978 African-American adults [23]. Walking was measured by self-reported frequency, and depressive symptoms were measured with modified versions of the CES-D scale. In this study, women who reported walking often presented lower odds for depressive symptoms than women who reported never walking (OR = 0.56, 95% CI: 0.38–0.82); however, no significant results were found for men.

In the same year, Kuwahara et al. [24] published a cohort study of 29,082 Japanese workers, examining the prospective associations of physical activity during commuting with the risk of depressive symptoms. During a mean follow-up of 4.7 years, 6177 adults developed depressive symptoms. Physical activity and depressive symptoms (similar to the CES-D scale) were assessed by a self-reported questionnaire. The hazard ratio (HR) for individuals who stand or walk during work was 0.86 (95% CI: 0.81–0.92) compared with sedentary workers. However, walking to and from work was not found to be associated with the risk of depressive symptoms.

More recently, Knott et al. [25] examined whether changes in commute mode were associated with differences in the severity of depressive symptoms in 5474 working adults from the United Kingdom in a population-base prospective cohort study (mean follow-up, 4.65 years). Mode, frequency, and distance of commuting to work were self-reported. The severity of depressive symptoms was assessed using the two-item Patient Health Questionnaire. Baseline asymptomatic adults who altered from inactive to active commuting to work reported less severe symptoms at follow-up than those who remained inactive (β = −0.10, 95% CI: −0.20–0.00). However, among baseline symptomatic adults, longer trips for work were associated with worse symptoms at follow-up (β = 0.64, 95% CI: 0.13–1.16).

The most recent study examined the cross-sectional associations between commute patterns and mental health in 5438 adults using survey data from 11 Latin American cities [26]. Commuting was self-reported, and depression was measured using the CES-D scale. No association was found between non-motorised modes of travel and depression.

Table 1. Characteristics of the studies.

Author, Year	Study Design	Sample and Country	Depression Measure	Active Commuting Measure	Observations	Main Results	Methodological Quality
Smith et al., 2010	Prospective cohort.	n = 3196 Japanese-American men who were involved in the Honolulu Heart Program aged 71–93 years; mean age 77 years. United States.	Center for Epidemiologic Studies Depression Scale (CES-D 11)	Participants reported how many city blocks they walked each day. Blocks were converted into miles using 12 blocks per mile as a conversion factor. This assessment was developed from the Harvard Alumni Survey.	Walking distance included leisure-time and active commuting.	Those who walked more had significantly lower rates of prevalent depressive symptoms in cross-sectional analyses. Elderly men, without chronic diseases, who walked longer distances per day were less likely to develop new depressive symptoms over eight years of follow-up.	Moderate
Kai et al., 2011	Prospective (1-year follow-up).	n = 634: 536 men, 98 women aged 20–60 years; 36.7 ± 9.2 years. Japan.	Center for Epidemiologic Studies Depression Scale (CES-D)	The duration of leisure-time physical activity and commuting by walking were measured using a self-report questionnaire.	Walking distance included leisure-time physical activity and commuting to work.	The adjusted odds ratio (OR) of depressive symptoms in the highest tertile of leisure-time physical activity was 50% lower (OR = 0.50, 95% CI: 0.26–0.97) than those in the lowest tertile. In contrast, no significant association was found between the risk of depressive symptoms and duration of commuting by walking.	Moderate
Julien et al., 2013	Prospective (5-years follow-up). VoisiNuAge Study.	n = 498: 236 men, 262 women aged 68–84 years (74.86 ± 4.18 men and 74.90 ± 3.97 women). Canada.	Geriatric Depression Scale (GDS)	Physical Activity Scale for the Elderly (PASE).	Walking distance included leisure-time and active commuting.	Depressive symptoms predicted walking frequency (higher depressive symptoms were related to fewer walking days), but walking frequency did not predict depressive symptoms at subsequent time points.	Moderate
Torres at el., 2015	Cross-sectional. National Survey of American Life (NSAL).	n = 2978: 1903 men, 1075 women aged ≥18 years. United states.	Center for Epidemiologic Studies Depression Scale (CES-D)	Walking was measured with responses to one question from the Americans' Changing Lives questionnaire.	Walking distance included leisure-time and active commuting.	Women who reported often walking had lower odds for depressive symptoms than women who reported never walking (OR = 0.56, 95% CI: 0.38–0.82). Walking frequency was not related to depressive symptoms in men.	Moderate

Table 1. *Cont.*

Author, Year	Study Design	Sample and Country	Depression Measure	Active Commuting Measure	Observations	Main Results	Methodological Quality
Kuwahara et al., 2015	Prospective (5-year follow-up). Japan Epidemiology Collaboration on Occupational Health (J-ECOH) Study.	n = 29,082 workers: 24,676 men, 4406 women aged 20–64 years; mean age 42.7 years. Japan.	Epidemiologic Studies Depression Scale (CES-D), Self-Rating Depression Scale (SDS)	Participants were asked whether they regularly engaged in any physical activity during leisure. Duration of walking to and from work was self-reported and categorised as <20 minutes, 20–40 min, and ≥ 40 min.	It assessed leisure-time physical activity, physical activity at work, and active commuting.	Leisure exercise showed a U-shaped association with the risk of depressive symptoms. Walking to and from work was not associated with depressive symptoms.	Moderate
Knott et al., 2018	Population-based prospective cohort. UK Biobank.	n = 5474, aged 37–73 years. United Kingdom.	Patient Health Questionnaire (PHQ-2)	Participants reported the frequency of trips from home to work (trips/week); the distance travelled (miles); and the mode of transport used ("car or motor vehicle" (hereafter "car" for simplicity), "public transport", and "walk" and/or "cycle").	Paper was focused on modes of travel to work.	Participants who were asymptomatic at baseline and switched to more active modes of commuting tended to report a lower severity of symptoms at follow-up than those who continued to travel inactively (β = −0.10, 95% CI: −0.20–0.00). Among commuters who were symptomatic at baseline, longer journeys were associated with worse symptoms at follow-up (β = 0.64, 95% CI: 0.13–1.16). Shifting from exclusive car use towards more active commuting may help prevent and attenuate depressive symptoms in working adults.	Moderate
Wang et al., 2019	Cross-sectional. La Encuesta CAF 2016.	n = 5438. Argentina, Bolivia, Brazil, Colombia, Ecuador, México, Panamá, Peru, Uruguay, and Venezuela.	Center for Epidemiologic Studies Depression Scale (CES-D)	Participants reported commuting time during a "normal day", uncongested commuting time, and travel mode commonly used for the commute.	Different modes of travel were assessed.	Every 10 more minutes of commuting time is associated with a 0.5% (p = 0.011) higher probability of screening positively for depression. There were not found any significant associations between non-motorised modes of travel and depression.	Moderate

4. Discussion

This review summarises studies, published up to December 2019, which met the defined criteria. Seven studies were systematically reviewed to address the relationship between active commuting and depression symptoms. In general, although some studies demonstrate that active commuting might be negatively related to depression symptoms, the evidence suggests that the active commuting and depression relationship is unclear.

From the seven studies screened, only two presented a significant relationship between active commuting and depression symptoms. In those two studies [20,25], switching to more active modes of travel and walking long distances were negatively related to the likelihood of developing new depressive symptoms. When examining the effect of walking on incident depressive symptoms in older men, Smith et al. [20] observed that those who walked more had lower rates of prevalent depressive symptoms and that those with chronic diseases who walked longer distances per day were less likely to develop eight-year incident depressive symptoms. Furthermore, the authors suggested that there seems to be a threshold effect in the protective effect of walking on the development of incident depressive symptoms, as few differences were found between the intermediate and high walking groups. This finding is of importance, especially for older adults who have more difficulties in engaging in high volumes of physical activity. More recently, using data from the UK Biobank, a study investigated whether changes in commute mode were associated with differences in the severity of depressive symptoms [25]. It was found that adults who altered from inactive to active commuting to work reported less severe symptoms at follow-up than those who remained inactive. This suggests that commuting behaviours change matters, and thus, active commuting may be used as an intervention strategy to prevent the development of depressive symptoms. Previous investigations in physical activity have shown that, for health purposes, present behaviours may be more important than past behaviours [27]. Active travel offers a suitable way of integrating PA into daily life, and those who use active modes of commuting have higher levels of PA [12,13]. As a result, people who often use more active ways to travel might have better health status [15–17]. Hypothetically, it means that active commuting can also have a protective effect on depression symptomology or reduce depression symptoms [9,10]. However, different types of PA have different effects on mental health status.

Among adults, there is evidence that leisure-time PA is more related to mental health problems, and specifically to depression, than other forms of PA [28–30]. In five out of seven articles, a significant relationship between active commuting and depression symptoms was not found [21–24,26]. Cross-sectional evidence from two studies showed that the association between active commuting and depression is not consistent. In one study, performed among Latin American adults, it was found that non-motorised modes of travel were not associated with depression [26]. On the other hand, a study among African-American adults reported that, while women who reported walking often presented a lower probability for depressive symptoms than women who reported never walking, the same pattern was not observed in men [23]. In order to prevent an increase in depressive symptoms, physical activity may need to improve fitness [31]. However, walking in many cases is probably not performed at a high enough intensity to improve fitness. This difference between sexes may be due to a large percentage of African-American women being obese and, thus, having lower exercise capacity [23]. This can lead to walking being a more intense physical activity among African-American women compared to African-American men. The other three studies had a longitudinal design and, in general, concluded that walking was not associated with depressive symptoms at follow-up [21,22,24]. In a one-year follow-up longitudinal survey performed among Japanese workers, it was found that depressive symptoms were not associated with tertiles of walking to work durations [21]. Similarly, in a cohort study with a mean follow-up of 4.7 years also among Japanese workers, walking to and from work was not related to the risk of depressive symptoms [24]. Lastly, a study among Canadian older adults verified that, while depressive symptoms predicted walking frequency at subsequent time points, walking frequency did not predict depressive symptoms [22]. The lack of a significant relationship between active commuting and depression symptoms in these articles are in agreement with previous studies among men and women, which showed that walking distance was not related to depression symptoms [32–34]. For those who use an active mode of transportation, transit connectivity matters more for mental health than active travel [26,34]. Furthermore, there is a difference between walking and cycling as a mode of active transportation. Most studies focus on walking as a way of active transportation. Those who usually walk as an active mode of transportation undertake at a lower intensity than cycling [34,35]. This is of particular importance, because PA intensity is a determinant of health. Thus, perhaps in some studies, the level of PA intensity while walking was too low to cause effects on mental health and depression symptoms.

Inconsistent findings identified in this systematic review can be a reflection of the different methodologies used and the different geographical areas and social contexts examined. Measures of active commuting widely varied from study to study, although all were self-reported. Some studies focused on volume [20,21,24], others on frequency [22,23]; one study focused only on the mode of commuting [26] and another one examined the transition from non-active commuting to active commuting [25]. The type of active commuting also differed among studies. Most investigated only walking [20–24], while two studies investigated active commuting without specifying the type [25,26]. Additionally, the context of the commuting was different among studies. Three studies referred to commuting to and from work [21,24,25]. The others did not specify the context of commuting. Due to this, comparability among studies is very limited. Regarding physical activity and active commuting volume and frequency are important information. Results may differ based on these variables. Although some studies examined volume or frequency, they used different time frames. Studies rarely consider both volume and frequency together. Another important aspect for comparability of the results is the type of active commuting, mainly because different types of commuting (e.g., walking versus cycling) have different intensities and volumes associated to them. Future studies should include frequency and volume and be as specific as possible when analysing active commuting. Preferably, similar methods should be used among studies to improve comparability. In addition to the studies being undertaken in different geographic areas and using different ways to measure active transport, it is important to mention that different scales were used to assess symptoms of depression. The use of different scales between the articles may also have contributed to the inconsistency of the results that were observed.

The social and built environment is an important factor to be considered in mental health. The neighbourhood socioeconomic level and built-environment characteristics are associated with a higher probability of screening positively for depression [36]. Walking or cycling in some built-environments can contribute to the development of depression symptoms [26,36]. Furthermore, for some people, active transportation is the only mode of transportation, because they do not have a car or access to mass transit options. In these cases, an active mode of transportation is not an option, it is a mandatory condition. As a result, transport exclusion is associated with social exclusion, which might increment potential mental health problems such as depression [37].

These study review findings should be considered in light of some limitations. Firstly, in all screened articles, the information on commuting and depression was self-reported, which may be subject to bias. Moreover, self-reported PA may have led to overestimates of total PA. Secondly, several articles do not make a clear distinction between active transport as a form of displacement and active transport as a form of leisure (e.g., walking for leisure). This lack of distinction precludes a more rigorous analysis of the relationship between active transport and depression symptoms. Thirdly, some studies were focused on specific populations, such as Japanese-American older men in Hawaii, African-American adults, or workers. This may compromise the generalisability of the results to the general population. Finally, two studies were cross-sectional, which makes it impossible to infer causality. Finally, search terms were selected to identify articles that associate active transportation and depression symptoms. Nevertheless, several articles were subsequently excluded, because neither the title nor abstract contained terms that could be associated with active travel or active commuting.

5. Conclusions

This systematic review shows that the relationship between active commuting and depression symptoms in adults and older adults is inconsistent. Overall, out of seven studies, only two found beneficial effects of active commuting on depression symptoms. Active commuting improves daily PA levels, which is known to be related to depression symptoms. Thus, hypothetically, active commuting could be related to depression. However, five studies did not find a significant relationship between active commuting and depression symptoms. More studies on this topic are necessary in order to understand if active commuting can be used as a public health strategy to tackle mental health problems such as depression. Future studies should include frequency and volume and be as specific as possible when analysing active commuting. Preferably, similar methods should be used among studies to improve comparability. Furthermore, future studies should be more specific regarding the context of commuting.

Author Contributions: Conceptualization, A.M., M.P. and D.H.-N.; methodology, A.M., M.P. and D.H.-N.; software, M.P. and D.H.-N.; validation, A.M. and D.G.-B.; formal analysis, A.M. and D.F.; investigation, A.M. and M.P.; data curation, A.M., M.P. and D.H.-N.; writing—original draft preparation, A.M. and D.F.; writing—review and editing, D.F., É.R.G. and D.G.-B.; and supervision, É.R.G. and D.G.-B. All authors have read and agreed to the published version of the manuscript.

Funding: This research received no external funding.

Conflicts of Interest: The authors declare no conflict of interest.

References

1. WHO. *Depression and Other Common Mental Disorders. Global Health Estimates*; World Health Organization: Geneva, Switzerland, 2017.
2. Chapman, D.P.; Perry, G.S. Depression as a major component of public health for older adults. *Prev. Chronic Dis.* **2008**, *5*, A22. [PubMed]
3. Vancampfort, D.; Correll, C.U.; Galling, B.; Probst, M.; De Hert, M.; Ward, P.B.; Rosenbaum, S.; Gaughran, F.; Lally, J.; Stubbs, B. Diabetes mellitus in people with schizophrenia, bipolar disorder and major depressive disorder: A systematic review and large scale meta-analysis. *World Psychiatry* **2016**, *15*, 166–174. [CrossRef] [PubMed]
4. Ferrari, A.J.; Charlson, F.J.; Norman, R.E.; Patten, S.B.; Freedman, G.; Murray, C.J.; Vos, T.; Whiteford, H.A. Burden of depressive disorders by country, sex, age, and year: Findings from the global burden of disease study 2010. *PLoS Med.* **2013**, *10*, e1001547. [CrossRef] [PubMed]
5. Walker, E.R.; McGee, R.E.; Druss, B.G. Mortality in mental disorders and global disease burden implications: A systematic review and meta-analysis. *JAMA Psychiatry* **2015**, *72*, 334–341. [CrossRef] [PubMed]
6. Karyotaki, E.; Smit, Y.; Holdt Henningsen, K.; Huibers, M.J.; Robays, J.; de Beurs, D.; Cuijpers, P. Combining pharmacotherapy and psychotherapy or monotherapy for major depression? A meta-analysis on the long-term effects. *J. Affect. Disord.* **2016**, *194*, 144–152. [CrossRef] [PubMed]
7. Khan, A.; Faucett, J.; Lichtenberg, P.; Kirsch, I.; Brown, W.A. A systematic review of comparative efficacy of treatments and controls for depression. *PLoS ONE* **2012**, *7*, e41778. [CrossRef]
8. Olfson, M.; Amos, T.B.; Benson, C.; McRae, J.; Marcus, S.C. Prospective service use and health care costs of Medicaid beneficiaries with treatment-resistant depression. *J. Manag. Care Spec. Pharm.* **2018**, *24*, 226–236. [CrossRef]
9. Schuch, F.B.; Vancampfort, D.; Firth, J.; Rosenbaum, S.; Ward, P.B.; Silva, E.S.; Hallgren, M.; Ponce De Leon, A.; Dunn, A.L.; Deslandes, A.C.; et al. Physical activity and incident depression: A meta-analysis of prospective cohort studies. *Am. J. Psychiatry* **2018**, *175*, 631–648. [CrossRef]
10. Rebar, A.L.; Stanton, R.; Geard, D.; Short, C.; Duncan, M.J.; Vandelanotte, C. A meta-meta-analysis of the effect of physical activity on depression and anxiety in non-clinical adult populations. *Health Psychol. Rev.* **2015**, *9*, 366–378. [CrossRef]
11. Tasci, G.; Baykara, S.; Gurok, M.G.; Atmaca, M. Effect of exercise on therapeutic response in depression treatment. *Psychiatry Clin. Psychopharmacol.* **2019**, *29*, 137–143. [CrossRef]

12. Sahlqvist, S.; Song, Y.; Ogilvie, D. Is active travel associated with greater physical activity? The contribution of commuting and non-commuting active travel to total physical activity in adults. *Prev. Med.* **2012**, *55*, 206–211. [CrossRef] [PubMed]
13. Yang, L.; Panter, J.; Griffin, S.J.; Ogilvie, D. Associations between active commuting and physical activity in working adults: Cross-sectional results from the Commuting and Health in Cambridge study. *Prev. Med.* **2012**, *55*, 453–457. [CrossRef] [PubMed]
14. Hillsdon, M.; Thorogood, M. A systematic review of physical activity promotion strategies. *Br. J. Sports Med.* **1996**, *30*, 84–89. [CrossRef] [PubMed]
15. Berglund, E.; Lytsy, P.; Westerling, R. Active traveling and its associations with self-rated health, BMI and physical activity: A comparative study in the adult Swedish population. *Int. J. Environ. Res. Public Health* **2016**, *13*, 455. [CrossRef] [PubMed]
16. Humphreys, D.K.; Goodman, A.; Ogilvie, D. Associations between active commuting and physical and mental wellbeing. *Prev. Med.* **2013**, *57*, 135–139. [CrossRef]
17. Chapman, R.; Keall, M.; Howden-Chapman, P.; Grams, M.; Witten, K.; Randal, E.; Woodward, A. A cost benefit analysis of an active travel intervention with health and carbon emission reduction benefits. *Int. J. Environ. Res. Public Health* **2018**, *15*. [CrossRef]
18. Moher, D.; Liberati, A.; Tetzlaff, J.; Altman, D.G.; Group, P. Preferred reporting items for systematic reviews and meta-analyses: The PRISMA statement. *Ann. Intern. Med.* **2009**, *151*, 264–269. [CrossRef]
19. National Collaborating Centre for Methods and Tools. Quality Assessment Tool for Quantitative Studies Method. Available online: http://www.nccmt.ca/resources/search/14 (accessed on 1 July 2016).
20. Smith, T.L.; Masaki, K.H.; Fong, K.; Abbott, R.D.; Ross, G.W.; Petrovitch, H.; Blanchette, P.L.; White, L.R. Effect of walking distance on 8-year incident depressive symptoms in elderly men with and without chronic disease: The Honolulu-Asia Aging Study. *J. Am. Geriatr. Soc.* **2010**, *58*, 1447–1452. [CrossRef]
21. Kai, Y.; Nagamatsu, T.; Yamaguchi, Y.; Tokushima, S. Effect of leisure-time physical activity and commuting by walking on depressive symptoms among Japanese workers. *Bull. Phys. Fit. Res. Inst.* **2011**, *109*, 1–8.
22. Julien, D.; Gauvin, L.; Richard, L.; Kestens, Y.; Payette, H. Longitudinal associations between walking frequency and depressive symptoms in older adults: Results from the VoisiNuAge study. *J. Am. Geriatr. Soc.* **2013**, *61*, 2072–2078. [CrossRef]
23. Torres, E.R.; Sampselle, C.M.; Neighbors, H.W.; Ronis, D.L.; Gretebeck, K.A. Depressive Symptoms and Walking in African-Americans. *Public Health Nurs.* **2015**, *32*, 381–387. [CrossRef] [PubMed]
24. Kuwahara, K.; Honda, T.; Nakagawa, T.; Yamamoto, S.; Akter, S.; Hayashi, T.; Mizoue, T. Associations of leisure-time, occupational, and commuting physical activity with risk of depressive symptoms among Japanese workers: A cohort study. *Int. J. Behav. Nutr. Phys. Act.* **2015**, *12*, 119. [CrossRef] [PubMed]
25. Knott, C.S.; Panter, J.; Foley, L.; Ogilvie, D. Changes in the mode of travel to work and the severity of depressive symptoms: A longitudinal analysis of UK Biobank. *Prev. Med.* **2018**, *112*, 61–69. [CrossRef] [PubMed]
26. Wang, X.; Rodriguez, D.A.; Sarmiento, O.L.; Guaje, O. Commute patterns and depression: Evidence from eleven Latin American cities. *J. Transp. health* **2019**, *14*. [CrossRef]
27. Marques, A.; Peralta, M.; Martins, J.; de Matos, M.G.; Brownson, R.C. Cross-sectional and prospective relationship between physical activity and chronic diseases in European older adults. *Int. J. Public Health* **2017**, *62*, 495–502. [CrossRef]
28. Lampinen, P.; Heikkinen, R.L.; Ruoppila, I. Changes in intensity of physical exercise as predictors of depressive symptoms among older adults: An eight-year follow-up. *Prev. Med.* **2000**, *30*, 371–380. [CrossRef]
29. Siefken, K.; Junge, A.; Laemmle, L. How does sport affect mental health? An investigation into the relationship of leisure-time physical activity with depression and anxiety. *Hum. Mov.* **2019**, *20*, 62–74. [CrossRef]
30. Joshi, S.; Mooney, S.J.; Kennedy, G.J.; Benjamin, E.O.; Ompad, D.; Rundle, A.G.; Beard, J.R.; Cerda, M. Beyond METs: Types of physical activity and depression among older adults. *Age Ageing* **2016**, *45*, 103–109. [CrossRef]
31. Dishman, R.K.; Sui, X.; Church, T.S.; Hand, G.A.; Trivedi, M.H.; Blair, S.N. Decline in cardiorespiratory fitness and odds of incident depression. *Am. J. Prev. Med.* **2012**, *43*, 361–368. [CrossRef]
32. McKercher, C.M.; Schmidt, M.D.; Sanderson, K.A.; Patton, G.C.; Dwyer, T.; Venn, A.J. Physical activity and depression in young adults. *Am. J. Prev. Med.* **2009**, *36*, 161–164. [CrossRef]

33. Kull, M.; Ainsaar, M.; Kiive, E.; Raudsepp, L. Relationship between low depressiveness and domain specific physical activity in women. *Health Care Women Int.* **2012**, *33*, 457–472. [CrossRef]
34. Mytton, O.T.; Panter, J.; Ogilvie, D. Longitudinal associations of active commuting with wellbeing and sickness absence. *Prev. Med.* **2016**, *84*, 19–26. [CrossRef]
35. Costa, S.; Ogilvie, D.; Dalton, A.; Westgate, K.; Brage, S.; Panter, J. Quantifying the physical activity energy expenditure of commuters using a combination of global positioning system and combined heart rate and movement sensors. *Prev. Med.* **2015**, *81*, 339–344. [CrossRef] [PubMed]
36. Sampson, L.; Martins, S.S.; Yu, S.; Chiavegatto Filho, A.D.P.; Andrade, L.H.; Viana, M.C.; Medina-Mora, M.E.; Benjet, C.; Torres, Y.; Piazza, M.; et al. The relationship between neighborhood-level socioeconomic characteristics and individual mental disorders in five cities in Latin America: Multilevel models from the World Mental Health Surveys. *Soc. Psychiatry Psychiatr. Epidemiol.* **2019**, *54*, 157–170. [CrossRef] [PubMed]
37. Lucas, K. Transport and social exclusion: Where are we now? *Transp. Policy* **2012**, *20*, 105–113. [CrossRef]

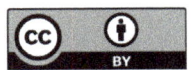

© 2020 by the authors. Licensee MDPI, Basel, Switzerland. This article is an open access article distributed under the terms and conditions of the Creative Commons Attribution (CC BY) license (http://creativecommons.org/licenses/by/4.0/).

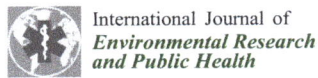

Article

Does Environmental Walkability Matter? The Role of Walkable Environment in Active Commuting

Eun Jung Kim [1], Jiyeong Kim [1] and Hyunjung Kim [2,*]

1. Department of Urban Planning, Keimyung University, 1095 Dalgubeol-daero, Dalseo-gu, Daegu 42601, Korea; kimej@kmu.ac.kr (E.J.K.); th154@naver.com (J.K.)
2. Department of Civil and Environmental Engineering, Seoul National University, Gwanak-ro 1, Gwanak-gu, Seoul 08826, Korea
* Correspondence: urbanistar@snu.ac.kr; Tel.: +82-2-880-8903

Received: 22 January 2020; Accepted: 14 February 2020; Published: 15 February 2020

Abstract: Since walkability plays an important role in active commuting, several cities are actively promoting its integration into urban and environmental planning policies. This study examined the association between walkability and active commuting in Seoul, Korea. A multilevel logistic regression model was used to examine the correlation between Walkability Score and the probability of active commuting after controlling for individual variables. The analysis used 129,044 individual samples nested within 424 administrative districts (dongs). In this study, three models were tested: Model 1 contained only individual variables, Model 2 contained individual variables and Walkability Score, and Model 3 included neighborhood-level variables in addition to the variables of Model 2. The results showed that the Walkability Score was significantly correlated with the odds of active commuting. Specifically, every additional one-point increase in Walkability Score was associated with 0.3% higher odds of active commuting (Model 2: odds ratio (OR) = 1.003, 95% confidence interval (CI) = 1.001–1.005; Model 3: OR = 1.003, 95% CI = 1.001–1.006). Additionally, public transportation density was also positively correlated with the odds of active commuting. The odds of active commuting were positively correlated with younger age, female, lower-income, and having no car. Based on the findings, policy recommendations in urban planning and design, transport engineering, and environmental planning are provided.

Keywords: active commuting; walking; cycling; Walk Score; Walkability Score, multilevel logistic regression model; geographic information system (GIS); Seoul

1. Introduction

Active commuting (e.g., walking and cycling to work or school) has numerous advantages. It is a cost-effective transportation mode, being an affordable means of transportation with little maintenance required [1]. Reduced car use due to active commuting can lead to a decrease in air pollution and traffic congestion, and more efficient use of urban land due to a reduction in parking lots [2–4]. Moreover, active commuting has several health benefits, including increasing physical activity [5] and promoting mental health [6–8], and reducing obesity [9], cardiovascular diseases [10–12], type 2 diabetes [13], cancers [10,12], and all-cause mortality [10,14,15]. Avila-Palencia et al. have examined the relationship between bicycle commuters and perceived stress in Barcelona, Spain. After controlling for individual and environmental variables, their study found that bicycle commuters who commuted by bicycle for more than four days a week were less stressed than non-bicycle commuters [6]. Avila-Palencia extended her study with colleagues to test transport mode and mental health and social cohesion in seven European cities. She found that walking was associated with good self-perceived health, higher vitality, and more frequent contact with family/friends, and cycling was correlated with good self-perceived health, higher vitality, less perceived stress and loneliness [7]. Likewise, a study conducted by Zijlema et al. has examined the association between active commuting through natural environments and mental health. They collected data using questionnaires from Spain, the Netherlands, Lithuania, and the United Kingdom, and used multilevel models at the city and neighborhood levels. They found a strong association between active commuting through natural environments and mental health [8].

Several studies have used health outcome variables rather than mental health measures as health indicators. Celis-Morales et al. examined the relationship between active commuting and cardiovascular disease, cancer, and all-cause mortality. They used data from UK Biobank, which was recruited from 22 sites across the UK. They found that active commuting was associated with a lower risk of cardiovascular diseases, cancer, and mortality [10]. Blond and Rasmussen with their colleagues focused on the effects of cycling on health promotion and conducted two empirical studies. They conducted their studies in Danish adults and collected data from the prospective cohort study, "Diet, Cancer, and Health". They found that cycling was associated with lower risks of coronary heart disease [11] and type 2 diabetes [13]. Andersen and colleagues have also focused on cycling as active commuting in Copenhagen, Denmark, and found cycling to work was associated with a lower risk of mortality [14].

Meanwhile, there have been studies that calculated the benefits of active commuting in monetary values. One report from Public Health England estimated that the economic cost of physical inactivity to the National Health Service in England is more than £450 million (approximately US $586 million) a year [16]. The British government has also reported that achieving their policy targets for walking and cycling could save £567 million (approximately US $740 million) a year on air quality [17].

Seoul is the most urbanized city in Korea. It has chronic urban problems typical of several megacities, such as long commuting distance and times, heavy traffic congestion, and severe air pollution, which are mainly caused by high levels of car dependence. The active commuting (e.g., walking and cycling) of Seoul was 28.0% in 2015 of the total commuting trip [18,19], which indicates the majority of commuting in Seoul is dependent on motorized commuting. This is causing societal costs in various areas, including environmental and public health, as discussed earlier. To address this, the city of Seoul recently proposed a number of urban policies to promote walking and cycling. Specifically, Seoul suggested a project titled, "Walkable City, Seoul" and "Two-wheel Seoul", whose main objective is to create a safe and convenient walking and cycling environment not only for reducing social costs by decreasing the number of cars but also to enhance citizens' health. A lot of projects have been promoted since 2016 including "Safe Walking Street for Children" to expend Children Protection Zone and Speeding Warning Signs, and a "Road Diet" project to reduce roadway and expanding the pedestrian road. Also, the city of Seoul is creating a pedestrian-oriented traffic environment thorough maintaining and connecting pedestrian roads. To promote cycling, Seoul is expanding bike-related infrastructure such as cycle lanes and bike-rental stations, and also operating Seoul's public bicycle sharing system, "Ddareungi", to encourage the greater use of bikes as a means of transportation [20].

It is often said that the neighborhood environment is important for promoting active commuting. Some evidence suggests that the built environment is associated with walking and cycling for transportation. A higher level of active commuting is associated with higher levels of street connectivity, population density, mixed land use, and public transportation density [21–26]. More specifically, walkability is positively correlated with walking and cycling by commuters. The walkable environment can help encourage people who commute short distances to walk or cycle. The walkable environment also induces people who commute using public transport to walk or cycle to where they access transportation (e.g., bus stops and subway stations) [25,27,28].

Numerous studies have focused on the measurement of environmental walkability, using objectively measured indices in particular [29–36]. These indices are all measured using geographic information systems (GIS), and the typical ones are Walkability Index, Moveability Index, Walk Score, Pedshed, and Pedestrian Environment Index. The Walkability Index included elements such as residential density, retail floor area ratio, street connectivity, and land-use mix [33,35]. Moveability

Index derived from the concept of the Walkability Index, an index that has been widely used in recent years. This includes elements of street connectivity, destination density, and the level of urbanization [31,32]. Pedshed is another index of walkability for the pedestrian catchment, calculated from the network/Euclidean buffer ratio [30]. The Pedestrian Environment Index is a newly developed index to measure pedestrian friendliness, calculated with four components including land-use mix, population density, commercial density, and intersection density [36].

One such index, Walk Score, is a popular measure which several empirical studies have used [37–40]. The Walk Score calculates access to nine types of utilitarian destinations including grocery stores, restaurants, shopping centers, coffee shops, banks, parks, schools, bookstores, and places of entertainment in a given area. In addition, the area may receive a penalty for having poor pedestrian friendliness (e.g., intersection density and average block length). The final score ranges from 0 (car-dependent) to 100 (walker's paradise) [41]. The Walk Score has the disadvantage of mainly measuring the accessibility of amenities and not measuring the qualitative factors of the urban environment. Therefore, some studies have conducted analyses comparing the Walk Score to other indices to verify its validity and reliability, and found that the Walk Score is suitable for use as a measure of environmental walkability [39,42].

A growing body of literature has found that Walk Score had positive associations with walking in communities [43–48]. Most of these studies have been conducted in the United States and Canada, where Walk Score data is available [49]. Some studies have been conducted to develop data in areas where no data is currently available on the Walk Score website [50]. Reyer et al. assessed the level of walkability in Stuttgart, Germany, using the Walk Score algorithm. They found a significantly positive relationship between Walk Score and active transportation (e.g., the walked distance for transport per week, the minutes of walking for transport per week, and the number of walking trips per week) after controlling for socioeconomic factors at the individual level [48]. Recently, Kim et al. also assessed the walkability level of Seoul, Korea by adapting the Walk Score methodology [51]. They found a positive association between Walk Score (in their study, "Walkability Score") and pedestrian satisfaction.

As in the empirical studies of the United States, Canada, and Germany [43–48], do people who live in areas with a higher level of walkability walk and bike more than those who live in areas with a lower level of walkability in Seoul, Korea? There are some previous studies from Asian countries similar to this topic, however, most focused on either promoting physical activity for older adults [52–55], or using survey/interview-based measurement of walkable environments [56,57]. Most importantly, there has been little research on the association between walkable environments and active commuting. Like Seoul, many Asian cities are in highly dense urban form, and most of the population is concentrated in big cities which leads to lacking space for physical activity. Especially for highly dense cities, promoting active commuting could be a realistic way to prevent physical inactivity. However, objectively measured indices measuring the level of walkability based on the built environment are mostly developed from Western countries, therefore works in Asian countries are lacking in spite of the necessity of investigation. Therefore, we consider our research question is timely and appropriate as the importance of walkable neighborhood environments on promoting a daily based physical activity is arising in literature. The purpose of this study is to examine if the walkable environment correlates with active commuting (e.g., walking and cycling) in Seoul. It also acts as a validation check on the applicability of the Walkability Score for assessing the level of neighborhood walkability in Seoul. In this study, the following hypothesis is tested: *Areas with more walkable environments have correlation with higher odds of walking and cycling to work and school (e.g., active commuting) than areas with less walkable environments.*

2. Materials and Methods

2.1. Study Area

Seoul is the capital of Korea, located in the northwest of the country. It has the highest population density (16,364 persons/km^2) in Korea [58]. Therefore, solving its transportation problems including traffic congestion, air pollution due to heavy traffic is of primary importance. Recently, the city of Seoul has been heavily promoting policies to encourage walking and cycling as one of the city's major issues under the project called "Walkable City, Seoul" [20]. Meanwhile, a recent study has measured the Walkability Score in Seoul [51], while there have been no such cities that have assessed the walkability levels in Korea yet. In other words, since there exists a walkability dataset for Seoul, it is straightforward to conduct research on the city. In addition, it has been more than 3 years since the city of Seoul promoted "Walkable City, Seoul" as one of the major policies, however, there is little research on the correlation between environmental walkability and active commuting in Seoul.

2.2. Variables: Data

2.2.1. Individual-Level Variables

- Outcome measure: travel mode of commuting (non-motorized /motorized commuting)

This study used the 'travel mode to work and school' data from the 2016 Household Travel Diary Survey of the Korea Transport Database as its dependent variable (Table 2). This mode includes commuting transport and is extracted by home-based origin or destination [59]. The Household Travel Diary Survey defines four types of travel purpose: work, school, shopping, and leisure. Only the cases of travel to work and school were extracted, which include walking, cycling, public transit (e.g., bus, subway), and private automobile. This study excluded the cases of a commuter using multiple modes in a trip. We dichotomized the variable into 1 for non-motorized transport ("walking" and "cycling") and 0 for motorized transport ("public transit" and "private automobile"). In total, 129,044 commuter trips were analyzed. Approximately 44.0% of respondents took walking and cycling trips for commuting purposes while the remaining 56.0% used public transport and private automobiles.

- Socioeconomic status

Individual variables included were age, gender (male/female), income level, and car ownership (no/yes), also sourced from the 2016 Household Travel Diary Survey [59]. The mean age was 37.6 (standard deviation (SD) = 15.5) and the mean income level was 4.0, which equates to a monthly income of 3–5 million won (approximately US $2727–4545). Approximately 56.3% of the respondents were male (female: 43.7%), and 71.9% of respondents owned a private automobile.

2.2.2. Neighborhood-Level (Dong-Level) Variables

- Walkability Score (key independent variable)

This study used the Walkability Score from Kim et al. [51] as an independent variable, which measures Seoul's walkability level using the Walk Score algorithm. The Walkability Score was derived by dividing the entirety of Seoul, except for the greenbelt and the Han River, into 100 × 100 m grid cells and calculating the score for a center point of each grid cell. As shown in Table 1, the Walkability Score is derived by considering accessibility to nine amenity facilities and pedestrian friendliness. Information on details such as the calculation method and descriptive statistics of outputs can be found in the study by Kim et al. [51].

Table 1. Categories, measures, and data source for the Walkability Score calculation.

Category	Measure	Data Source
Distance to amenity	Grocery	Seoul Open Data Plaza [60]
	Restaurants	
	Shopping	Road Name Address [61]
	Coffee	Seoul Open Data Plaza [60]
	Banks	National Spatial Data Infrastructure Portal [62]
	Parks	Road Name Address [61]
	Schools	
	Books	
	Entertainment	Website of three major cinemas [63–65], Open Data Portal [66], and Road Name Address [61]
Pedestrian Friendliness	Intersection density	National Spatial Data Infrastructure Portal [62]
	Average block length	

The original contents of this table are came from Walk Score methodology [41] and Table 1 of Kim et al. [51], and they were newly edited here.

Seoul consists of 424 administrative districts ("dong" in Korean), which are used as the neighborhood-level units in this study. The Walkability Score, measured at the grid point-level (N = 44,000), was then aggregated at the dong level (N = 424) for analysis (Figure 1). The mean Walkability Score of the 424 dongs was 68.2 (SD = 9.8; Table 2).

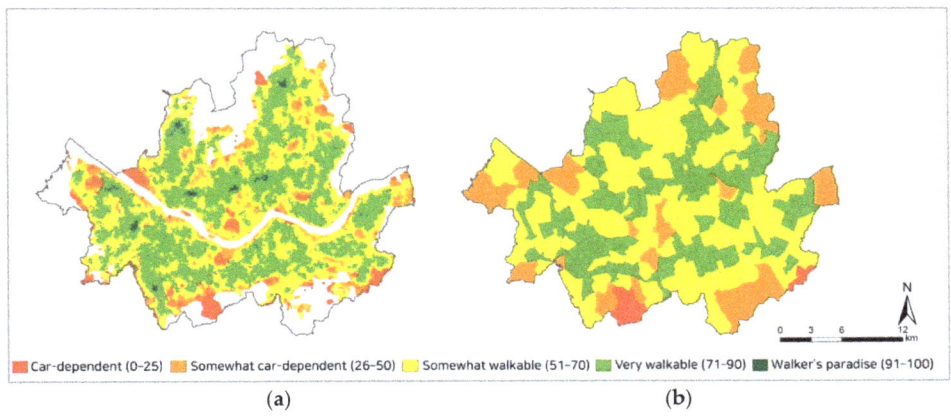

Figure 1. Walkability Score of Seoul: (a) Walkability Score at grid point-level (N = 44,000; Source: [51]); (b) Walkability Score at dong level (N = 424); Areas marked with null values in Figure 1a (greenbelt and Han River) are not included when calculating the Walkability Score for each dong in Figure 1b.

- Additional neighborhood environmental factors

Additional environmental variables analyzed include land use mix, residential density, and public transport density. Some studies have found that land-use mix is significantly associated with walking for transport [26,67]. Therefore, this study included the land-use mix variable that measures the mixture of residential, commercial, industrial, and greenspace. It is measured by an entropy index ranging from 0 to 1, where 0 is single land use and 1 is perfect mixing within the land-use types. Residential density (i.e., number of residential units per square meter) is considered an environmental factor because it is the most commonly used index to measure urban form that is correlated with walking and physical activity [26,68–71]. Public transport use has also been found to contribute to enhanced physical activity [25]. Therefore, public transport destination density (i.e., the number of bus stops and subway stations per square kilometer) was also included as an additional neighborhood environmental factor. Since the density of Seoul is very high, a lot of traffic occurs especially during commuting. Therefore, the city of Seoul has built a very tightly knitted public transportation network in and between bus and subway, and since 2004, the transfer fee between public transportations (e.g., subway to bus, bus to subway) is free of charge [72]. This had led to results in the use of public transportation trips in Seoul; a combination of buses and subways. Therefore, in this study, we calculated public transport density by combining bus stops and subway stations. All environmental variable data were collected in 2017, measured at dong level, and captured using ArcGIS 10.6 (ESRI, Redlands, CA, USA).

Table 2. Measurement, data source, and descriptive statistics of variables.

Variable	Measurement	Data Source	Frequency (%)	Mean (SD)
Dependent Variable				
Travel mode to work and school	Binary: 0 = Motorized commuting (public transport and private automobile), 1 = Non-motorized commuting (walking and cycling)	Household Travel Diary Survey from the Korea Transport Database [59]	56,724 (44.0%) 72,320 (56.0%)	
Individual Variables (Level 1)				
Age	Continuous: Age			37.6 (15.5)
Gender	Binary: 0 = male, 1 = female	Household Travel Diary Survey from the Korea Transport Database [59]	72,638 (56.3%) 56,406 (43.7%)	
Income	Continuous: 1 = less than 1 million won, 2 = 1–2 million won, 3 = 2–3 million won, 4 = 3–5 million won, 5 = 5–10 million won, 6 = more than 10 million won			4.0 (1.0)
Car ownership	Binary: 0 = no, 1 = yes		36,321 (28.1%) 92,723 (71.9%)	
Neighborhood Variables (Level 2; Dong level)				
Walkability Score	Continuous: Walkability Score	Kim et al. [51]		68.2 (9.8)
Land use mix [1]	Continuous: 0 (single use) – 1 (perfect mixing)	National Spatial Data Infrastructure Portal [62]		0.50 (0.3)
Residential density [1]	Continuous: Number of residential units per square kilometer	Statistical Geographic Information Service [73]		94.1 (24.9)
Public transport density [1]	Continuous: Number of public transport destinations (bus stops and subway stations) per square kilometer	Seoul Transport Operation and Information Service [74], Road Name Address [61]		8.3 (2.2)

[1] square root-transformed, SD: standard deviation.

2.3. Analytical Methods

Bivariate analysis was used to compare the differences between variables at the individual level and neighborhood level by Walkability Score. Specifically, the *t*-test was employed for comparison of travel mode types and urban forms between areas with higher walkability and areas with lower walkability. A multilevel logistic model was used to examine the probability of non-motorized commuting transport (e.g., walking and cycling for commuting trips) by considering both individual-level and neighborhood-level (dong-level) variables. The analysis includes 129,044 individual commuters nested within 424 dongs using a two-level structure (individual: level 1, dong: level 2). Two-level logistic regression analysis was performed using R (version 3.6.1).

3. Results

3.1. Bivariate Analyses of Walkability Score and Individual-Level and Neighborhood-Level Variables

3.1.1. Travel Mode Comparison between Groups by Level of Walkability Score

Figure 2 shows the proportion of non-motorized (walking and cycling) and motorized (public transport and private automobile) commuters by the level of Walkability Score in Seoul. As shown in Figure 2a, 56.3% of residents were walkers in very walkable areas, whereas only 52.2% were walkers in car-dependent areas. Similar to this, almost 1.0% of people used a bicycle for commuting in very walkable areas, while nobody (0.0%) cycled in car-dependent areas. The figure shows that the higher the Walkability Score, the higher the proportion of people walking and cycling for commuting purposes.

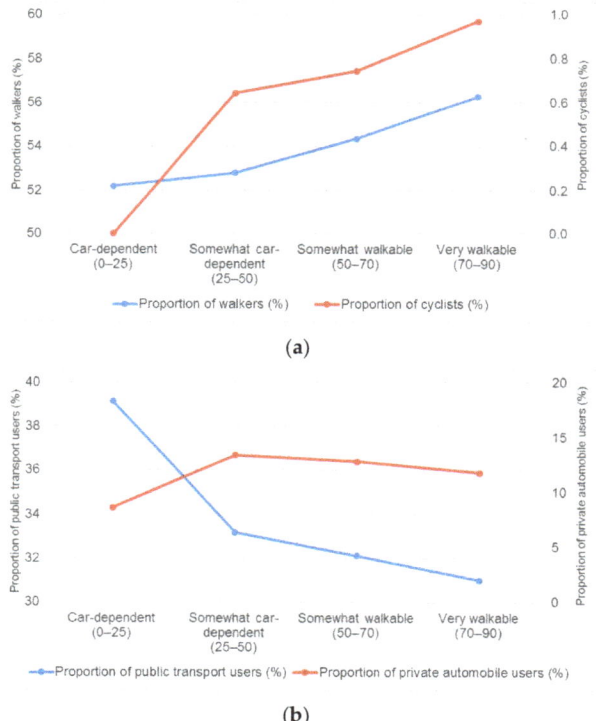

Figure 2. The proportion of (**a**) non-motorized commuters; (**b**) motorized commuters.

Conversely, Figure 2b illustrates that the proportion of public transit users in areas with higher Walkability Score is considerably less than in car-dependent areas. The proportion of public transit users dramatically decreased from 39.2% in car-dependent areas to 31.0% in very walkable areas. For the proportion of private automobile users, an increase from 8.6% in car-dependent areas to 13.3% in somewhat car-dependent areas, followed by a general decline to 11.7% in very walkable areas was found.

3.1.2. *t*-Test for the Comparison between Areas with High Walkability and Low Walkability Scores

As shown in Figure 2, higher proportions of walkers and cyclists in areas with higher Walkability Scores were found than in areas with lower Walkability Scores. However, these results were not statistically significant. Therefore, the mean difference between areas with higher walkability and lower walkability are compared.

To do so, we classified the entirety of Seoul as either more walkable or less walkable. More walkable areas were those with a Walkability Score ≥ 50 (i.e., somewhat walkable and very walkable); less walkable areas were those with a Walkability Score < 50 (i.e., car-dependent and somewhat car-dependent). We then calculated the mean value for each dong. Of the 424 dongs, 395 had a mean Walkability Score of 50 or more, and 29 dongs had a mean Walkability Score of less than 50.

Table 3 shows the results of the *t*-test between the two groups (high Walkability Score vs low Walkability Score). There were significantly more walking trips for commuting purposes in the more walkable areas (55.4%) than those with a less walkable environment (50.5%) at the 0.05 significance level. However, the other three travel modes (cycling, public transport, and private automobile) had no statistical mean differences between areas with high and low Walkability Scores.

Urban form variables of residential density and public transport density in the areas with a more walkable environment (Walkability Score ≥ 50) were significantly higher than those with a less walkable environment (Walkability Score < 50). This is consistent with the results of previous studies [25,26,68–71]. With respect to land use mix, this study found contrasting results with those of other studies [26,67]. Although proper land-use mix is generally known to increase the level of active transport (e.g., walking and cycling), there is some contrary evidence suggesting that mixed-use development in some high-density cities may not always produce a positive effect on walking and cycling activities [75–77]. This is because high-density cities would reduce the chance for people to undertake walking or cycling as people could move easily to another neighborhood by public transportation [75,77]. Seoul is one the high-density cities; while the total area of Seoul constitutes 0.60 % of Korea, the total population was almost 19.04% (the total population of Seoul was 9,857,426) of the national population as of 2017 [78], and having a good public transportation in the neighborhood. This might be applied to Seoul, and our finding could contribute to this contrary evidence showing the areas with higher Walkability Score had lower level of land use mix.

Table 3. *t*-Test results of the comparison between areas with Walkability Score equal or greater than 50 (N = 395) and areas with Walkability Score less than 50 (N = 29).

Variables	Dongs with Walkability Score ≥50 (N = 395)		Dongs with Walkability Score <50 (N = 29)		*p*-Values for Difference	
	Mean	SD	Mean	SD	t	*p*-Value
Travel Mode						
Walking	55.4%	5.9%	50.5%	12.9%	2.1	0.049
Cycling	0.9%	1.0%	0.7%	1.0%	1.1	0.255
Public transport	30.7%	5.3%	32.2%	6.2%	−1.4	0.149
Private automobile	13.0%	6.4%	16.7%	14.8%	−1.3	0.196
Urban Forms						
Land use mix [1]	0.5	0.3	0.6	0.1	−6.4	0.000
Residential density [1]	94.7	25.2	55.1	16.8	11.8	0.000
Public transport density [1]	8.4	2.2	5.9	1.7	7.8	0.000

[1] square root-transformed.

3.2. Multilevel Analysis for Predictor of Non-Motorized Commuting Trips

To investigate the role of the walkable environment on the incidence of active commuting trips, we employed a multilevel logistic regression model using two levels of data: individual commuter (level 1) and dong (level 2). A total of 129,044 individuals nested within 424 dongs were used. Individuals living in the same area (dong) share the same environmental conditions.

The results of the multilevel logistic regression model for the odds of non-motorized (walking and cycling) commuting are presented in Table 4. Model 1 is the unconditional model with only individual-level predictors, while models of 2 and 3 include neighborhood-level variables. As a neighborhood-level variable, only the Walkability Score is considered in Model 2, and additional urban form variables, as well as the Walkability Score, are included in Model 3. The Intraclass Correlation Coefficient (ICC) shows that 2.1% of the total variance was at the neighborhood level from models 2 and 3. Based on Akaike Information Criterion (AIC) and Bayesian Information Criterion (BIC) values, Model 3 is preferred.

The findings of the analyses are three-fold. First, the neighborhood-level Walkability Score had a significantly positive relationship with the individual-level odds of non-motorized trips at the 0.01 significance level. People who lived in areas (dongs) with a higher Walkability Score were much more likely to undertake walking and cycling trips for commuting purposes. Specifically, every additional one-point increase in Walkability Score was associated with 0.3% higher odds of walking and cycling trips for commuting purposes from both Model 2 and Model 3 (Model 2: odds ratio (OR) = 1.003, 95% confidence interval (CI) = 1.001–1.005; Model 3: OR = 1.003, 95% CI = 1.001–1.006). This result empirically supports the hypothesis that areas with more walkable environments have correlation with higher odds of walking and cycling to work and school (i.e., active commuting) more than areas with a less walkable environment.

Second, public transport density was positively correlated with the odds of non-motorized trips at the 0.05 significance level (OR = 1.012, CI = 1.001–1.023). This result is similar to that of previous studies, which found that access to public transportation was positively correlated with walking and cycling [25,27,28]. Other neighborhood-level variables had no statistical relationship with the odds of non-motorized trips from Model 3.

Third, the effects of all individual variables are fairly consistent across all models. The odds of non-motorized transport were positively correlated with the female gender (reference group: male), while it was negatively associated with age, level of income, and car ownership (reference group: no). Thus, those who were female, younger, on a lower income, and had no car were more likely to walk and bike for commuting purposes.

Table 4. Multilevel logistic models for odds of non-motorized (walking and cycling) commuting.

Variables	Model 1				Model 2				Model 3			
	OR	p-Value	95% CI Lower	95% CI Upper	OR	p-Value	95% CI Lower	95% CI Upper	OR	p-Value	95% CI Lower	95% CI Upper
Intercept.	3.090 ***	<0.001	3.026	3.154	2.511 ***	<0.001	2.358	2.664	2.387 ***	<0.001	2.218	2.557
Individual Variables (Level 1)												
Age	0.987 ***	<0.001	0.987	0.988	0.987 ***	<0.001	0.985	0.989	0.987 ***	<0.001	0.985	0.988
Gender (reference: male)	1.340 ***	<0.001	1.317	1.363	1.340 ***	<0.001	1.316	1.364	1.336 ***	<0.001	1.312	1.361
Income	0.932 ***	<0.001	0.919	0.945	0.936 ***	<0.001	0.922	0.950	0.936 ***	<0.001	0.922	0.951
Car ownership (reference: no)	0.713 ***	<0.001	0.684	0.742	0.707 ***	<0.001	0.674	0.740	0.707 ***	<0.001	0.673	0.741
Neighborhood Variables (Level 2; Dong level)												
Walkability Score					1.003 **	0.002	1.001	1.005	1.003 **	0.008	1.001	1.006
Land use mix [1]									1.021	0.615	0.939	1.103
Residential density [1]									0.999	0.136	0.998	1.000
Public transport density [1]									1.012 *	0.031	1.001	1.023
AIC	173690.1				173218.1				170807.0			
BIC	173748.7				173423.3				171041.1			
ICC					2.1%				2.1%			
N					129,044							

*** $p < 0.001$, ** $p < 0.01$, * $p < 0.05$; [1] square root-transformed; OR = Odds Ratio; CI = Confidence Interval; AIC = Akaike Information Criterion; BIC = Bayesian Information Criterion; ICC = Intraclass Correlation Coefficient.

4. Discussion

Encouraging active commuting is one of the most important agendas in the fields of urban planning and design, transportation planning and engineering, environmental planning, and even public health. Several studies have identified individual health benefits of active commuting [5–15], and a report from Public Health England also identified its benefits for the wider population including reductions in air pollution, noise, and economic costs [79]. Thus, efforts are being made by policymakers from a multitude of countries to change citizens' commuting behaviors toward active commuting, and Seoul is no exception [20].

The quality of the environment is one of the most important factors influencing the level of walking and cycling taking place in a city. Therefore, this study examined the role of environmental walkability on active commuting. Specifically, it tested the hypothesis that areas with more walkable environments have correlation with higher odds of walking and cycling to work and school (i.e., active commuting) more than areas with less walkable environments.

In this study, we found that the level of walkability was positively correlated with the probability of walking and cycling for commuting purposes in Seoul. This finding supports the hypothesis that the walkable environment has a strong role in the incidence of active commuting. Second, public transportation density had a significantly positive relationship with the probability of walking and cycling. This indicates that public transportation destinations, including subway stations and bus stops, encourages walking and cycling. As discussed earlier, some studies have shown that easy access to public transportation leads people to walk and bike to public transport facilities [25,27,28]. In other words, more people can walk and bike in areas with a higher density of public transportation. Third, other individual variables were correlated with active commuting, which is consistent with the results of previous empirical studies [39,80]. Individual factors such as age, gender, income, and car ownership were strongly correlated with active commuting. The odds of active commuting were strongly associated with younger age, female, lower income, and having no car.

Based on the findings of this study, some suggestions for future policymaking can be made. First, creating walkable environments could be considered a measure for sustainable development indicators within local and national urban and environmental policies. Policy actions to promote active commuting will directly contribute to achieving the third goal of the United Nations 2030 Sustainable Development Goals (SDGs), i.e., good health and well-being [81]. Creating a walkable environment could be tied to the SDGs and put forward as a city-wide policy. Second, neighborhood- and city-level efforts seem necessary for encouraging active commuting. Our findings clearly indicate that the level of neighborhood walkability can play an important role in promoting walking and cycling in daily life. Actions by the city government of Seoul should include creating its own customized strategies in order to more effectively promote active commuting. The city of Seoul should earmark investments for building walkable and cyclable environments. In particular, since Seoul Metropolitan Government is promoting the "Walkable City, Seoul" project as one of the major projects for urban planning and design, the city of Seoul is creating a pedestrian-oriented traffic environment to maintain pedestrian roads and form pedestrian walkways that connect to one another by linking the disconnected pedestrian paths [20]. From our findings, the city of Seoul can consider maintaining and connecting pedestrian pathways not only for leisure walking but also for active commuting in terms of promoting citizens' daily physical activities.

This study has several limitations, and directions for future study to address them are as follows. First, although this study could examine the overall correlation between walkability and active commuting throughout the entire Seoul, it could not include different characteristics by sub-regions. In further research, the areas with low levels of walkability and/or active commuting in particular should be examined. Second, this study dichotomized travel purpose into motorized and non-motorized transport for the use of a multilevel logistic model. For this reason, it was somewhat difficult to find and discuss the results for each transportation purpose. In a future study, it may be necessary to use a multilevel analysis for categorical outcomes. Third, the study only examined the correlation between walkability and active commuting. Further research could go beyond active commuting to empirically analyze how environmental walkability plays a role in reducing diseases (e.g., obesity, cardiovascular disease, and type 2 diabetes) and in improving health conditions (e.g., self-reported health status and mental health). Fourth, the Walkability Score used was adapted from the popular Walk Score index; however, walkability level using another objectively measured index can be considered. According to previous empirical literature on Seoul, other indices such as Walkability Index, Pedshed, and Moveability Index could be examined [42]. Lastly, the Walkability Score used in this study does not include elements that evaluate the quality of the environment. The behavior of walking and cycling depends on the quality of the environment (e.g., the level of greenness of parks, the quality of pedestrian streets, etc.). For example, some studies found that cognitive perception of urban form or urban design qualities is important for pedestrians [82,83]. In future studies, it is necessary to use a walkability index that considers variables related to environmental quality.

Despite these limitations, this study has the following implications. First, we used a relatively large amount of data including 129,044 covering all administrative units (N = 424) in Seoul. Therefore, the study was able to meaningfully look at the overall associations between active commuting and environmental walkability in Seoul. Second, we employed an objectively measured environmental walkability index, which can more reliably stand for environmental walkability, and thus be more useful for policy purposes, than a subjective index. Third, because the correlation of environmental walkability and active commuting was analyzed using a multilevel logistic model, factors from both individual and neighborhood levels could be taken into account. Furthermore, because individual-level variables were nested within the neighborhood, the multilevel analysis allowed the impact of multilevel factors on the dependent variable (active commuting) to be examined. Lastly, this study empirically investigated the relationship between environmental walkability and active commuting in Seoul. Although it has been several years since the city of Seoul implemented the "Walkable City, Seoul" project, no studies have examined how the creation of walkable environment correlates with walking and cycling. In this aspect, we believe this study is significant in that we explored the relationship between the level of neighborhood walking environment and walking and cycling in Seoul.

5. Conclusions

This study found a positive correlation between objectively-measured environmental walkability and active commuting outcomes using a multilevel logistic regression model in a Korean context. In general, personal behavior variables such as walking and cycling are highly influenced by individual characteristics (e.g., gender, age, income, etc.). Nevertheless, this study found a significant correlation between Walkability Score and the odds of active commuting. Based on the results of this study, we can expect several related policies to promote active commuting in the fields of urban regeneration, environmental planning, and transportation engineering. Furthermore, it is expected that health-promotion policies would benefit from the encouragement of active commuting.

Author Contributions: Conceptualization, E.J.K. and H.K.; methodology, E.J.K. and H.K.; software, E.J.K. and J.K.; validation, E.J.K., J.K. and H.K.; formal analysis, E.J.K. and J.K.; investigation, E.J.K.; resources, E.J.K.; data curation, E.J.K. and J.K.; writing—original draft preparation, E.J.K., J.K. and H.K.; writing—review and editing, E.J.K. and H.K.; visualization, J.K.; supervision, E.J.K.; project administration, E.J.K.; funding acquisition, E.J.K. All authors have read and agreed to the published version of the manuscript.

Funding: This work was supported by the National Research Foundation of Korea (NRF) grant funded by the Korea government (MSIT) (No. NRF-2017R1A2B4005440).

Conflicts of Interest: The authors declare no conflict of interest. The funders had no role in the design of the study; in the collection, analyses, or interpretation of data; in the writing of the manuscript; or in the decision to publish the results.

References

1. Castillo-Manzano, J.I.; Sánchez-Braza, A. Can anyone hate the bicycle? The hunt for an optimal local transportation policy to encourage bicycle usage. *Environ. Politics* **2013**, *22*, 1010–1028. [CrossRef]
2. Heinen, E.; van Wee, B.; Maat, K. Commuting by bicycle: An overview of the literature. *Transp. Rev.* **2010**, *30*, 59–96. [CrossRef]
3. Pucher, J.; Dill, J.; Handy, S. Infrastructure, programs, and policies to increase bicycling: An international review. *Prev. Med.* **2010**, *50*, S106–S125. [CrossRef] [PubMed]
4. Woodcock, J.; Edwards, P.; Tonne, C.; Armstrong, B.G.; Ashiru, O.; Banister, D.; Beevers, S.; Chalabi, Z.; Chowdhury, Z.; Cohen, A.; et al. Public health benefits of strategies to reduce greenhouse-gas emissions: Urban land transport. *Lancet* **2009**, *374*, 1930–1943. [CrossRef]
5. Mueller, N.; Rojas-Rueda, D.; Cole-Hunter, T.; de Nazelle, A.; Dons, E.; Gerike, R.; Götschi, T.; Int Panis, L.; Kahlmeier, S.; Nieuwenhuijsen, M. Health impact assessment of active transportation: A systematic review. *Prev. Med.* **2015**, *76*, 103–114. [CrossRef] [PubMed]
6. Avila-Palencia, I.; de Nazelle, A.; Cole-Hunter, T.; Donaire-Gonzalez, D.; Jerrett, M.; Rodriguez, D.A.; Nieuwenhuijsen, M.J. The relationship between bicycle commuting and perceived stress: A cross-sectional study. *BMJ Open* **2017**, *7*, e013542. [CrossRef] [PubMed]
7. Avila-Palencia, I.; Int Panis, L.; Dons, E.; Gaupp-Berghausen, M.; Raser, E.; Götschi, T.; Gerike, R.; Brand, C.; de Nazelle, A.; Orjuela, J.P.; et al. The effects of transport mode use on self-perceived health, mental health, and social contact measures: A cross-sectional and longitudinal study. *Environ. Int.* **2018**, *120*, 199–206. [CrossRef]
8. Zijlema, W.L.; Avila-Palencia, I.; Triguero-Mas, M.; Gidlow, C.; Maas, J.; Kruize, H.; Andrusaityte, S.; Grazuleviciene, R.; Nieuwenhuijsen, M.J. Active commuting through natural environments is associated with better mental health: Results from the phenotype project. *Environ. Int.* **2018**, *121*, 721–727. [CrossRef]
9. Steell, L.; Garrido-Méndez, A.; Petermann, F.; Díaz-Martínez, X.; Martínez, M.A.; Leiva, A.M.; Salas-Bravo, C.; Alvarez, C.; Ramirez-Campillo, R.; Cristi-Montero, C.; et al. Active commuting is associated with a lower risk of obesity, diabetes and metabolic syndrome in Chilean adults. *J. Public Health* **2018**, *40*, 508–516. [CrossRef]
10. Celis-Morales, C.A.; Lyall, D.M.; Welsh, P.; Anderson, J.; Steell, L.; Guo, Y.; Maldonado, R.; Mackay, D.F.; Pell, J.P.; Sattar, N.; et al. Association between active commuting and incident cardiovascular disease, cancer, and mortality: Prospective cohort study. *BMJ* **2017**, j1456. [CrossRef]
11. Blond, K.; Jensen, M.K.; Rasmussen, M.G.; Overvad, K.; Tjønneland, A.; Østergaard, L.; Grøntved, A. Prospective study of bicycling and risk of coronary heart disease in Danish men and women. *Circulation* **2016**, *134*, 1409–1411. [CrossRef] [PubMed]
12. Matthews, C.E.; Jurj, A.L.; Shu, X.O.; Li, H.L.; Yang, G.; Li, Q.; Gao, Y.T.; Zheng, W. Influence of exercise, walking, cycling, and overall nonexercise physical activity on mortality in Chinese women. *Am. J. Epidemiol.* **2007**, *165*, 1343–1350. [CrossRef] [PubMed]
13. Wareham, N.J.; Rasmussen, M.G.; Grøntved, A.; Blond, K.; Overvad, K.; Tjønneland, A.; Jensen, M.K.; Østergaard, L. Associations between recreational and commuter cycling, changes in cycling, and type 2 diabetes risk: A cohort study of Danish men and women. *PLoS Med.* **2016**, *13*, e1002076. [CrossRef]
14. Andersen, L.B.; Schnohr, P.; Schroll, M.; Hein, H.O. All-cause mortality associated with physical activity during leisure time, work, sports, and cycling to work. *Arch. Intern. Med.* **2000**, *160*, 1621. [CrossRef]
15. Andersen, L.B.; Cooper, A.R. Commuter cycling and health. In *Transport and health issues 2011*; Verlag MetaGISInfosysteme: Mannheim, Germany, 2011; pp. 9–19.
16. Physical Inactivity: Economic Costs to NHS Clinical Commissioning Group. Available online: https://assets.publishing.service.gov.uk/government/uploads/system/uploads/attachment_data/file/524234/Physical_inactivity_costs_to_CCGs.pdf (accessed on 13 January 2020).
17. The Role of Walking and Cycling in Solving the UK's Air Quality Crisis. Available online: https://www.sustrans.org.uk/media/2914/2914.pdf (accessed on 13 January 2020).
18. Statistics of Walking Modal Share. Available online: https://www.koti.re.kr/user/bbs/BD_selectBbs.do?q_clCode=&q_searchKeyTy=&q_searchVal=%EC%88%98%EB%8B%A8%EB%B6%84%EB%8B%B4%EB%A5%A0&q_bbsCode=1012&q_bbscttSn=20181231140927838&q_rowPerPage=10&q_currPage=1&q_bbsSortType=& (accessed on 9 January 2020).

19. Statistics of Biking Modal Share. Available online: https://www.koti.re.kr/user/bbs/BD_selectBbs.do?q_clCode=&q_searchKeyTy=&q_searchVal=%EC%88%98%EB%8B%A8%EB%B6%84%EB%8B%B4%EB%A5%A0&q_bbsCode=1012&q_bbscttSn=20181231135535997&q_rowPerPage=10&q_currPage=3&q_bbsSortType=& (accessed on 8 January 2020).
20. Walkable City, Seoul. Available online: http://english.seoul.go.kr/policy-information/urban-planning/walkable-city-seoul/you-walk-more-seoul-becomes-happier/ (accessed on 3 December 2019).
21. Saelens, B.E.; Sallis, J.F.; Frank, L.D. Environmental correlates of walking and cycling: Findings from the transportation, urban design, and planning literatures. *Ann. Behav. Med.* **2003**, *25*, 80–91. [CrossRef]
22. Panter, J.R.; Jones, A. Attitudes and the environment as determinants of active travel in adults: What do and don't we know? *J. Phys. Act. Health* **2010**, *7*, 551–561. [CrossRef]
23. Van Holle, V.; Deforche, B.; Van Cauwenberg, J.; Goubert, L.; Maes, L.; Van de Weghe, N.; De Bourdeaudhuij, I. Relationship between the physical environment and different domains of physical activity in European adults: A systematic review. *BMC Public Health* **2012**, *12*. [CrossRef]
24. Humpel, N. Environmental factors associated with adults' participation in physical activity a review. *Am. J. Prev. Med.* **2002**, *22*, 188–199. [CrossRef]
25. Rissel, C.; Curac, N.; Greenaway, M.; Bauman, A. Physical activity associated with public transport use—a review and modelling of potential benefits. *Int. J. Environ. Res. Public Health* **2012**, *9*, 2454–2478. [CrossRef]
26. Rodríguez, D.A.; Evenson, K.R.; Diez Roux, A.V.; Brines, S.J. Land use, residential density, and walking. *Am. J. Prev. Med.* **2009**, *37*, 397–404. [CrossRef]
27. Besser, L.; Dannenberg, A. Walking to public transitsteps to help meet physical activity recommendations. *Am. J. Prev. Med.* **2005**, *29*, 273–280. [CrossRef] [PubMed]
28. Lachapelle, U. Walk, bicycle, and transit trips of transit-dependent and choice riders in the 2009 United States national household travel survey. *J. Phys. Act. Health* **2015**, *12*, 1139–1147. [CrossRef]
29. Lefebvre-Ropars, G.; Morency, C.; Singleton, P.A.; Clifton, K.J. Spatial transferability assessment of a composite walkability index: The pedestrian index of the environment (pie). *Transp. Res. Part D Transp. Environ.* **2017**, *57*, 378–391. [CrossRef]
30. Porta, S.; Renne, J.L. Linking urban design to sustainability: Formal indicators of social urban sustainability field research in Perth, Western Australia. *Urban Des. Int.* **2005**, *10*, 51–64. [CrossRef]
31. Buck, C.; Pohlabeln, H.; Huybrechts, I.; De Bourdeaudhuij, I.; Pitsiladis, Y.; Reisch, L.; Pigeot, I. Development and application of a moveability index to quantify possibilities for physical activity in the built environment of children. *Health Place* **2011**, *17*, 1191–1201. [CrossRef] [PubMed]
32. Buck, C.; Tkaczick, T.; Pitsiladis, Y.; De Bourdehaudhuij, I.; Reisch, L.; Ahrens, W.; Pigeot, I. Objective measures of the built environment and physical activity in children: From walkability to moveability. *J. Urban Health* **2014**, *92*, 24–38. [CrossRef] [PubMed]
33. Frank, L.D.; Sallis, J.F.; Saelens, B.E.; Leary, L.; Cain, K.; Conway, T.L.; Hess, P.M. The development of a walkability index: Application to the neighborhood quality of life study. *Br. J. Sports Med.* **2009**, *44*, 924–933. [CrossRef]
34. Stockton, J.C.; Duke-Williams, O.; Stamatakis, E.; Mindell, J.S.; Brunner, E.J.; Shelton, N.J. Development of a novel walkability index for London, United Kingdom: Cross-sectional application to the whitehall ii study. *BMC Public Health* **2016**, *16*. [CrossRef]
35. Frank, L.D.; Sallis, J.F.; Conway, T.L.; Chapman, J.E.; Saelens, B.E.; Bachman, W. Many pathways from land use to health: Associations between neighborhood walkability and active transportation, body mass index, and air quality. *J. Am. Plan. Assoc.* **2006**, *72*, 75–87. [CrossRef]
36. Peiravian, F.; Derrible, S.; Ijaz, F. Development and application of the pedestrian environment index (pei). *J. Transp. Geogr.* **2014**, *39*, 73–84. [CrossRef]
37. Nykiforuk, C.I.J.; McGetrick, J.A.; Crick, K.; Johnson, J.A. Check the score: Field validation of street smart walk score in Alberta, Canada. *Prev. Med. Rep.* **2016**, *4*, 532–539. [CrossRef] [PubMed]
38. Gilderbloom, J.I.; Riggs, W.W.; Meares, W.L. Does walkability matter? An examination of walkability's impact on housing values, foreclosures and crime. *Cities* **2015**, *42*, 13–24. [CrossRef]
39. Manaugh, K.; El-Geneidy, A. Validating walkability indices: How do different households respond to the walkability of their neighborhood? *Transp. Res. Part D Transp. Environ.* **2011**, *16*, 309–315. [CrossRef]

40. Duncan, D.T.; Aldstadt, J.; Whalen, J.; Melly, S.J.; Gortmaker, S.L. Validation of walk score® for estimating neighborhood walkability: An analysis of four US metropolitan areas. *Int. J. Environ. Res. Public Health* **2011**, *8*, 4160–4179. [CrossRef]
41. Walk Score Methodology. Available online: http://pubs.cedeus.cl/omeka/files/original/b6fa690993d59007784a7a26804d42be.pdf (accessed on 15 December 2017).
42. Kim, E.J.; Kim, Y.-J. A reliability check of walkability indices in Seoul, Korea. *Sustainability* **2019**, *12*, 176. [CrossRef]
43. Chiu, M.; Shah, B.R.; Maclagan, L.C.; Rezai, M.-R.; Austin, P.C.; Tu, J.V. *Walk Score and the Prevalence of Utilitarian Walking and Obesity Among Ontario Adults: A Cross-Sectional Study*; Statistics Canada: Ottawa, ON, Canada, 2015.
44. Chudyk, A.M.; Winters, M.; Moniruzzaman, M.; Ashe, M.C.; Gould, J.S.; McKay, H. Destinations matter: The association between where older adults live and their travel behavior. *J. Transp. Health* **2015**, *2*, 50–57. [CrossRef]
45. Hirsch, J.A.; Moore, K.A.; Evenson, K.R.; Rodriguez, D.A.; Roux, A.V.D. Walk score® and transit score® and walking in the multi-ethnic study of atherosclerosis. *Am. J. Prev. Med.* **2013**, *45*, 158–166. [CrossRef]
46. Hirsch, J.A.; Diez Roux, A.V.; Moore, K.A.; Evenson, K.R.; Rodriguez, D.A. Change in walking and body mass index following residential relocation: The multi-ethnic study of atherosclerosis. *Am. J. Public Health* **2014**, *104*, e49–e56. [CrossRef]
47. Wasfi, R.A.; Dasgupta, K.; Eluru, N.; Ross, N.A. Exposure to walkable neighbourhoods in urban areas increases utilitarian walking: Longitudinal study of canadians. *J. Transp. Health* **2016**, *3*, 440–447. [CrossRef]
48. Reyer, M.; Fina, S.; Siedentop, S.; Schlicht, W. Walkability is only part of the story: Walking for transportation in Stuttgart, Germany. *Int. J. Environ. Res. Public Health* **2014**, *11*, 5849–5865. [CrossRef]
49. Walk Score Professional. Available online: https://www.walkscore.com/professional/research.php (accessed on 28 May 2019).
50. Walk Score. Available online: https://www.walkscore.com/ (accessed on 15 December 2017).
51. Kim, E.J.; Won, J.; Kim, J. Is Seoul walkable? Assessing a walkability score and examining its relationship with pedestrian satisfaction in Seoul, Korea. *Sustainability* **2019**, *11*, 6915. [CrossRef]
52. Hanibuchi, T.; Kawachi, I.; Nakaya, T.; Hirai, H.; Kondo, K. Neighborhood built environment and physical activity of japanese older adults: Results from the aichi gerontological evaluation study (ages). *BMC Public Health* **2011**, *11*. [CrossRef] [PubMed]
53. Soma, Y.; Tsunoda, K.; Kitano, N.; Jindo, T.; Tsuji, T.; Saghazadeh, M.; Okura, T. Relationship between built environment attributes and physical function in japanese community-dwelling older adults. *Geriatr. Gerontol. Int.* **2017**, *17*, 382–390. [CrossRef] [PubMed]
54. Koohsari, M.; Nakaya, T.; Oka, K. Activity-friendly built environments in a super-aged society, japan: Current challenges and toward a research agenda. *Int. J. Environ. Res. Public Health* **2018**, *15*, 2054. [CrossRef]
55. Ying, Z.; Ning, L.D.; Xin, L. Relationship between built environment, physical activity, adiposity, and health in adults aged 46–80 in Shanghai, China. *J. Phys. Act. Health* **2015**, *12*, 569–578. [CrossRef]
56. Ani, R.; Zheng, J. Proximity to an exercise facility and physical activity in China. *Southeast Asian J. Trop. Med. Public Health* **2014**, *45*, 1483–1491.
57. Cerin, E.; Sit, C.H.P.; Barnett, A.; Johnston, J.M.; Cheung, M.-C.; Chan, W.-M. Ageing in an ultra-dense metropolis: Perceived neighbourhood characteristics and utilitarian walking in Hong Kong elders. *Public Health Nutr.* **2012**, *17*, 225–232. [CrossRef]
58. Statistics of Population Density. Available online: http://kosis.kr/statHtml/statHtml.do?orgId=101&tblId=DT_1B08024&vw_cd=MT_ZTITLE&list_id=A1_13&seqNo=&lang_mode=ko&language=kor&obj_var_id=&itm_id=&conn_path=MT_ZTITLE (accessed on 10 January 2020).
59. Korea Transport Database. Available online: https://www.ktdb.go.kr/www/selectPbldataChargerWebList.do?key=12 (accessed on 15 May 2019).
60. Seoul open data plaza. Available online: http://data.seoul.go.kr/dataList/datasetList.do (accessed on 10 March 2019).
61. Road Name Address. Available online: http://www.juso.go.kr/addrlink/addressBuildDevNew.do?menu=mainJusoLayer (accessed on 1 March 2018).
62. National Spatial Data Infrastructure Portal. Available online: http://data.nsdi.go.kr/dataset (accessed on 15 March 2018).

63. CGV. Available online: http://www.cgv.co.kr/ (accessed on 15 December 2017).
64. Lotte Cinema. Available online: http://www.lottecinema.co.kr/LCHS/index.aspx (accessed on 15 December 2017).
65. Megabox. Available online: http://www.megabox.co.kr/ (accessed on 15 December 2017).
66. Open Data Portal. Available online: https://www.data.go.kr/search/index.do (accessed on 15 May 2018).
67. Duncan, M.J.; Winkler, E.; Sugiyama, T.; Cerin, E.; Du Toit, L.; Leslie, E.; Owen, N. Relationships of land use mix with walking for transport: Do land uses and geographical scale matter? *J. Urban Health* **2010**, *87*, 782–795. [CrossRef]
68. Saelens, B.E.; Sallis, J.F.; Frank, L.D.; Cain, K.L.; Conway, T.L.; Chapman, J.E.; Slymen, D.J.; Kerr, J. Neighborhood environment and psychosocial correlates of adults' physical activity. *Med. Sci. Sports Exerc.* **2012**, *44*, 637–646. [CrossRef]
69. Chaudhury, H.; Mahmood, A.; Michael, Y.L.; Campo, M.; Hay, K. The influence of neighborhood residential density, physical and social environments on older adults' physical activity: An exploratory study in two metropolitan areas. *J. Aging Stud.* **2012**, *26*, 35–43. [CrossRef]
70. Saelens, B.E.; Handy, S.L. Built environment correlates of walking. *Med. Sci. Sports Exerc.* **2008**, *40*, S550–S566. [CrossRef] [PubMed]
71. Forsyth, A.; Michael Oakes, J.; Lee, B.; Schmitz, K.H. The built environment, walking, and physical activity: Is the environment more important to some people than others? *Transp. Res. Part D Transp. Environ.* **2009**, *14*, 42–49. [CrossRef]
72. Pubic Transportation of Seoul. Available online: http://english.seoul.go.kr/life-information/transportation-information/public-transportation/1-bus/ (accessed on 12 February 2020).
73. Statistical Geographic Information Service. Available online: https://sgis.kostat.go.kr/view/index (accessed on 15 May 2019).
74. Seoul Transport Operation & Information Service. Available online: http://topis.seoul.go.kr/ (accessed on 15 March 2018).
75. Wang, Y.; Chau, C.K.; Ng, W.Y.; Leung, T.M. A review on the effects of physical built environment attributes on enhancing walking and cycling activity levels within residential neighborhoods. *Cities* **2016**, *50*, 1–15. [CrossRef]
76. Brown, B.B.; Yamada, I.; Smith, K.R.; Zick, C.D.; Kowaleski-Jones, L.; Fan, J.X. Mixed land use and walkability: Variations in land use measures and relationships with bmi, overweight, and obesity. *Health Place* **2009**, *15*, 1130–1141. [CrossRef]
77. Cerin, E.; Lee, K.-Y.; Barnett, A.; Sit, C.H.P.; Cheung, M.-C.; Chan, W.-M.; Johnston, J.M. Walking for transportation in Hong Kong chinese urban elders: A cross-sectional study on what destinations matter and when. *Int. J. Behav. Nutr. Phys. Act.* **2013**, *10*, 78. [CrossRef]
78. KOSIS. Available online: http://kosis.kr/statisticsList/statisticsListIndex.do?menuId=M_01_01&vwcd=MT_ZTITLE&parmTabId=M_01_01#SelectStatsBoxDiv (accessed on 27 May 2019).
79. Cycling and Walking for Individual and Population Health Benefits. Available online: https://assets.publishing.service.gov.uk/government/uploads/system/uploads/attachment_data/file/757756/Cycling_and_walking_for_individual_and_population_health_benefits.pdf (accessed on 13 January 2020).
80. Boisjoly, G.; Wasfi, R.; El-Geneidy, A. How much is enough? Assessing the influence of neighborhood walkability on undertaking 10-minutes walks. *J. Transp. Land Use* **2018**, *11*. [CrossRef]
81. World Health Organization. *Global Action Plan on Physical Activity 2018–2030: More Active People for a Healthier World*; World Health Organization: Geneva, Switzerland, 2018.
82. D'Acci, L. Aesthetical cognitive perceptions of urban street form. Pedestrian preferences towards straight or curvy route shapes. *J. Urban Des.* **2019**, *24*, 896–912. [CrossRef]
83. Ewing, R.; Handy, S. Measuring the unmeasurable: Urban design qualities related to walkability. *J. Urban Des.* **2009**, *14*, 65–84. [CrossRef]

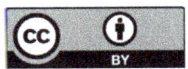

© 2020 by the authors. Licensee MDPI, Basel, Switzerland. This article is an open access article distributed under the terms and conditions of the Creative Commons Attribution (CC BY) license (http://creativecommons.org/licenses/by/4.0/).

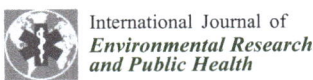 International Journal of *Environmental Research and Public Health*

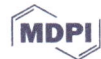

Article

Active Commuting to School and Physical Activity Levels among 11 to 16 Year-Old Adolescents from 63 Low- and Middle-Income Countries

Miguel Peralta [1,2], Duarte Henriques-Neto [1], Joana Bordado [3], Nuno Loureiro [2,4], Susana Diz [3] and Adilson Marques [1,2,*]

[1] CIPER, Faculdade de Motricidade Humana, Universidade de Lisboa, 1499-002 Lisboa; Portugal; mperalta@fmh.ulisboa.pt (M.P.); duarteneto@campus.ul.pt (D.H.-N.)
[2] ISAMB, Universidade de Lisboa, 1649-028 Lisboa, Portugal; nloureiro@ipbeja.pt
[3] Faculdade de Motricidade Humana, Universidade de Lisboa, 1499-002 Lisboa; Portugal; joanabordado@gmail.com (J.B.), sucris.diz@gmail.com (S.D.)
[4] Escola Superior de Educação, Instituto Politécnico de Beja, 7800-295 Beja, Portugal
* Correspondence: amarques@fmh.ulisboa.pt; Tel.: +351-214-149-100

Received: 21 January 2020; Accepted: 14 February 2020; Published: 17 February 2020

Abstract: Background: Global physical activity levels are low. Active commuting to school is a low-cost and sustainable behaviour that promotes adolescents' physical activity levels. Despite its importance, data on low- and middle-income countries is scarce. This study aimed to assess the relationship between active commuting to school and physical activity (PA) levels among 11–16 years-old adolescents from 63 low- and middle-income countries and six world regions. Methods: Data were from the GSHS database. Participants were 187,934 adolescents (89,550 boys), aged 11–16 years-old, from 63 low- and middle-income countries. Active commuting to school and PA were self-reported as the number of days adolescents walked or cycled to school and engaged in physical activity for at least 60 min in the past 7 days. Results: Boys and girls who actively commuted to school presented higher prevalence of attaining the PA recommendations, but only for the 13–14 (boys: 16.6% versus 22.0%; girls: 9.8% versus 14.6%) and 15–16 (boys: 16.3% versus 21.6%; girls: 8.0% versus 14.0%) year-old age groups. Only for Oceania, Central Asian, Middle Eastern, and North African girls and Sub-Saharan African boys no difference was found in the prevalence of attaining the PA recommendations between those who actively commuted to school and those who did not. Boys who actively commuted to school were 42% (95% CI: 1.37, 1.46) more likely to achieve the PA recommendations, while girls were 66% (95% CI: 1.59, 1.73) more likely to achieve the PA recommendations. Conclusions: Active commuting to school is associated with the adolescents' physical activity levels. However, it may have a lesser influence in helping younger adolescents attaining physical activity recommendations. Public health authorities should promote active commuting to school among adolescents in order to improve the PA levels and promote health.

Keywords: active travel; physical inactivity; region; school-aged children

1. Introduction

Global physical activity levels are low. Even though the World Health Organization (WHO) recommends adolescents to engage in at least 60 min of daily moderate-to-vigorous physical activity [1], it is estimated that 77.6% of boys and 84.7% of girls, aged 11 to 17 years old are physically inactive [2]. This is a worrying fact, as physical activity is associated with several health benefits, including cardiovascular, bone, metabolic, and mental health [3].

There are several strategies with the potential to increase adolescents' physical activity levels. Active commuting to school (e.g., walking or cycling) is one of them [4]. It is a low-cost and sustainable behaviour that several studies suggest to be an effective strategy to increase adolescents overall physical activity [5,6]. Active commuting to school by walking contributes to increased daily physical activity in both boys and girls [4]. Findings from randomized control trials have demonstrated that those in the active commuting walking group (experimental group) increased the number of minutes in moderate-to-vigorous physical activity [7,8]. Similarly, those who cycle to school are more active than those who do not [9]. Whether assessing physical activity through a questionnaire, accelerometer or pedometer, studies have observed that active commuting to school is positively associated with physical activity. This relationship is further supported by evidence demonstrating that active commuters have higher physical activity levels on weekdays [10,11]. Furthermore, among adolescents living in urban contexts, it was found that more than half of their daily physical activity was due to active commuting [12].

As an intervention strategy to promote physical activity, a recent systematic review concluded that active commuting is effective [6]. Furthermore, from an educational perspective, active transportation stimulated at early ages [10] can help to consolidate this behaviour throughout life [13]. However, despite the effectiveness of active commuting as a strategy to promote physical activity, the number of adolescents active commuting to school in high-income countries has been decreasing [14–16]. Among low- and middle-income countries, data are limited. Notwithstanding, investigations from Brazil [17], Mozambique [18] and Vietnam [19] have shown that in these countries a downward trend in active commuting to school is also observed.

Although there is strong evidence for the relationship between active commuting to school and physical activity levels in adolescents, the majority of the studies were conducted in high-income countries. Thus, in low- and middle-income countries, data on this relationship is limited [20]. International studies using comparable methods are important to establish trends or generalization of the associations, support decision making and inform global efforts on the promotion of physical activity and sustainable transport. For that reason, and from a public health perspective, more data about active commuting on low- and middle-income countries is required. This information should allow to better support public health policies and decision making regarding the promotion of physical activity in these countries. Therefore, the aim of this study was to assess the relationship between active commuting to school and physical activity levels among 11–16 years-old adolescents from 63 low- and middle-income countries and six world regions.

2. Materials and Methods

2.1. Participants and Procedures

This study is based on the Global School-Based Student Health Survey (GSHS), a cross-sectional survey aimed primarily at students aged between 13 and 17 years old from several low- and middle-income countries worldwide. The GSHS uses a standardized scientific sample selection process, common school-based methodology and self-administered questionnaire supported by the WHO with the collaboration of the United Nations' UNICEF, UNESCO, and UNAIDS, and the technical assistance from the Centers for Disease Control and Prevention. The questionnaire includes validated survey items selected from 10 core modules, including: alcohol use, dietary behaviours, drug use, hygiene, mental health, physical activity, protective factors, sexual behaviours, tobacco use, and violence and unintentional injury. More information about the GSHS can be found elsewhere [21].

Publicly available GSHS data, collected from 2007 to 2015, for low- and middle-income countries was used. Data collected in the surveys were self-reported. For this study, adolescents aged between 11 and 16 years-old were considered, as this was the age range that guaranteed participants in each age from all the available countries. Furthermore, only adolescents who reported data on sex, active commuting to school, and physical activity were considered. The final sample consisted of 187,934 adolescents (89,550 boys, 98,384 girls), aged 11 to 16 years-old (mean age 14.3 ± 1.2), from 63 countries (1841 Afghanistan, 4350 Algeria, 1177 Antiqua and Barbuda, 26,636 Argentina, 1299 Bahamas,

2857 Bangladesh, 1548 Barbados, 1993 Belize, 3378 Bolivia, 1616 British Virgin Islands, 2283 Brunei Darussalam, 2313 Cambodia, 1591 Chile, 2622 Costa Rica, 1735 Curacao, 1512 Dominica, 2424 Egypt, 1833 El Salvador, 1590 Fiji, 1763 Ghana, 3866 Guatemala, 2269 Guyana, 1696 Honduras, 1944 Iraq, 1551 Kiribati, 2460 Kuwait, 2522 Laos, 2162 Lebanon, 20672 Malaysia, 1921 Mauritania, 2135 Mauritius, 2744 Myanmar, 4431 Mongolia, 2760 Morocco, 1015 Mozambique, 2604 Namibia, 477 Nauru, 137 Niue, 2360 Oman, 5054 Pakistan, 4281 Palestinian territory, 2811 Peru, 7730 Philippines, 1675 Saint Kitts and Nevis, 2067 Samoa, 2389 Seychelles, 1262 Solomon Islands, 2040 Sudan, 1620 Suriname, 3027 Syria, 3193 Tanzania, 4745 Thailand, 2241 Timor-Leste, 110 Tokelau, 2148 Tonga, 2639 Trinidad and Tobago, 865 Tuvalu, 2461 United Arab Emirates, 3415 Uruguay, 1080 Vanuatu, 2267 Vietnam, 855 Wallis and Futuna, and 1872 Yemen) and six world regions (Central Asia, Middle East, North Africa, East and Southeast Asia, Latin America and Caribbean, Oceania, South Asia, and Sub-Saharan Africa) defined by the World Bank as low- and middle-income countries at the time of data collection.

2.2. Measures

Participants filled a self-administered questionnaire during a school lesson (questionnaires were country-specific and translated to the country official language). Active commuting to school was self-reported as the number of days adolescents walked or cycled to school in the past week ('During the past 7 days, on how many days did you walk or ride a bicycle to or from school?'). Those who reported active commuting at least 1 day in the past week were considered to active commute to school. Adolescents were asked to report the number of days they engaged in physical activity for at least 60 min in the past 7 days ('During the past 7 days, on how many days were you physically active for a total of at least 60 min per day?'). Answers were given on an 8-point scale (0 = none to 7 = daily). This has been shown to be a valid and reliable question for assessing adolescents' physical activity in epidemiological research [22].

2.3. Data Analysis

The mean frequency of physical activity (days/week) and the prevalence of attaining the physical activity recommendations for those who actively commuted to school and those who did not, according to age group (11–12, 13–14 and 15–16 years old) and region (Central Asia, Middle East, and north Africa, East and southeast Asia, Latin America and Caribbean, Oceania, South Asia, Sub-Saharan Africa) were calculated and the 95% confidence intervals (CI) were estimated. Logistic regression was performed to analyse the relationship between active commuting to school and attaining the physical activity recommendations. Unadjusted and adjusted analyses for age and region were tested. Attaining the physical activity recommendations was defined, using the WHO criteria, as engaging in moderate-to-vigorous physical activity for at least 60 min every day [1]. All analyses were stratified by sex. Data analysis was performed using IBM SPSS Statistics version 25 (IBM Corp., Armonk, NY, USA).

3. Results

Participants' characteristics are presented in Table 1. Most adolescents were aged between 13 and 15 years old and only 15.6% (19.5% boys, 12.0% girls) engaged in at least 60 min of physical activity every day. More than half of the adolescents (56.1%) active commuted to school.

Table 1. Adolescents characteristics, including age, region, physical activity, and active commuting to school, by sex.

Adolescents' Characteristics	Total (n = 187,934)		Boys (n = 89,550)		Girls (n = 98,384)	
	n	% (95% CI)	n	% (95% CI)	n	% (95% CI)
Age (years)						
11	1843	1.0 (0.5, 1.4)	827	0.9 (0.3, 1.6)	1016	1.0 (0.4, 1.7)
12	11,296	6.0 (5.6, 6.4)	4965	5.5 (4.9, 6.2)	6331	6.4 (5.6, 7.0)
13	39,403	21.0 (20.6, 21.4)	18,160	20.3 (19.7, 20.9)	21,243	21.6 (21.0, 22.1)
14	51,392	27.3 (27.0, 27.7)	24,488	27.3 (26.8, 27.9)	26,904	27.3 (26.8, 27.9)
15	49,720	26.5 (26.1, 26.8)	24,132	26.9 (26.4, 27.5)	25,588	26.0 (25.5, 26.5)
16	34,280	18.2 (17.8, 18.6)	16,978	19.0 (18.4, 19.5)	17,302	17.6 (17.0, 18.2)
Region						
Central Asia, Middle East, and north Africa	34,532	18.4 (18.0, 18.8)	16,243	18.1 (17.5, 18.7)	18,289	18.6 (18.0, 19.2)
East and southeast Asia	44,773	23.8 (23.4, 24.2)	21,158	23.6 (23.1, 24.2)	23,615	24.0 (23.5, 24.5)
Latin America and Caribbean	66,931	35.6 (35.3, 36.0)	31,938	35.7 (35.1, 36.2)	34,993	35.6 (35.1, 36.1)
Oceania	12,142	6.5 (6.0, 6.5)	5450	6.1 (5.5, 6.7)	6692	6.8 (6.2, 7.4)
South Asia	12,496	6.6 (6.2, 7.1)	7016	7.8 (7.2, 8.5)	5480	5.6 (5.0, 6.2)
Sub-Saharan Africa	17,060	9.1 (8.6, 9.5)	7745	8.6 (8.0, 9.3)	9315	9.5 (8.9, 10.1)
Physical activity (days/week)						
0	47,611	25.3 (24.9, 25.7)	20,574	23.0 (22.4, 23.5)	27,037	27.5 (26.9, 28.0)
1	38,660	20.6 (20.2, 21.0)	16,411	18.3 (17.7, 18.9)	22,249	22.6 (22.1, 23.2)
2	26,817	14.3 (13.9, 14.7)	11,617	13.0 (12.4, 13.6)	15,200	15.4 (14.9, 16.0)
3	18,642	9.9 (9.5, 10.3)	9036	10.1 (9.5, 10.7)	9606	9.8 (9.2, 10.4)
4	10,898	5.8 (5.4, 6.2)	5792	6.5 (5.8, 7.1)	5106	5.2 (4.6, 5.8)
5	10,630	5.7 (5.2, 6.1)	5602	6.3 (5.6, 6.9)	5028	5.1 (4.5, 5.7)
6	5360	2.9 (2.4, 3.3)	3033	3.4 (2.7, 4.0)	2327	2.4 (1.7, 3.0)
7	29,316	15.6 (15.2, 16.0)	17,485	19.5 (18.9, 20.1)	11,831	12.0 (11.4, 12.6)
Active commuting to school						
No	82,423	43.9 (43.5, 44.2)	37,380	41.7 (41.2, 42.2)	45,043	45.8 (45.3, 46.2)
Yes	10,5511	56.1 (55.8, 56.4)	52,170	58.3 (57.8, 58.7)	53,341	54.2 (53.8, 54.6)

CI: confidence interval.

In both boys and girls, active commuting to school was related to the physical activity levels (Table 2). For every age group, those who actively commuted to school had a higher frequency of physical activity (days/week). The oldest age group showed the biggest (boys, 0.61 days/week, 95% CI: 0.56, 0.61; girls, 0.66 days/week, 95% CI: 0.62, 0.70) mean difference, whereas the youngest age group presented the lowest (boys, 0.47 days/week, 95% CI: 0.34, 0.60; girls, 0.42 days/week, 95% CI: 0.31, 0.53). Furthermore, those who actively commuted to school presented higher prevalence of attaining the physical activity recommendations, but only for the 13–14 (boys: 16.6% versus 22.0%; girls: 9.8% versus 14.6%) and 15–16 (boys: 16.3% versus 21.6%; girls: 8.0% versus 14.0%) year-old age groups.

Table 2. Mean frequency of physical activity (day/week) and the prevalence of attaining the physical recommendations according to active commuting by age group.

Active Commuting to School	Physical Activity (Days/Week) Mean (95% CI)		
	11–12 year-olds	13–14 year-olds	15–16 year-olds
Boys			
No	2.43 (2.34, 2.53)	2.51 (2.48, 2.55)	2.59 (2.55, 2.63)
Yes	2.90 (2.80, 2.99)	3.10 (3.07, 3.13)	3.20 (3.16, 3.23)
Girls			
No	1.98 (1.90, 2.05)	2.00 (1.98, 2.03)	1.88 (1.85, 1.91)
Yes	2.40 (2.32, 2.48)	2.58 (2.55, 2.61)	2.54 (2.51, 2.56)

Active Commuting to School	% Attaining Physical Activity Recommendations% (95% CI)		
	11–12 year-olds	13–14 year-olds	15–16 year-olds
Boys			
No	16.7 (13.3, 20.0)	16.6 (15.2, 17.9)	16.3 (14.9, 17.7)
Yes	21.1 (17.9, 24.3)	22.0 (20.9, 23.1)	21.6 (20.5, 22.7)
Girls			
No	12.0 (9.0, 15.0)	9.8 (8.6, 11.0)	8.0 (6.6, 9.4)
Yes	14.9 (11.9, 18.0)	14.6 (13.5, 15.8)	14.0 (12.8, 15.2)

CI: confidence interval.

The relationship between active commuting to school and physical activity according to region is shown in Table 3. For every region, boys and girls that active commuted to school had higher frequency of physical activity. South Asia (boys, 1.05 days/week, 95% CI: 0.91, 1.19; girls, 1.01 days/week, 95% CI: 0.86, 1.01) and Oceania (boys, 0.74 days/week, 95% CI: 0.60, 0.88; girls, 0.92 days/week, 95% CI:

0,80, 1,04) were the regions with the biggest mean difference in the frequency of physical activity between those who actively commuted to school and those who did not, while Central Asia, Middle East, and North Africa (boys, 0.43 days/week, 95% CI: 0.35, 0.51; girls, 0.29 days/week, 95% CI: 0.22, 0.36) had the lowest. Only for Oceania, Central Asian, Middle Eastern, and North African girls and Sub-Saharan African boys no difference was found in the prevalence of attaining the physical activity recommendations between those who actively commuted to school and those who did not.

Table 3. Mean frequency of physical activity (days/week) and the prevalence of attaining the physical activity recommendations according to active commuting by regions.

Active Commuting to School	Physical Activity (Days/Week) Mean (95% CI)					
	Central Asia, Middle East, and north Africa	East and southeast Asia	Latin America and Caribbean	Oceania	South Asia	Sub-Saharan Africa
Boys						
No	2.71 (2.65, 2.77)	2.34 (2.29, 2.39)	2.82 (2.78, 2.87)	2.29 (2.19, 2.39)	1.66 (1.56, 1.76)	2.36 (2.27, 2.44)
Yes	3.14 (3.09, 3.19)	2.95 (2.90, 3.00)	3.43 (3.39, 3.46)	3.03 (2.94, 3.12)	2.71 (2.63, 2.78)	2.90 (2.82, 2.99)
Girls						
No	2.01 (1.97, 2.06)	1.72 (1.68, 1.75)	2.13 (2.10, 2.17)	1.98 (1.90, 2.06)	1.94 (1.83, 2.06)	1.81 (1.74, 1.87)
Yes	2.30 (2.25, 2.35)	2.23 (2.19, 2.26)	2.75 (2.72, 2.78)	2.90 (2.82, 2.99)	2.95 (2.86, 3.04)	2.45 (2.38, 2.53)
Active Commuting to School	% Attaining Physical Activity Recommendations % (95% CI)					
	Central Asia, Middle East, and north Africa	East and southeast Asia	Latin America and Caribbean	Oceania	South Asia	Sub-Saharan Africa
Boys						
No	19.2 (17.1, 21.3)	14.3 (12.5, 16.2)	18.4 (16.8, 20.0)	13.9 (10.2, 17.7)	8.1 (3.7, 12.5)	15.6 (12.6, 18.6)
Yes	23.3 (21.5, 25.1)	20.4 (18.8, 22.1)	23.4 (22.2, 24.7)	17.0 (13.8, 20.2)	19.4 (16.9, 21.8)	20.7 (18.0, 23.5)
Girls						
No	10.9 (8.9, 12.9)	5.5 (3.8, 7.3)	10.1 (8.6, 11.6)	10.9 (7.6, 14.1)	12.5 (8.3, 16.7)	9.9 (7.2, 12.5)
Yes	13.3 (11.5, 15.2)	10.1 (8.4, 11.7)	15.5 (14.3, 16.8)	15.9 (12.9, 18.9)	21.7 (18.8, 24.6)	16.2 (13.4, 18.9)

CI: confidence interval.

Table 4 presents the odds ratio for attaining the physical activity recommendations according to active commuting to school. In the adjusted analysis, boys who actively commuted to school were 42% (95% CI: 1.37, 1.46) more likely to achieve the physical activity recommendations, and girls who actively commuted to school were 66% (95% CI: 1.59, 1.73) more likely to achieve the physical activity recommendations.

Table 4. Odds ratio for attaining the physical activity recommendations according to active commuting to school.

Active Commuting to School	Attaining Physical Activity Recommendations OR (95% CI)			
	Boys		Girls	
	Unadjusted	Adjusted	Unadjusted	Adjusted
No	1.00 (ref)	1.00 (ref)	1.00 (ref)	1.00 (ref)
Yes	1.41 (1.36, 1.46)	1.42 (1.37, 1.47)	1.65 (1.58, 1.71)	1.66 (1.59, 1.73)

OR: odds ratio; CI: confidence interval. Analysis adjusted for age and region.

4. Discussion

This study aimed to assess the relationship between active commuting to school and the physical activity levels of 11–16 year-olds from 63 low- and middle-income countries and six world regions. It was found that both boys and girls who actively commuted to school engaged more frequently in physical activity and were more likely to attain the WHO physical activity recommendations. However, age and region differences were found.

Physical activity is an important health behaviour associated to several health benefits [3]. A previous systematic review found that adolescents who actively commuted to school are more physically active and that active school travel interventions often lead to increases in adolescents' physical activity levels [5] and can help to consolidate this behaviour throughout life [13]. In accordance with previous results from mainly high-income countries, this study showed that in low- and middle-income countries, active commuting to school is also associated to physical activity, and that boys and girls who actively commuted to school were, respectively, 42% and 66% more likely to attain the physical activity recommendations. This is a relevant finding, as active commuting to school is an effective strategy to increase the globally low physical activity levels [2,5]. Furthermore, active commuting to school is also associated with lower measures of adiposity and better cardiorespiratory fitness [5,20]. Globally, international, regional and national public health authorities should promote active commuting to school among adolescents in order to improve the physical activity levels and promote health.

Although boys and girls from all age groups (11–12, 13–14 and 15–16 years-old) who actively commuted to school engaged more frequently in physical activity, the prevalence of attaining the physical activity recommendations was only higher for those who actively commuted in the 13–14 and 15–16 years-old age groups. This may be due to several reasons. On the one hand, the difference in the prevalence of attaining the physical activity recommendations between active commuters and non-active commuters was the smallest in the youngest age group. This suggests that for the 11–12 years-old age group, active commuting to school may not be a significant contributor to achieve the recommended physical activity levels, as it is for the 13–14 and 15–16 years-old age groups. On the other hand, the 11–12 years-old sample was much smaller than the other age groups, which may have led to less accuracy in determining significant statistical differences. Notwithstanding, physical activity levels are known to decrease across adolescence, thus younger adolescents are more physically active than their older peers [23,24]. Because of this, active commuting to school may have a lesser influence in helping younger adolescents attain physical activity recommendations, although it contributes to the overall physical activity levels.

A systematic review, performed mainly with studies from high-income countries in Europe, North America and Oceania, indicated that active commuting to school is positively associated with the physical activity levels of school-aged children and adolescents [5]. In this study, with data from low- and middle-income countries, similar findings were observed. However, the prevalence of boys and girls from Oceania; girls from Central Asia, Middle East, and North Africa; and boys from Sub-Saharan Africa attaining the physical activity recommendations was similar for active commuters and non-active commuters. These findings show that regional differences in the relationship between active commuting and physical activity may exist. Future research should try to explore possible reasons for this. Nonetheless, in all regions, boys and girls who actively commuted engaged more frequently in physical activity. Therefore, active commuting to school should be used as a strategy to promote physical activity across all regions.

The interpretation of this study's findings warrants some public health policy implications for low- and middle-income countries. Active commuting to school seems to contribute to the overall physical activity levels of adolescents from low- and middle-income countries, as it does for high-income countries. Taking into account the global levels of insufficient physical activity [2], public health authorities from these countries are recommended to use active commuting to school as a strategy to promote physical activity and health among adolescents. Additionally, the contribution of active commuting to school for achieving the physical activity recommendations appears to be more relevant for adolescents aged 13 and over. Thus, active commuting may be a more suitable strategy to promote physical activity among adolescents aged 13 and older than for their younger peers.

The present study has several limitations that are important to mention. Data was collected at the school setting, resulting in the exclusion of adolescents that do not attend schools. Also, data represented only adolescents aged 11–16 years-old and the GSHS focuses mainly on adolescents aged 13–17 years. Thus, the 11–12 years-old sample was small, in comparison to the other age groups, and adolescents aged 17 were not included. Data on active commuting to school and physical activity were self-reported and therefore subject to bias. Nevertheless, because of the large samples used in each national or regional survey, self-report was the most feasible methodology and is still the backbone of surveillance studies [25]. Furthermore, intensity is an important part of the WHO physical activity recommendations, as children and adolescents should engage in at least 60 moderate-to-vigorous intensity physical activity daily. However, in the GSHS questionnaire, used in this study, the question regarding physical activity does not consider intensity (only duration and frequency). This limitation could lead to bias in the classification of adolescents attaining the physical activity recommendations. There is still no consensus regarding the optimal cut-off criteria for dichotomizing active commuting [26]. In this study, a cut-off value of 1 day was used as the aim of the study was to compare those who did not actively commute to school (i.e., 0 days of active commuting) and those who did, even if only on 1 day. Additionally, because this study used a sample of 63 countries with different cultural and administrative settings, the number of days adolescents went to school could vary between countries. Thus, establishing a cut-off value different than one could lead to bias. Also, the question regarding active commuting does not allow to differentiate the type of active commuting, such as walking or cycling. It would be interesting to compare whether walking and cycling have similar or different contributions for the physical activity levels.

5. Conclusions

Active commuting to school is associated with the adolescents' physical activity levels. However, some sex, age and regional differences were observed. Active commuting seems to have a greater effect among girls, as girls who actively commuted to school were 66% more likely to attain the physical activity recommendations, while boys were only 42%. Also, active commuting to school may have a lesser influence in helping younger adolescents attain the physical activity recommendations, as no differences were found in the 11–12 years-old group, although it contributes to the overall physical activity levels. Therefore, public health authorities should promote active commuting to school among adolescents in order to improve the physical activity levels and promote health, especially among adolescents aged 13 years old and over.

Author Contributions: Conceptualization, M.P. and D.H.-N.; methodology, M.P. and A.M.; formal Analysis, M.P. and D.H.-N; Writing—Original draft preparation, M.P. and J.B.; Writing—Review and editing, A.M., N.L. and S.D.; supervision, A.M. All authors have read and agreed to the published version of the manuscript.

Funding: This research received no external funding.

Conflicts of Interest: The authors declare no conflict of interest.

References

1. WHO. *Global Recommendations on Physical Activity for Health*; 978-92-4-159-997-9; World Health Organization: Geneva, Switzerland, 2010.
2. Guthold, R.; Stevens, G.A.; Riley, L.M.; Bull, F.C. Global trends in insufficient physical activity among adolescents: A pooled analysis of 298 population-based surveys with 1.6 million participants. *Lancet Child Adolesc. Health* **2019**. [CrossRef]
3. USDHHS. *2018 Physical Activity Guidelines Advisory Committee Scientific Report*; US Department of Health and Human Services: Washington, DC, USA, 2018.
4. Aparicio-Ugarriza, R.; Mielgo-Ayuso, J.; Ruiz, E.; Avila, J.M.; Aranceta-Bartrina, J.; Gil, A.; Ortega, R.M.; Serra-Majem, L.; Varela-Moreiras, G.; Gonzalez-Gross, M. Active Commuting, Physical Activity, and Sedentary Behaviors in Children and Adolescents from Spain: Findings from the ANIBES Study. *Int. J. Environ. Res. Public Health* **2020**, *17*, 668. [CrossRef] [PubMed]
5. Larouche, R.; Saunders, T.J.; Faulkner, G.; Colley, R.; Tremblay, M. Associations between active school transport and physical activity, body composition, and cardiovascular fitness: A systematic review of 68 studies. *J. Phys. Act. Health* **2014**, *11*, 206–227. [CrossRef] [PubMed]
6. Larouche, R.; Mammen, G.; Rowe, D.A.; Faulkner, G. Effectiveness of active school transport interventions: A systematic review and update. *BMC public health* **2018**, *18*, 206. [CrossRef]
7. Sirard, J.R.; Alhassan, S.; Spencer, T.R.; Robinson, T.N. Changes in physical activity from walking to school. *J. Nutr. Educ. Behav.* **2008**, *40*, 324–326. [CrossRef]

8. Mendoza, J.A.; Watson, K.; Baranowski, T.; Nicklas, T.A.; Uscanga, D.K.; Hanfling, M.J. The walking school bus and children's physical activity: A pilot cluster randomized controlled trial. *Pediatrics* **2011**, *128*, e537–e544. [CrossRef]
9. Panter, J.; Jones, A.; Van Sluijs, E.; Griffin, S. The influence of distance to school on the associations between active commuting and physical activity. *Pediatr. Exerc. Sci.* **2011**, *23*, 72–86. [CrossRef]
10. Duncan, E.K.; Scott Duncan, J.; Schofield, G. Pedometer-determined physical activity and active transport in girls. *Int. J. Behav. Nutr. Phys. Act.* **2008**, *5*, 2. [CrossRef]
11. Sirard, J.R.; Riner, W.F., Jr.; McIver, K.L.; Pate, R.R. Physical activity and active commuting to elementary school. *Med. Sci. Sports Exerc.* **2005**, *37*, 2062–2069. [CrossRef]
12. Rainham, D.G.; Bates, C.J.; Blanchard, C.M.; Dummer, T.J.; Kirk, S.F.; Shearer, C.L. Spatial classification of youth physical activity patterns. *Am. J. Prev. Med.* **2012**, *42*, e87–e96. [CrossRef]
13. Dora, C. A different route to health: Implications of transport policies. *BMJ* **1999**, *318*, 1686–1689. [CrossRef] [PubMed]
14. Gray, C.E.; Larouche, R.; Barnes, J.D.; Colley, R.C.; Bonne, J.C.; Arthur, M.; Cameron, C.; Chaput, J.P.; Faulkner, G.; Janssen, I.; et al. Are we driving our kids to unhealthy habits? Results of the active healthy kids Canada 2013 report card on physical activity for children and youth. *Int. J. Environ. Res. Public Health* **2014**, *11*, 6009–6020. [CrossRef] [PubMed]
15. Tremblay, M.S.; Gray, C.E.; Akinroye, K.; Harrington, D.M.; Katzmarzyk, P.T.; Lambert, E.V.; Liukkonen, J.; Maddison, R.; Ocansey, R.T.; Onywera, V.O.; et al. Physical activity of children: A global matrix of grades comparing 15 countries. *J. Phys. Act. Health* **2014**, *11* (suppl. 1), S113–S125. [CrossRef] [PubMed]
16. Grize, L.; Bringolf-Isler, B.; Martin, E.; Braun-Fahrlander, C. Trend in active transportation to school among Swiss school children and its associated factors: Three cross-sectional surveys 1994, 2000 and 2005. *Int. J. Behav. Nutr. Phys. Act.* **2010**, *7*, 28. [CrossRef] [PubMed]
17. Costa, F.F.; Silva, K.S.; Schmoelz, C.P.; Campos, V.C.; de Assis, M.A. Longitudinal and cross-sectional changes in active commuting to school among Brazilian schoolchildren. *Prev. Med.* **2012**, *55*, 212–214. [CrossRef]
18. dos Santos, F.K.; Maia, J.A.; Gomes, T.N.; Daca, T.; Madeira, A.; Damasceno, A.; Katzmarzyk, P.T.; Prista, A. Secular trends in habitual physical activities of Mozambican children and adolescents from Maputo City. *Int. J. Environ. Res. Public Health* **2014**, *11*, 10940–10950. [CrossRef]
19. Trang, N.H.; Hong, T.K.; Dibley, M.J. Active commuting to school among adolescents in Ho Chi Minh City, Vietnam: Change and predictors in a longitudinal study, 2004 to 2009. *Am. J. Prev. Med.* **2012**, *42*, 120–128. [CrossRef]
20. Sarmiento, O.L.; Lemoine, P.; Gonzalez, S.A.; Broyles, S.T.; Denstel, K.D.; Larouche, R.; Onywera, V.; Barreira, T.V.; Chaput, J.P.; Fogelholm, M.; et al. Relationships between active school transport and adiposity indicators in school-age children from low-, middle- and high-income countries. *Int. J. Obes. Suppl.* **2015**, *5*, S107–S114. [CrossRef]
21. GSHS. Available online: https://www.who.int/ncds/surveillance/gshs/en/ (accessed on 8 December 2019).
22. Ridgers, N.D.; Timperio, A.; Crawford, D.; Salmon, J. Validity of a brief self-report instrument for assessing compliance with physical activity guidelines amongst adolescents. *J. Sci. Med. Sport* **2012**, *15*, 136–141. [CrossRef]
23. Corder, K.; Sharp, S.J.; Atkin, A.J.; Griffin, S.J.; Jones, A.P.; Ekelund, U.; van Sluijs, E.M. Change in objectively measured physical activity during the transition to adolescence. *Br. J. Sports Med.* **2015**, *49*, 730–736. [CrossRef]
24. Farooq, M.A.; Parkinson, K.N.; Adamson, A.J.; Pearce, M.S.; Reilly, J.K.; Hughes, A.R.; Janssen, X.; Basterfield, L.; Reilly, J.J. Timing of the decline in physical activity in childhood and adolescence: Gateshead Millennium Cohort Study. *Br. J. Sports Med.* **2018**, *52*, 1002–1006. [CrossRef] [PubMed]
25. Pedisic, Z.; Bauman, A. Accelerometer-based measures in physical activity surveillance: Current practices and issues. *Br. J. Sports Med.* **2015**, *49*, 219–223. [CrossRef] [PubMed]
26. Zaragoza, J.; Corral, A.; Estrada, S.; Abos, A.; Aibar, A. Active or Passive Commuter? Discrepancies in Cut-off Criteria among Adolescents. *Int. J. Environ. Res. Public Health* **2019**, *16*, 3796. [CrossRef] [PubMed]

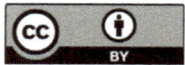

© 2020 by the authors. Licensee MDPI, Basel, Switzerland. This article is an open access article distributed under the terms and conditions of the Creative Commons Attribution (CC BY) license (http://creativecommons.org/licenses/by/4.0/).

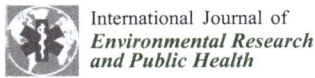 International Journal of *Environmental Research and Public Health*

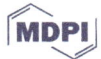

Review

A Scoping Review of Children and Adolescents' Active Travel in Ireland

João Costa [1,*], Manolis Adamakis [1], Wesley O'Brien [1] and João Martins [2,3,4]

1. Sports Studies and Physical Education Programme, School of Education, 2 Lucan Place, Western Road, Cork T12 KX72, Ireland; emmanouil.adamakis@ucc.ie (M.A.); wesley.obrien@ucc.ie (W.O.)
2. Laboratório de Pedagogia, Faculdade de Motricidade Humana e UIDEF, Instituto de Educação, University of Lisbon, 1499-002 Cruz Quebrada—Dafundo, Portugal; jmartins@fmh.ulisboa.pt
3. Environmental Health Institute, Lisbon Medical School, University of Lisbon, 1649-028 Lisbon, Portugal
4. Centro Interdisciplinar do Estudo da Performance Humana (CIPER), Faculdade de Motricidade Humana, Universidade de Lisboa, 1499-002 Cruz Quebrada—Dafundo, Portugal
* Correspondence: joao.costa@ucc.ie; Tel.: +353-21-490-2537

Received: 7 February 2020; Accepted: 13 March 2020; Published: 18 March 2020

Abstract: There appears to be a lack of existing data that comprehensively summarizes the evidence of children and adolescents' active travel in the Republic of Ireland. In lieu of this, a scoping review was conducted to map the existing literature (2000–2020) on children and adolescents' active travel in the Republic of Ireland. A scoping review design extracted a total of 19 publications, which show a consistent focus on the identified population's active travel patterns, mainly to and from school, mostly self-report and cross-sectional research study designs; however, there are few longitudinal data, intervention and participatory studies. Key issues from these identified scoping review studies are discussed with the potential to better inform policy makers, practitioners and researchers to delineate programmes and strategies for promoting active travel among children and adolescents in the Republic of Ireland.

Keywords: Republic of Ireland; review; active transport; active commuting; youth; physical activity

1. Introduction

Regular physical activity (PA) participation reduces the risk of disease, in addition to providing a multitude of benefits that help individuals sleep better, feel better, and perform daily tasks more easily [1]. These benefits can be achieved through a variety of PA modalities, and active travel (i.e., using self-propelled mediums, such as walking or cycling, some or all the way to a destination) can contribute as much as 30% towards meeting the recommended daily levels of PA for health [2,3]. A recent PA review [4] identified positive associations between active travel and health outcomes across 68 studies. Specifically, active travel through cycling was clearly linked with improvements in cardiorespiratory fitness.

In terms of PA participation, children and youth, however, are failing to meet the recommended guidelines for health [5,6], and active travel needs to become more integrated in society as an important additional source of PA participation [7]. Compared with other modalities of PA, active travel has the additional advantage of being convenient and free of monetary costs [8]. Yet, data show a significant decline in active travel over the past 30 years such as the prevalence of active travel for children which was almost 48% in the 1970s but had declined to 13% by 2009 in the United States [9], with similar downward trends observed in Canada [10,11], Switzerland [12], the United Kingdom [13], Australia [14,15], and New Zealand [16].

1.1. Summary of Past Reviews on Active Travel of Children and Adolescents

Past reviews sustain that the existing strength of the evidence for active travel is still debatable, warranting continuing research [17–20]. To promote walking, Carlin et al.'s [17] review concluded that school-based interventions show meaningful potential. A key supporting argument for school-based active travel interventions is that children and adolescents go to school every day, and this environment is a natural and ongoing opportunity to develop active travel behaviours [17]. Other elements that show good promise in promoting active travel are interventions with a systematic design, including intermittent approaches of short bouts of active travel, as well as other settings [17,18,20]. Moreover, past reviews highlight other key factors that contribute to sustain active travel as a behaviour, such as parental involvement, longitudinal trends of youth as they progress through school, peer relationships, urban safety, distance and schedule convenience [17,20].

In terms of how research on active travel is conducted, a large portion of the research is conducted with cross-sectional designs, primarily from walking-based research, and using self-reported data from children and youth [20]. Most of this research also tends to be developed in Europe. Apparently, research with adolescents falls short compared to that with children [17]. Saunders and colleagues [19] argue that there appears to be no standardised way of addressing active travel, where Schoeppe and colleagues [20] state that: "The definition of active school travel varied in terms of frequency and duration of active travel, and journey to and/or from school. Moreover, most included studies did not employ reliable and valid active travel." (p.317).

1.2. Overview of Irish Data on Active Travel of Children and Adolescents

For clarification purposes, the island of Ireland comprises two different national jurisdictions, i.e., Northern Ireland which (along with Scotland, Wales, and England) belongs to the United Kingdom, and the Republic of Ireland as part of the European Union. Each jurisdiction has a respective government, hence its own ministries.

Most recent nationally representative data across the island of Ireland ($N = 6651$; age range 10–18 years old; 53% female) indicates that 42% of primary and 40% of secondary school children self-report walking or cycling to and from school [21]. In comparison to the previously disseminated active travel data [22], this represents an 11% increase in active travel among Irish primary school children since 2010 [21]. In combating the widely accepted age-related decline in PA participation [23,24], specifically during adolescence [25], it is concerning, however, that the most recent 40% figure of secondary school children actively commuting [21] to and from school in Ireland has not increased since 2010 [22]. It could be argued, based on the data of Woods et al. [21] that there is a lack of safe places to crossroads, and the distance to schools are significant barriers preventing Irish adolescents from increasing their levels of active travel.

At a government policy level, in the Republic of Ireland, it has been promising to observe the National Physical Activity Plan [26]. This policy specifically addresses under action area four of the "Environment" that the promotion of active transport is one of the most practical and sustainable ways to increase population levels of PA. For example, one of the specific action four areas from this National Physical Activity Plan is to 'ensure that the planning, development and design of towns, cities and schools promotes cycling and walking … ' (p.24). While gender and location (urban versus rural) inequalities in active transport are still in existence for Irish children and adolescents [27], the data from Woods et al. [21] has put the promotion of active travel on the map for this population, and recommends that the island of Ireland must now set a realistic and meaningful target for increasing the percentage of children and adolescents walking and cycling to school between 2019 and 2027.

1.3. Purpose of This Review

To our knowledge, no review has been published that comprehensively summarises the evidence in relation to children and adolescents' active travel in the Republic of Ireland. This raised our research question of: "What is the nature and content of research on the active travel of children and adolescents conducted in the Irish context, and what type of implications are (not) being addressed?" Therefore, the purpose of this scoping review is to undertake the following: a) to map and summarize the existing literature findings from the past two decades (2000–2020), specifically relating to contextual study factors, such as age and gender, for active travel in children and adolescents from the Republic of Ireland; b) to document the existing study design, supporting theories, measurement protocol and prevalence of active travel in these identified scoping review studies; and c) to identify current barriers, gaps and areas of opportunity for active travel promotion in the literature. This scoping review can contribute to mapping the key concepts underpinning the active travel research field and evaluating the specific types of evidence-based data available [28]. Ultimately, this scoping review study has the potential to better inform policy makers, practitioners and researchers in order to delineate programmes and strategies for promoting active travel among children and adolescents in the Republic of Ireland.

2. Materials and Methods

Given the aforementioned aims, the selection of a scoping review process was identified as the most suitable methodological approach to undertake this study, following relevant literature on the methods of conducting this type of review [28,29]. Guided by the research questions presented above, the following evidence-informed scoping review framework, as proposed by Arksey and O'Malley [28], was implemented:

1. Identifying relevant studies—a PubMed and Scopus database search was conducted. While these different databases provided existing published research evidence, Google Scholar and the Open Access to Irish Research database (RIAN) were also used in the context of this scoping review for identifying outstanding grey literature, such as theses, policies and reports.
2. Study selection—by screening and assessing the data based on the inclusion and exclusion criteria, a set of publications was filtered down to a final selection of 19 studies eligible for the current review.
3. Charting the data—each relevant document was screened and summarised, as the research team achieved consensus on the final list of references for the research.

Each of these three identified stages are described and justified in further detail below.

2.1. Establishing Search Terms and Criteria to Identify Relevant Studies

The design of the literature search strategy started with breaking down the research question into an initial set of keywords, such as "active travel", "Ireland" or "Irish", "children", "adolescents" or "adolescence". With supporting evidence from the literature informed by previous reviews [17–20], further keywords were added, namely "active transport" or "active commuting". Having selected the search tools and terms, the chosen databases' advanced search options and different combinations with Boolean operators (e.g., ("active travel" OR "active transport" OR "active commuting") AND ("youth" OR "children" OR "adolescence" OR "adolescents") AND ("Ireland" OR "Irish")) were employed for the selection of potentially relevant documents.

The main objective and inclusion criteria of this search strategy was to collect all potential sources that specifically investigated and reported elements of active travel as PA of children and adolescents in the Irish context, across a range of publications (e.g., theses and dissertations, statistics, research and policy papers, research reports, conference abstracts and proceedings), regardless of the methodological decisions employed. As the research context for three of the authorship team relates to the Republic of Ireland, and considering that some works presented data in aggregate for the whole island of Ireland, it was decided that only publications with a clear presentation or breakdown of data from the Republic of Ireland were to be included. Finally, an a priori timeframe for the charting of included documents was set to the last two decades, specifically as it appeared that the oldest study was published after 2000. As such, the search strategy was conducted between December 2019 and January 2020 to capture the most recent publications from the last two decades.

As for exclusion criteria, broader concepts such as "independent mobility" were not considered as part of this scoping review, as this research domain typically comprises more elements beyond active travel, such as free play (e.g., [30]). Also, active travel literature from fields outside of the PA domain (e.g., earth sciences such as geography) was excluded.

After establishing essential search terms and criteria, the research team proceeded to extract documents. The choice of the Scopus and PubMed databases sought to include core research fields to the topic of study, namely social sciences and sport/health sciences. With the screening of each document, attention was given to the reference list, specifically in order to identify if a potentially relevant document was missed by the initial search strategy.

2.2. Study Selection

With the input of the identified terms in each search tool and database, the entries provided through Scopus and PubMed had the title and abstract checked. Furthermore, Google Scholar and RIAN were included as search tools to find other potentially relevant grey literature as theses and reports. Based on this process (cf. Figure 1), and after removing duplicates, 43 publications were identified for screening according to the inclusion and exclusion criteria mentioned in the previous stage and reduced to a total of 32 potentially relevant publications for the scoping review exercise. All 32 documents' data were summarised to assess their full eligibility, leading to a total of 19 studies being included in the review. All the research team were involved in this process. Where questions arose, they were discussed as a team and a collective decision was made. For example, O'Keeffe and O'Beirne [30] present active travel data but because such data is aggregated for all of the island of Ireland, without a specific breakdown for the Republic of Ireland, this document was excluded.

2.3. Charting the Data

The process of charting the data was prepared through the design of an online review summary, by assigning each author a balanced set of documents for populating the relevant content. This process started with the 32 potentially eligible documents and concluded with 19 included documents in the review. The evaluation of the document eligibility was facilitated by organising the dimensions and charting guidelines as per Table 1 below:

Table 1. Charting dimensions and guidelines.

Charting Dimension	Charting Guideline
Study Design	Refer if research was intervention, multiple baseline, case-study, etc.
Population/Sample	Refer sample size, key demographics, and highlight if cohort is primary or secondary education level.
Method	Refer if data were self-reported or objectively measured, with the specific tools if relevant.
Active Travel concept(s) and theoretical frameworks	Identify which concept was used (e.g., Active Travel, Active Transport, Active Commuting) and what theoretical frameworks explicitly informed the study.
Summary of Findings	Summarise only disaggregated data related to active travel in the context of the Republic of Ireland.

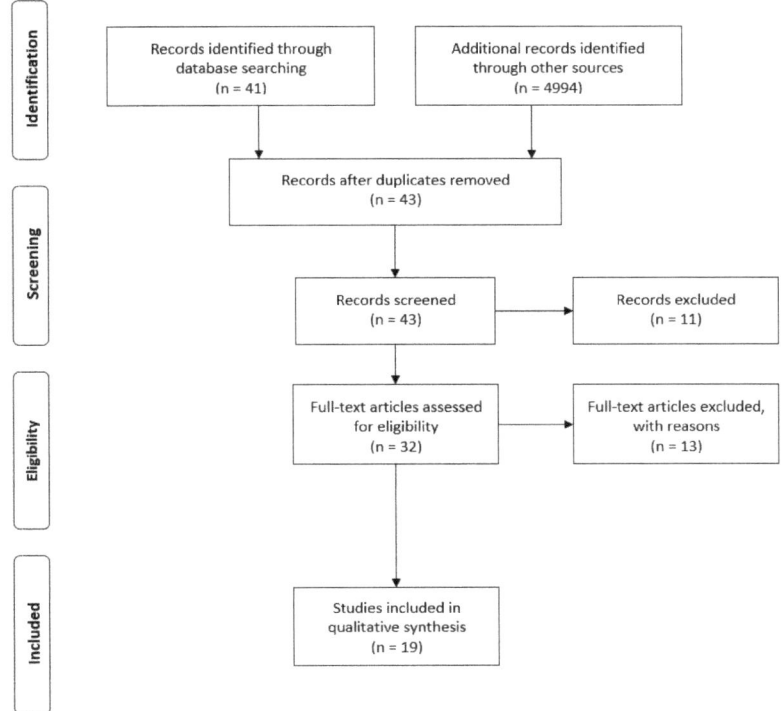

Figure 1. Scoping review flow diagram of reviewed studies from the combined databases and search tools based on the PRISMA protocol. The volume of "additional records identified through other sources" is highly increased from the Google Scholar results which returned 4940 links.

3. Results

An overview of the scoping review process is presented in accordance with the PRISMA protocol as shown in Figure 1.

Table 2 summarises the findings and specifically identifies the study, study design, population/sample, methods used for data collection, the concept of active travel used and theoretical framework, and main findings. The results are presented according to the following themes: methodological characteristics and main findings of the studies.

Table 2. Review summary

Document	Study Design	Population/Sample (n; % of Girls; Mean Age, Age Range; Other)	Method	Active Travel Concept(s) and Theoretical Frameworks	Summary of Findings
Nelson et al. (2008) [31]	Cross-sectional	$n = 4,013$ adolescents; 48.1% girls; 16.1 years, 15–17 years.	Self-report questionnaires.	Active commuting; Mode of transport, barriers, distance. No theoretical framework mentioned.	33% walked or cycled to school; A higher proportion of males than females commuted actively (41.0% vs. 33.8%); Adolescents living in more densely populated areas had greater odds of active commuting than those in the most sparsely populated areas; Most walkers lived within 1.5 miles and cyclists within 2.5 miles of school; A 1-mile increase in distance decreased the odds of active commuting by 71%.
Nelson and Woods (2010) [32]	Cross-sectional (from Take PART study: PA research for teenagers)	$n = 2159$ adolescents; 47.1% girls; 16.0 years, 15–17 years.	Self-report questionnaires.	Active commuting (cycle, walking); Inactive commuting (car, bus or train); Duration, frequency. Mentions the Social-Ecological theory.	Most adolescents chose active modes of travel (61.3% walked, 8.7% cycled); boys were more likely to cycle to school (15.4% vs. 1.2%) and girls were more likely to travel by car (27.0% vs. 18.3%).
Woods et al. (2010) [22]	Cross-sectional (Children's Sport Participation and Physical Activity (CSPPA) study, Nationally representative Irish cluster sample)	n = 1275 primary school students; 45% female; 11.4 years, 10–13 years; $n = 4122$ post-primary school students; 52% female; 14.5 years, 12–18 years.	Self-report questionnaires; ActiGraph, accelerometers and pedometers.	Active travel; Type of transport, duration, distance. No theoretical framework mentioned.	38% (31% primary, 40% post-primary) of children and youth walked or cycled to school in 2009; journey durations were on average 15 min for active commuters; No gender differences existed for active commuting at primary school; post-primary females were less likely to actively commute than males (38% vs. 43%, $p < 0.01$); 1% of primary pupils and 3% of post-primary pupils cycled to school; Main barriers: Distance (37% primary, 54% post-primary); Time (13% and 19%); Traffic-related danger for primary (13%); and Convenience for post-primary (8%).

Table 2. Cont.

Document	Study Design	Population/Sample (n; % of Girls; Mean Age, Age Range; Other)	Method	Active Travel Concept(s) and Theoretical Frameworks	Summary of Findings
Coulter and Woods (2011) [33]	Cross-sectional	n = 605 students; 44% female; 8.8 years, 5–15 years. Other: All students from 1 single, large, urban, mixed primary school in Dublin.	Self-report questionnaires.	Active Commuting (as walking or cycling to school on the previous day); Inactive commuting (traveling by bus or car); Estimation of residential distance from School. No theoretical framework mentioned.	39.9% of children actively commuted to school (37.8% walk, 1.1% cycle); 40.7% of children actively commuting from school (39% walk, 1.7% cycle); 56.6% of primary aged children are driven to school; 28.9% live within 1 km of the school but are inactive commuters; Gender did not predict active commuting; Compared with younger children (5–6 years), the odds of inactively commuting for every year increase in age decreases by approximately 24%.
Gahan (2011) [34]	Cross-sectional	n = 89 adolescents; 6–15 years; 48.3% female (returned questionnaires) n = 44 adolescents; 6–15 years; 47.7% girls (participated in the workshop).	Self-report questionnaires; Workshop; Walkability audit.	Active travel; Type of transport, frequency. Mentions social ecological frameworks.	Most commonly used mode of transport by children and young people: 1. Parents' car (357 times); 2. Walking (205 times); 3. Cycling (80 times); Most commonly use of walking and cycling is going to school, shop, friend's house; Main barriers: no place to walk (56%); difficulty crossing the road (57%); drivers do not behave well (60%); neighbourhood is not a nice place to live (35%).
Murtagh and Murphy (2011) [35]	Cross-sectional	n = 140 children; 39.3% female; 9.9 years, 9–11 years.	Self-report questionnaires; Objective pedometers for step count.	Active travel; Active commute. No theoretical framework mentioned.	62.1% travelled by car, and 36.4% walked to school; Children who walked or cycled to school had higher daily step counts than those who travelled by passive modes (16,118 ± 5757 vs. 13,363 ± 5332 steps).
Sullivan and Nic Gabhainn (2012) [36]	Cross-sectional (From the national research study of Health Behaviour in School-aged Children (HBSC))	n = 16,060 students; 49% girls; 10–17 years. From 3rd class in primary school to 5th year in post-primary school. Other: Nationally representative Irish cluster sample.	Self-report questionnaires.	Active travel; Type of transport, duration, frequency (every day). No theoretical framework mentioned.	Walk: boys 23.9%, girls 23.5%; 10–11 years 26.0%, 12–14 years 23.7%, 15–17 years 22.6%; SC1–2 19.9%, SC3–4 23.2%, SC5–6 27.0%; Cycle: boys 3.7%, girls 0.8%; 10–11 years 4.0%, 12–14 years 2.5%, 15–17 years 1.6%; SC1–2 1.8%, SC3–4 2.5%, SC5–6 3.2%.
Clarke and The HBSC Ireland Team (2013) [37]	Cross-sectional (factsheet)	Sample from the HBSC research study; n = 12,661 (10–17 years).	Self-report questionnaires.	Travel to school by walking or cycling for the main part of their journey. No theoretical framework mentioned.	26.5% of schoolchildren in Ireland reported actively travelling to school, 28.1% boys, 24.7% girls; Boys, younger children, children from lower social classes, and children living in urban areas were more likely to report actively travelling to school; Children who reported actively travelling to school were more likely to report excellent health, to be very happy, to be more active.

Table 2. Cont.

Document	Study Design	Population/Sample (n; % of Girls; Mean Age, Age Range; Other)	Method	Active Travel Concept(s) and Theoretical Frameworks	Summary of Findings
Delaney (2013) [38]	Cross-sectional	$n = 2877$ participants; 53% girls; 12–20 years.	Self-report questionnaires.	Active travel; Distance to school. No theoretical framework mentioned.	24% used active transport as a means of travel to school; Most individuals, who use active transport, live within 1 mile of their school; The percentages of those using active travel dropped the further individuals live from their respective school; Those who were active in sport and recreation activities appeared to be greater users of active travel.
Daniels et al. (2014) [39]	Cross-sectional.	$n = 73$ children; 60.3% female; 11–13 years.	Self-report questionnaires; Workshop.	Active School Travel (walking and cycling). No theoretical framework mentioned.	Non-active travel = 69.9%; 54.5% who reported they actively travelled do so 4-5 days per week; 86.3% reported owning a bicycle; None of the active travellers reported travelling to school with parents; they were more likely to travel to school with friends compared to children who do not travel actively (59.1% vs. 9.8 %); **Main promoters:** 1. Company/Parents and Community; 2. School infrastructure/School; 3. Distance/Parents; 4. Physical Health/Parents, Self, Health Professionals; 5. Equipment/Parents, Self, School, Government; **Main barriers:** 1. Distance/Community and Parents; 2. Weather/Government and Weatherman; 3. Lifestyle/Parents; 4. Road infrastructure and planning/Government, School, Builders; 5. Strangers/Community, Parents, Government, Builders.
Harrington et al. (2014) [40]	Report (including both longitudinal and cross-sectional reports and studies)	HBSC: $n = 13,611$ (11–15 years; 2013–2014 waves—representative sample). Growing Up in Ireland (GUI) Infant and Child Cohorts: $n \approx 9,000$ children and their caregivers; (Wave 3 of the infant cohort, followed up at age 5 years); $n \approx 7400$ children; 2011–2012, from Wave 2 of the child cohort, followed up at age 13 years.	Children and parents self-report questionnaires.	Percentage of children reporting active transport to or from school each day. No theoretical framework mentioned.	Active transportation grade D (meaning 21% to 40% meet the defined benchmark); Data from larger studies provided evidence of children/adolescents succeeding with 20% to 29%; Sex gaps evident for other indicators may not be as obvious for active transport; Children from rural areas were less likely to active commute than their urban counterparts.

Table 2. Cont.

Document	Study Design	Population/Sample (n; % of Girls; Mean Age, Age Range; Other)	Method	Active Travel Concept(s) and Theoretical Frameworks	Summary of Findings
McMinn et al. (2014) [41]	Cross-sectional (including 5 countries)	n = 136; 8.7 years, 69.9 girls.	Self-report questionnaires.	Active commuting; Walkers. Mentions the Theory of Planned Behaviour.	Republic of Ireland 42.0% walkers (i.e. those participants who categorized themselves as being in the action or maintenance stages, according to Theory of Planned Behaviour).
Woods and Nelson (2014) [42]	Cross-sectional	n = 199 adolescents; 42.3% girls; 15.9 years, 15–17 years.	Self-report questionnaires; Objective distance (map-measured).	Distance, Time and Mode of active travel (walk, cycle, car, bus). No theoretical framework mentioned.	Mode of transport: walk 72.4%, car 21.1%, bus 6.5%; Distance travelled by active commuters 1.3 km - perceived distance 1.4 km; by inactive 1.4 km, perceived 2.7 km; Active commuters were accurate in their perception of distance travelled; For passive commuters, the average actual distance (1350 m) travelled to school was significantly shorter than their perception of this distance.
Lambe (2015) [43]	Community-wide intervention study collected at 2 time-points (May 2011 and May 2013).	Study 1: Primary Education: 5th–6th class students (n = 1457) in 21 primary schools (9 in intervention town 1; 5 in intervention town 2; and 7 in the control town). Study 2: Secondary Education: 1st, 2nd, the class students in 15 secondary schools (6 schools in intervention town 1; 5 in intervention town 2; and 4 in the control town).	Self-report questionnaires.	Travel mode to school; Actual and Preferred; Awareness of community interventions on active travel. Mentions ecological models.	Study 1: At baseline, 25.6% and 3.7% of the total sample walked or cycled to school; boys were more likely to cycle than girls; Greater proportions of students walked or cycled home from school than to school (39.3% vs. 29.3%); Car was the most common mode of travel to or from school in each town (60.8% and 49.1%, respectively); Overall, the intervention had no effect on active travel behaviour. Study 2: 17% of the total sample actively commuted to school and distance was a key factor; 64% of the total sample lived more than 3km from their school and of these, only 7% actively commuted to school; Boys were more likely to engage in active travel to school but car travel was still the most common (62%) and preferred (47%) mode of travel for all; Overall, awareness of the community-wide active travel campaign increased by 13% and 20% in intervention towns 1 and 2.
Central Statistics Office (2016) [44]	Cross-sectional (Census 2016, national population survey)	n = 896,575 commuters (546,614 primary commuters; 349,961 secondary commuters). Adult respondents.	Self-report questionnaires.	Self-propelled transport (walking - cycling). No theoretical framework mentioned.	Primary Education: Active transport decreased from 49.5% in 1986 to 24.8% in 2016. In 2016, 22% of Irish vs. 38% non-Irish walk; 1% of Irish and 2% of non-Irish cycle. Secondary Education: Walking decreased from 31.9% in 1986 to 21.2% in 2016; Cycling decreased from 15.3% in 1986 to 2.1% in 2016; Just over a fifth of secondary students walked to school (74,111) up slightly from 73,946 (0.2%) in 2011, but as a percentage of commuters, down almost 2% since 2011; 2016 saw the reversal of this trend with a 10.5% increase since 2011, bringing the numbers of secondary students taking to their bikes to over 7,000.

Table 2. Cont.

Document	Study Design	Population/Sample (n; % of Girls; Mean Age, Age Range; Other)	Method	Active Travel Concept(s) and Theoretical Frameworks	Summary of Findings
Harrington et al. (2016) [27]	Report (including both longitudinal and cross-sectional reports and studies)	Sample from: Ireland's 2016 Report Card Growing Up in Ireland (GUI) Infant and Child Cohorts; HBSC; Children's Sport Participation and Physical Activity (CSPPA Plus)/	Self-report questionnaires. Interviews.	Active transportation. No theoretical framework mentioned.	Active Transportation - Grade D (The grade for each indicator is based on the percentage of children and youth meeting a defined benchmark, D is 21% to 40%); 23% males, 25% females used of active transport in a local sample of 2877.
Murtagh, Dempster, and Murphy (2016) [45]	Cross-sectional	Sample from "Growing Up in Ireland" study; Wave 1 n = 8502 (9 years); Wave 2 n = 7479 (13 years).	Interviews. Self-report questionnaires. Anthropometric measures.	Active school travel (uptake and maintenance; dropped out); Walking and cycling classified as active; Travel mode. Mentions the Bioecological Model.	Within a 4 years period, active travel decreased from 25% to 20%; More likely to uptake or maintain if living in Urban; Less distance affected uptake and maintenance. Walking: Wave1 = 23.8% to Wave2 = 17.8% Cycling: Wave1 = 1.3% to Wave2 = 2.0%; At 9 years of age 75% of children travelled to school using passive travel modes; At 13 years 66% of students maintained passive commuting modes, 14% switched from active to passive commuting, 11% maintained active commuting, and 9% took up active commuting; Overall, at 13 years, 80.2% of the sample travelled to school using passive modes.
Lambe et al. (2017) [46]	Repeat cross-sectional study of a natural experiment	n = 1459 5th-6th class students from all the 21 schools in 3 towns (n = 1038 students in 2 intervention towns; n = 419 students in 1 control town).	Self-report questionnaires.	Actual and preferred mode of travel to and from school; Awareness of the active travel campaign in school and town; Percentage of children that walk or cycle to school. No theoretical framework mentioned.	Baseline: Total sample, car use (60.8%), cycle (3.7%), walk (25.6%); Walk or cycle from school (39.3%), to school (29.3%); Bicycle ownership (>85%); Preference for walking and cycling to school was considerably higher than preference for being driven. Intervention impact: There was no overall intervention effect detected for active travel to or from school. To school (Town1: pre 33.9%, post 31.2%; Town 2: pre 28.8%, post 33.0%); From school (Town1: pre 41.0%, post 39.5%, Town 2: pre 37.4%, post 38.4%). Some evidence of an effect for males in intervention town 2 (increase of 14% in active travel home from school).
Woods et al. (2018) [21]	Cross-sectional (CSPPA study - Nationally representative Irish cluster sample)	n = 1103 Primary school students, 56% female; 11.43 years (n = 3594 Post-primary school students; 54% female; 14.11 years; 45% male).	Self-report questionnaires ActiGraph accelerometers and pedometers.	Active travel and active commuting; Type of transport, duration, distance. No theoretical framework mentioned.	42% primary, 40% post-primary school children reported walking or cycling to or from school; 2.2% reported cycling to or from school; At primary school level, more 6th class pupils reported actively commuting than 5th class pupils (47% vs. 36%); At post primary school level, active commuting peaked during 4th year (61%), but was lowest among 6th year pupils (23%); Main barriers: 1. Not enough safe places to cross the road for primary school students (26%), distance being too far for post-primary students (32%); 2. Heavy schoolbags for primary and post-primary school students (22% and 28%, respectively).

3.1. Methodological Characteristics of the Studies

Overall, very few of the reviewed research items make explicit the theoretical underpinnings that inform the study design, mostly relying on ecological psychology models and frameworks [32,34,43,45]. McMinn et al. [41] present the sole study relying on a social psychology model with the Theory of Planned Behaviour (TPB) [47]. In that study, the Republic of Ireland data were only specifically reported for active travel descriptive statistics, and then aggregated in the Northwest European region to report on the tested TPB constructs. By using an ecological framework, Lambe [43] found similar results and has warned about the importance of differing intention from behaviour. Murtagh, Dempster, and Murphy's longitudinal study [45] make use of one of Bronfenbrenner's earlier versions of the bioecological model of human development (1979) [48], considering it to structure the layers of data from the individual (e.g., body mass index, BMI) to the context layers of the immediate settings (microsystems of family, neighbourhood, school, and others). The authors then analyse the associations of those factors with active school travel patterns. Such approach allowed the authors to identify and quantify the: 1) change in distance to school, 2) too much traffic (at baseline), and 3) rural setting (at baseline), as significantly associated to active school travel upkeep, uptake or drop out.

The publications presented in the current scoping review included a minimum sample size of 73 children [39] to a maximum of 16,060 children [36]. Some of the included studies combined data from more than one project [27,40,43,45] subsequently leading to an increased combined number of participants (e.g., Harrington et al. [27,40] with a total sample from both studies ≈30,000 participants). Of special interest is the Census statement document [44], which included commuter data from all Irish primary and secondary students (896,575 commuters). In total, 10 of the identified studies had more than 2000 participants as a sample size.

Most studies focused on children in 5th to 6th class (10–12 years of age) of primary school, while few studies included students at a younger age (i.e., <10 years of age) [33,34,41,45]. Regarding other demographic information provided, more than half of the studies reported participants' gender (almost even distribution between boys and girls), and a few further studies reported the area of residence and socioeconomic status (i.e., [32,38,39]).

As for the research design, most studies were cross-sectional and used national representative samples [21,22,36,37,44] or non-national representative samples [31–35,38,39,42]. Two studies pertained to the same context and were defined, by the authors, as a community-wide intervention study [43], and a repeated cross-sectional study of a natural experiment [46]. Only one piece of research used a nationally representative sample in a longitudinal study [45].

In terms of data collection procedures, many studies used self-reported questionnaires (only) to assess the active travel data of children and adolescents [31,33,36–38,41,43,44,46]. Mode of transportation, frequency, duration and distance were indicators often asked. Other studies used mixed methodological approaches, such as questionnaires and interviews [45]; questionnaires and consultation with young people [39]; and questionnaires, interviews and workshops [34]. A minority of studies used a combination of self-reported data (questionnaires) and objective data (accelerometer and/or pedometers) [21,22,35].

3.2. Main Findings of the Studies

The percentage of active travel reported for most studies ranged between 20.0%–40.0%, while some studies reported a higher prevalence of active travel (i.e., 70.0% in Nelson and Woods [32]; 72.4% in Woods and Nelson [42]). In general, there was a higher percentage of children and adolescents who preferred walking, instead of cycling to a destination. The nationally representative studies included found a trend towards the increase of active transport during the last decade, for both children and adolescents [21,22,44]. Two of the intervention studies had no effect on the active travel behaviours to or from school for children and adolescents [43,46].

Based on gender analysis, no active travel differences existed for primary school participants, although secondary school female students were less likely to actively commute than their male counterparts [21,22,31,36,37,40,46], especially when considering cycling [32,36]. It was evident from all studies that active travel is declining with age. For example, Sullivan and Nic Gabhainn [36] reported that the walking percentage was reduced by 3.4% and cycling by 2.4% between the 10- to 11-year age bracket and the 15- to 17-year age bracket. Also, children and adolescents from lower socioeconomic backgrounds were more likely to report active travel to school [36,37].

The main barriers reported in 9 studies that prevented children and adolescents from active travel to various destinations were distance, location (urban vs rural), weather, road, general safety issues, time constraints and heavy school bags. Specifically, for location and distance, it was evident that urban status [21,22,31,37,40,45] and the decrease of distance from the destination [39,45] positively influenced the likelihood of active travel for children and adolescents. The optimal estimated distance for facilitating active travel was 1 mile [31,38].

Finally, only two studies reported on the health benefits of active travel. Murtagh and Murphy [44] found that children who walked or cycled to school had higher daily step counts than those who travelled by passive modes. Clarke and The HBSC Ireland Team [37] concluded that children who reported higher incidences of active travel to school were more likely to report excellent health, as well as increased happiness and overall physical activity levels.

4. Discussion

The present scoping review sought to map and summarize the existing literature (2000–2020) regarding active travel amongst children and adolescents from the Republic of Ireland and identify points of future development. This discussion will address the paper's objectives, namely regarding the a) main findings; b) research methods; and c) current gaps and areas of opportunity.

4.1. Main Findings from Research in the Republic of Ireland

Main results showed that the time-trends in active travel, based across the data from various Irish studies, has increased during the last decade; however, in terms of modality, a significant decrease in the proportion of children and adolescents (especially females) cycling to school was noted. The reported levels of active travel in the current scoping review were similar to those of other western countries (e.g., [10,12]), apart from the United States [9].

The age-related decline in active travel was evident in all studies identified. In the Republic of Ireland context, older students tended to walk or cycle less, when compared to their younger peers (adolescents vs. children), and this is a consistent trend globally [6,21,24]. Also, female adolescents had the lowest rates of active travel, which is in accordance with overall PA trends by gender during adolescence [6,49,50]. Apart from the perceived barriers highlighted in various surveys, the decline in girls' active travel levels may be related to their advanced pubertal maturation compared with boys, though the relative importance of biological and environmental influences on general PA remains unclear [51]. Considering that most studies focused on children above 10 years of age, these studies do not span across both childhood and adolescence, and there is little empirical evidence on the active travel levels of children below 10 years of age. It is possible that the decline in active travel commences in early childhood, even before adolescence, so more longitudinal studies targeting younger children are warranted.

An interesting finding was the particularly low levels of cycling noted in all studies, usually below 3% [21,22,43–46]. While parental safety concerns and distances travelled are barriers to children's active travel [21,22,39], other factors include children's lack of competence in terms of cycling [31,52]. Since active travel through cycling is linked with improvements in cardiorespiratory fitness [4], more high-quality intervention studies, such as longitudinal research study designs with robust methodological procedures could be developed to promote children's cycling skills, active travel pursuits and the dissemination of evidence surrounding the existing health benefits.

The major barriers that prevented Irish children and adolescents from active travel to various destinations were distance, location (urban vs. rural), and general safety issues. The optimal estimated distance for facilitating active travel was 1 mile [31,38], while most of the adolescents who perceived distance as a barrier to actively commuting lived further than 2.5 miles from school [31]. Similarly, in Switzerland, the large prevalence of children living within 1 mile of school did not change significantly between 1994 and 2005, and this contributed to the relatively high proportion of children actively commuting to school [12]. Also, children and adolescents living in rural areas reported lower active travel levels, mainly because the infrastructure has not been adequately developed, leading to an increased popularity of motorized transportation in those areas [34].

4.2. Trends and Contributions of the Active Travel Research Methods in the Irish Context

Of the 19 references included and analysed in this review, a large majority had a cross-sectional research design (e.g., [33,42]), while only a few adopted a longitudinal (e.g., [45]) or intervention approach (e.g., [43]). Most of this is aligned to what previous reviews have observed regarding the research methods on active travel [17–20]. Given these findings and the need to have quality evidence-based protocols towards the promotion of active travel (walking and cycling) in young people, future research should consider the importance of longitudinal randomized controlled trials [53–55]. Cohort studies might be of critical importance to further understand the patterns and predictors of change for active travel throughout childhood and adolescence. Cross-sectional and large-scale representative studies, that use self-reported data collection methods might also be an efficient approach to the continuation of active travel surveillance and identifying the possible associated factors at population level. A distinctive feature found in many of the analysed studies from this scoping review is the inclusion of nationally representative samples (e.g., [21,22,37,45]). Even though, in the last decade, there have been some national studies carried out in the Republic of Ireland (e.g., [21,22]), the vast majority of this research has been with secondary-level adolescents, requiring more of a research emphasis to be placed on primary school children (e.g., [33,39]), and particularly under the age of 10 where data are clearly missing.

As for the data collection procedures, many studies focused on the use of self-report questionnaires (e.g., [31,36,43]). Self-reported data may be subject to social desirability bias [56], and this limitation has been acknowledged in the analysed studies. A few, however, have used a combination of self-report questionnaires and interviews/workshops (e.g., [34,39,45]). Daniels et al. [39] and Lambe [43] align in their need for more qualitative methodologies to better explore the experiences of children and adolescents. Inclusively, Daniels and colleagues [39] demonstrated that participative research methodologies on active travel can be implemented successfully with primary school-level children. A mixed methodology approach for measurement procedures might be more suitable to further understand the perspectives of young people and their parents on active travel, as well as to give young people's voice and co-construct meaningful solutions to increase their active travel behaviour [57]. A limited number of studies used objective PA data, such as accelerometers or pedometers [21,22,35]. This specific approach might be suitable to capture PA data related to walking, but not cycling. Therefore, future studies should be creative in their technological-based strategies (e.g., Global Positioning System (GPS) use) to better capture objective cycling behaviour.

At a deeper critical level, the reviewed research also refers to issues surrounding research quality. Lambe [43] highlights the critical concerns of: 1) avoiding type 2 errors by stratifying the analysis according to criterion distances and gender for walking and cycling; 2) enhancing data validity to include a "preferred type of active travel" item (given differences between actual and preferred); and c) more accurately measuring active travel when using the Children's Sport Participation and Physical Activity (CSPPA) [22] self-report survey. Nelson and Woods [32] also consider that research should focus on the perceptions of specific characteristics of the environment related to contextual awareness, such as the 'presence of pedestrian crossings', rather than generic statements relating to 'perceptions of pedestrian safety'. These considerations from Nelson and Woods [32], and from Lambe [43], resonate with Saunders and colleagues [19] on issues relating to active travel definitions and measurement. As discussed above, most of the reviewed studies addressed active travel related to school, based on the recurrent fact that most children and adolescents go to school every day [37]. However, this observation might be too narrow an approach, as school-related active travel mainly contributes to overall quantities of PA participation [2,3], and only a minority of the research analysed in the present review included active travel from a broader perspective beyond the school commute or explicitly considered other modes of active travel used by children such as scooters and skates.

While national policies (e.g., [26,58]) and local authorities are beginning to show alignment and acknowledge the main research recommendations, one of the primary barriers for the near null effect on active travel in the two communities found by Lambe [43] and colleagues [46] was parental gatekeeping. According to the author(s), attenuating the secular trend for the declining levels of active travel to school presents a considerable challenge for local authorities in Ireland. Woods et al. [22] previously stated that active commuters who live in urban areas tend to be more involved in sport and PA, however, overall government departments of transport and sport need to work together to address the issue of non-participation in sport and active commuting. This further concurs with Delaney et al.'s [38] findings, specifically that active participants in sport and recreation events are more likely to use active travel.

4.3. Gaps and Areas of Opportunity for Active Travel Research in the Irish Context

The previous discussion sections highlighted essential issues from the reviewed documentation, as the need to use mixed and more robust methods, the overall enhancement of methods quality, the need to widen the sample demographics in the younger cohorts, or considering the issues of definition and measurement of active travel not only to other destinations than school but also considering other mediums of active travel than walking and cycling.

To a much lesser extent, only five [32,34,41,43,45] of the analysed documents in this scoping review highlighted their theoretical underpinnings, raising this as a notable area of opportunity in active travel research. Those works provide examples of contribution to their main theories and can extend the impact towards increasing levels of active travel with children and adolescents. McMinn et al.'s [41] study is an example of how this might be more clearly integrated by using the TPB [47] as a model that explains an intention (represented by the motivation and willingness) towards a given behaviour. According to Ajzen, a behaviour intention is informed by the interconnection of the attitude (referring to the affective evaluation of the relevance of the behaviour), the subjective norm (referring to the perceived positive or negative social pressure on the behaviour) and the perceived behavioural control (referring to the perception of how successful the behaviour can be in a given context). However, McMinn's study did not present this specific data for the Irish population and, instead, aggregated it in the Northwest region.

While TPB is indeed a valuable theoretical framework to explore the individual attitudes, in the Irish context there is more awareness to ecological frameworks which help to explain the relation between the person and the environment through agency. Two such frameworks are those of Gibson's Affordance Theory [59], which was not considered by any of the reviewed studies, and Bronfenbrenner's Bioecological Model of Human Development (also presented as the Process–Person–Context–Time model) [60] which was considered by most of the reviewed research.

Building on Murtagh, Dempster, and Murphy's [45] use of Bronfenbrenner's model, it must be noted that this framework has been developed and refined from its earlier versions used by Murtagh and colleagues. According to Bronfenbrenner [60], the proximal processes in the micro- and mesosystem are essential to connect the person to the environment on a developmental perspective, but the research reviewed in our study does not explicitly explore what processes are (in)effective for active travel, and mainly asks about patterns, and contextual facilitators and inhibitors. One such process identified in the reviewed literature can be parental modelling (e.g., [43]) but the specific elements of this (and others) proximal process(es) as being (un)successful need to be better explored and explained. Moreover, if active travel is to be promoted as a desired lifelong behaviour, research needs to more strongly consider not only the immediate settings (microsystems of family, neighbourhood, school, and others) but also their mesosystemic interdependence (e.g., school–family) to provide more sustained, and potentially more effective, implications.

At the same time, as explored by Murtagh, Dempster, and Murphy [45], the personal factors need to be addressed to understand why active travel intentions do not fully, or more regularly, translate into actual active travel behaviour. This dilemma is where the notion of affordances from Gibson [59] may be most important, as a given contextual feature might drive away the active travel behaviour in one person but might make it present in another person. In short, Gibson considered that subject and environment are an inextricable behavioural dyad to present the idea that behaviour emerges from the physical properties of the environment in interaction with the subject's dispositions and resources. For example, while urban children tend to engage more with active travel, Lambe [43] showed that the contextual changes of the communities did not promote the expected increase in active travel which would be theoretically explained due to the affordance as perception of urban traffic did not change. Lambe [43] also showed that rural area children are more likely to identify the lack of resources as a reason (an affordance) to not engage with active travel. This means that the affordances are very much contextual and situational as a child might be able to cycle in a space where confidence and safety are perceived (e.g., neighbourhood) but not perform that ability/behaviour in a more contextually challenging environment, which could explain at a more theoretical level Nelson and colleagues' [31] findings of low perceived cycling ability in low active travel patterns. Based on Gibson's [59] theory, and from a research example provided by Kyttä, Oliver, Ikeda, Ahmadi, Omiya, and Laatikainen's [61] research with a sample of Finnish and Japanese children, it could be hypothesised that affordances related to active travel are strongly dependent on affordances of independent mobility and this might prove to be an effective focus to the future designs of interventions and active travel research in general.

4.4. Strengths and Limitations

A strong point of this review is that it has a clear scope as it attempts to draw a picture of the current research and main findings on active travel in Ireland with children and adolescents. We have tried to point out the factors that are important determinants of active travel according to the existing literature, without making selections or excluding any studies because of their lower quality, or for being published in academic outputs (e.g., journals). Additionally, the search and inclusion process (not only databases but also contextually relevant databases as Irish universities' repositories), which included developing a search strategy in consultation with a literature review expert and having four reviewers for a proportion of the entire source texts, is a strong point.

One limitation of this review is that its scope may not be broad enough because only studies reporting walking and cycling as means of, mainly, school-related active travel were included. Furthermore, most of the included studies focused on children above 10 years of age, as there is little empirical evidence regarding children below 10 years of age. Additionally, the range of data collection and analysis techniques used in the studies under review makes them hard to compare and makes the mixed results more difficult to interpret. As for the data collection procedures, most studies used self-report questionnaires, which may be subject to social desirability bias. A related issue is that this scoping review did not conduct a quality assessment of reviewed sources. The results should, therefore, be interpreted with some caution. Nevertheless, we believe that the current review provides a thorough survey of the available Irish literature on active travel and the range of research conducted into the subject with valuable insights.

5. Conclusions

This paper aimed to map the existing documentation (research, reports, policy) addressing children and adolescents active travel with regards to PA in the context of the Republic of Ireland, between 2000 and 2020, through a scoping review.

Although the levels of active travel among children and adolescents in the Republic of Ireland are higher than in other countries, the existing low levels of cycling to and from a destination, in conjunction with distance and safety barriers, are potentially contributing factors which might explain the difficulty in adopting active travel lifestyle behaviours for children and adolescents. To better approach this, policy needs to keep supporting and building on current evidence, but also ensure cross-sector collaboration and guidelines. Future data collection strategies relating to the surveillance of active travel behaviours for children and adolescents in the Republic of Ireland should consider the suggestions to use and enhance robust methodological instruments (accelerometers, GPS tracking devices, validated PA wearable devices etc.), with scientifically rigorous longitudinal research designs. At an underpinning level, research designs need to carefully consider the issues of active travel definition and measurement, and make more explicit use of, and contribute to, the underpinning theoretical frameworks that support active travel research.

Author Contributions: Conceptualization, J.C., M.A., and W.O.; methodology, J.C., M.A., W.O., and J.M.; validation, J.C., M.A., W.O., and J.M.; formal analysis, J.C., M.A., W.O., and J.M.; data curation, J.C.; writing—original draft preparation, J.C., M.A., W.O., and J.M.; writing—review and editing, W.O., and J.C. All authors have read and agreed to the published version of the manuscript.

Funding: This research received no external funding.

Conflicts of Interest: The authors declare no conflict of interest.

References

1. Physical Activity Guidelines Advisory Committee. *Physical Activity Guidelines Advisory Committee Scientific Report*; Department of Health and Human Services: Washington, DC, USA, 2018.
2. Sluijs, E.V.; Fearne, V.; Mattocks, C.; Riddoch, C.; Griffin, S.; Ness, A. The contribution of active travel to children's physical activity levels: Cross-sectional results from the ALSPAC study. *Prev. Med.* **2009**, *48*, 519–524. [CrossRef] [PubMed]
3. Voss, C.; Winters, M.; Frazer, A.; McKay, H. School-travel by public transit: Rethinking active transportation. *Prev. Med. Rep.* **2015**, *2*, 65–70. [CrossRef] [PubMed]
4. Larouche, R.; Saunders, T.J.; Faulkner, G.E.J.; Colley, R.; Tremblay, M. Associations Between Active School Transport and Physical Activity, Body Composition, and Cardiovascular Fitness: A Systematic Review of 68 Studies. *J. Phys. Act. Health* **2014**, *11*, 206–227. [CrossRef] [PubMed]
5. Dumith, S.; Hallal, P.; Reis, R.; Kohl, H.W., 3rd. Worldwide prevalence of physical inactivity and its association with human development index in 76 countries. *Prev. Med.* **2011**, *53*, 24–28. [CrossRef]
6. Hallal, P.; Andersen, L.; Bull, F.; Guthold, R.; Haskell, W.; Ekelund, U.; Lancet Physical Activity Series Working Group. Global physical activity levels: Surveillance progress, pitfalls, and prospects. *Lancet* **2012**, *380*, 247–257. [CrossRef]
7. Faulkner, G.; Buliung, R.; Flora, P.; Fusco, C. Active school transport, physical activity levels and body weight of children and youth: A systematic review. *Prev. Med.* **2009**, *48*, 3–8. [CrossRef]
8. Rosenberg, D.; Sallis, J.; Conway, T.; Cain, K.; McKenzie, T. Active Transportation to School Over 2 Years in Relation to Weight Status and Physical Activity. *Obesity* **2006**, *14*, 1771–1776. [CrossRef]
9. McDonald, N.; Brown, A.; Marchetti, L.; Pedroso, M. U.S. school travel, 2009: An assessment of trends. *Am. J. Prev. Med.* **2011**, *41*, 146–151. [CrossRef]
10. Buliung, R.N.; Mitra, R.; Faulkner, G. Active school transportation in the Greater Toronto Area, Canada: an exploration of trends in space and time (1986-2006). *Prev. Med.* **2009**, *48*, 507–512. [CrossRef]
11. Mammen, G.; Stone, M.; Faulkner, G.; Ramanathan, S.; Buliung, R.; O'Brien, C.; Kennedy, J. Active school travel: An evaluation of the Canadian school travel planning intervention. *Prev. Med.* **2014**, *60*, 55–59. [CrossRef]
12. Grize, L.; Bringolf-Isler, B.; Martin, E.; Braun-Fahrländer, C. Trend in active transportation to school among Swiss school children and its associated factors: Three cross-sectional surveys 1994, 2000 and 2005. *Int. J. Behav. Nutr. Phys. Act.* **2010**, *7*, 28. [CrossRef] [PubMed]
13. Timperio, A.; Ball, K.; Salmon, J.; Roberts, R.; Giles-Cort, B.; Simmons, D.; Baur, L.A.; Crawford, D. Personal, Family, Social, and Environmental Correlates of Active Commuting to School. *Am. J. Prev. Med.* **2006**, *30*, 45–51. [CrossRef] [PubMed]

14. Tudor-Locke, C.; Ainsworth, B.E.; Popkin, B.M. Active commuting to school: An overlooked source of childrens' physical activity? *Sports Med.* **2001**, *31*, 309–313. [CrossRef] [PubMed]
15. van der Ploeg, H.P.; Merom, D.; Corpuz, G.; Bauman, A.E. Trends in Australian children traveling to school 1971-2003: Burning petrol or carbohydrates? *Prev. Med.* **2008**, *46*, 60–62. [CrossRef]
16. Smith, M.; Ikeda, E.; Hinckson, E.; Duncan, S.; Maddison, R.; Meredith-Jones, K.; Walker, C.; Mandic, S. Results from New Zealand's 2018 Report Card on Physical Activity for Children and Youth. *J. Phys. Act. Health* **2018**, *15*, S390–S392. [CrossRef]
17. Carlin, A.; Murphy, M.H.; Gallagher, A.M. Do Interventions to Increase Walking Work? A Systematic Review of Interventions in Children and Adolescents. *Sports Med.* **2016**, *46*, 515–530. [CrossRef]
18. Salmon, J.; Booth, M.; Phongsavan, P.; Murphy, N.; Timperio, A. Promoting Physical Activity Participation among Children and Adolescents. *Epidemiol. Rev.* **2007**, *29*, 144–159. [CrossRef]
19. Saunders, L.; Green, J.; Petticrew, M.; Steinbach, R.; Roberts, H. What Are the Health Benefits of Active Travel? A Systematic Review of Trials and Cohort Studies. *PLoS ONE* **2013**, *8*, e69912. [CrossRef]
20. Schoeppe, S.; Duncan, M.; Badland, H.; Oliver, M.; Curtis, C. Associations of children's independent mobility and active travel with physical activity, sedentary behaviour and weight status: A systematic review. *J. Sci. Med. Sport* **2013**, *16*, 312–319. [CrossRef]
21. Woods, C.; Powell, C.; Saunders, J.; O'Brien, W.; Murphy, M.; Duff, C.; Farmer, O.; Johnston, A.; Connolly, S.; Belton, S. *The Children's Sport Participation and Physical Activity Study 2018 (CSPPA 2018)*; Department of Physical Education and Sport Sciences, University of Limerick: Limerick, Ireland; Sport Ireland, and Healthy Ireland: Dublin, Ireland; Sport Northern Ireland: Belfast, Northern Ireland, 2018.
22. Woods, C.; Moyna, N.; Quinlan, A.; Tannehill, D.; Walsh, J. *The Children's Sport Participation and Physical Activity Study (CSPPA). Research Report No 1*; School of Health and Human Performance, Dublin City University and The Irish Sports Council: Dublin, Ireland, 2010.
23. Graf, C.; Beneke, R.; Bloch, W.; Bucksch, J.; Dordel, S.; Eiser, S.; Ferrari, N.; Koch, B.; Krug, S.; Lawrenz, W.; et al. Recommendations for Promoting Physical Activity for Children and Adolescents in Germany. A Consensus Statement. *Obes. Facts* **2014**, *7*, 178–190. [CrossRef]
24. WHO. *Growing up Unequal: Gender and Socioeconomic Differences in Young People's Health and Well-Being. Health Behaviour in School-Aged Children Study: International Report from the 2013/14 Survey*; World Health Organization: Copenhagen, Denmark, 2016.
25. Farooq, M.; Parkinson, K.; Adamson, A.; Pearce, M.; Reilly, J.; Hughes, A.; Janssen, X.; Basterfield, L.; Reilly, J. Timing of the decline in physical activity in childhood and adolescence: Gateshead Millennium Cohort Study. *Br. J. Sports Med.* **2018**, *52*, 1002. [CrossRef]
26. Department of Health & Department of Transport, Tourism and Sport. *Healthy Ireland: Get Ireland Active—National Physical Activity Plan for Ireland*; Department of Health & Department of Transport, Tourism and Sport: Dublin, Ireland, 2016.
27. Harrington, D.; Murphy, M.; Carlin, A.; Coppinger, T.; Donnelly, A.; Dowd, K.; Keating, T.; Murphy, N.; Murtagh, E.; O'Brien, W.; et al. Results From Ireland North and South's 2016 Report Card on Physical Activity for Children and Youth. *J. Phys. Act. Health* **2016**, *13*, S183–S188. [CrossRef] [PubMed]
28. Arksey, H.; O'Malley, L. Scoping studies: Towards a methodological framework. *Int. J. Soc. Res. Methodol.* **2005**, *8*, 19–32. [CrossRef]
29. Munn, Z.; Peters, M.; Stern, C.; Tufanaru, C.; McArthur, A.; Aromataris, E. Systematic review or scoping review? Guidance for authors when choosing between a systematic or scoping review approach. *BMC Med. Res. Methodol.* **2018**, *18*, 143. [CrossRef] [PubMed]
30. O'Keeffe, B.; O'Beirne, A. *Children's Independent Mobility on the island of Ireland*; Get Ireland Active and Mary Immaculate College University of Limerick: Limerick, Ireland, 2015.
31. Nelson, N.; Foley, E.; O'Gorman, D.; Moyna, N.; Woods, C. Active commuting to school: How far is too far? *Int. J. Behav. Nutr. Phys. Act.* **2008**, *5*, 1. [CrossRef] [PubMed]
32. Nelson, N.; Woods, C. Neighborhood Perceptions and Active Commuting to School Among Adolescent Boys and Girls. *J. Phys. Act. Health* **2010**, *7*, 257–266. [CrossRef]
33. Coulter, M.; Woods, C. An Exploration of Children's Perceptions and Enjoyment of School-Based Physical Activity and Physical Education. *J. Phys. Act. Health* **2011**, *8*, 645–654. [CrossRef]
34. Gahan, R.-A. *Perceptions of the Built Environment and Active Travel in Children and Young People*; Waterford Institute of Technology: Waterford, Ireland, 2011.

35. Murtagh, E.; Murphy, M. Active Travel to School and Physical Activity Levels of Irish Primary Schoolchildren. *Pediatric Exerc. Sci.* **2011**, *23*, 230–236. [CrossRef]
36. Sullivan, L.; Nic Gabhainn, S. *HBSC Ireland 2010: Physical Activity, Active Travel and Exercise among Schoolchildren in Ireland 2010. Galway: Health Promotion Research Centre, NUI Galway. Short Report to Department of Children and Youth Affairs for the National Strategy for Research and Data on Children's Lives 2011–2016*; HBSC and Department of Health and Health Promotion Research Centre and NUI Galway: Galway, Ireland, 2012.
37. Clarke, N. ; The HBSC Ireland Team. *Active Travel among Schoolchildren in Ireland. HBSC Ireland Research Factsheet No. 22*; HBSC and Department of Health and Health Promotion Research Centre and NUI Galway: Galway, Ireland, 2013.
38. Delaney, P. *Sport and Recreation Participation and Lifestyle Behaviours in Waterford City Adolescents*; Coaching Ireland: Limerick, Ireland, 2013.
39. Daniels, N.; Kelly, C.; Molcho, M.; Sixsmith, J.; Byrne, M.; Gabhainn, S.N. Investigating active travel to primary school in Ireland. *Health Educ.* **2014**, *114*, 501–515. [CrossRef]
40. Harrington, D.M.; Belton, S.; Coppinger, T.; Cullen, M.; Donnelly, A.; Dowd, K.; Keating, T.; Layte, R.; Murphy, M.; Murphy, N.; et al. Results from Ireland's 2014 Report Card on Physical Activity in Children and Youth. *J. Phys. Act. Health* **2014**, *11*, S63–S68. [CrossRef]
41. McMinn, D.; Rowe, D.A.; Murtagh, S.; Nelson, N.M.; Čuk, I.; Atiković, A.; Peček, M.; Breslin, G.; Murtagh, E.M.; Murphy, M.H. Psychosocial factors related to children's active school travel: A comparison of two European regions . *Int. J. Exerc. Sci.* **2014**, *7*, 75–86.
42. Woods, C.; Nelson, N. An evaluation of distance estimation accuracy and its relationship to transport mode for the home-to-school journey by adolescents. *J. Transp. Health* **2014**, *1*, 274–278. [CrossRef]
43. Lambe, B. *The Effectiveness of Active Travel Initiatives in Irish Provincial Towns: An Evaluation of a Quasi-Experimental Natural Experiment*; Waterford Institute of Technology: Waterford, Ireland, 2015.
44. CSO. Census of Population 2016—Profile 6 Commuting in Ireland. Available online: https://www.cso.ie/en/releasesandpublications/ep/p-cp6ci/p6cii/p6stp/ (accessed on 1 December 2019).
45. Murtagh, E.; Dempster, M.; Murphy, M. Determinants of uptake and maintenance of active commuting to school. *Health Place* **2016**, *40*, 9–14. [CrossRef] [PubMed]
46. Lambe, B.; Murphy, N.; Bauman, A. Active Travel to Primary Schools in Ireland: An Opportunistic Evaluation of a Natural Experiment. *J. Phys. Act. Health* **2017**, *14*, 448–454. [CrossRef] [PubMed]
47. Ajzen, I. The theory of planned behavior. *Organ. Behav. Hum. Decis. Process.* **1991**, *50*, 179–211. [CrossRef]
48. Bronfenbrenner, U. *The Ecology of Human Development: Experiments by Nature and Design*; Harvard University Press: Cambridge, MA, USA, 1979.
49. Corder, K.; Sharp, S.; Atkin, A.; Griffin, S.; Jones, A.; Ekelund, U.; Sluijs, E.V. Change in objectively measured physical activity during the transition to adolescence. *Br. J. Sports Med.* **2015**, *49*, 730. [CrossRef]
50. Dumith, S.; Gigante, D.; Domingues, M.; Kohl, H.W., 3rd. Physical activity change during adolescence: A systematic review and a pooled analysis. *Int. J. Epidemiol.* **2011**, *40*, 685–698. [CrossRef]
51. Sherar, L.B.; Cumming, S.P.; Eisenmann, J.C.; Baxter-Jones, A.D.G.; Malina, R.M. Adolescent Biological Maturity and Physical Activity: Biology Meets Behavior. *Pediatric Exerc. Sci.* **2010**, *22*, 332–349. [CrossRef]
52. Larsen, K.; Gilliland, J.; Hess, P.; Tucker, P.; Irwin, J.; He, M. The Influence of the Physical Environment and Sociodemographic Characteristics on Children's Mode of Travel to and From School. *Am. J. Public Health* **2009**, *99*, 520–526. [CrossRef]
53. Ginja, S.; Arnott, B.; Araujo-Soares, V.; Namdeo, A.; McColl, E. Feasibility of an incentive scheme to promote active travel to school: A pilot cluster randomised trial. *Pilot Feasibility Stud.* **2017**, *3*, 57. [CrossRef]
54. Larouche, R.; Mammen, G.; Rowe, D.A.; Faulkner, G. Effectiveness of active school transport interventions: A systematic review and update. *BMC Public Health* **2018**, *18*, 206. [CrossRef] [PubMed]
55. Wen, L.M.; Fry, D.; Merom, D.; Rissel, C.; Dirkis, H.; Balafas, A. Increasing active travel to school: Are we on the right track? A cluster randomised controlled trial from Sydney, Australia. *Prev. Med.* **2008**, *47*, 612–618. [CrossRef] [PubMed]
56. Klesges, L.M.; Baranowski, T.; Beech, B.; Cullen, K.; Murray, D.M.; Rochon, J.; Pratt, C. Social desirability bias in self-reported dietary, physical activity and weight concerns measures in 8- to 10-year-old African-American girls: Results from the Girls health Enrichment Multisite Studies (GEMS). *Prev. Med.* **2004**, *38*, 78–87. [CrossRef] [PubMed]

57. O'Sullivan, M.; MacPhail, A. *Young People's Voices in Physical Education and Youth Sport*; Routledge: London, UK, 2010.
58. Institute of Public Health in Ireland. *Active Travel—Healthy Lives*; Institute of Public Health in Ireland: Dublin, Ireland, 2011.
59. Gibson, J. The Ecological Approach to Visual Perception. Lawrence Erlbaum Associates, Inc.: Hillsdale, NJ, USA, 1986; (Original work published 1979).
60. Bronfenbrenner, U. *Making Human Beings Human*; Sage: Thousand Oaks, CA, USA, 2005.
61. Kyttä, M.; Oliver, M.; Ikeda, E.; Ahmadi, E.; Omiya, I.; Laatikainen, T. Children as urbanites: Mapping the affordances and behavior settings of urban environments for Finnish and Japanese children. *Child. Geogr.* **2018**, *16*, 319–332. [CrossRef]

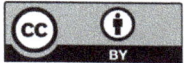

© 2020 by the authors. Licensee MDPI, Basel, Switzerland. This article is an open access article distributed under the terms and conditions of the Creative Commons Attribution (CC BY) license (http://creativecommons.org/licenses/by/4.0/).

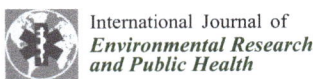 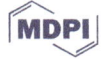

Article

Neighborhood Walkability and Active Transportation: A Correlation Study in Leisure and Shopping Purposes

Eun Jung Kim [1], Jiyeong Kim [1] and Hyunjung Kim [2,*]

[1] Department of Urban Planning, Keimyung University, 1095 Dalgubeol-daero, Dalseo-gu, Daegu 42601, Korea; kimej@kmu.ac.kr (E.J.K.); th154@naver.com (J.K.)
[2] Department of Civil and Environmental Engineering, Seoul National University, Gwanak-ro 1, Gwanak-gu, Seoul 08826, Korea
* Correspondence: urbanistar@snu.ac.kr; Tel.: +82-2-880-8903

Received: 28 February 2020; Accepted: 24 March 2020; Published: 25 March 2020

Abstract: A walkable environment is a crucial factor for promoting active transportation. The purpose of this study is to examine the association between neighborhood walkability and active transportation for noncommuting purposes (leisure and shopping) in Seoul, Korea. The Walkability Score is used as a measure of walkability, and a multilevel logistic regression model is employed to measure the odds of active transportation (i.e., walking and cycling; nonmotorized trips) at two levels: individual (level 1) and neighborhood (level 2). The results of the study showed that the Walkability Score was significantly correlated with higher odds of active transportation in shopping models. Specifically, every one-point increase in the Walkability Score was associated with 1.5%–1.8% higher odds of active transportation in shopping models. However, there was no significant correlation between the two in leisure models. Meanwhile, individual characteristics associated with the odds of active transportation differed in the leisure and shopping models. Older age was positively correlated with the odds of active transportation in the leisure model, while females showed a positive correlation in the shopping model. Based on the study, urban and transportation planners can recommend urban policies to promote active transportation in an urban setting.

Keywords: active transportation; walking; cycling; leisure trip; shopping trip; Walk Score; Walkability Score; multilevel logistic regression model; Seoul

1. Introduction

An increase in sedentary behavior and a proportionate growth in chronic diseases have been considered the most critical public health issues in the modern world, prompting several researchers in the public health and urban planning fields to investigate the environmental impact of promoting higher levels of physical activity [1,2]. As a means to promote physical activity, walking and cycling can be considered feasible daily activities for most people [3–5]. Among the different types of physical activities, walking and cycling are considered suitable for all age groups, given that they do not require special skills or facilities, and allow people to manage the intensity of their own movements [5]. Therefore, efforts to enhance walking and cycling within the community have been gaining momentum lately [5].

Promoting physical activity can help prevent a rise in the overweight and obese population and reduce the risk of potential chronic ailments such as respiratory diseases and Type 2 diabetes, as well as mortality risk from cardiovascular diseases and cancer [3,6–10]. Enhanced physical activity can also benefit mental health as it can improve emotions and the sense of recognition [11], reduce pressure [12,13], and depression [14]. From the urban and transportation planning perspective, walking and cycling, usually termed as "nonmotorized transport" or "active transportation," can be considered an important means for promoting sustainable cities and for providing social, environmental, and economic benefits [4,15]. Therefore, there is a growing emphasis on the importance of active transportation in light of urban problems such as traffic congestion, environmental pollution, energy shortage, and an increase in the obese population.

It is imperative to promote environmental and policy approaches to encourage physical activity considering that it can benefit all citizens in the neighborhood [16–18]. Accordingly, efforts to find an adequate built environment for physical activity, especially a walkable environment, has attracted the attention of policymakers, urban and transportation researchers, and public health scientists. Several studies have identified built environmental factors that most significantly influence walking behavior in urban and suburban areas [4,7,19–21], and efforts were made to develop a methodology to objectively measure the level of walkability. Consequently, several indices such as the Walk Score, Walkability Index, and Pedestrian Index of the Environment were developed combining various built environmental variables that influence walking behavior [7,19–32]. The Walk Score is one of the popular indices that objectively measures neighborhood walkability, taking into account the accessibility of amenities in the vicinity (e.g., grocery stores, restaurants, shopping centers, coffee shops, parks, schools) and pedestrian friendliness (e.g., intersection density and average block length) [25], and is currently used in various fields, including public health, real estate, and urban planning [33–37]. Studies have verified whether the Walk Score is appropriate to describe the level of walkability, and correspondingly, several works of the literature showed that a higher level of Walk Score is positively correlated with walking behavior [7,26,29,30,38–42].

A number of studies have investigated the association between walkability and health indicators using the Walk Score [42–44]. Xu and Wang examined the impact of the neighborhood environment on physical inactivity and obesity in Washington, D.C. in the United States. Using a multilevel regression model, they found that street connectivity was negatively associated with obesity, while Walk Score was negatively associated with physical inactivity. They also found that the obesity risk varied depending on urbanicity levels and gender, with a higher Walk Score linked to a lower risk of obesity in urban areas for females [43]. Wasfi et al. examined the influence of neighborhood walkability on the Body Mass Index (BMI) of urban Canadians using the Walk Score and the National Population Health Survey of Canada, and found that neighborhood walkability influences BMI trajectories for males [42]. McCormack et al. explored the relationship between walkability and waist circumference, waist-to-hip ratio, and BMI in Calgary, Alberta, Canada. Correspondingly, they found that a higher Walk Score was associated with lower odds of having a large waist circumference; neighborhoods with a lower Walk Score had higher odds of a high waist circumference, BMI, and waist circumference–BMI risk [44]. In short, previous studies have shown that developing a walkable environment can influence physical activity, which can lead to a significant population health impact.

2. Research Background

Over the past several decades, rapid industrialization and urbanization have led to significant lifestyle changes resulting in an increasing overweight and obese population, creating a significant public health burden in many countries [5,45]. A practical way to encourage physical activity on a daily basis is to promote active transportation. Therefore, several studies identified that a walkable environment has a positive association with active transportation [7,21,26–32]. For example, Reyer et al. used the Walkability Index and the Walk Score to explore the link to active transportation and found a tendency toward more active travel in more walkable neighborhoods [7]. Likewise, Knuiman et al. examined the relationship of neighborhood walkability and accessibility to a destination using walking as transportation in Perth, Australia. They found that accessibility to local destination, land use mix, and street connectivity are important determinants for promoting walking as a means of transportation [32].

Studies regarding the relationship between walkability and noncommuting active trips mainly considered the leisure purpose of walking or cycling. Investigating the neighborhood walkability in Canada, de Sa and Arden found that respondents living in highly walkable 500 m buffer zones (upper quartiles of the walkability index) were more likely to walk or cycle for leisure than those living in low-walkable buffer zones. When a 1000 m buffer zone was applied, respondents in more walkable neighborhoods were more likely to walk or cycle for both leisure and transport-related purposes [27]. Dyck et al. examined the association between leisure-time physical activity and perceived neighborhood environmental walkability in Belgium, Australia, and the United States. Except for the city of Ghent, Belgium, there was a positive linear association with recreational walking and leisure time physical activity [28]. Thielman et al. estimated the association between walkability and physical activity by transport walking and leisure time physical activity in Canada at the national level. They found that walkability was associated with transport walking in all age groups and city sizes. However, it had an inverse association with leisure-time physical activity among young adults and in large cities [29]. Some studies examined walkability for shopping purposes [21,30,31], but there are few studies that examined both leisure and shopping trips depending on the neighborhood walkability. For example, Habibian and Hosseinzadeh examined walkability across trip purposes including commuting, educational, and shopping, although they did not consider trips for leisure [31]. Manaugh and El-Geneidy examined the relationship between the trip purpose and walkability in nonmotorized mode of transportation; however, they considered noncommuting trip purposes mainly for shopping [30]. Lefebvre-Ropars et al. examined the association between walking time and the built environment using the Pedestrian Index of the Environment (PIE). They considered both shopping and leisure as noncommuting trips, and found that the PIE was more strongly correlated to the choice of walking for work, leisure, or shopping in very short trips [21]. However, they did not consider cycling as active transportation. In sum, previous studies on noncommuting active trips mainly focused on leisure walking/cycling, or investigated either leisure or shopping trips, or mainly focused on walking.

Korea is facing a severe health problem related to physical inactivity [45]. According to the Community Health Survey of Korea, the walking rate (the percentage of people who walked more than five days a week for more than 30 min a day in a week) in the country decreased overall during the past decade, from 50.6% in 2008 to 42.9% in 2018, while the proportion of individuals who are obese increased from 21.6% in 2008 to 31.8% in 2018 [46]. This increase in physical inactivity and obesity can be considered a social problem in Korea, which underscores the importance of developing pedestrian-friendly urban environments [47–50]. Accordingly, the city of Seoul is promoting "Walkable City, Seoul" as a major urban policy to enhance citizens' health and reduce traffic congestion [51]. A pedestrian-oriented traffic environment is being modeled with increasing safe walking zones and connecting touristic spots. Furthermore, bicycling is being promoted by expanding bike-related infrastructure, such as a sharing bike system.

A recent study by Kim et al. examined the association between walkability and active commuting (i.e., walking and cycling to work or school) in Seoul using the Walkability Score, and empirically found a positive correlation between walkability and active commuting [52]. This raises another question as to whether walkability will also have a significant positive association in the case of noncommuting trips (e.g., leisure and shopping trips) with active transportation (i.e., walking and cycling). In addition, based on trip purposes, would a walkable environment associate similarly or differently within leisure and shopping trips? Especially, noncommuting trips are an intentional trip that may more likely depend on the neighborhood environment than a commuting trip [30]. Some studies found that the distance and duration of noncommuting walking were substantially longer than they were for commuting purpose, as well as the importance of urban forms on noncommuting trips [21,53]. In particular, compared to commuting, a noncommuting trip can induce more walking and cycling if an adequate walkable and bikeable built environment is provided in the neighborhood. This study expands the scope of Kim et al.'s [52] research by considering the Walkability Score and active transportation differentiating the trip purposes to noncommuting. The purpose of this study is to examine the association between the level of walkability measured by the Walkability Score and active transportation for noncommuting trips in Seoul, Korea. Specifically, the relationship between the walkability level and active transportation (i.e., walking and cycling) in noncommuting trips (i.e., shopping and leisure trip) will be examined considering both individual characteristics and the built environment of the neighborhood by conducting a multilevel analysis in Seoul.

3. Materials and Methods

3.1. Study Area

The study focuses on the city of Seoul, and uses travel mode data from the Household Travel Diary Survey adapted from the Korea Transport Database [54]. The total number of home-based trips for leisure and shopping purposes in the survey were 9998 and 8578, respectively. The city of Seoul consists of 424 neighborhoods with their own administrative offices. The neighborhood is referred to as "dong" in Korea, which is the most disaggregated administrative unit. Of the 424 neighborhoods, some had very few sample numbers in the survey. For example, in the case of Jamwon-dong, only four individuals responded to the survey. Neighborhoods that had notably few samples such as Jamwon-dong were excluded from the multilevel modeling, given that ensuring a sufficient number of samples is one of the most important issues in multilevel analyses [55–57]. For unbiased results, some studies suggested "30/30" and "20/50" rules that indicated the minimum number of observations per group/minimum number of groups. Kreft recommended the "30/30" [58], while Hox recommended the "'20/50" rule [59]. To prevent biased estimate of parameters, we employed a minimum of 30 respondents per neighborhood for the study. Out of the 424 neighborhoods, the number of corresponding neighborhoods was 129 and 91 in the leisure and shopping models, respectively. Overall, the study used 5742 individuals nested within 129 neighborhoods and 3722 individuals nested within 91 neighborhoods in the leisure and shopping trip models, respectively, as shown in Figure 1.

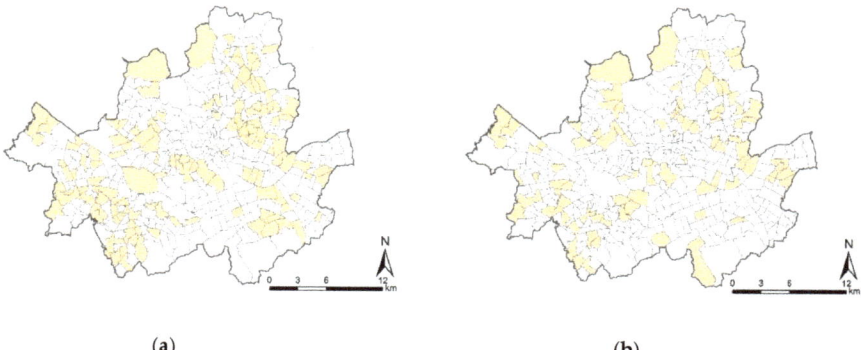

Figure 1. Study area: (**a**) Neighborhoods with at least 30 individual respondents for leisure trips (N = 129); (**b**) Neighborhoods with at least 30 individual respondents for shopping trips (N = 91).

3.2. Measures

As mentioned earlier, this research expands on a study by Kim et al. [52]. In this study, an investigation of the correlation between noncommuting active trips (i.e., leisure and shopping) and the Walkability Score was conducted. Accordingly, independent variables were basically derived from related data sources and methodology from Kim et al. [52], differentiating the trip purposes used as the dependent variables. The measurements and data sources of variables used in this study are shown in Table 1.

3.2.1. Individual-level Variables (Level 1)

All individual-level variables of this study were acquired from the 2016 Household Travel Diary Survey from the Korea Transport Database [54], which is a traffic-related survey conducted every five years across the country and considered as a nationwide passenger survey in Korea. This survey examines the travel diary of household members aged five and older on weekdays, and is conducted through home visits and online using a self-reported questionnaire [60].

- Dependent variables: Travel mode (motorized vs. nonmotorized modes)

As dependent variables, this study used active transportation (e.g., walking and cycling) separately for leisure and shopping purposes. From the Household Travel Diary Survey, there are four travel modes—walking, bicycling, public transport, and private automobile. For the analysis, they were coded as binaries—1 for nonmotorized modes (walking and cycling) and 0 for motorized modes (public transport and private automobile).

- Individual socioeconomic status variable

At the individual level, several socioeconomic status variables were considered as confounding factors, including age, gender, household income, and car ownership. These individual variables were also acquired from the 2016 Household Travel Diary Survey from the Korea Transport Database [54].

3.2.2. Neighborhood-level Variables (Level 2)

This study employed the neighborhood as a spatial unit for multilevel modeling at level 2. All neighborhood-level variables in this study used the mean values of each neighborhood.

- Walkability Score

As a key independent variable, this study employed the Walkability Score, which was assessed in Seoul by Kim et al. [61]. Moreover, a recent study found that the Walkability Score is a reliable index to measure environmental walkability in the city [62]. The value of the Walkability Score is calculated by the Walk Score algorithm, which basically calculates the accessibility of utilitarian destinations with a distance decay function. They include nine amenities essential to everyday life—grocery stores, restaurants, shopping centers, coffee shops, banks, parks, schools, books, and entertainment. The Walkability Score calculates the closest network distance from each amenity and then awards 100% of the maximum points to amenities located within a network distance of 400 m, 75% within 800 m, 40% within 1.2 km, and 12.5% within 1.6 km of a given location [61]. By combining the accessibility of nine types of utilitarian destinations, the scores are normalized on a scale of 0 to 100. Additionally, poor pedestrian friendliness is considered as a penalty element. It considers the intersection density and average block length as factors of pedestrian friendliness. Areas with lower intersection density (no penalty: intersections per square mile > 200) and longer average block length (no penalty: average block length < 120 m) receive penalties up to 10% of the total score. The Walk Score ranges from 0 (car-dependent) to 100 (walkers' paradise) [25]. Geospatial data used for assessing the Walkability Score in Seoul were collected from both governmental websites and private companies. More detailed information on measures, data sources, and calculation methods is found in Kim et al. [61].

- Neighborhood environmental variables

The Walkability Score is adapted from the Walk Score, which is an index that combines various variables that represent urban form such as density, diversity, and destination accessibility [21,62]. Since the Walk Score itself is a composite index of neighborhood walkability, there are some studies that include only itself as a neighborhood environmental variable [7,63]. However, one study found that there are some urban form elements such as land use diversity and walking route supply that the Walk Score does not include [21]. Therefore, this study considered land use mix and sidewalk length as additional neighborhood environmental variables. Land use mix is an important urban environmental variable for promoting walking and cycling. Some studies have shown that the higher the land use mix, the more people walk and/or are physically active [31,32,64,65]. The entropy index was used to measure a land use mixture of residential, commercial, industrial, and greenspaces. It ranges from 0 (single use) to 1 (perfect mixing). Moreover, sidewalk length (i.e., total length of sidewalks per square kilometer) was considered in this study, given that it was positively associated with the minutes of neighborhood-based walking for transportation [66]. The data used in the analysis were obtained from the public source of the National Spatial Data Infrastructure Portal [67], while the neighborhood environmental variables were captured by ArcGIS.

Table 1. Measurement, data source, and descriptive statistics of variables.

Variable	Measurement	Data Source
Dependent Variable		
Travel mode	Binary: 0 = Motorized mode, 1 = Nonmotorized mode	Household Travel Diary Survey from the Korea Transport Database [54]
Individual Variables (Level 1)		
Age	Continuous: Age	
Gender	Binary: 0 = male, 1 = female	
Income	Ordinal: 1 = less than 1 million won, 2 = 1–2 million won, 3 = 2–3 million won, 4 = 3–5 million won, 5 = 5–10 million won, 6 = more than 10 million won	Household Travel Diary Survey from the Korea Transport Database [54]
Car ownership	Binary: 0 = no, 1 = yes	
Neighborhood Variables (Level 2)		
Walkability Score	Continuous: Walkability Score	Kim et al. [61]
Land use mix [1]	Continuous: 0 (single use)–1 (perfect mixing)	National Spatial Data Infrastructure Portal [67]
Sidewalk length	Continuous: Length of sidewalk per square kilometer	

[1] Land Use Mix $= -1 \left(\sum_{i=1}^{n} p_i \times \ln(p_i) \right) / \ln(n)$, where p_i is the proportion of the land use type of i, i = residential, commercial, industrial, and greenspaces, n = total number of land uses in the mix (=4).

3.3. Data Analysis

A multilevel logistic regression model was used, with the two odds of nonmotorized trips (walking and cycling) for (1) leisure purposes and (2) shopping purposes. An odds ratio (OR) is a statistic that quantified the association between an outcome and exposure. When calculating a logistic regression analysis, the regression coefficient is an estimated increase in the log probability of the outcome according to a unit increase in the exposure value [68]. If the OR is exactly 1, there is no correlation between outcome and exposure. When the OR is greater than 1, then there is a positive association, conversely if the OR is less than 1, then there is a negative correlation between outcome and exposure. Applying this concept here, this study examined the correlation between outcome (odds of nonmotorized trips for noncommuting) and exposure (individual and neighborhood variables). The multilevel data included two levels: individual (level 1) and neighborhood (level 2). Individuals living in the same neighborhood shared the same Walkability Score and the neighborhood environmental characteristics including land use mix and sidewalk length at the corresponding level. R software was used for the analysis in this study.

4. Results

4.1. Descriptive Statistics of Variables

As shown in Table 2, the proportions of individuals using nonmotorized modes of transportation for leisure and shopping purposes were 81.8% and 76.8%, respectively. In both the samples, the ratio of the motorized mode to nonmotorized mode was approximately 1 to 4. From the individual variables, the participants for the leisure and shopping trips reported a mean age of 61.1 and 53.5 years, respectively. The median income level of households per month was 4 and 3, respectively, for each subsample; the value of 3 corresponds to 2–3 million won while 4 corresponds to 3–5 million won. The variable of household income ranged from 1 (less than 1 million won) to 6 (more than 10 million won). In the leisure and shopping trip group, the proportion of female participants was 61.4% and 90.9%, and the proportion of car ownership was 54.8% and 63.3%, respectively.

Table 2. Descriptive statistics of variables.

Variable	Measurement	Leisure Purpose		Shopping Purpose	
		%	Mean (SD)	%	Mean (SD)
Dependent Variable					
Travel mode	Binary: 0 = Motorized mode 1 = Nonmotorized mode	18.2% 81.8%		23.2% 76.8%	
Individual Variables (Level 1)					
Age	Continuous: Age		61.1 (16.7)		53.5 (15.1)
Gender	Binary: 0 = male 1 = female	38.7% 61.4%		9.1% 90.9%	
Income	Ordinal: Household income level		4 [1]		3 [2]
Car ownership	Binary: 0 = no 1 = yes	45.2% 54.8%		36.7% 63.3%	
Neighborhood Variables (Level 2)					
Walkability Score	Continuous: Walkability Score		67.55 (9.0)		67.71 (9.8)
Land use mix [3]	Continuous: 0 (single use)–1 (perfect mixing)		0.52 (0.3)		0.53 (0.3)
Sidewalk length [3]	Continuous: Length of sidewalk per square kilometer		1.99 (0.6)		1.95 (0.6)

[1] This is a median value and it corresponds to 3–5 million won, [2] this is a median value and it corresponds to 2–3 million won, [3] square root-transformed, SD: standard deviation.

The mean values of the neighborhood environmental variables were slightly different because the target areas (number of neighborhoods for leisure model = 129, number of neighborhoods for shopping model = 91) varied between leisure and shopping travels, although it was basically similar in the two samples. In the samples of leisure and shopping purposes, the mean value of Walkability Score was 67.55 (SD = 9.0) and 67.71 (SD = 9.8), respectively. Meanwhile, the mean value of land use mix was 0.52 (SD = 0.3) and 0.53 (SD = 0.3), and the mean value of sidewalk length was 1.99 (SD = 0.6) and 1.95 (SD = 0.6), respectively. Both variables of land use mix and sidewalk length were square root-transformed for use in the multilevel analysis.

4.2. Results of Multilevel Logistic Models: Odds of Active Transportation for Leisure and Shopping Purposes

This study conducted a multilevel logistic model because individual variables were nested within neighborhoods. Generally, there are three phases of procedure for multilevel logistic regression: (step 1) an empty model without predictors to assess variation of log-odds between clusters, (step 2) an intermediate model to assess the variation of the lower-level effects between clusters, and (step 3) a final model to test a research hypothesis [69]. Based on the procedure, this study first ran a model without predictors and found it was necessary to employ the multilevel analysis. In the second phase, we tested which variables were associated with the odds of outcome (active transportation) by performing a likelihood-ratio test. The final model was then presented according to theoretical importance as well as the statistical significance of variables. There are two final models each in the leisure and shopping models. Model 1 considers individual and neighborhood variables, but only considered the Walkability Score as a neighborhood variable, while Model 2 included additional neighborhood-level variables in Model 1. Specifically, the dependent variable is binary, for example, an individual using nonmotorized transportation (=1, and 0 otherwise) for leisure and shopping purposes. Model 1 included age, gender, income, and car ownership as individual variables (level 1) and the Walkability Score as a neighborhood variable (level 2). Meanwhile, Model 2 basically included all variables used in Model 1, but added land use mix and sidewalk length as neighborhood variables (level 2). The results of multilevel logistic models are shown in Table 3. Since Models L–2 and S–2 contained theoretically important neighborhood environmental variables such as land use mix and sidewalk length, the results from both Model 1 (L–1 and S–1) and Model 2 (L–2 and S–2) are reported in this section.

4.2.1. Odds of Active Transportation for Leisure Purposes

The results of the analysis are as follows. First, the Walkability Score was insignificant in both Models L–1 and L–2. At the 0.1 significance level, there was no evidence of statistical interaction between the Walkability Score and the odds of nonmotorized trips in both Model L–1 ($p = 0.145$) and Model L–2 ($p = 0.178$). Second, age was positively associated with the odds of nonmotorized trips in this model. Older adults were more likely to use active transportation for leisure purposes. The results are similar to a previous study, which found that young adults had a negative association with leisure physical activity [29]. Third, car ownership was a statistically significant predictor of nonmotorized trips. Individuals having a car are much less likely to walk or cycle for leisure purpose. Fourth, gender and household income were not associated with the odds of nonmotorized trips in both the models. Previous studies also showed different associations on gender and the Walk Score (e.g., positive association of lower risk of obesity for females in urban areas [43], while showing no significant influence on BMI for females [42]). With respect to income level, a previous study showed that lower income individuals were more likely to walk and cycle for commuting purposes [52]. For economic reason, the lower the income, the more likely it is to commute by walking and cycling. On the other hand, because travel for leisure and shopping purposes are less sensitive to income than commuting travel, it is understandable that there no significant correlation between income level and the odds of nonmotorized trips in this study. Fifth, unlike previous studies [31,32,64–66], additional neighborhood environmental variables, including land use mix and sidewalk length, had no statistical relationships with the odds of nonmotorized trips in Model L–2.

Table 3. Results of the multilevel logit regression analyses for estimating environmental correlates of active transportation in leisure and shopping purposes.

Variable	Odds of Nonmotorized Trip for Leisure Purpose								Odds of Nonmotorized Trip for Shopping Purpose							
	Model L-1				Model L-2				Model S-1				Model S-2			
	OR	p-Value	95% CI Lower	Upper	OR	p-Value	95% CI Lower	Upper	OR	p-Value	95% CI Lower	Upper	OR	p-Value	95% CI Lower	Upper
Intercept	1.662	0.266	0.766	2.557	1.540	0.375	0.587	2.493	0.879	0.785	−0.051	1.809	0.871	0.789	−0.138	1.881
Individual Variables (Level 1)																
Age	1.012 ***	<0.001	1.008	1.017	1.013 ***	0.000	1.008	1.017	1.004	0.227	0.997	1.011	1.003	0.374	0.996	1.010
Gender (reference: male)	1.043	0.600	0.885	1.202	1.050	0.547	0.892	1.208	1.755 ***	<0.001	1.473	2.036	1.735 ***	0.000	1.444	2.026
Income	1.044	0.248	0.971	1.117	1.043	0.263	0.969	1.116	0.996	0.925	0.904	1.087	0.983	0.731	0.886	1.080
Car Ownership (reference: no)	0.519 ***	<0.001	0.301	0.736	0.523 ***	0.000	0.306	0.739	0.646 ***	<0.001	0.407	0.885	0.652 ***	0.001	0.410	0.894
Neighborhood Variables (Level 2)																
Walkability Score	1.009	0.145	0.997	1.020					1.015 *	0.013	1.003	1.026				
Land use mix [1]					1.082	0.699	0.681	1.483					0.944	0.789	0.518	1.369
Sidewalk length [1]					1.000	1.000	0.797	1.203					0.949	0.646	0.727	1.172
ICC	9.3%				9.2%				4.5%				4.7%			
N	5742								3722							

*** $p < 0.001$, ** $p < 0.01$, * $p < 0.05$; [1] square root-transformed; OR = Odds Ratio; CI = Confidence Interval; ICC = Intraclass Correlation Coefficient.

4.2.2. Odds of Active Transportation for Shopping Purposes

The results for the shopping model can be summarized as follows. First, similar to previous studies [30,31], the Walkability Score was significantly associated with the odds of nonmotorized trips in both Model S–1 and Model S–2. Every one-point increase in the Walkability Score was associated with 1.5% and 1.8% higher odds of nonmotorized trips in Model S–1 (OR: 1.015, 95% CI = 1.003–1.026) and Model S–2 (OR: 1.018, 95% CI = 1.005–1.031), respectively. Second, the female gender was positively correlated with the odds of nonmotorized trips in both models, as they tended to walk and cycle more for shopping purposes. Third, as with leisure models, car ownership was significantly associated with nonmotorized trips. Individuals with cars were associated with lower odds of nonmotorized trips for shopping. Fourth, there were contradictory results depending on individual variables. For example, age was a significant predictor in leisure models similar to the previous study [29]; however, it was insignificant in shopping models. Income level had no significance in both leisure and shopping models. Fifth, similar to leisure models, there were no significant correlations between the odds of nonmotorized trips and neighborhood variables such as land use mix and sidewalk length. Finally, according to the intraclass correlation coefficient (ICC) value, about 4.5% of the total variance in the odds of nonmotorized trips for shopping purposes was accounted for by differences of the Walkability Scores between neighborhoods in Model S–1. The ICC represents the proportion of the between-group variance compared to the total variance [70]. The interpretation of the ICC is the expected correlation between randomly selected observations from the same group [71]. In this study, the ICC is the proportion of variance in the odds of nonmotorized trips (outcome variable) that is explained by the neighborhood (level 2). It indicated that neighborhood walkability was one of the most important factors affecting individuals' behavior of active transportation for shopping purposes. Model S–2 showed about 4.7% explanatory power of neighborhood variables (level 2), but the significance of additional neighborhood environmental variables, such as land use mix and sidewalk length, were not guaranteed. There are some arguments that if ICC is close to zero (typically less than 4%–5%), there is lesser need to use a multilevel analysis [72,73]. However, it is still necessary to use multilevel analysis in nested data [73].

5. Discussion

This study examined the correlation between the level of walkability and noncommuting trips by conducting multilevel logistic regression analysis with the two odds of active transportation (i.e., walking and cycling) for leisure and shopping purposes. It is an expansion of a prior study that revealed a positive correlation between neighborhood walkability and active commuting in Seoul [52], since it is likely that noncommuting trips are more influenced by the neighborhood environment than commuting trips when people walk or cycle [30]. As a result, we empirically discovered that the walkability level of Seoul's neighborhoods was positively correlated with the probability of active transportation for shopping purposes while showing no statistical correlation in leisure purposes.

Discussions based on the findings are presented as follows. First, the correlation between the Walkability Score and the nonmotorized trips varied in the leisure and shopping models. In the shopping models, the Walkability Score was positively correlated with the odds of nonmotorized trips (Model S–1: OR = 1.015, 95% CI = 1.003–1.026; Model S–2: OR = 1.018, 95% CI = 1.005–1.031). However, there was no significant correlation between the Walkability Score and the odds of nonmotorized trips for leisure purposes. This differs from the findings of previous literature that showed that the odds ratios of walking for the Pedestrian Index of the Environment (PIE) were 1.05 for leisure and 1.04 for shopping purposes [21]. This difference is interpreted based on the indicators included in the walkability index. While the PIE considers the 5Ds of urban form, including density, diversity, design, destination accessibility, and distance to transit [21], the Walkability Score mainly considers destination accessibility [25]. As mentioned earlier, the Walkability Score was assessed based on the accessibility of amenities including grocery stores, restaurants, shopping centers [61]. Therefore, it can be demonstrated that the Walkability Score is an index based on the accessibility of amenities that are more suitable for shopping than for leisure purposes. Second, other neighborhood-level variables had no significant correlation with the odds of nonmotorized trips both in the leisure and shopping models. From Models L–2 and S–2, no variable was significant among land use mix and sidewalk length. This result is different from those of previous studies in which active transport (e.g., walking) and/or physical activity was positively correlated with land use mix [31,64,65]. Meanwhile, some studies showed mixed-use development may not provide a positive effect on walking and cycling in some high-density cities because these cities would reduce the chance for people walking or cycling as they can move easily to another area by public transportation [5,74,75]. This might be applied to Seoul because it is one of the high-density cities [76] and has good public transportation in its neighborhoods. Regarding sidewalk length, this analysis showed a similar result to the previous study that estimated the association between sidewalk length and walking for different trip purposes [66]. It found that neighborhood-based walking for transportation had a positive association with sidewalk length but had no association in recreation walking, which was in line with our research on active transportation for leisure and shopping purposes. Third, the types of individual variables that were significantly associated with the odds of nonmotorized trips differ in the leisure and shopping models. Specifically, older age was positively correlated with the odds of nonmotorized trips for leisure purposes, while female gender had a positive correlation with the odds of nonmotorized trips for shopping purposes. These results can be used to develop various urban policies. For example, older people were more likely to have higher odds of nonmotorized trips for leisure purposes in this study. This finding presents an important issue for further research on age-friendly community design. Environmental factors that promote leisure walking (e.g., greener landscape, well-designed street furniture, wide pedestrian roads, safer pathway) in the development of age-friendly communities may be considered. In addition, a higher Walk Score was correlated to a lower risk of obesity for females in urban areas [43]. As noted from the result, the female gender tends to walk and cycle for shopping purposes; therefore, planning a wider choice of commercial facilities in a walkable and bikeable distance in urban areas or creating a more walkable environment for shopping could induce more physical activity for females. Finally, according to ICC values, the level of walkability of the neighborhood was an important factor in influencing individuals' odds of nonmotorized trips for shopping purposes. From the results of the multilevel analyses, the proportion accounted for by the Walkability Score in the odds of nonmotorized trips for shopping purposes was about 4.5%. Although the ICC value was high at 9.3% in the leisure model (Model L–1), the Walkability Score was insignificant; therefore, it was not discussed. Additionally, compared to the results of the previous study by Kim et al. [52] (ICC was 2.1% for active commuting model), active trips for shopping had a higher ICC value (4.5%) in this study. This indicates that the Walkability Score is a walkability index that responds more sensitively and effectively to the odds of nonmotorized trips for shopping purposes when compared to commuting purposes.

This study has several limitations; directions for future studies to address them follow. At the outset, even though this study found a significant correlation between the walkability and odds of active transportation for shopping purposes, it showed no correlation between them for leisure models. This may be due to the Walkability Score's sensitive nature toward walking and cycling for shopping purposes. For further direction of the study, the Walkability Score can be developed and customized based on trip purposes. For example, it will be possible to develop a walkability index, "Walkability Score for Leisure," where people can search for environmental conditions for leisure purposes in their daily lives by considering the characteristics and contents of each facility that can attract and affect leisure trips. Second, this study examined the correlation of neighborhood walkability with active transportation in Seoul. The city of Seoul is promoting policies regarding walking and cycling, and the neighborhood environment is being developed toward a more walkable environment [51]. Future research will be able to experiment with other cities in Korea, which could help identify practical policies in urban design and transportation planning that can be used across the country. Third, since we focused on active transportation for noncommuting trips, this study combined walking and cycling into nonmotorized transportation. However, walkers and cyclists can have different characteristics of shopping and leisure trips. In a further study, an analysis comparing walking and cycling behavior on each trip's purposes could be discussed. Fourth, the mean ages of the participants for leisure and shopping purposes were relatively high, corresponding to middle-aged and older adults. This can reflect that retired people may have more time for recreational and shopping activities, and thus they are likely to spend their time on the active mode of the trip. Nevertheless, the older age of respondents remains a limitation. Future studies need to properly extract samples and use them for analysis so that respondents are not biased at a specific age group. Finally, this study is a cross-sectional design that cannot identify causal relationship over time. Cross-sectional analysis cannot identify whether individuals walk frequently because of its walkable environmental conditions or whether the individuals who walk a lot more choose to live in walkable neighborhoods. For further study, a longitudinal analysis can be performed to examine the causality between walkable environment and active transportation.

Despite these limitations, this study is significant in several aspects. First, since the correlation of environmental walkability and active trips was analyzed using a multilevel logistic model, factors from both individual and neighborhood levels were taken into account. Although the ICC values were generally low at 4.5% in Model S–1 and 4.7% in Model S–2, it is suggested that multilevel modeling is required when dealing with nested data [73]. That is, because individual-level variables were nested within the neighborhood, the multilevel analysis allowed an examination of the impact of multilevel factors on the dependent variable (active transportation). Second, there are few studies that comprehensively examined active transportation for both leisure and shopping purposes. In this study, we compared the probability of active transportation (i.e., walking and cycling) for each travel purpose (i.e., leisure and shopping purposes) depending on the Walkability Score. Based on our findings, a tailored policy guideline can be provided based on trip purposes. Finally, we found that the Walkability Score, measured in Seoul, had a significant validity for examining the odds of active transportation for shopping purposes. However, this study demonstrated that more variables should be considered when assessing active transportation, especially for leisure purposes, as they affect not just accessibility to local destinations but also other urban form factors such as density, diversity, and design, and the quality of urban environments. From the findings of this study, policymakers and researchers from the urban and transportation planning and public health fields can obtain a comprehensive understanding of enhancing active travel in leisure and shopping, based on the primary concerns.

6. Conclusions

Walking and cycling have attracted the attention of urban planners and policymakers not only as a means of sustainable transport but also to boost individuals' physical activity levels [5]. The built environment plays a crucial role in promoting active transportation, and various efforts have been made to measure the correlation between neighborhood walkability and active trips. Meanwhile, it is often said that a walkable neighborhood environment can promote the use of active transportation in noncommuting trips [30]. Accordingly, this study identified the correlation between neighborhood walkability and active transportation for leisure and shopping purposes. The results of this study showed that the association between walkability and active transportation varies depending on trip purposes. The results remind urban policymakers of the need to differentiate policy remedies while promoting active transportation. Based on this study, various policy suggestions for promoting active transportation were established, and it is expected that citizens will be encouraged to walk and cycle and increase physical activity to enjoy a better quality of life.

Author Contributions: Conceptualization, E.J.K. and H.K.; Methodology, E.J.K. and H.K.; Software, E.J.K. and J.K.; Validation, E.J.K., J.K., and H.K.; Formal Analysis, E.J.K. and J.K.; Investigation, E.J.K.; Resources, E.J.K.; Data Curation, E.J.K. and J.K.; Writing—Original Draft Preparation, E.J.K., J.K., and H.K.; Writing—Review and Editing, E.J.K. and H.K.; Visualization, J.K.; Supervision, E.J.K.; Project Administration, E.J.K.; Funding Acquisition, E.J.K. All authors have read and agreed to the published version of the manuscript.

Funding: This work was supported by the National Research Foundation of Korea (NRF) grant funded by the Korea government (MSIT) (No. NRF-2017R1A2B4005440).

Conflicts of Interest: The authors declare no conflict of interest.

References

1. Carr, L.J.; Dunsiger, S.I.; Marcus, B.H. Validation of walk score for estimating access to walkable amenities. *Br. J. Sports Med.* **2010**, *45*, 1144–1148. [CrossRef] [PubMed]
2. Shashank, A.; Schuurman, N. Unpacking walkability indices and their inherent assumptions. *Health Place* **2019**, *55*, 145–154. [CrossRef] [PubMed]
3. Nykiforuk, C.I.J.; McGetrick, J.A.; Crick, K.; Johnson, J.A. Check the Score: Field Validation of Street Smart Walk Score in Alberta, Canada. *Prev. Med. Rep.* **2016**, *4*, 532–539. [CrossRef] [PubMed]
4. Moura, F.; Cambra, P.; Gonçalves, A.B. Measuring walkability for distinct pedestrian groups with a participatory assessment method: A case study in Lisbon. *Landsc. Urban Plan.* **2017**, *157*, 282–296. [CrossRef]
5. Wang, Y.; Chau, C.K.; Ng, W.Y.; Leung, T.M. A review on the effects of physical built environment attributes on enhancing walking and cycling activity levels within residential neighborhoods. *Cities* **2016**, *50*, 1–15. [CrossRef]
6. Powell, K.E.; Paluch, A.E.; Blair, S.N. Physical activity for health: What kind? How much? How intense? On top of what? *Annu. Rev. Public Health* **2011**, *32*, 349–365. [CrossRef]
7. Reyer, M.; Fina, S.; Siedentop, S.; Schlicht, W. Walkability is only part of the story: Walking for transportation in Stuttgart, Germany. *Int. J. Environ. Res. Public Health* **2014**, *11*, 5849–5865. [CrossRef]
8. Hakim, A.A.; Petrovitch, H.; Burchfiel, C.M.; Ross, G.W.; Rodriguez, B.L.; White, L.R.; Yano, K.; Curb, J.D.; Abbott, R.D. Effects of walking on mortality among nonsmoking retired men. *N. Engl. J. Med.* **1998**, *338*, 94–99. [CrossRef]
9. Manson, J.E.; Hu, F.B.; Rich-Edwards, J.W.; Colditz, G.A.; Stampfer, M.J.; Willett, W.C.; Speizer, F.E.; Hennekens, C.H. A prospective study of walking as compared with vigorous exercise in the prevention of coronary heart disease in women. *N. Engl. J. Med.* **1999**, *341*, 650–658. [CrossRef]
10. Brownson, R.C.; Housemann, R.A.; Brown, D.R.; Jackson-Thompson, J.; King, A.C.; Malone, B.R.; Sallis, J.F. Promoting physical activity in rural communities. *Am. J. Prev. Med.* **2000**, *18*, 235–241. [CrossRef]
11. Ohmatsu, S.; Nakano, H.; Tominaga, T.; Terakawa, Y.; Murata, T.; Morioka, S. Activation of the serotonergic system by pedaling exercise changes anterior cingulate cortex activity and improves negative emotion. *Behav. Brain Res.* **2014**, *270*, 112–117. [CrossRef] [PubMed]
12. Kario, K.; Schwartz, J.E.; Davidson, K.W.; Pickering, T.G. Gender differences in associations of diurnal blood pressure variation, awake physical activity, and sleep quality with negative affect. *Hypertension* **2001**, *38*, 997–1002. [CrossRef] [PubMed]
13. Vancampfort, D.; Probst, M.; Adriaens, A.; Pieters, G.; De Hert, M.; Stubbs, B.; Soundy, A.; Vanderlinden, J. Changes in physical activity, physical fitness, self-perception and quality of life following a 6-month physical activity counseling and cognitive behavioral therapy program in outpatients with binge eating disorder. *Psychiatry Res.* **2014**, *219*, 361–366. [CrossRef] [PubMed]
14. Dunn, A.L.; Trivedi, M.H.; O'Neal, H.A. Physical activity dose-response effects on outcomes of depression and anxiety. *Med. Sci. Sports Exerc.* **2001**, *33*, S587–S597. [CrossRef]
15. Sallis, J.F.; Frank, L.D.; Saelens, B.E.; Kraft, M.K. Active transportation and physical activity: Opportunities for collaboration on transportation and public health research. *Transp. Res. Part A Policy Pract.* **2004**, *38*, 249–268. [CrossRef]
16. Schmid, T.L.; Pratt, M.; Howze, E. Policy as intervention: Environmental and policy approaches to the prevention of cardiovascular disease. *Am. J. Public Health* **1995**, *85*, 1207–1211. [CrossRef]
17. King, A.C.; Jeffery, R.W.; Fridinger, F.; Dusenbury, L.; Provence, S.; Hedlund, S.A.; Spangler, K. Environmental and policy approaches to cardiovascular disease prevention through physical activity: Issues and opportunities. *Health Educ. Q.* **2016**, *22*, 499–511. [CrossRef]
18. Sallis, J.; Bauman, A.; Pratt, M. Environmental and policy interventions to promote physical activity. *Am. J. Prev. Med.* **1998**, *15*, 379–397. [CrossRef]
19. Frank, L.D.; Schmid, T.L.; Sallis, J.F.; Chapman, J.; Saelens, B.E. Linking objectively measured physical activity with objectively measured urban form. *Am. J. Prev. Med.* **2005**, *28*, 117–125. [CrossRef]

20. Frank, L.D.; Sallis, J.F.; Saelens, B.E.; Leary, L.; Cain, K.; Conway, T.L.; Hess, P.M. The development of a walkability index: Application to the neighborhood quality of life study. *Br. J. Sports Med.* **2009**, *44*, 924–933. [CrossRef]
21. Lefebvre-Ropars, G.; Morency, C.; Singleton, P.A.; Clifton, K.J. Spatial transferability assessment of a composite walkability index: The pedestrian index of the environment (pie). *Transp. Res. Part D Transp. Environ.* **2017**, *57*, 378–391. [CrossRef]
22. Porta, S.; Renne, J.L. Linking urban design to sustainability: Formal indicators of social urban sustainability field research in Perth, Western Australia. *Urban Des. Int.* **2005**, *10*, 51–64. [CrossRef]
23. Kuzmyak, J.R.; Baber, C.; Savory, D. Use of walk opportunities index to quantify local accessibility. *Transp. Res. Rec. J. Transp. Res. Board* **2006**, *1977*, 145–153. [CrossRef]
24. Buck, C.; Pohlabeln, H.; Huybrechts, I.; De Bourdeaudhuij, I.; Pitsiladis, Y.; Reisch, L.; Pigeot, I. Development and application of a moveability index to quantify possibilities for physical activity in the built environment of children. *Health Place* **2011**, *17*, 1191–1201. [CrossRef]
25. Walk Score Methodology. Available online: http://pubs.cedeus.cl/omeka/files/original/b6fa690993d59007784a7a26804d42be.pdf (accessed on 15 December 2017).
26. Hirsch, J.A.; Moore, K.A.; Evenson, K.R.; Rodriguez, D.A.; Roux, A.V.D. Walk score® and transit score® and walking in the multi-ethnic study of atherosclerosis. *Am. J. Prev. Med.* **2013**, *45*, 158–166. [CrossRef]
27. de Sa, E.; Ardern, C.I. Neighbourhood walkability, leisure-time and transport-related physical activity in a mixed urban–rural area. *PeerJ* **2014**, *2*, e440. [CrossRef]
28. Van Dyck, D.; Cerin, E.; Conway, T.L.; De Bourdeaudhuij, I.; Owen, N.; Kerr, J.; Cardon, G.; Frank, L.D.; Saelens, B.E.; Sallis, J.F. Perceived neighborhood environmental attributes associated with adults' leisure-time physical activity: Findings from Belgium, Australia and the USA. *Health Place* **2013**, *19*, 59–68. [CrossRef]
29. Thielman, J.; Rosella, L.; Copes, R.; Lebenbaum, M.; Manson, H. Neighborhood walkability: Differential associations with self-reported transport walking and leisure-time physical activity in canadian towns and cities of all sizes. *Prev. Med.* **2015**, *77*, 174–180. [CrossRef]
30. Manaugh, K.; El-Geneidy, A. Validating walkability indices: How do different households respond to the walkability of their neighborhood? *Transp. Res. Part D Transp. Environ.* **2011**, *16*, 309–315. [CrossRef]
31. Habibian, M.; Hosseinzadeh, A. Walkability index across trip purposes. *Sustain. Cities Soc.* **2018**, *42*, 216–225. [CrossRef]
32. Knuiman, M.W.; Christian, H.E.; Divitini, M.L.; Foster, S.A.; Bull, F.C.; Badland, H.M.; Giles-Corti, B. A longitudinal analysis of the influence of the neighborhood built environment on walking for transportation: The reside study. *Am. J. Epidemiol.* **2014**, *180*, 453–461. [CrossRef] [PubMed]
33. Liao, Y.; Lin, C.-Y.; Lai, T.-F.; Chen, Y.-J.; Kim, B.; Park, J.-H. Walk score®and its associations with older adults' health behaviors and outcomes. *Int. J. Environ. Res. Public Health* **2019**, *16*, 622. [CrossRef] [PubMed]
34. Mazumdar, S.; Learnihan, V.; Cochrane, T.; Phung, H.; O'Connor, B.; Davey, R. Is walk score associated with hospital admissions from chronic diseases? Evidence from a cross-sectional study in a high socioeconomic status Australian city-state. *BMJ Open* **2016**, *6*, e012548. [CrossRef] [PubMed]
35. Rauterkus, S.Y.; Miller, N. Residential land values and walkability. *J. Sustain. Real Estate* **2011**, *3*, 23–43. [CrossRef]
36. Washington, E.; Dourado, E. The premium for walkable development under land use regulations. *SSRN Electron. J.* **2018**. [CrossRef]
37. Pivo, G. Walk score: The significance of 8 and 80 for mortgage default risk in multifamily properties. *J. Sustain. Real Estate* **2014**, *6*, 187–210. [CrossRef]
38. Winters, M.; Barnes, R.; Venners, S.; Ste-Marie, N.; McKay, H.; Sims-Gould, J.; Ashe, M.C. Older adults' outdoor walking and the built environment: Does income matter? *BMC Public Health* **2015**, *15*. [CrossRef]
39. Towne, S.D.; Won, J.; Lee, S.; Ory, M.G.; Forjuoh, S.N.; Wang, S.; Lee, C. Using walk score™ and neighborhood perceptions to assess walking among middle-aged and older adults. *J. Community Health* **2016**, *41*, 977–988. [CrossRef]
40. Wasfi, R.A.; Dasgupta, K.; Eluru, N.; Ross, N.A. Exposure to walkable neighbourhoods in urban areas increases utilitarian walking: Longitudinal study of Canadians. *J. Transp. Health* **2016**, *3*, 440–447. [CrossRef]
41. Méline, J.; Chaix, B.; Pannier, B.; Ogedegbe, G.; Trasande, L.; Athens, J.; Duncan, D.T. Neighborhood walk score and selected cardiometabolic factors in the French record cohort study. *BMC Public Health* **2017**, *17*. [CrossRef]

42. Wasfi, R.A.; Dasgupta, K.; Orpana, H.; Ross, N.A. Neighborhood walkability and body mass index trajectories: Longitudinal study of canadians. *Am. J. Public Health* **2016**, *106*, 934–940. [CrossRef] [PubMed]
43. Xu, Y.; Wang, F. Built environment and obesity by urbanicity in the U.S. *Health Place* **2015**, *34*, 19–29. [CrossRef] [PubMed]
44. McCormack, G.; Blackstaffe, A.; Nettel-Aguirre, A.; Csizmadi, I.; Sandalack, B.; Uribe, F.; Rayes, A.; Friedenreich, C.; Potestio, M. The independent associations between walk score® and neighborhood socioeconomic status, waist circumference, waist-to-hip ratio and body mass index among urban adults. *Int. J. Environ. Res. Public Health* **2018**, *15*, 1226. [CrossRef] [PubMed]
45. Park, S.; Kim, Y.; Shin, H.-R.; Lee, B.; Shin, A.; Jung, K.-W.; Jee, S.H.; Kim, D.H.; Yun, Y.H.; Park, S.K.; et al. Population-attributable causes of cancer in Korea: Obesity and physical inactivity. *PLoS ONE* **2014**, *9*, e90871. [CrossRef] [PubMed]
46. A Glance at Local Health Statistics. Available online: https://chs.cdc.go.kr/chs/stats/statsMain.do (accessed on 20 March 2018).
47. Kim, E.J. Development and application of healthy city indicators and index: Case of Seoul metropolitan area. *Korea Spat. Plan. Rev.* **2012**, *72*, 161–180. [CrossRef]
48. Kim, E.J.; Kang, M. Effects of built environmental factors on obesity and self-reported health status in Seoul metropolitan area using spatial regression model. *Korea Spat. Plan. Rev.* **2011**, *68*, 85–98. [CrossRef]
49. Kim, T.; Kim, E. Healthy-friendly environmental correlates of population health. *Korea Spat. Plan. Rev.* **2014**, *81*, 185–200.
50. Kim, T.H.; Kim, E.J.; Jun, H.S. Directions of establishing a guideline for healthy cities. *J. Korea Plan. Assoc.* **2014**, *49*, 127. [CrossRef]
51. Walkable City, Seoul. Available online: http://english.seoul.go.kr/policy-information/urban-planning/walkable-city-seoul/you-walk-more-seoul-becomes-happier/ (accessed on 3 December 2019).
52. Kim, E.J.; Kim, J.; Kim, H. Does environmental walkability matter? The role of walkable environment in active commuting. *Int. J. Environ. Res. Public Health* **2020**, *17*, 1261. [CrossRef]
53. Yang, Y.; Diez-Roux, A.V. Walking distance by trip purpose and population subgroups. *Am. J. Prev. Med.* **2012**, *43*, 11–19. [CrossRef]
54. Korea Transport Database. Available online: https://www.ktdb.go.kr/www/selectPbldataChargerWebList.do?key=12 (accessed on 15 May 2019).
55. Maas, C.J.; Hox, J.J. Robustness issues in multilevel regression analysis. *Stat. Neerl.* **2004**, *58*, 127–137. [CrossRef]
56. Maas, C.J.; Hox, J.J. Sufficient sample sizes for multilevel modeling. *Methodology* **2005**, *1*, 86–92. [CrossRef]
57. Łaszkiewicz, E. Sample size and structure for multilevel modelling: Monte carlo investigation for the balanced design. *Metod. Ilościowe W Bad. Ekon.* **2013**, *14*, 19–28.
58. Kreft, I. *Are Multilevel Techniques Necessary? An Overview, Including Simulation Studies*; California State University: Los Angeles, CA, USA, 1996.
59. Hox, J. Multilevel modeling: When and why. In *Classification, Data Analysis, and Data Highways*; Springer: Berlin/Heidelberg, Germany, 1998; pp. 147–154.
60. 2016 Passenger Travel Surveys. Available online: https://www.ktdb.go.kr/common/pdf/web/viewer.html?file=/DATA/pblcte/20170529040735516.pdf (accessed on 15 March 2019).
61. Kim, E.J.; Won, J.; Kim, J. Is seoul walkable? Assessing a walkability score and examining its relationship with pedestrian satisfaction in Seoul, Korea. *Sustainability* **2019**, *11*, 6915. [CrossRef]
62. Kim, E.J.; Kim, Y.-J. A reliability check of walkability indices in Seoul, Korea. *Sustainability* **2019**, *12*, 176. [CrossRef]
63. Boisjoly, G.; Wasfi, R.; El-Geneidy, A. How much is enough? Assessing the influence of neighborhood walkability on undertaking 10-minutes walks. *J. Transp. Land Use* **2018**, *11*. [CrossRef]
64. Rodríguez, D.A.; Evenson, K.R.; Diez Roux, A.V.; Brines, S.J. Land use, residential density, and walking. *Am. J. Prev. Med.* **2009**, *37*, 397–404. [CrossRef]
65. Duncan, M.J.; Winkler, E.; Sugiyama, T.; Cerin, E.; duToit, L.; Leslie, E.; Owen, N. Relationships of land use mix with walking for transport: Do land uses and geographical scale matter? *J. Urban Health* **2010**, *87*, 782–795. [CrossRef]

66. McCormack, G.R.; Shiell, A.; Giles-Corti, B.; Begg, S.; Veerman, J.; Geelhoed, E.; Amarasinghe, A.; Emery, J.C. The association between sidewalk length and walking for different purposes in established neighborhoods. *Int. J. Behav. Nutr. Phys. Act.* **2012**, *9*, 92. [CrossRef]
67. National Spatial Data Infrastructure Portal. Available online: http://data.nsdi.go.kr/dataset (accessed on 15 March 2018).
68. Szumilas, M. Explaining odds ratios. *J. Can. Acad. Child Adolesc. Psychiatry* **2010**, *19*, 227–229.
69. Sommet, N.; Morselli, D. Keep calm and learn multilevel logistic modeling: A simplified three-step procedure using stata, r, mplus, and spss. *Int. Rev. Soc. Psychol.* **2017**, *30*, 203–218. [CrossRef]
70. Heck, R.H.; Tomas, S.L. *An Introduction to Multilevel Modeling Techniques: Mlm and Sem Approaches Using Mplus*, 3rd ed.; Routledge/Taylor & Francis Group: New York, NY, USA, 2015.
71. Hox, J.J.; Moerbeek, M.; Van de Schoot, R. *Multilevel Analysis: Techniques and Applications*; Routledge: New York, NY, USA, 2010.
72. Hughes, L.C.; Anderson, R.A. Issues regarding aggregation of data in nursing systems research. *J. Nurs. Meas.* **1994**, *2*, 79–101. [CrossRef] [PubMed]
73. Hayes, A.F. A primer on multilevel modeling. *Hum. Commun. Res.* **2006**, *32*, 385–410. [CrossRef]
74. Brown, B.B.; Yamada, I.; Smith, K.R.; Zick, C.D.; Kowaleski-Jones, L.; Fan, J.X. Mixed land use and walkability: Variations in land use measures and relationships with bmi, overweight, and obesity. *Health Place* **2009**, *15*, 1130–1141. [CrossRef] [PubMed]
75. Cerin, E.; Lee, K.-Y.; Barnett, A.; Sit, C.H.P.; Cheung, M.-C.; Chan, W.-M.; Johnston, J.M. Walking for transportation in Hong Kong Chinese urban elders: A cross-sectional study on what destinations matter and when. *Int. J. Behav. Nutr. Phys. Act.* **2013**, *10*, 78. [CrossRef] [PubMed]
76. KOSIS. Available online: http://kosis.kr/statisticsList/statisticsListIndex.do?menuId=M_01_01&vwcd=MT_ZTITLE&parmTabId=M_01_01#SelectStatsBoxDiv (accessed on 27 May 2019).

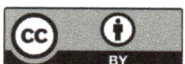

© 2020 by the authors. Licensee MDPI, Basel, Switzerland. This article is an open access article distributed under the terms and conditions of the Creative Commons Attribution (CC BY) license (http://creativecommons.org/licenses/by/4.0/).

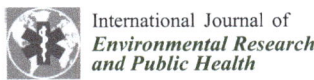

Review

Active Commuting and Physical Fitness: A Systematic Review

Duarte Henriques-Neto [1], Miguel Peralta [1,2], Susana Garradas [3], Andreia Pelegrini [4], André Araújo Pinto [4], Pedro António Sánchez-Miguel [5] and Adilson Marques [1,2,*]

1. CIPER, Faculdade de Motricidade Humana, Universidade de Lisboa, 1649-004 Lisbon and Portugal; duarteneto13@gmail.com (D.H.-N.); mperalta@fmh.ulisboa.pt (M.P.)
2. ISAMB, Faculty of Medicine, University of Lisbon, 1649-004 Lisbon, Portugal
3. Faculdade de Motricidade Humana, Universidade de Lisboa, 1649-004 Lisbon, Portugal; susanamartinsgarradas@gmail.com
4. Health and Sport Sciences Center, State University of Santa Catarina, 3664-8600 Coqueiros - Florianopolis, Brazil; pelegrini.andreia@gmail.com (A.P.); andrefsaude@hotmail.com (A.A.P.)
5. Department of Didactics of Music, Plastic and Body Expression, Teacher Training College, University of Extremadura, 10003 Cáceres, Spain; pesanchezm@unex.es
* Correspondence: amarques@fmh.ulisboa.pt; Tel.: +351-21-414-9100

Received: 24 March 2020; Accepted: 12 April 2020; Published: 15 April 2020

Abstract: Physical fitness (PF) is considered an excellent biomarker of health. One possible strategy to improve PF levels is active commuting. This review, performed accordingly to the Preferred Reporting Items for Systematic Reviews guidelines includes scientific articles published in peer-reviewed journals up to December 2019 that aim at examining the relationship between active travel/commuting and PF. The search was performed in three databases (PubMed, Scopus, and Web of Science). Sixteen studies were included in this review. Findings from the 16 studies were unclear. From the eleven studies on children and adolescents screened, eight were cross-sectional, one prospective cohort, one quasi-experimental, and one experimental. From the five studies on adults, four were experimental and one cross-sectional. Body mass, waist circumference, skinfolds, fat mass, cardiorespiratory fitness, upper and lower strength tests were performed in children, adolescents, and adults. Agility and speed tests were performed only in the young age groups. Majority of the investigations on young ages and adults have shown positive effects or relationships between active commuting and several attributes of PF. However, to avoid misconceptions, there is a need for future robust investigation to identify potential mediators or confounders in this relationship. More robust investigations are essential to understand how and whether decision-makers and public health authorities can use active travel/commuting as a strategy to improve PF in all ages.

Keywords: active commuters; active travel; walking; cycling; physical fitness

1. Introduction

Physical inactivity is one of the main risk factors for mortality worldwide [1,2]. Therefore, there is a global need to promote strategies to increase physical activity (PA) levels. PA can be performed in several contexts such as work, organized sports, recreational activities, home activities, and active travel/commuting [2–5]. Active travel/commuting is an ecological and non-motorized transport mode for all ages, which can be characterized by a form of displacement through PA from/to home and workplace/school. Active commuting increases individual energy expenditure and is easy to incorporate in normal daily routines [6,7]. Active travel/commuting, such as cycling or walking, seems to be an effective strategy to improve daily PA levels; however, it might also improve physical fitness (PF) levels, in addition to promoting health [8–10]. Previous studies have demonstrated a strong association between active travel/commuting and PA levels; moreover, higher cardiorespiratory fitness (CRF), strength levels, and lower obesity indicators values have been associated with cycling and walking to school/work in young and adult populations [11–13].

PF is considered a biomarker of health, and the most common health-related attributes of PF are CRF, muscular fitness (MF), and body composition [14,15]. Assessing body composition, CRF, and/or MF attributes allows one to monitor an individual's PA levels and health status, through the performance of most human systems [14]. Previous reviews have examined the relationships between active commuting and several attributes of PF at young ages [16–19]. Although some positive associations were observed between active commuting and CRF, MF, and body composition, the results are not consistent [20–22]. Furthermore, even though there are some studies among adults, there are no systematic reviews examining associations between PF and active travel/commuting in adults [23,24]. For that reason, the relationship between active travel/commuting and PF among several age groups is, thus far, unclear. The aim of this study was to systematically review the evidence on the association between PF and active travel/commuting in both young and adult populations.

2. Materials and Methods

This systematic review was performed in accordance to the Preferred Reporting Items for Systematic Reviews and Meta-Analysis (PRISMA) guidelines [25].

2.1. Inclusion Criteria

This review includes scientific articles published in peer-reviewed journals until December 31 2019 that aim at examining the relationship between active travel/commuting and PF. Inclusion criteria for articles to be eligible for this review were the following: (1) having a cross-sectional, prospective, observational, cohort, or experimental study design (study design criteria); (2) presenting outcomes of PF, including body composition, CRF, and MF (outcome criteria); (3) examining the association between PF and active travel/commuting (data analysis criteria); (4) focusing on young or adult population (participants criterion); (5) being published in English, Portuguese, or Spanish (language criteria); (6) not having been included in a previous systematic review on the same topic. Articles not meeting all of the inclusion criteria were excluded from the systematic review (exclusion criteria).

2.2. Search Strategy

Three international databases were screened, including PubMed, Scopus, and Web of Science, with scientific articles published in peer-reviewed journals until 31 December 2019 aiming at examining the association between active travel/commuting and PF being identified. In each database, a search was performed through a pre-defined combination of keywords sought in the title and abstract of articles. The combination of keywords used was the following: travel* OR transport* OR commut* OR cycle OR cycling OR bicycl* OR bik* OR walk* OR AND fitness* OR physical function OR physiological function OR physical health OR physiological health*. After the search, identified articles were screened for duplicates and were removed if there were duplicates. Then, title and abstract of identified articles were screened by two authors (D.H.-N.; M.P.) in order to identify studies that met all the inclusion criteria. After screening, articles identified as relevant were retrieved for full text analysis. Full text articles were examined by three authors (D.H.-N.; M.P.; A.M.) for inclusion in the systematic review, and the decision to include or exclude articles from the systematic review was made by consensus. The review protocol was not registered in PROSPERO due to organizational constraints.

2.3. Data Extraction and Harmonization

Based on PRISMA, a data extraction form was developed [25]. The following information was obtained from each manuscript: authors' name and year of publication, study design, country, sample characteristics (number of participants, gender, age), the instruments for assessing PF levels, the instruments for assessing active travel or active commuting, main results, and investigation quality.

The extraction was achieved by one author (D.H.-N.), and coding was verified by two authors. (S.G.; P.S.-M.)

2.4. Study Quality and Risk of Bias

The Quality Assessment Tool for Quantitative Studies checklist was used to assess the articles' quality [26]. This checklist includes 19 items, which assessed the following criteria: selection bias, study design, confounders, blinding, data collection methods, withdrawals and dropouts, intervention integrity, and analyses. The 19 items were divided in the 8 sections listed above and for each section a score of strong, moderate, or weak methodological quality was given. From the interpretation of the scores of each section, an overall score was given to each article. The study quality and risk-of-bias procedure was performed by two authors (S.G.; A.M.).

2.5. Synthesis of Results

This systematic review examined the association between PF and active travel/commuting in young and adult populations. A synthesis of the results and characteristics (such as, design, participant characteristics and sample size, measures, main results, and investigation quality) of each included article are presented. A narrative review of the included studies was performed.

3. Results

3.1. Search Results

A total of 1313 articles were identified during the search. Of those, 683 were identified as duplicates, resulting in 603 articles for the title and abstract screening. In this phase, 27 articles were extracted for full text read, from which 11 were excluded for not meeting the inclusion criteria, namely: three were not focused in active travel/commuting, two were systematic reviews, four were cited in previous systematic reviews, and two were written in Korean or Japanese. Thus, 16 articles were identified as relevant. The flow chart of study selection is presented in Figure 1.

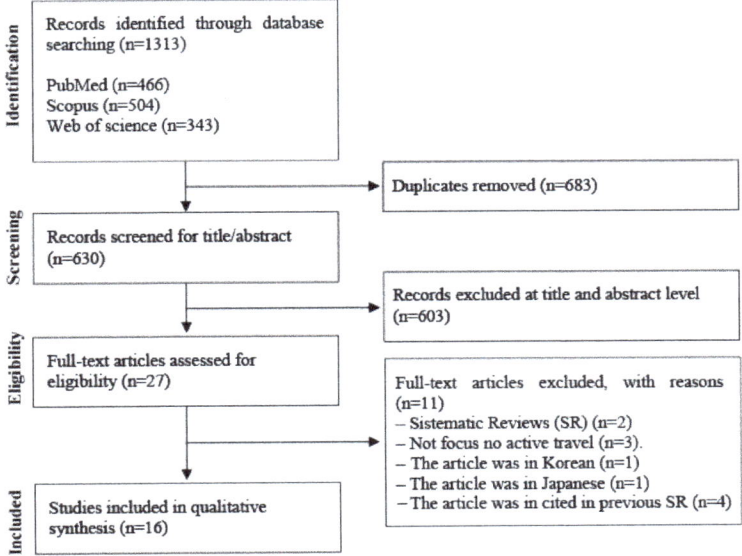

Figure 1. Flow diagram of investigation selection.

3.2. Investigation Characteristics

Tables 1 and 2 present the characteristics of the studies for children/adolescents and adults, respectively. Seventeen articles were included for final qualitative analysis, with 11 studies targeting the young population, i.e., children (up to 13 years old) and adolescents (up to 18 years old), and five studies that focused on the adult population. Every study was either focused on children/adolescents or on adults. None of the included studies were focused on children/adolescents and adults at the same time. All studies were mainly completed in Europe, for both populations.

3.2.1. Children/Adolescent

From the 11 studies focused on children/adolescents, four were performed in Spain, two in England, two in Norway, one in Sweden, one in Brazil, and one in Colombia. Furthermore, eight were cross-sectional [3,12,27–32], one prospective cohort [33], one quasi-experimental [34], and one experimental [35]. The CRF was the PF attribute assessed the most (nine studies), while MF was assessed in three studies [3,27], and agility in two studies [3,31]. Only one study assessed the speed [31]. Active commuting was reported by the participants in most studies (ten studies), except for one study in which the parents reported how their child usually went to school [29]. Distance from house to school, used in one study, was calculated by Google Maps. Seven studies showed a positive association between PF levels and active commuting, mainly in participants who cycled. Two studies observed a positive effect of active commuting on PF attributes assessed in girls but not in boys, and the other five studies found no relationship between active commuting with body composition, CRF, upper strength, and lower strength. Only two studies reported results related to body composition variables. From 11 investigations subjected to methodological quality analysis, one strong, nine moderate, and one weak investigation were identified (Table 1).

In six studies activity, commuting was positively associated with PF [12,27,28,30,33,35]. Active commuting by cycling improves CRF [12,30,35], body composition [12], and muscular strength [27]. One experimental investigation [35] concluded that active commuting improves the CRF, while another quasi-experimental investigation [34] did not find associations between active commuting and PF. The only prospective investigation screened showed that active commuting by cycling in children over a span of six years, increased the PF in 14% [33]. On the other hand, in four studies an association between active commuting and PF was not observed [3,29,32,34]. In one study, mixed results were observed. Girls who actively commuted to school showed better levels of upper limb strength and velocity. However, non-significant associations were observed in boys [31].

3.2.2. Adults

Results of the studies in adult are presented in Table 2. For adults, five studies were identified: two in Denmark, one in Belgium, one in Finland, and one in Switzerland. From these five studies, four were experimental and two cross-sectional. The CRF was assessed in all studies, while MF was assessed in only one study. Variables of active commuting were assessed mainly by self-report, GPS (global position system), and Google Maps. From the 5 studies with adults, two were classified as having strong methodological quality, one moderate, and two weak methodological qualities. In general, a positive effect of active commuting on PF attributes was observed. Cycling to work has the potential to increase physical performance in an untrained people [36], and bicycle commuting improve CRF and reduced body fat [13,24,37]. Four weeks of active commuting can lead to improvements in CFR [38].

4. Discussion

The aim of this systematic review was to examine the association between PF and active travel/commuting in young and adult populations. Studies published until December 2019 were identified according to the inclusion criteria. A total of 16 studies were systematically reviewed. Some studies, in young and adult samples, demonstrated that active commuting is related to PF levels. However, in young populations, four studies did not find positive effects of active commuting on

PF levels. Overall, the results between active commuting and PF levels in adults seem to be more consistent than those at young ages.

4.1. Children/Adolescents

Firstly, CRF is an attribute with a higher genetic component and increases only 8%–9% with three weekly bouts of 20 min of PA, at 80%–90% of maximum heart rate, for 10–12 weeks [39]. Secondly, some tests are flawed, with respect to the estimation of peak VO_2 in mL/kg/min at young ages [40]. Other factors that can explain the non-association between active commuting and CRF in young ages are as follows: The age of participants, mode of active commuting (e.g., walking or cycling), lower active commuting distance, high-deprivation neighborhoods, frequency of commuting, and the overall amount of time spent being an active commuter [12,28,30,33]. When examining the association between active commuting and MF, the authors observed that cyclists had higher handgrip strength and walkers had higher vertical jump peak power when compared with non-active commuters [27]. Furthermore, positive association was observed between active commuting and upper limb strength in girls but not in boys [31]. This result is crucial to retain, in order to understand the various impacts of active commuting on girls and boys. Different results in PF between girls and boys can be explained because the girls usually have lower levels of PA and MF than boys. The specific type of physical exercise (walking or cycling) promotes specific physiologic adaptations, which act in several intensities on several attributes of PF [41,42].

The positive association between active commuting and CRF in prospective study [35] is in accordance with previous investigations, which concluded that promoting active commuting to school among children and adolescents may be a useful strategy to improve CRF and other health outcomes [11,43,44]. Our discoveries highlighted the variability of the investigations' results, which can be explained by different methodologies applied and/or non-control of other confounders. The social environment and the neighborhood characteristics are crucial factors to be considered when promoting active commuting in youth [30]. Overall, active commuting is associated with healthier levels of PF among youth. The findings from this systematic review concur with those from previous systematic reviews [18,19].

4.2. Adults

From the five studies screened, a positive association between active commuting and several PF attributes was observed. A cross-sectional investigation showed a positive association between active commuting and metabolic health, along with the beneficial impact on the promotion of the PA levels in adults. However, no association between active commuting and CRF and MF was found [13].

Four intervention investigations used cycling to analyze the potential positive effects of active commuting on PF levels. After one year of experimental investigation, the authors concluded that cycling to work had a positive effect on CRF levels on the intervention group [36]. The experimental investigation, performed over six months, showed active bike commuters presented better CRF than the non-active commuting group, but not when compared with the group that performed vigorous PA in leisure time [24]. Both active groups had similar improvements [24]. However, it seems that for the same period of intervention, the intensity of PA plays an essential role in the improvement of CRF [45]. The majority of studies performed in adults indicated that active commuters had greater cardiovascular fitness, especially those who cycled to and from work. Cycling to and from work seems to be an essential tool to reduce the time required to expend a given quantity of energy. Additionally, high-intensity physical exercises seem to be a fundamental exercise component to increase CRF, and they serve as a protective factor against several metabolic diseases [24,45,46]. Active commuting improved the cardiometabolic health and CRF in both groups, but with slow effects in the active commuting group when compared with the leisure-time vigorous-intensity group [24]. Previous investigations have shown the impact of lifestyle exercise on adiposity, while the changes in CRF seem to be more dependent on the exercise intensity [45,47].

Table 1. Characteristics of the studies in children and adolescents.

Author, Year	Study Design	Country	Sample	Physical Fitness Attribute (Measure)	Active Commuting Measure	Observation	Main Results	Study Quality
Borrestad et al., 2012 [35]	Experimental	Norway	Total n = 204 IG, 26 (10.8 ± 0.7 years), Boys (53.9%) CG, 27 (10.9 ± 0.7 years), boys (51.9%)	CRF: Peak oxygen consumption (VO_{2peak}, mL O_2/min/kg), HR_{peak} (h/min), BMI (kg/m^2)	Participants reported how many days a week they traveled to/from school in the last 3 months by walking, cycling, car, or public transport. Distance to school (km).	Active commuting; Cycle ergometer test	Active commuting by cycling in both groups (IG and CG) improves the CRF in children.	Moderate
Chillón et al., 2012 [33]	Prospective cohort	Sweden	Total n = 262 120 boys, 142 girls Swedish children who were involved in the European Youth Heart Study (EYHS)	CRF: (VO_{2max}) expressed in absolute terms (L/min); BMI (kg/m^2); WC (cm); Skinfolds (mm)	Participants reported how they go to school. Passive: car, bus, train or Active: bicycle or walk (%).	Active commuting; Cycle ergometer test; calipers	Bicycling to school in childhood was related to improvements in fitness 6 years later. Children who became bicyclists in adolescence improved their fitness levels. No changes were observed for fatness.	Moderate
Østergaard et al., 2013 [12]	Cross-sectional	Norway	Total n = 1694, aged 9–15 years, 577 Boys, 482 Girls Norwegian who were participated in the Physical Activity among Norwegian Children Study	CRF: (VO_{2max}, mL/kg/min); Functional strength (cm), Muscular endurance (n) (s); BMI (kg/m^2); Skinfolds (mm)	Participants reported how they go to school: passively (car/motorcycle or bus/train) or actively (bicycle or walk).	Active commuting Time of travel (minutes); Cycle ergometer test; Standing jump, Sit-ups, Biering–Sørensen test, Harpenden calipers	Active commuting, especially cycling, is positively associated with body composition, CRF, and MF when compared to passive commuting.	Strong

Table 1. *Cont.*

Author, Year	Study Design	Country	Sample	Physical Fitness Attribute (Measure)	Active Commuting Measure	Observation	Main Results	Study Quality
Ropero et al., 2014 [27]	Cross-sectional	England	Total n = 6829, aged 10–16 years; (53% males, age 12.9 ± 1.2 years) English adolescent who participated in the East of England Healthy Hearts Study	Muscular fitness: upper strength (kg), lower strength (cm) and (W·kg^{-1}); BMI (kg/m^2)	Participants reported how they go to school: passively (car or public transport) or actively (bicycle or walk). Distance to school (km).	Active commuting: Distance from home to school calculated by Google Maps. MF: Handgrip test, Vertical jump	When compared with passive travelers, cyclists had higher handgrip strength and walkers had higher vertical jump peak power.	Moderate
Villa-González et al., 2015 [28]	Cross-sectional	Spain	Total n = 494, aged 8–11 (9.2 ± 0.6) years, 577 Boys (9.3 ± 0.6 years), 229 (9.2 ± 0.6 years) Girls.	CRF (VO$_{2max}$ mL·min^{-1}·kg^{-1}, stage); MF (cm, kg), Agility (s).	Participants reported how they go to school: passively (car or public transport) or actively (bicycle or walk).	Active commuting Weekly frequency: (0–2 active travels vs. 3–7 active travels vs. 8–10 active travels); PACER test, Push-up test, Handgrip test, Standing long jump, Leg extension test.	No associations were found between active commuting with CRF and upper body MF. Positive associations between active commuting with agility and lower body MF in girls and boys.	Weak
Noonan et al., 2017 [30]	Cross-sectional	England	Total n = 194, aged 8–11 (9.2 ± 0.6) years, 87 Boys (9.97 ± 0.30 years), 107 Girls (9.95 ± 0.30 years).	CRF (laps); MF: upper strength (kg), lower strength (cm) and (W·kg^{-1}); BMI (kg·m^{-2})	Participants reported by how they go to the school: passively (scooter, bus, car, train, taxi, other) or actively (bicycle or walk).	Active commuting; distance (km) calculated by Google Maps; PACER test, Push-up test, Handgrip test, Standing long jump, Leg extension test.	Active commuters, who live further away from school had better cardiorespiratory fitness.	Moderate

Table 1. Cont.

Author, Year	Study Design	Country	Sample	Physical Fitness Attribute (Measure)	Active Commuting Measure	Observation	Main Results	Study Quality
Pires et al., 2017 [31]	Cross-sectional	Brazil	Total n = 751, aged 7–17; 312 Boys and 349 Girls.	MF: upper strength (m), lower strength (m); Speed (s); Agility (s) BMI (kg/m^2)	Participants reported how they go to school. Passive: car, bus, train or active-bicycle, walk (%)	Active commuting (%); Medicinal ball throw; Standing long jump; Square test.	Girls who actively commute to school showed better levels of upper limb strength and velocity. No significant difference was observed for the physical fitness between transport groups in boys.	Moderate
Villa-González et al., 2017 [34]	Quasi-experimental	Spain	Total n = 251, aged 8–11 (9.2 ± 0.6) years, IG: 73 boys and 68 girls; CG: 54 boys and 56 girls.	CRF (VO$_{2max}$ mL/kg/min, stage), MF (cm, kg), Agility (s).	Participants reported how they go to school. Passively (car, bus, train) or actively (bicycle, walk).	Weekly frequency (0–2 active travels vs. 3–7 active travels vs. 8–10 active travels); PACER test, Push-up test, Handgrip test, Standing long jump, Leg extension test.	No associations between active commuters and health-related fitness.	Moderate
Ramirez-Velez et al., 2017 [3]	Cross-sectional	Colombia	Total n = 2877, aged 7–17, 312 boys, 349 girls.	CRF Peak oxygen consumption (VO$_{2peak}$ mL/O$_2$/min/kg); MF: upper strength (kg), lower strength (kg); Flexibility (cm); Agility (s); BMI (kg/m^2), WC (cm).	Participants reported how they go to school: by car, public transportation or actively (walking, cycling).	Active commuting (days per week); PACER test; Handgrip test; Standing long jump test; 4 × 10 m shuttle run.	Regular cycling to school may be associated with better physical fitness, especially in girls.	Moderate

Table 1. Cont.

Author, Year	Study Design	Country	Sample	Physical Fitness Attribute (Measure)	Active Commuting Measure	Observation	Main Results	Study Quality
Muntaner-Mas et al., 2018 [32]	Cross-sectional	Spain	Total n = 2518, aged 10–16 years (13.0 ± 2.1).	CRF (VO$_{2\,peak}$, mL kg min^{-1}); BMI (kg/m^2).	Participants reported how they go to school. Passively (car, bus, train) or actively (by bicycle, walk, by riding skate).	Active commuting (%); PACER test.	No relationship between active commuting to school and CRF in children and adolescents.	Moderate
Ruiz-Hermosa et al., 2018 [29]	Cross-sectional	Spain	Total n = 2518, aged 4–7 years (13.0 ± 2.1).	CRF (VO$_2$ peak, mL kg min^{-1}); MF: lower strength (cm); BMI (kg/m^2), WC (cm), Skinfolds (mm).	Children's parents reported how they go to school. Passive (car, bus, train) or Active (bicycle, walk).	Active commuting (time); Course-Navette or PACER test; Standing long jump test; Holtain Ltd. Caliper	No relationship between walking to school with adiposity indicators, physical fitness.	Moderate

BMI, body mass index; CG, control group; CRF, cardiorespiratory fitness; IG, intervention group; MF, muscular fitness; MOD, moderate activity; PACER, Progressive Aerobic Cardiovascular Endurance Run; VIG, vigorous activity; WC, waist circumference.

Table 2. Characteristics of the studies in adult.

Author, Year	Study Design	Country	Sample	Physical Fitness Attribute (Measure)	Active Commuting Measure	Observation	Main Results	Study Quality
De Geus et al., 2009 [36]	Experimental	Belgium	Total n = 80 IG, 30 males (43 ± 6 years), 35 females (43 ± 3); CG, 7 males (50 ± 8 years), 8 females (48 ± 6 years)	CRF (Maximal external power [P_{max} (/kg)]; Peak oxygen uptake [VO_{2peak} (/kg)], Absolute maximal external power (P_{max}), Relative peak oxygen uptake (VO_{2peak}/kg), Heart ratio max (beats/min), respiratory exchange ratio (VCO_2/VO_2)	Participants reported a weekly diary. Distance and the time spend on each trip by car/motorcycle; bus/train; bicycle; walk to work.	Measured the distance and the time spend on each trip; cycle ergometer test.	The maximal external power and peak oxygen uptake increased significantly in IG (Male and Female). Cycling to work has the potential to increase physical performance in an untrained study population.	Moderate

Table 2. *Cont.*

Author, Year	Study Design	Country	Sample	Physical Fitness Attribute (Measure)	Active Commuting Measure	Observation	Main Results	Study Quality
Moller et al., 2011 [37]	Experimental	Denmark	Total n = 48 IG 13 males (43 ± 8.9 years), 6 females (44.4 ± 8); CG, 16 males (46.1 ± 9.9 years), 7 females (46 ± 9.1 years)	CRF (VO_{2max} ml/kg/min); Heart ratio max (beats/min); Respiratory exchange ratio (VCO_2/VO_2); BMI (kg/m^2); Skinfolds (mm)	Participants used their bicycle and registered the cycling distance	Active commuting was calculated by (Mavic M-Tech 7) Cycle ergometer test; Harpenden calipers	CRF was significantly improved and body fat reduced in 8 weeks of commuter cycling.	Strong
Vaara, et al, 2014 [13]	Cross-sectional	Finland	Total n = 781, aged 18–90 years (47.1 ± 8.7 years); Male (81.9%)	CRF: VO_{2max}, mL/kg/min. MF: reps/min, kg and N). WC (cm), body fat: bioelectrical impedance.	Participants reported a weekly diary. The time spend per day by bicycle or walk to work	Active commuting was classified by total time. CRF was assessed by cycle ergometer, and VO_{2max} estimated from HR and maximal power.	The high active commuting group showed better results in CRF, some MF tests and WC with other active commuting groups.	Weak
Hochsmann et al., 2018 [38]	Experimental	Switzerland	Total n = 32 adults, aged 18–50 years. 28 males and 2 females	CRF: ($VO_{2\,peak}$, mL kg min^{-1}); BMI (kg/m^2).	E-bike group and bike group reported a typical route to work.	Active commuting (km and elevation calculated by Google Maps, Google Inc, Mountain View, California). CRF was assessed by cycle ergometer.	A period of 4 weeks of active commuting can lead to improvements in VO_{2peak} in both groups. Moreover, no significant difference in VO_{2peak} and maximal ergometric workload gain.	Weak

Table 2. *Cont.*

Author, Year	Study Design	Country	Sample	Physical Fitness Attribute (Measure)	Active Commuting Measure	Observation	Main Results	Study Quality
Blond et al., 2019 [24]	Experimental	Denmark	Total n = 130 adults, aged 20–45 years. CG 18 (male 9, female 9); IG bike 35 (male 16, female 19); IG/MOD 39 (male 19, female 20); IG/VIG 38 (male 20, female 18)	CRF: (VO$_{2\,peak}$, mL kg min^{-1}); BMI (kg/m^2).	The daily distance was calculated for participants in bike based on their energy expenditure while cycling from/to work/school.	The active commuting distance was monitored using Polar RC3 GPS (Polar, Finland). CRF was determined using an electronically braked cycle and open circuit indirect respiratory calorimetry.	CRF increased in all exercise active commuting groups compared with non-active commuting.	Strong

BMI, body mass index; CG, control group; CRF, cardiorespiratory fitness; IG, intervention group; MF, muscular fitness; MOD, moderate activity; VIG, vigorous activity; WC, waist circumference.

Several limitations have been identified in these investigations, which can explain the results. However, it was possible to identify potential mediators or confounders, which can influence the relationship between active commuting and the results of several attributes of PF [13,23]. Although most studies examined the effects of active commuting and non-active commuting, an experimental investigation analyzed the effect of E-Bike versus bike commuting on CRF in overweight adults, which concluded that both bike systems increased CRF levels, even if the bikes were electrically assisted [38].

Ambiguous or inconsistent results observed mainly among children and adolescents in this systematic review can be the result of the several methodologies used to access PF attributes, the type of active commuting, the type of population, the geographic area, and the environmental context. Additionally, the measures of active commuting extensively varied (e.g., frequency, duration, and distance) among the investigations screened in this systematic review. Due to all these factors, rigorous comparison among investigations is highly limited.

This systematic review is not without some limitations. Firstly, active travel/commuting was self-reported in all the included studies. This may be subject to bias, especially at young ages. Secondly, most investigations do not control the intensity of active commuting. Thirdly, studies were mainly focused on a specific world area in high- or mid-income countries. Finally, the terms selected to identify investigations that examined active commuting and PF could have excluded several articles (e.g., ones in which the predefined terms were found neither in the title nor the abstract).

Overall, the results seem to indicate that active travel/commuting and PF are positively associated in young and adult population. Walking and cycling are common modes used by young active commuters. Young cyclists had higher CRF level, while walkers had better MF levels. In adults, cycling is the principal mode of active commuting and is associated with greater PF levels, especially CRF. Active commuting by cycling increases the intensity level of physical activity and seems to be an excellent strategy to improve the PF levels. These findings highlight that active commuting promotes health status. However, for all entities who promote active commuting, it is essential considering factors such as age, sex, and environment at the moment to select the adequate active commuting mode.

5. Conclusions

Findings from this review suggest that among younger ages, active travel/commuting is inconsistently related to PF and that several factors should be considered to compare the effectiveness of active commuting in improving PF outcomes in children and adolescents. Findings of studies in adults demonstrated the positive effect of active commuting on CRF and body composition. Overall, most studies have shown a positive relationship between active commuting and several attributes of PF. Additionally, active commuting, by cycling, seems to have a more positive impact on several PF attributes. However, there is a need to identify potential mediators or confounders in this relationship, in order to avoid misconceptions. More investigations on this topic are essential to understand how and whether decision makers and public health authorities can use active travel/commuting as a strategy to improve PF in all ages. In order to achieve that, it is important that future investigation pursue a more detailed approach when examining active travel/commuting, especially taking into account its context and specificity.

Author Contributions: Conceptualization, A.M., M.P., and D.H.-N.; methodology, A.M., M.P., and D.H.-N.; software, M.P. and D.H.-N.; validation, A.M., S.G., A.P., and P.A.S.-M.; formal analysis, D.H-N., A.P., and M.P.; investigation, D.H.-N., P.A.S.-M., and M.P.; data curation, A.M., M.P., and D.H.-N.; writing—original draft preparation, A.M. and D.H.-N.; writing—review and editing, S.G., A.P., P.A.S.-M., A.A.P., and M.P.; and supervision, A.M., A.A.P.,and M.P. All authors have read and agreed to the published version of the manuscript.

Funding: This research received no external funding.

Conflicts of Interest: The authors declare no conflict of interest.

References

1. WHO. *Physical Activity Strategy for the WHO European Region 2016–2025*; Europe, R.C.F., Ed.; World Helath Organization: Vilnus, Lithuania, 2015.
2. Committee, P.A.G.A. *2018 Physical Activity Guidelines Advisory Committee Scientific Report*; U.S. Department of Health and Human Services: Washington, DC, USA, 2018.
3. Ramirez-Velez, R.; Correa-Bautista, J.E.; Lobelo, F.; Izquierdo, M.; Alonso-Martinez, A.; Rodriguez-Rodriguez, F.; Cristi-Montero, C. High muscular fitness has a powerful protective cardiometabolic effect in adults: Influence of weight status. *BMC Public Health* **2016**, *16*, 1012. [CrossRef] [PubMed]
4. Australian Sports Commission. *Addressing the Decline in Sport Participation in Secondary Schools*; Australian Sports Commission: Bruce, Australia, 2017.
5. Canada, P.H.A.O. *A Common Vision for Increasing Physical Activity and Reducing Sedentary Living in Canada*; Federal, P.A.T.G., Ed.; Diabetes Action Canada: Toronto, ON, Canada, 2018.
6. Page, N.C.; Nilsson, V.O. Active Commuting: Workplace Health Promotion for Improved Employee Well-Being and Organizational Behavior. *Front. Psychol.* **2017**, *7*. [CrossRef] [PubMed]
7. Aparicio-Ugarriza, R.; Mielgo-Ayuso, J.; Ruiz, E.; Ávila, J.M.; Aranceta-Bartrina, J.; Gil, Á.; Ortega, R.M.; Serra-Majem, L.; Varela-Moreiras, G.; González-Gross, M. Active Commuting, Physical Activity, and Sedentary Behaviors in Children and Adolescents from Spain: Findings from the ANIBES Study. *Int. J. Environ. Res. Public Health* **2020**, *17*, 668. [CrossRef] [PubMed]
8. Pizarro, A.N.; Ribeiro, J.C.; Marques, E.A.; Mota, J.; Santos, M.P. Is walking to school associated with improved metabolic health? *Int. J. Behav. Nutr. Phys. Act.* **2013**, *10*, 12. [CrossRef] [PubMed]
9. Garcia-Hermoso, A.; Quintero, A.P.; Hernandez, E.; Correa-Bautista, J.E.; Izquierdo, M.; Tordecilla-Sanders, A.; Prieto-Benavides, D.; Sandoval-Cuellar, C.; Gonzalez-Ruiz, K.; Villa-Gonzalez, E.; et al. Active commuting to and from university, obesity and metabolic syndrome among Colombian university students. *BMC Public Health* **2018**, *18*, 523. [CrossRef] [PubMed]
10. Steell, L.; Garrido-Mendez, A.; Petermann, F.; Diaz-Martinez, X.; Martinez, M.A.; Leiva, A.M.; Salas-Bravo, C.; Alvarez, C.; Ramirez-Campillo, R.; Cristi-Montero, C.; et al. Active commuting is associated with a lower risk of obesity, diabetes and metabolic syndrome in Chilean adults. *J. Public Health* **2018**, *40*, 508–516. [CrossRef]
11. Cooper, A.R.; Wedderkopp, N.; Jago, R.; Kristensen, P.L.; Moller, N.C.; Froberg, K.; Page, A.S.; Andersen, L.B. Longitudinal associations of cycling to school with adolescent fitness. *Prev. Med.* **2008**, *47*, 324–328. [CrossRef]
12. Ostergaard, L.; Kolle, E.; Steene-Johannessen, J.; Anderssen, S.A.; Andersen, L.B. Cross sectional analysis of the association between mode of school transportation and physical fitness in children and adolescents. *Int. J. Behav. Nutr. Phys. Act.* **2013**, *10*, 91. [CrossRef]
13. Vaara, J.P.; Kyrolainen, H.; Fogelholm, M.; Santtila, M.; Hakkinen, A.; Hakkinen, K.; Vasankari, T. Associations of leisure time, commuting, and occupational physical activity with physical fitness and cardiovascular risk factors in young men. *J. Phys. Act. Health* **2014**, *11*, 1482–1491. [CrossRef] [PubMed]
14. Ortega, F.B.; Ruiz, J.R.; Castillo, M.J.; Sjostrom, M. Physical fitness in childhood and adolescence: A powerful marker of health. *Int. J. Obes.* **2008**, *32*, 1–11. [CrossRef]
15. Bouchard, C.; Blair, S.N.; Haskell, W. *Physical Activity and Health*, 2nd ed.; Human Kinetics: Champaign, IL, USA, 2012.
16. Lee, M.C.; Orenstein, M.R.; Richardson, M.J. Systematic Review of Active Commuting to School and Children's Physical Activity and Weight. *J. Phys. Act. Health* **2008**, *5*, 930–949. [CrossRef]
17. Faulkner, G.E.J.; Buliung, R.N.; Flora, P.K.; Fusco, C. Active school transport, physical activity levels and body weight of children and youth: A systematic review. *Prev. Med.* **2009**, *48*, 3–8. [CrossRef] [PubMed]
18. Lubans, D.R.; Boreham, C.A.; Kelly, P.; Foster, C.E. The relationship between active travel to school and health-related fitness in children and adolescents: A systematic review. *Int. J. Behav. Nutr. Phys. Act.* **2011**, *8*, 5. [CrossRef] [PubMed]
19. Larouche, R.; Saunders, T.J.; Faulkner, G.; Colley, R.; Tremblay, M. Associations between active school transport and physical activity, body composition, and cardiovascular fitness: A systematic review of 68 studies. *J. Phys. Act. Health* **2014**, *11*, 206–227. [CrossRef]
20. Gordon-Larsen, P.; Nelson, M.C.; Beam, K. Associations among Active Transportation, Physical Activity, and Weight Status in Young Adults. *Obes. Res.* **2005**, *13*, 868–875. [CrossRef]

21. Cooper, A.R.; Wedderkopp, N.; Wang, H.A.N.; Andersen, L.B.; Froberg, K.; Page, A.S. Active Travel to School and Cardiovascular Fitness in Danish Children and Adolescents. *Med. Sci. Sports Exerc.* **2006**, *38*, 1724–1731. [CrossRef]
22. Andersen, L.B.; Lawlor, D.A.; Cooper, A.R.; Froberg, K.; Anderssen, S.A. Physical fitness in relation to transport to school in adolescents: The Danish youth and sports study. *Scand. J. Med. Sci. Sports* **2009**, *19*, 406–411. [CrossRef]
23. Hoehner, C.M.; Barlow, C.E.; Allen, P.; Schootman, M. Commuting distance, cardiorespiratory fitness, and metabolic risk. *Am. J. Prev. Med.* **2012**, *42*, 571–578. [CrossRef]
24. Blond, M.B.; Rosenkilde, M.; Gram, A.S.; Tindborg, M.; Christensen, A.N.; Quist, J.S.; Stallknecht, B.M. How does 6 months of active bike commuting or leisure-time exercise affect insulin sensitivity, cardiorespiratory fitness and intra-abdominal fat? A randomised controlled trial in individuals with overweight and obesity. *Br. J. Sports Med.* **2019**, *53*, 1183–1192. [CrossRef] [PubMed]
25. Moher, D.; Liberati, A.; Tetzlaff, J.; Altman, D.G.; Group, P. Preferred reporting items for systematic reviews and meta-analyses: The PRISMA statement. *Ann. Intern. Med.* **2009**, *151*, 264–269. [CrossRef] [PubMed]
26. Tools, N.C.C.f.M.A. Quality Assessment Tool for Quantitative Studies Method. 2008. Available online: http://www.nccmt.ca/resources/search/14 (accessed on 1 July 2016).
27. Ropero, A.B.; Nadal, A.; Mora, C.; Cohen, D.; Ogunleye, A.A.; Taylor, M.; Voss, C.; Micklewright, D.; Sandercock, G.R. Association between habitual school travel and muscular fitness in youth. *Prev. Med.* **2014**, *67*, 216–220. [CrossRef]
28. Villa-Gonzalez, E.; Ruiz, J.R.; Chillon, P. Associations between Active Commuting to School and Health-Related Physical Fitness in Spanish School-Aged Children: A Cross-Sectional Study. *Int. J. Environ. Res. Public Health* **2015**, *12*, 10362–10373. [CrossRef] [PubMed]
29. Ruiz-Hermosa, A.; Martinez-Vizcaino, V.; Alvarez-Bueno, C.; Garcia-Prieto, J.C.; Pardo-Guijarro, M.J.; Sanchez-Lopez, M. No Association Between Active Commuting to School, Adiposity, Fitness, and Cognition in Spanish Children: The MOVI-KIDS Study. *J. Sch. Health* **2018**, *88*, 839–846. [CrossRef] [PubMed]
30. Noonan, R.J.; Boddy, L.M.; Knowles, Z.R.; Fairclough, S.J. Fitness, fatness and active school commuting among liverpool schoolchildren. *Int. J. Environ. Res. Public Health* **2017**, *14*, 995. [CrossRef] [PubMed]
31. Pires, A.L.; Soares, S.S.; Welser, L.; da Silva, C.F.; Sehn, A.P.; Kern, D.G.; Valim, A.; Reuter, C.P.; Burgos, M.S. Association between commuting to school and physical fitness related to motor performance in schoolchildren. *Rev. Epidemiol. Control. Infecc.* **2017**, *7*, 9.
32. Muntaner-Mas, A.; Herrador-Colmenero, M.; Borras, P.A.; Chillon, P. Physical activity, but not active commuting to school, is associated with cardiorespiratory fitness levels in young people. *J. Transp. Health* **2018**, *10*, 297–303. [CrossRef]
33. Chillon, P.; Ortega, F.B.; Ruiz, J.R.; Evenson, K.R.; Labayen, I.; Martinez-Vizcaino, V.; Hurtig-Wennlof, A.; Veidebaum, T.; Sjostrom, M. Bicycling to school is associated with improvements in physical fitness over a 6-year follow-up period in Swedish children. *Prev. Med.* **2012**, *55*, 108–112. [CrossRef]
34. Villa-Gonzalez, E.; Ruiz, J.R.; Mendoza, J.A.; Chillon, P. Effects of a school-based intervention on active commuting to school and health-related fitness. *BMC Public Health* **2017**, *17*, 20. [CrossRef]
35. Borrestad, L.A.; Ostergaard, L.; Andersen, L.B.; Bere, E. Experiences from a randomised, controlled trial on cycling to school: Does cycling increase cardiorespiratory fitness? *Scand. J. Public Health* **2012**, *40*, 245–252. [CrossRef]
36. de Geus, B.; Joncheere, J.; Meeusen, R. Commuter cycling: Effect on physical performance in untrained men and women in Flanders: Minimum dose to improve indexes of fitness. *Scand. J. Med. Sci. Sports* **2009**, *19*, 179–187. [CrossRef]
37. Moller, N.C.; Ostergaard, L.; Gade, J.R.; Nielsen, J.L.; Andersen, L.B. The effect on cardiorespiratory fitness after an 8-week period of commuter cycling—a randomized controlled study in adults. *Prev. Med.* **2011**, *53*, 172–177. [CrossRef] [PubMed]
38. Hochsmann, C.; Meister, S.; Gehrig, D.; Gordon, E.; Li, Y.; Nussbaumer, M.; Rossmeissl, A.; Schafer, J.; Hanssen, H.; Schmidt-Trucksass, A. Effect of E-Bike Versus Bike Commuting on Cardiorespiratory Fitness in Overweight Adults: A 4-Week Randomized Pilot Study. *Clin. J. Sport Med. Off. J. Can. Acad. Sport Med.* **2018**, *28*, 255–265. [CrossRef]
39. Armstrong, N.; Welsman, J. Youth cardiorespiratory fitness: Evidence, myths and misconceptions. *Bull. World Health Organ.* **2019**, *97*, 777–782. [CrossRef] [PubMed]

40. Welsman, J.; Armstrong, N. The 20 m shuttle run is not a valid test of cardiorespiratory fitness in boys aged 11–14 years. *BMJ Open Sport Exerc. Med.* **2019**, *5*, e000627. [CrossRef] [PubMed]
41. Marta, C.C.; Marinho, D.A.; Barbosa, T.M.; Izquierdo, M.; Marques, M.C. Physical Fitness Differences Between Prepubescent Boys and Girls. *J. Strength Cond. Res.* **2012**, *26*, 1756–1766. [CrossRef] [PubMed]
42. Buchowski, M.; Telford, R.M.; Telford, R.D.; Olive, L.S.; Cochrane, T.; Davey, R. Why Are Girls Less Physically Active than Boys? *Findings from the LOOK Longitudinal Study. PLoS ONE* **2016**, *11*, e0150041. [CrossRef]
43. Aires, L.; Mendonça, D.; Silva, G.; Gaya, A.R.; Santos, M.P.; Ribeiro, J.C.; Mota, J. A 3-Year Longitudinal Analysis of Changes in Body Mass Index. *Int. J. Sports Med.* **2009**, *31*, 133–137. [CrossRef]
44. Pabayo, R.; Gauvin, L.; Barnett, T.A.; Nikiéma, B.; Séguin, L. Sustained Active Transportation is associated with a favorable body mass index trajectory across the early school years: Findings from the Quebec Longitudinal Study of Child Development birth cohort. *Prev. Med.* **2010**, *50*, S59–S64. [CrossRef]
45. Ross, R.; Hudson, R.; Stotz, P.J.; Lam, M. Effects of Exercise Amount and Intensity on Abdominal Obesity and Glucose Tolerance in Obese Adults. *Ann. Intern. Med.* **2015**, *162*, 325. [CrossRef]
46. Wen, D.; Utesch, T.; Wu, J.; Robertson, S.; Liu, J.; Hu, G.; Chen, H. Effects of different protocols of high intensity interval training for VO2max improvements in adults: A meta-analysis of randomised controlled trials. *J. Sci. Med. Sport* **2019**, *22*, 941–947. [CrossRef]
47. Verheggen, R.J.H.M.; Maessen, M.F.H.; Green, D.J.; Hermus, A.R.M.M.; Hopman, M.T.E.; Thijssen, D.H.T. A systematic review and meta-analysis on the effects of exercise training versus hypocaloric diet: Distinct effects on body weight and visceral adipose tissue. *Obes. Rev.* **2016**, *17*, 664–690. [CrossRef] [PubMed]

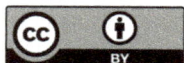

© 2020 by the authors. Licensee MDPI, Basel, Switzerland. This article is an open access article distributed under the terms and conditions of the Creative Commons Attribution (CC BY) license (http://creativecommons.org/licenses/by/4.0/).

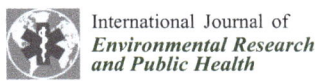 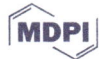

Article

Prevalence of Physical Activity among Adolescents from 105 Low, Middle, and High-Income Countries

Adilson Marques [1,2,*], **Duarte Henriques-Neto** [1], **Miguel Peralta** [1,2], **João Martins** [1,2,3], **Yolanda Demetriou** [4], **Dorothea M. I. Schönbach** [4] and **Margarida Gaspar de Matos** [2,5]

1. Centro Interdisciplinar de Estudo da Performance Humana, Faculdade de Motricidade Humana, Universidade de Lisboa, 1499-002 Lisboa, Portugal; duarteneto@campus.ul.pt (D.H.-N.); mperalta@fmh.ulisboa.pt (M.P.); jmartins@fmh.ulisboa.pt (J.M.)
2. Instituto de Saúde Ambiental, Universidade de Lisboa, 1649-028 Lisboa, Portugal; mmatos@fmh.ulisboa.pt
3. Laboratório de Pedagogia, Faculdade de Motricidade Humana e UIDEF, Instituto de Educação, Universidade de Lisboa, 1649-013 Lisboa, Portugal
4. Department of Sport and Health Sciences, Technical University of Munich, 80333 Munich, Germany; yolanda.demetriou@tum.de (Y.D.); dorothea.schoenbach@tum.de (D.M.I.S.)
5. Faculdade de Motricidade Humana, Universidade de Lisboa, 1499-002 Lisboa, Portugal
* Correspondence: amarques@fmh.ulisboa.pt; Tel.: +351-214-149-100

Received: 11 April 2020; Accepted: 29 April 2020; Published: 30 April 2020

Abstract: Introduction: Physical activity (PA) is a beneficial health behaviour, however most adolescents worldwide are physically inactive. Updated information on the prevalence and trends of PA is important to inform national and international authorities and support countries' public health policies and actions. This study aimed to present the worldwide, regional, and national prevalence of PA participation according to its frequency in adolescents. Methods: This study is based on cross-sectional surveys of adolescents' populations from several countries and all regions worldwide. The sample comprised 520,533 adolescents (251,788 boys; 268,745 girls), from 105 countries and regions. Results: Most adolescents engaged in PA up to 3 days/week (57.1%; 95% CI: 56.9; 57.2). The prevalence of engaging in PA every day decreases over the age from 28.2% at age of 11–12 years (95% CI: 27.4; 29.0) to 21.2% at age of 16–17 years (95% CI: 20.3; 22.0) among boys; and from 19.4% (95% CI: 18.5; 20.2) to 11.1% (95% CI: 10.1; 12.0) among girls. For boys and girls who engaged in PA 5-6 days/week, the prevalence increases from countries with the lowest human development index to countries with the highest. Cambodia (7.3%, 95% CI: 3.8; 10.8), Philippines (7.7%, 95% CI: 5.6; 9.7), Sudan (8.8%, 95% CI: 4.7; 12.9), Timor-Leste (8.9%, 95% CI: 5.5; 12.3), and Afghanistan (10.1%, 95% CI: 6.1; 14.1) were the countries with the lowest prevalence of sufficient PA. Conclusions: National, regional, and worldwide data on the prevalence of physical activity in adolescents highlights the importance of improving the global levels of PA, especially in girls. Identifying the factors causing the age-related decrease in physical activity levels will permit public health entities to define priority actions and policies against physical inactivity.

Keywords: sports; physical exercise; young people; physical inactivity

1. Introduction

Physical activity (PA) is an important health behaviour. Among children and adolescents, PA has a significant impact on cardiovascular, bone, and metabolic health, improving fitness, weight status, and sleep [1]. Besides physical health benefits, there is increasing evidence on the cognitive, psychological, and social benefits of PA [2]. Furthermore, PA benefits obtained during adolescence can be transferred into adulthood [1,3]. To achieve these benefits, adolescents are recommended to engage in moderate-to-vigorous intensity PA at least 60 min every day [4].

Promoting PA is of importance to public health. Even if PA recommendations are not attained, major improvements in health can be achieved from modest increases in regular PA [5]. Furthermore, some evidence suggests that those who are below the current public health recommendations benefit more from increases in PA than those who are already within the recommendations [1]. Thus, the public health impact of PA and the potential benefits of even small population-wide increases are considerable [1].

Despite all the health benefits of PA, most adolescents worldwide are physically inactive. It is estimated that 77.6% of boys and 84.7% of girls aged 11 to 17 years old are physically inactive [6]. The evidence also suggests that PA declines during adolescent years [6,7]. Updated information on the prevalence and trends of physical inactivity is important to inform national and international authorities and support countries' public health policies and actions. Nonetheless, previous studies focused on the percentage of adolescents who did not practice enough PA to achieve PA recommendations [6–8]. Thus, all adolescents who did not achieve the PA recommendations were grouped in the same group. However, considering in the same group adolescents who do not practice enough PA on any day of the week with adolescents who practice 3 or more days/week for at least 60 min of PA may not be useful for policymakers and public health promoters. Knowledge of PA participation prevalence according to frequency, i.e., times practiced per week, is also crucial as it presents more detailed data and allows for further action and tailored public health strategies in each country. Thus, the aim of this study, using cross-sectional survey data, was to present the worldwide, regional, and national prevalence of PA participation according to its frequency in adolescents aged 11 to 17 years.

2. Materials and Methods

2.1. Participants and Procedures

This study is based on cross-sectional surveys of adolescents' populations from several countries, from all regions worldwide. Data were collected from representative national sample sizes of at least 100 adolescents, from 105 countries. Data were from national and international surveys, namely the Health Behaviour in School-aged Children (HBSC), the Global School-Based Student Health Survey (GSHS), the Youth Risk Behavior Surveillance (YRBS), the Pesquisa Nacional de Saúde do Escolar (PENSE), and the Encuesta Nacional de Salud y Nutrición (ENSNUT). The final database, with data from all surveys, consisted of 558,443 adolescents. As the surveys did not collect data from adolescents within the same age range, only adolescents aged 11 to 17 years were selected to allow comparison between countries. Adolescents with missing data/non-response on PA were removed from the sample. The final sample comprised 520,533 adolescents (251,788 boys, 268,745 girls) from 105 countries and eight regions.

Data collected in surveys were self-reported. Adolescents were asked to report the number of days they were physically active for a total of at least 60 min per day in the last 7 days. Answers were given on an 8-point scale (0 = none to 7 = daily). This is a valid and reliable question assessing adolescents' PA at an epidemiological level [9,10], and it has been used in several studies [6,11–13]. Although the data came from different surveys (HBSC, GSHS, YRBS, PENSE, ENSANUT), it should be noted that in all surveys the same question was used to assess the adolescents' PA levels. Adolescents were provided with a definition of PA accompanied by examples of some age-relevant activities (e.g., running, cycling, dancing, playing football, basketball).

2.2. Data Analysis

For the entire sample, descriptive statistics were calculated (percentages and 95% confidence interval). To estimate the prevalence of PA levels, data were stratified by sex, age (11 to 12 years, 13 to 15 years, 16 to 17 years), eight world regions (1. Central and Eastern Europe, 2. Central Asia, the Middle East, and North Africa, 3. East and southeast, Asia, 4. High-income Western countries, 5. Oceania, 6. Sub-Saharan Africa, 7. South Asia, 8. Latin America and the Caribbean), adapted from the World Bank and previous studies [6,14], human development index (HDI) (low, middle, high, very high), and countries [15]. PA was recoded into 1 to 2 days/week, 3 to 4 days/week, 5 to 6 days/week, and every day. The daily practice of moderate to vigorous PA of at least 60 min was defined as reaching the PA recommendation [4]. Descriptive data are presented as percentages. The prevalence of PA levels was calculated along with a 95% confidence interval (CI). Data analysis was performed using IBM SPSS Statistics version 25.

3. Results

Table 1 presents the sample distribution according to age, HDI, and PA levels. Boys and girls presented different figures. About half of the boys (50.1%; 95% CI: 49.8, 50.2) engaged in PA up to 3 days/week and for girls, the prevalence was 63.6% (95% CI: 63.4, 63.8). For every day PA, boys presented a higher prevalence than girls (22.1%; 95% CI: 21.7, 22.4 vs. 12.6%, 95% CI: 12.2, 12.9).

Table 1. Participants' characteristics.

	Total (n = 520,533)		Boys (n = 25,1788)		Girls (n = 268,745)	
	n	% (95% CI)	n	% (95% CI)	n	% (95% CI)
Age						
11 years	55,782	10.7 (10.5, 11.0)	27,153	10.8 (10.4, 11.2)	28,629	10.7 (10.3, 11.0)
12 years	25,609	4.9 (4.7, 5.2)	12,246	4.9 (4.5, 5.2)	13,363	5.0 (4.6, 5.3)
13 years	116,031	22.3 (22.1, 22.5)	54,536	21.7 (21.3, 22.0)	61,495	22.9 (22.6, 23.2)
14 years	116,894	22.5 (22.2, 22.7)	55,184	21.9 (21.6, 22.3)	61,710	23.0 (22.6, 23.3)
15 years	131,520	25.3 (25.0, 25.5)	64,961	25.8 (25.5, 26.1)	66,559	24.8 (24.4, 25.1)
16 years	53,582	10.3 (10.0, 10.6)	27,251	10.8 (10.5, 11.2)	26,331	9.8 (9.4, 10.2)
17 years	21,115	4.1 (3.8, 4.3)	10,457	4.2 (3.8, 4.5)	10,658	4.0 (3.6, 4.3)
HDI						
Very high	225,408	43.3 (43.1, 43.5)	110,258	43.8 (43.5, 44.1)	115,150	42.8 (42.6, 43.1)
High	185,430	35.6 (35.4, 35.8)	89,604	35.6 (35.3, 35.9)	95,826	35.7 (35.4, 36.0)
Middle	87,088	16.7 (16.5, 17.0)	40,249	16.0 (15.6, 16.3)	46,839	17.4 (17.1, 17.8)
Low	22,607	4.3 (4.1, 4.6)	11,677	4.6 (4.3, 5.0)	10,930	4.1 (3.7, 4.4)
PA						
Never	94,279	18.1 (17.9, 18.4)	37,395	14.9 (14.5, 15.2)	56,884	21.2 (20.8, 21.5)
1 days/week	69,607	13.4 (13.1, 13.6)	29,089	11.6 (11.2, 11.9)	40,518	15.1 (14.7, 15.4)
2 days/week	68,091	13.1 (12.8, 13.3)	29,280	11.6 (11.3, 12.0)	38,811	14.4 (14.1, 14.8)
3 days/week	64,870	12.5 (12.2, 12.7)	30,111	12.0 (11.6, 12.3)	34,759	12.9 (12.6, 13.3)
4 days/week	50,501	9.7 (9.4, 10.0)	25,403	10.1 (9.7, 10.5)	25,098	9.3 (9.0, 9.7)
5 days/week	51,611	9.9 (9.7, 10.2)	27,098	10.8 (10.4, 11.1)	24,513	9.1 (8.8, 9.5)
6 days/week	32,193	6.2 (5.9, 6.4)	17,855	7.1 (6.7, 7.5)	14,338	5.3 (5.0, 5.7)
Every day	89,381	17.2 (16.9, 17.4)	55,557	22.1 (21.7, 22.4)	33,824	12.6 (12.2, 12.9)

Abbreviation: HDI, Human development index; PA, physical activity.

In Table 2, the prevalence of PA levels stratified by age groups is presented. The prevalence of the lowest level of PA (never) increases from 11 to 12 years to 16 to 17 years among boys and girls. Overall, the biggest increase is from 11 to 12 years to 13 to 15 years. From the ages of 13 to 15 to 16 to 17 years, the increase is slight. On the other hand, the prevalence of engaging in PA every day decreases over the age from 28.2% (95% CI: 27.4, 29.0) to 21.2% (95% CI: 20.3, 22.0) among boys, and from 19.4% (95% CI: 18.5, 20.2) to 11.1% (95% CI: 10.1, 12.0) among girls. The prevalence of PA 3 to 4 days/week and 5 to 6 days/week also decreases with age among boys and girls.

Table 2. Physical activity levels according to age, stratified by sex.

	Age		
	11–12 Years	13–15 Years	16–17 Years
Boys	% (95% CI)	% (95% CI)	% (95% CI)
Never	6.7 (5.8, 7.7)	16.0 (15.6, 16.5)	17.9 (17.0, 18.9)
1–2 days/week	16.7 (15.8, 17.6)	23.6 (23.2, 24.0)	28.0 (27.1, 28.9)
3–4 days/week	24.9 (24.1, 25.8)	22.0 (21.6, 22.4)	19.1 (18.2, 20.0)
5–6 days/week	23.4 (22.6, 24.3)	17.5 (17.0, 17.9)	13.8 (12.9, 14.7)
Every day	28.2 (27.4, 29.0)	20.9 (20.5, 21.3)	21.2 (20.3, 22.0)
Girls	% (95% CI)	% (95% CI)	% (95% CI)
Never	8.4 (7.5, 9.4)	23.1 (22.7, 23.5)	25.6 (24.7, 26.5)
1–2 days/week	21.9 (21.0, 22.7)	30.0 (29.6, 30.4)	35.7 (34.8, 36.5)
3–4 days/week	28.3 (27.5, 29.1)	21.9 (21.5, 22.3)	17.3 (16.4, 18.3)
5–6 days/week	22.1 (21.2, 22.9)	13.6 (13.2, 14.0)	10.4 (9.4, 11.3)
Every day	19.4 (18.5, 20.2)	11.4 (11.0, 11.8)	11.1 (10.1, 12.0)

The levels of PA according to the HDI is presented in Table 3. The prevalence of never engaging in PA of at least 60 min/day is more pronounced in countries with the lowest HDI. For boys and girls, the prevalence decreases moderately among low HDI countries to high HDI countries. However, there is a very sharp decrease in countries with very high HDI. In boys and girls who engaged in PA 5 to 6 days/week, the prevalence increases from the countries with the lowest HDI to the countries with the highest HDI. For PA every day, boys from countries with very high HDI presented a slightly higher prevalence (24.7%, 95% CI: 24.2, 25.2) compared to those from countries with high, middle and low HDI. For the girls, no clear pattern was observed. The highest prevalence for achieving PA recommended levels were from the countries with the lowest HDI (16.5%, 95% CI: 14.8, 18.2) and highest HDI (14.7%, 95% CI: 14.2, 15.2).

Table 3. Physical activity levels according to the human development index, stratified by sex.

	Human Development Index			
	Low	Middle	High	Very High
Boys	% (95% CI)	% (95% CI)	% (95% CI)	% (95% CI)
Never	30.2 (28.7, 31.7)	25.3 (24.5, 26.2)	19.1 (18.6, 19.7)	5.9 (5.3, 6.5)
1–2 days/week	32.1 (30.7, 33.6)	31.9 (31.1, 32.7)	24.2 (23.7, 24.8)	18.2 (17.7, 18.7)
3–4 days/week	12.0 (10.3, 13.7)	14.8 (13.9, 15.7)	20.7 (20.1, 21.3)	26.9 (26.4, 27.4)
5–6 days/week	6.8 (5.0, 8.6)	9.6 (8.6, 10.5)	15.1 (14.5, 15.7)	24.3 (23.8, 24.8)
Every day	18.9 (17.3, 20.5)	18.4 (17.5, 19.3)	20.8 (20.2, 21.4)	24.7 (24.2, 25.2)
Girls	% (95% CI)	% (95% CI)	% (95% CI)	% (95% CI)
Never	36.4 (34.9, 37.9)	30.2 (29.5, 31.0)	31.0 (30.5, 31.6)	7.8 (7.2, 8.4)
1–2 days/week	30.9 (29.3, 32.4)	35.6 (34.9, 36.3)	29.9 (29.3, 30.4)	26.6 (26.1, 27.1)
3–4 days/week	9.8 (8.0, 11.6)	14.0 (13.1, 14.8)	18.3 (17.7, 18.9)	30.1 (29.6, 30.6)
5–6 days/week	6.4 (4.6, 8.2)	8.3 (7.5, 9.2)	10.8 (10.2, 11.4)	20.7 (20.2, 21.3)
Every day	16.5 (14.8, 18.2)	11.8 (11.0, 12.7)	10.0 (9.4, 10.6)	14.7 (14.2, 15.2)

The prevalence of PA levels according to regions is presented in Table 4. Across all regions, girls were less active than boys. For boys and girls, the lowest prevalence of never doing PA was observed in Central and Eastern Europe, and in high-income Western countries. Conversely, South Asian countries presented the highest prevalence. The regions that showed the highest prevalence of never doing PA are the same that showed the highest prevalence for doing PA daily. Among girls, the results were quite different. Girls from South Asia were the ones that had the highest prevalence in achieving PA recommended levels.

Table 4. Physical activity levels according to regions, stratified by sex.

	Region							
	Central and Eastern Europe	Central Asia, Middle East, and North Africa	East and Southeast Asia	High-Income Western Countries	Oceania	Sub-Saharan Africa	South Asia	Latin America and Caribbean
Boys	% (95% CI)	% (95% CI)	% (95% CI)	% (95% CI)	% (95% CI)	% (95% CI)	% (95% CI)	% (95% CI)
Never	3.3 (2.4, 4.3)	19.0 (17.8, 20.3)	23.5 (22.4, 24.6)	3.5 (2.7, 4.2)	26.4 (24.2, 28.6)	27.5 (25.7, 29.3)	35.1 (33.1, 37.2)	22.3 (21.7, 22.9)
1–2 days/week	15.0 (14.1, 15.9)	32.4 (31.3, 33.6)	34.0 (33.0, 35.0)	16.2 (15.5, 16.9)	31.0 (28.8, 33.2)	30.9 (29.2, 32.6)	28.6 (26.4, 30.7)	25.4 (24.9, 26.0)
3–4 days/week	27.2 (26.3, 28.0)	18.1 (16.8, 19.4)	16.0 (14.9, 17.1)	28.8 (28.1, 29.4)	13.9 (11.5, 16.4)	15.1 (13.2, 17.0)	9.8 (7.4, 12.3)	19.2 (18.6, 19.8)
5–6 days/week	25.9 (25.1, 26.7)	8.7 (7.3, 10.0)	8.7 (7.5, 9.9)	26.8 (26.2, 27.5)	12.9 (10.5, 15.4)	8.2 (6.2, 10.2)	6.3 (3.8, 8.8)	14.0 (13.3, 14.6)
Every day	28.6 (27.8, 29.4)	21.7 (20.5, 23.0)	17.8 (16.6, 18.9)	24.7 (24.0, 25.4)	15.7 (13.3, 18.1)	18.3 (16.4, 20.1)	20.2 (17.9, 22.5)	19.1 (18.5, 19.7)
Girls	% (95% CI)	% (95% CI)	% (95% CI)	% (95% CI)	% (95% CI)	% (95% CI)	% (95% CI)	% (95% CI)
Never	4.5 (3.6, 5.4)	26.3 (25.2, 27.5)	26.8 (25.8, 27.8)	4.4 (3.6, 5.1)	30.0 (28.0, 32.0)	34.9 (33.3, 36.4)	37.0 (34.7, 39.4)	35.6 (35.1, 36.2)
1–2 days/week	21.7 (20.9, 22.6)	39.2 (38.2, 40.3)	44.1 (43.2, 45.0)	24.2 (23.6, 24.9)	31.3 (29.4, 33.3)	33.5 (31.9, 35.1)	22.6 (20.0, 25.2)	29.9 (29.3, 30.4)
3–4 days/week	31.9 (31.1, 32.7)	15.2 (13.9, 16.4)	15.3 (14.2, 16.4)	33.6 (33.0, 34.2)	13.8 (11.6, 16.0)	13.1 (11.3, 14.9)	8.0 (5.1, 10.8)	15.5 (14.9, 16.1)
5–6 days/week	23.4 (22.6, 24.2)	6.8 (5.6, 8.1)	6.0 (4.8, 7.1)	23.4 (22.7, 24.0)	11.5 (9.3, 13.7)	6.0 (4.1, 7.9)	8.4 (5.5, 11.3)	9.6 (8.9, 10.2)
Every day	18.5 (17.6, 19.3)	12.5 (11.2, 13.7)	7.9 (6.8, 9.0)	14.4 (13.7, 15.1)	13.4 (11.2, 15.6)	12.5 (10.7, 14.4)	24.0 (21.4, 26.6)	9.4 (8.7, 10.0)

Cambodia (7.3%, 95% CI: 3.8, 10.8), Philippines (7.7, 95% CI: 5.6, 9.7), Sudan (8.8, 95% CI: 4.7, 12.9), Timor-Leste (8.9, 95% CI: 5.5, 12.3), and Afghanistan (10.1, 95% CI: 6.1, 14.1) were the countries with the lowest prevalence of sufficient PA. Three of those countries are from East and Southeast Asia (Cambodia, Philippines, and Timor-Leste). From the other regions, the countries with the lowest prevalence of sufficient PA were Italy from the High-income Western countries (10.3%, 95% CI: 7.3, 13.2), Syria from Central Asia, Middle East, and North Africa (10.6%, 95% CI: 7.2, 13.9), Vanuatu from Oceania (11%, 95% CI: 5.4, 16.6), Curaçao from Latin America and the Caribbean (11.7, 95% CI: 7.7, 15.8), Mauritania from Sub-Sharan Africa (12.1%, 95% CI: 7.9, 16.3), and Estonia from Central and Eastern Europe (16.4%, 95% CI: 13.6, 19.3). Countries that presented the highest prevalence of PA every day, achieving the PA recommended levels, were Finland (27.9, 95% CI: 25.7, 30.0), Albania (28.0, 95% CI: 25.6, 30.3), Bulgaria (28.6, 95% CI: 26.2, 31.0), the United States (32.3, 95% CI: 30.9, 33.8), and Bangladesh (48.2, 95% CI: 45.6, 50.8). Considering PA ≥5 days per week, countries that presented the highest prevalence were Iceland (53.7, 95% CI: 52.3, 55.0), the United States (56.7, 95% CI: 55.6, 57.9), Canada (58.0, 95% CI: 56.9, 59.1), Finland (58.7, 95% CI: 57.0, 60.3), and Bangladesh (59.7, 95% CI: 57.4, 62.1). Table A1 shows the physical activity levels by regions and countries (Appendix A).

4. Discussion

This study found that the prevalence of adolescents doing sufficient PA was low. Less than 20% of the adolescents engaged in PA every day and almost 20% never engaged in PA. Regardless of the country, region, HDI, or age group, adolescent girls revealed consistently lower PA levels than boys. These results reinforce the urgent need for worldwide international, national, and local agencies to take action to promote PA, especially among girls. Interventions conducted for improving girls' PA have shown small but significant effects [16]. Successful strategies for changing girls' PA were found for interventions that were theory-driven, multi-component in design, school-based, and that also offer physical education, which addresses the unique needs of girls and targeting girls only [16,17]. Engagement with young people, such as active listening to their voices, has also been identified as an important way of developing meaningful PA opportunities [18,19].

The scaling up of implementing known effective policies and programs as well as social marketing campaigns combined with community-based interventions have been suggested for increasing PA in adolescents, particularly in girls [6]. Overall, recent evidence of PA trend studies indicates that the percentage of physically active adolescent girls has not increased over the years [6,20]. This suggests that programs and policies to promote PA among adolescent girls are having limited success. Nevertheless, in another trend study, an increase in the prevalence of PA among girls has been found aged 11 to 15 years from 10 out of 32 countries [21]. Understanding why these countries succeed in improving girls' PA levels might be important in helping to define and implement more effective policies and strategies.

Another major finding from our study was that sufficient PA decreases with age among boys and girls, which is in line with previous literature [22]. In our study, a decrease with age seems to be similar in both sexes, i.e., around 7% to 8% from 11 to 12 years to 16 to 17 years. However, the biggest decrease in meeting the PA levels is from 11 to 12 years to 13 to 15 years. Therefore, early adolescence seems to be a critical period for either preventing the PA decline or promoting PA. Furthermore, considering that PA decline starts at ages 6 to 7 [22], that PA may track from childhood to adolescence [23], that childhood is a critical period for developing the basic motor competencies [24], and the fact that in our study 11-year-old boys and girls had already low levels of PA, there is a need for a greater emphasis on promoting PA from an early age (and not only in adolescence).

It was found that the prevalence of never engaging in PA of at least 60 min per day was more pronounced in countries with the lowest HDI and decreased for countries with higher HDI. Additionally, the prevalence of engaging in PA 5 to 6 days/week was higher in countries with the highest HDI. A similar trend was observed among low- and middle-income countries, where increased HDI values were associated with decreased levels of physical inactivity [25]. In contrast, the analyses based on the

2018 Activity Report Card for children and youth showed higher PA levels in the low and medium HDI countries [8]. Additionally, the prevalence of insufficient PA in analysis with adults was more than twice as high in high-income countries as in low-income countries [26]. Finally, less economically developed countries had the lowest prevalence of physical inactivity, while physical inactivity was more prevalent among the most developed economic countries [7]. The different findings between studies can be in part explained based on compositional differences in the study sample and PA measurement method. For instance, in Activity Report Cards the PA assessment used indicators that included 5 behaviors (overall PA, organized sports participation, active play, active transportation, sedentary behavior) [8], while for the present study a single-item indicator of total PA was used. Furthermore, the fact that PA also varies across countries suggests that the factors influencing PA lie mostly at the national community level [26]. Nevertheless, these conflicting results highlight an area for future research to better understand the factors affecting the relationship between PA and HDI.

The results of this investigation have several implications for national and international public health policies. Overall, this investigation reinforces the World Health Organization's recommendation for countries to develop or update national policy and implementation plans on PA [27] as findings suggest an urgent need to improve PA levels among adolescents. One critical aspect is the necessity of allocating the necessary political priority and resources to enable the implementation of PA policies [6].

For every single country, age and sex were factors associated with PA participation. In this regard, national public health policies aiming to promote PA should also focus on reducing the gap between sexes and age groups. Thus, effectively promoting PA among adolescents requires identifying, understanding, and intervening on the causes and inequities [6]. Furthermore, because of the low levels of PA, countries would benefit and should invest in the promotion of PA in all its forms (including recreational PA, sports participation, physical education, and active travel) and in all sectors. This multisectoral approach, leading to the involvement of health authorities, schools, sports clubs and federations, regional planners, and political leaders on PA promoting strategies, is considered effective and commended in the WHO Global action plan on PA 2018-2030 [28].

Several limitations of this study are important to mention. Data were collected at the school setting resulting in the exclusion of adolescents that do not attend schools. In addition, data were from adolescents aged 11 to 17 years. However, data from the HBSC survey were collected among those who attended the grades 6, 8, and 10. Thus, adolescents from the HBSC survey were mostly aged 11, 13, and 15 years, whereas the GSHS focuses on adolescents aged 13 to 17 years. Furthermore, data were self-reported and subject to bias. Despite large samples used in each national or regional survey, self-report was the most feasible methodology and is still the backbone of surveillance studies [29].

5. Conclusions

Monitoring PA levels in adolescents allows the identification of specific needs and inequities within and between countries, and consequently promotes informed decisions and actions. Findings show that worldwide PA levels among adolescents are low, as 14.9% of boys and 21.2% of girls report to never practice PA, and that the situations get worse with aging. Identifying and understanding the main factors related to the insufficient and decreased PA levels, will permit international and national public health entities to define priority actions and policies against physical inactivity. Reducing the gender gap, specifically improving girls' PA levels should be considered a priority in public health-related actions. This process, initiated with national or regional surveillance of PA, ultimately aims to improve PA levels and promotes healthy lifestyles among adolescents as well as carrying them forward into adulthood.

Author Contributions: Conceptualization, A.M. and M.P.; methodology, M.P. and D.H.-N.; software, A.M. and J.M.; formal analysis, A.M., J.M., Y.D. and D.M.I.S.; investigation, A.M. and M.P.; resources, M.G.d.M.; data curation, D.H.-N. and M.P.; writing—original draft preparation, A.M., M.P.; writing—review and editing, J.M.; visualization, Y.D., D.M.I.S. and M.G.d.M.; supervision, M.G.d.M. All authors have read and agreed to the published version of the manuscript.

Funding: This research received no external funding.

Acknowledgments: The authors would like to thank all the adolescents who participated in the study. The authors would also like to thank the researchers who made the databases available through free access.

Conflicts of Interest: The authors declare no conflict of interest.

Appendix A

Table A1. Physical activity levels by region and countries.

Region	Country	Physical Activity (%)				
		Never	1–2 Days/Week	3–4 Days/Week	5–6 Days/Week	Every Day
Central and eastern Europe	Albania	3.1	21.0	30.2	17.8	28.0
	Bulgaria	4.5	18.4	26.5	22.0	28.6
	Canada	3.7	12.7	25.6	33.0	25.0
	Croatia	2.6	17.7	27.5	26.5	25.6
	Czech Republic	2.5	17.7	32.9	25.7	21.3
	Estonia	3.6	21.1	35.1	23.8	16.4
	Greenland	10.7	31.7	22.7	16.8	18.0
	Hungary	5.1	18.8	29.0	24.5	22.6
	Latvia	3.1	20.8	33.6	24.0	18.4
	Macedonia	2.7	14.7	31.1	24.6	26.9
	Moldova	3.7	23.8	24.6	21.8	26.0
	Poland	4.3	16.3	27.9	27.6	24.0
	Romania	9.6	26.8	23.7	18.7	21.3
	Russia	5.0	19.8	38.6	18.7	17.9
	Slovakia	3.2	17.8	29.6	24.1	25.3
	Slovenia	3.1	20.1	32.4	25.9	18.5
	Ukraine	4.5	16.5	32.0	20.8	26.3
Central Asia, Middle East, and north Africa	Algeria	11.4	53.7	14.0	5.8	15.1
	Armenia	4.9	19.9	34.6	17.8	22.9
	Egypt	30.4	40.9	10.7	3.6	14.5
	Iraq	37.1	31.4	11.9	5.0	14.6
	Kuwait	22.6	32.8	19.5	9.6	15.5
	Lebanon	16.3	29.3	18.1	11.7	24.6
	Mongolia	13.9	30.4	19.5	11.0	25.2
	Morocco	22.0	49.0	11.0	4.8	13.1
	Oman	27.9	36.8	19.5	4.1	11.7
	Palestinian territory	33.8	33.3	11.4	5.8	15.7
	Syria	35.6	39.2	10.7	3.9	10.6
	United Arab Emirates	19.0	32.8	20.3	9.9	18.0
	Yemen	38.8	35.2	9.7	4.4	11.9
East and southeast Asia	Brunei Darussalam	16.4	38.9	23.5	9.2	12.1
	Cambodia	38.2	42.8	8.3	3.3	7.3
	Laos	24.3	43.5	11.5	5.5	15.2
	Malasya	17.9	39.0	19.1	9.1	14.9
	Philippines	44.3	34.6	8.8	4.6	7.7
	Thailand	23.7	38.7	17.8	8.1	11.9
	Timor-Leste	30.2	49.6	8.2	3.2	8.9
	Viet Nam	27.6	38.8	14.2	6.2	13.1

Table A1. Cont.

Region	Country	Physical Activity (%)				
		Never	1–2 Days/Week	3–4 Days/Week	5–6 Days/Week	Every Day
High-income western countries	Austria	2.4	20.1	32.9	25.0	19.4
	Belgium	3.6	23.3	34.1	22.5	16.6
	Denmark	4.9	23.1	35.6	23.2	13.1
	England	2.4	17.1	33.5	28.5	18.5
	Finland	1.8	11.3	28.2	30.8	27.9
	France	4.8	27.2	35.0	20.1	12.9
	Germany	3.7	22.7	37.4	20.8	15.4
	Greece	6.5	23.2	34.3	22.6	13.4
	Iceland	4.6	13.9	27.9	31.2	22.4
	Ireland	3.4	14.3	29.6	29.1	23.6
	Israel	16.3	34.9	24.3	12.1	12.4
	Italy	8.3	28.7	33.8	18.9	10.3
	Luxembourg	2.8	19.6	30.4	24.4	22.8
	Malta	7.3	24.3	28.2	22.3	17.9
	Netherlands	3.2	15.5	31.8	31.3	18.3
	Norway	3.0	16.6	33.7	27.9	18.9
	Portugal	3.6	28.7	32.9	19.0	15.8
	Scotland	3.1	16.7	34.0	28.7	17.5
	Spain	3.0	15.0	30.2	25.9	25.9
	Sweden	4.5	19.2	34.4	27.8	14.1
	Switzerland	2.1	18.4	36.0	29.1	14.4
	United States		22.2	21.1	24.4	32.3
	Wales	4.0	20.6	35.5	23.5	16.3
Oceania	Fiji	26.0	27.3	14.7	13.5	18.5
	Kiribati	28.0	32.9	12.5	8.8	17.8
	Nauru	49.2	19.3	11.0	7.9	12.6
	Niue	27.7	21.9	19.0	19.0	12.4
	Samoa	28.3	32.5	18.3	9.0	11.8
	Solomon Islands	18.9	38.9	15.4	10.5	16.4
	Tokelau	33.1	17.4	11.6	14.0	24.0
	Tonga	32.4	31.1	11.6	11.1	13.8
	Tuvalu	47.0	26.7	9.4	5.4	11.6
	Vanuatu	17.7	29.2	8.1	34.0	11.0
	Wallis and Futuna	20.7	37.3	19.5	9.1	13.3
Sub-Sharan Africa	Ghana	32.7	32.6	14.8	6.9	13.0
	Mauritania	41.1	34.3	8.0	4.5	12.1
	Mauritius	18.0	31.3	19.1	12.4	19.2
	Mozambique	21.4	45.4	13.8	6.0	13.4
	Namibia	41.4	26.3	11.8	6.5	14.1
	Seychelles	31.3	28.1	16.5	7.2	16.9
	Sudan	33.0	40.5	14.2	3.5	8.8
	Tanzania	27.3	30.5	14.0	8.1	20.2
South Asia	Afghanistan	30.1	36.5	14.7	8.6	10.1
	Bangladesh	23.1	9.9	7.3	11.6	48.2
	Pakistan	45.7	30.8	7.7	4.1	11.7

Table A1. Cont.

Region	Country	Physical Activity (%)				
		Never	1–2 Days/Week	3–4 Days/Week	5–6 Days/Week	Every Day
Latin America and Caribbean	Antiqua and Barbuda	30.1	21.1	16.2	9.8	22.7
	Argentina	15.1	35.0	20.2	11.5	18.2
	Bahamas	31.9	28.8	15.8	8.9	14.6
	Barbados	28.1	27.6	16.7	9.4	18.3
	Belize	32.4	21.8	15.4	9.5	20.9
	Bolivia	22.3	38.9	15.9	9.4	13.5
	Brasil	34.2	24.1	16.8	12.9	12.0
	British Virgin Islands	31.3	26.9	16.2	7.7	18.0
	Chile	16.5	32.0	23.9	12.4	15.2
	Costa Rica	18.0	35.1	19.2	9.6	18.1
	Curaçao	32.3	31.9	16.5	7.6	11.7
	Dominica	35.1	28.7	13.3	6.8	16.1
	El Salvador	28.6	35.4	13.7	8.5	13.8
	Guatemala	26.9	35.9	15.9	7.2	14.0
	Guyana	39.2	26.2	11.8	7.2	15.6
	Honduras	28.9	37.3	12.3	5.8	15.7
	Mexico	17.5	38.5	16.8	9.3	17.8
	Peru	17.8	37.7	19.3	9.8	15.4
	Saint Kitts and Nevis	32.7	26.9	15.3	7.2	18.0
	Suriname	26.0	30.8	16.6	7.4	19.2
	Trinidad and Tobago	29.8	26.4	15.6	8.3	19.9
	Uruguay	20.7	31.0	20.7	12.4	15.2

References

1. USDHHS. *2018 Physical Activity Guidelines Advisory Committee Scientific Report*; U.S. Department of Health and Human Services: Washington, DC, USA, 2018.
2. Rodriguez-Ayllon, M.; Cadenas-Sanchez, C.; Estevez-Lopez, F.; Munoz, N.E.; Mora-Gonzalez, J.; Migueles, J.H.; Molina-Garcia, P.; Henriksson, H.; Mena-Molina, A.; Martinez-Vizcaino, V.; et al. Role of Physical Activity and Sedentary Behavior in the Mental Health of Preschoolers, Children and Adolescents: A Systematic Review and Meta-Analysis. *Sports Med.* **2019**, *49*, 1383–1410. [CrossRef] [PubMed]
3. Reiner, M.; Niermann, C.; Jekauc, D.; Woll, A. Long-term health benefits of physical activity–a systematic review of longitudinal studies. *BMC Public Health* **2013**, *13*, 813. [CrossRef] [PubMed]
4. WHO. *Global Recommendations on Physical Activity for Health*; World Health Organization: Geneva, Switzerland, 2010.
5. Wen, C.P.; Wai, J.P.; Tsai, M.K.; Yang, Y.C.; Cheng, T.Y.; Lee, M.C.; Chan, H.T.; Tsao, C.K.; Tsai, S.P.; Wu, X. Minimum amount of physical activity for reduced mortality and extended life expectancy: A prospective cohort study. *Lancet* **2011**, *378*, 1244–1253. [CrossRef]
6. Guthold, R.; Stevens, G.A.; Riley, L.M.; Bull, F.C. Global trends in insufficient physical activity among adolescents: A pooled analysis of 298 population-based surveys with 1.6 million participants. *Lancet Child. Adolesc. Health* **2020**, *4*, 23–35. [CrossRef]
7. Dumith, S.C.; Hallal, P.C.; Reis, R.S.; Kohl, H.W., 3rd. Worldwide prevalence of physical inactivity and its association with human development index in 76 countries. *Prev. Med.* **2011**, *53*, 24–28. [CrossRef]
8. Aubert, S.; Barnes, J.D.; Abdeta, C.; Abi Nader, P.; Adeniyi, A.F.; Aguilar-Farias, N.; Andrade Tenesaca, D.S.; Bhawra, J.; Brazo-Sayavera, J.; Cardon, G.; et al. Global Matrix 3.0 Physical Activity Report Card Grades for Children and Youth: Results and Analysis from 49 Countries. *J. Phys. Act. Health* **2018**, *15*, S251–S273. [CrossRef]
9. Ridgers, N.D.; Timperio, A.; Crawford, D.; Salmon, J. Validity of a brief self-report instrument for assessing compliance with physical activity guidelines amongst adolescents. *J. Sci. Med. Sport* **2012**, *15*, 136–141. [CrossRef]

10. Prochaska, J.J.; Sallis, J.F.; Long, B. A physical activity screening measure for use with adolescents in primary care. *Arch. Pediatr. Adolesc. Med.* **2001**, *155*, 554–559. [CrossRef]
11. Marques, A.; Bordado, J.; Tesler, R.; Demetriou, Y.; Sturm, D.J.; de Matos, M.G. A composite measure of healthy lifestyle: A study from 38 countries and regions from Europe and North America, from the Health Behavior in School-Aged Children survey. *Am. J. Hum. Biol.* **2020**, e23419. [CrossRef]
12. Marques, A.; Loureiro, N.; Avelar-Rosa, B.; Naia, A.; Matos, M.G. Adolescents' healthy lifestyle. *J. Pediatr. (Rio. J.)* **2020**, *96*, 217–224. [CrossRef]
13. Marques, A.; Demetriou, Y.; Tesler, R.; Gouveia, E.R.; Peralta, M.; Matos, M.G. Healthy Lifestyle in Children and Adolescents and Its Association with Subjective Health Complaints: Findings from 37 Countries and Regions from the HBSC Study. *Int. J. Environ. Res. Public Health* **2019**, *16*, 3292. [CrossRef] [PubMed]
14. World Bank Country Classification. Available online: https://datahelpdesk.worldbank.org/knowledgebase/topics/19280-country-classification (accessed on 1 December 2019).
15. UNDP. *Human Development Report 2016. Human Development for Everyone*; United Nations Development Programme: New York, NY, USA, 2016.
16. Owen, M.B.; Curry, W.B.; Kerner, C.; Newson, L.; Fairclough, S.J. The effectiveness of school-based physical activity interventions for adolescent girls: A systematic review and meta-analysis. *Prev. Med.* **2017**, *105*, 237–249. [CrossRef] [PubMed]
17. Camacho-Minano, M.J.; LaVoi, N.M.; Barr-Anderson, D.J. Interventions to promote physical activity among young and adolescent girls: A systematic review. *Health Educ. Res.* **2011**, *26*, 1025–1049. [CrossRef] [PubMed]
18. Martins, J.; Marques, A.; Sarmento, H.; Carreiro da Costa, F. Adolescents' perspectives on the barriers and facilitators of physical activity: A systematic review of qualitative studies. *Health Educ. Res.* **2015**, *30*, 742–755. [CrossRef] [PubMed]
19. Corr, M.; McSharry, J.; Murtagh, E.M. Adolescent girls' perceptions of physical activity: A systematic review of qualitative studies. *Am. J. Health Promot.* **2019**, *33*, 806–819. [CrossRef]
20. Booth, V.M.; Rowlands, A.V.; Dollman, J. Physical activity temporal trends among children and adolescents. *J. Sci. Med. Sport* **2015**, *18*, 418–425. [CrossRef]
21. Kalman, M.; Inchley, J.; Sigmundova, D.; Iannotti, R.J.; Tynjala, J.A.; Hamrik, Z.; Haug, E.; Bucksch, J. Secular trends in moderate-to-vigorous physical activity in 32 countries from 2002 to 2010: A cross-national perspective. *Eur. J. Public Health* **2015**, *25* (Suppl. 2), 37–40. [CrossRef]
22. Farooq, M.A.; Parkinson, K.N.; Adamson, A.J.; Pearce, M.S.; Reilly, J.K.; Hughes, A.R.; Janssen, X.; Basterfield, L.; Reilly, J.J. Timing of the decline in physical activity in childhood and adolescence: Gateshead Millennium Cohort Study. *Br. J. Sports Med.* **2018**, *52*, 1002–1006. [CrossRef]
23. Telama, R.; Yang, X.; Leskinen, E.; Kankaanpaa, A.; Hirvensalo, M.; Tammelin, T.; Viikari, J.S.; Raitakari, O.T. Tracking of physical activity from early childhood through youth into adulthood. *Med. Sci. Sports Exerc.* **2014**, *46*, 955–962. [CrossRef]
24. Gallahue, D.L.; Ozmun, J.C.; Goodway, J.D. *Understanding Motor Development: Infants, Children, Adolescent and Adults*; McGraw-Hill: Boston, MA, USA, 2012.
25. Atkinson, K.; Lowe, S.; Moore, S. Human development, occupational structure and physical inactivity among 47 low and middle income countries. *Prev. Med. Rep.* **2016**, *3*, 40–45. [CrossRef]
26. Guthold, R.; Stevens, G.A.; Riley, L.M.; Bull, F.C. Worldwide trends in insufficient physical activity from 2001 to 2016: A pooled analysis of 358 population-based surveys with 1·9 million participants. *Lancet Glob. Health* **2018**, *6*, e1077–e1086. [CrossRef]
27. WHO. *ACTIVE: A Technical Package for Increasing Physical Activity*; World Health Organization: Geneva, Switzerland, 2018.
28. WHO. *Global Action Plan on Physical Activity 2018–2030: More Active People for a Healthier World*; World Health Organization: Geneva, Switzerland, 2018.
29. Pedisic, Z.; Bauman, A. Accelerometer-based measures in physical activity surveillance: Current practices and issues. *Br. J. Sports Med.* **2015**, *49*, 219–223. [CrossRef] [PubMed]

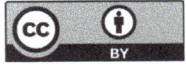

© 2020 by the authors. Licensee MDPI, Basel, Switzerland. This article is an open access article distributed under the terms and conditions of the Creative Commons Attribution (CC BY) license (http://creativecommons.org/licenses/by/4.0/).

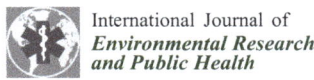 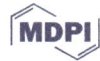

Article

A Combined Modal and Route Choice Behavioral Complementarity Equilibrium Model with Users of Vehicles and Electric Bicycles

Senlai Zhu [1,*], Jie Ma [2,*], Tianpei Tang [1,3] and Quan Shi [1]

1. School of Transportation and Civil Engineering, Nantong University, Nantong 226019, China; tangtianpei@ntu.edu.cn (T.T.); shi.q@ntu.edu.cn (Q.S.)
2. School of Transportation, Southeast University, Nanjing 210096, China
3. Business School, University of Shanghai for Science and Technology, Shanghai 200093, China
* Correspondence: zhusenlai@ntu.edu.cn (S.Z.); majie@seu.edu.cn (J.M.)

Received: 25 April 2020; Accepted: 21 May 2020; Published: 24 May 2020

Abstract: The popularity of electric bicycles in China makes them a common transportation mode for people to commute and move around. However, with the increase in traffic volumes for both vehicles and electric bicycles, urban traffic safety and congestion problems are rising due to traffic conflicts between these two modes. To regulate travel behavior, it is essential to analyze the mode choice and route choice behaviors of travelers. This study proposes a combined modal split and multiclass traffic user equilibrium model formulated as a complementarity problem (CP) to simultaneously characterize the mode choice behavior and route choice behavior of both vehicle and electric bicycle users. This model captures the impacts of route travel time and out-of-pocket cost on travelers' route choice behaviors. Further, modified Bureau of Public Roads (BPR) functions are developed to model the travel times of links with and without physical separation between vehicle lanes and bicycle lanes. This study also analyzes the conditions for uniqueness of the equilibrium solution. A Newton method is developed to solve the proposed model. Numerical examples with different scales are used to validate the proposed model. The results show that electric bicycles are more favored by travelers during times of high network congestion. In addition, total system travel time can be reduced significantly through physical separation of vehicle lanes from electric bicycle lanes to minimize their mutual interference.

Keywords: traffic behavior; user equilibrium; complementarity problem; electric bicycle; commute mode choice

1. Introduction

In recent years, electric bicycles (E-bikes) quickly became one of the main nonmotorized travel modes in some developing countries, especially in China [1–3]. E-bikes have many merits over both regular bikes and vehicles, including that they are much faster and can support longer trips compared with regular bikes. Further, despite the lower maximum speed, they are much more flexible and can run at higher speeds than vehicles in congested areas. E-bikes also have other advantages, such as high availability due to low price, efficient energy consumption, and no tailpipe emissions. Due to these characteristics, E-bikes are now one of the main transportation modes in China. Each year, over 35 million E-bikes are sold in China and the installed base of E-bike in use is over 100 million [4].

However, with the increase in traffic volumes for both vehicles and electric bicycles, due to traffic conflicts between these two modes, various urban traffic problems are rising, such as traffic safety, traffic congestion, and parking problems. Recently, extensive research efforts were devoted to address the multiple research needs related to E-bikes, such as estimating cycling capacity, the bicycle equivalent unit for E-bikes, consumption behavior of E-bikes users, and characteristics of traffic accident involving

E-bikes [5–7]. Existing research generally studied the operational characteristics of E-bike from the micro level, such as operations on links or intersections. However, as an important commute mode, few studies investigated the corresponding mode choice and route choice behaviors, which play important roles in designing management strategies and operational decisions related to E-bikes to alleviate the above traffic problems at the traffic-network level.

Similar to the Braess paradox [8], overall performance of the urban transportation network may decrease when improving the operational level of a certain link or intersection for vehicles and E-bikes. To address traffic problems caused by conflicts between vehicles and E-bikes, the mode choice and route choice behaviors of users at the network level require study, alongside the impact of various management strategies (such as separating bicycle lanes and vehicle lanes by physical separations, e.g., parterres and barriers on some links) on these travel behaviors.

Hence, to simultaneously estimate the mode choice and route choice behaviors of vehicles (cars/automobiles) and E-bikes, this paper proposes a combined modal split and route choice model, with the underlying assumption that all users own vehicles and E-bikes and can choose traffic modes based on the congestion level of each mode. Thus, the general flow pattern is estimated using an user equilibrium model which assumes that nobody can reduce their own travel cost by unilaterally shifting their route or mode at the equilibrium state. Considering the well-established complementarity theory, the proposed multimode traffic assignment model is developed as a complementarity problem (CP).

In reality, vehicle lanes and bicycle lanes on some links are separated by physical barriers, while some links have no physical separations. Link cost functions are different under these two cases. In the literature, the Bureau of Public Roads (BPR) cost function [9] was frequently adopted to analyze the link travel time characteristic of vehicles in congested networks. Without loss of generality, modified BPR functions of each mode are developed to capture the interference between vehicles and E-bikes in different scenarios. As discussed before, compared with vehicles, E-bikes can run at higher speeds in congested areas, even though their designed speeds are less than those of vehicles. This characteristic can be captured by setting different parameters in the modified BPR functions. Out-of-pocket costs are considered in the proposed model to capture impacts of factors such as fuel or electricity consumption, vehicle or E-bike depreciation, insurance, the environment, etc., on mode choice.

In summary, the contributions of this paper include:

(1) The proposal of a complementarity problem to model the multimode and traffic assignment problems regarding both vehicles and E-bikes, with the uniqueness of solution to this problem analytically discussed;
(2) The development of modified BPR functions to capture interactions between the two traffic modes and impacts of characteristics of each mode on link travel time;
(3) The consideration of out-of-pocket costs related to factors (such as security, environment, distance, fuel and electricity prices, etc.) affecting users' mode choice behaviors.

The rest of the paper is organized as follows. Related literature is reviewed in the next section. In Section 3, the CP model for the multimode traffic assignment problem is presented. Section 4 discusses the uniqueness of the equilibrium solution. In Section 5, a Newton method for solving the proposed model is developed. Section 6 applies the proposed method to two numerical examples. The last section concludes this study.

2. Literature Review

2.1. Traffic Assignment Model

Traffic assignment models are important tools in the design of effective management strategies and operational decisions to improve network performance, for example, they are usually leveraged to deploy infrastructures optimally to reduce traffic congestion [10–13] and to find optimal traffic signal settings to minimize total travel time [14,15]. Among various traffic assignment models, the user equilibrium problem is perhaps the most common due to its simple assumption of travelers' behavior and the close-form formulation. The user equilibrium problem assumes that at the equilibrium state, nobody can reduce their own travel cost by unilaterally shifting their travel route.

Given Origin–Destination (OD) flows, the user equilibrium problem is treated traditionally as two different methods, namely, deterministic user equilibrium [16] and stochastic user equilibrium [17]. In deterministic user equilibrium methods, all users are assumed to have perfect information about route costs and all choose the routes of minimum cost. In stochastic user equilibrium methods, the traffic costs are considered as random variables and route choices are different among different users. In this paper, the proposed CP model estimates the deterministic user equilibrium condition of traffic flow for both vehicles and E-bikes.

2.2. Traffic Assignment Model with Multiple Modes

In reality, various modes can be chosen by travelers, such as vehicle, public transportation (bus, metro, taxi), bike (E-bike, regular bike), and so on. To estimate the use ratio of each mode, various methods are proposed, such as discrete choice models [18,19]. After giving the ratio of each, to address the traffic assignment problem with multiple modes, many studies attempted to convert the traffic flows of all other modes into standard passenger cars, followed by conversion of total traffic volume to be used as the input of demand for the traffic assignment model. However, each mode has particular characteristics (such as speed, travel time, capacity, security), which may be ignored if all modes are converted to the standard passenger cars.

In the literature, several multimode and/or multiclass traffic assignment models [20,21] and combined modal split and traffic assignment models [22,23] were proposed to model heterogeneous travel behavior. To capture the characteristics of travel cost realistically, these studies used different link cost functions for different traffic modes. However, in this paper, due to interactions between E-bikes and vehicles, travel cost functions may be asymmetric, thereby increasing the difficulty to formulate a mathematical programming problem. In the literature, traffic assignment problems with asymmetry travel cost functions were usually modeled as variational inequality (VI), complementarity, fixed-points, and entropy maximization problems [24–30]. Despite all these efforts, the best approach to this multimode traffic assignment problem is still under debate.

In existing multimode traffic assignment models, the demand of each mode is normally determined (or assumed to be elastic). That is, these models do not consider mode choice behaviors of users. To address this problem, we first need to study factors affecting mode choice behaviors. This paper focuses on studying the travel behaviors considering users of vehicles and E-bikes. In fact, except for travel time, users choose to use vehicles or E-bikes based on factors such as security, weather, distance, fuel and electricity prices, and so on. Similar to Liu and Li [31], we define costs related to these factors as out-of-pocket costs.

In addition, modes such as buses and taxis use the same lanes as vehicles, and modes such as metros do not interfere with vehicles in space at all. Different from these modes, E-bikes are designed to run in bicycle lanes separated from vehicle lanes. On some links, bicycle lanes and vehicle lanes are physically separated, such as by parterres and barriers. However, bicycle lanes and vehicle lanes are separated only by traffic markings instead of physically on some links. In this case, vehicles and E-bikes may occupy each other's lanes. This interference should be considered in the traffic equilibrium problem, and the existing link travel time function cannot capture this interference.

To address the aforementioned gap in the existing research, this paper proposes a combined modal split and route choice model, in which out-of-pocket costs are considered in the mode route cost function and modified BPR functions are adopted to analyze the link travel time of vehicles and E-bikes for links with and without physical separation between vehicle lanes and bicycle lanes.

3. Model Formulation

Consider a strongly connected network [N, A], where N is the set of nodes and A is the set of directed links. Notations are first given as the following:

$T_a, \overline{T}_a$: Travel time on link $a \in A$ for vehicles and E-bikes, respectively; $T_a^0, \overline{T}_a^0$ are the corresponding free-flow travel times;

$v_a, \overline{v}_a$: Flow of vehicles and E-bikes on link a, respectively;

$C_a, \overline{C}_a$: Capacity of link a for vehicles and E-bikes, respectively;

$p_i^w, \overline{p}_i^w$: Travel time on route i between OD pair w for vehicles and E-bikes, respectively; $i \in P^w$, P^w is the set of routes connecting OD pair w;

$f_i^w, \overline{f}_i^w$: Flow of vehicles and E-bikes on route i between OD pair w, respectively;

f: $f = [\ldots, f^w, \ldots]^T$ with dimension n_1 equals the total number of routes in the network, $(\cdot)^T$ denotes the transpose of either a vector or a matrix, and $f^w = [\ldots, f_i^w, \ldots]$ is the vehicle route flow set of OD pair w;

$\overline{f}$: $\overline{f} = [\ldots, \overline{f}^w, \ldots]^T$ with dimension n_1, in which $\overline{f}^w = [\ldots, \overline{f}_i^w, \ldots]$ is the E-bike route flow set of OD pair w;

q^w: Demand between OD pair w, including demand of vehicles and E-bikes. $q^w > 0$

q: $q = [\ldots, q^w, \ldots]^T$ with dimension n_2 equals the total number of OD pairs in the network;

δ_{ia}^w: Link–route incidence indicator, which is 1 if link a belongs to route i between OD pair w, and 0 otherwise;

σ_i^w: Route–OD pair incidence indicator, which is 1 if route i belongs to OD pair w, and 0 otherwise;

σ: The route–OD pair incidence matrix with the dimensions $n_1 \times n_2$;

LL_a: Length of link a;

LR_i: Length of route i; $LR_i = \sum_a \delta_{ia}^w LL_a$;

π^w: Minimum (equilibrium) travel cost between OD pair w;

π: $\pi = [\ldots, \pi^w, \ldots]$ with dimension n_2;

$l_i^w, \overline{l}_i^w$: Out-of-pocket costs (costs related to factors such as weather, distance, fuel and electricity prices) of route i between OD pair w for users of vehicles and E-bikes, respectively;

$C_i^w, \overline{C}_i^w$: Costs (including travel time and out-of-pocket costs) of route i between OD pair w for users of vehicles and E-bikes, respectively;

C: $C = [\ldots, C^w, \ldots]^T$ with dimension n_1, in which $C^w = [\ldots, C_i^w, \ldots]$ is the vehicle route cost set of OD pair w;

$\overline{C}$: $\overline{C} = [\ldots, \overline{C}^w, \ldots]^T$ with dimension n_1, in which $\overline{C}^w = [\ldots, C_i^w, \ldots]$ is the E-bike route cost set of OD pair w.

Suppose route cost functions $C_i^w, \overline{C}_i^w$ of route i between OD pair w for users of both vehicles and E-bikes are given, respectively. The multiclass traffic equilibrium problem considering users of vehicles and E-bikes is formulated as the following mixed complementary problem (MCP):

$$0 \le f_i^w \perp C_i^w - \pi^w \ge 0, \forall i \tag{1}$$

$$0 \le \overline{f}_i^w \perp \overline{C}_i^w - \pi^w \ge 0, \forall i \tag{2}$$

$$\sum_{i \in P^w} \left(f_i^w + \overline{f}_i^w \right) = q^w, \forall w \tag{3}$$

Equations (1) and (2) are the complementary slackness conditions. That is, for each OD pair w, if the flow on route i satisfies $f_i^w \ge 0$ ($\overline{f}_i^w \ge 0$), the route cost C_i^w ($\overline{C}_i^w$) on route i is equal to the minimal route cost π^w, i.e., $C_i^w = \pi^w$ ($\overline{C}_i^w = \pi^w$). These complementary slackness conditions are consistent with the Wardrop's user equilibrium (UE) principle, i.e., all used routes have equal and minimum travel costs, and all unused routes have equal or higher travel costs. Equation (3) is the flow conservation constraint.

To reduce the MCP formulated by Equations (1)–(3) to a pure CP, Equation (3) is reformulated as follows (the proof of the equivalent of Equations (3) and (4) is given in Appendix A):

$$0 \leq \pi^w \perp \sum_{i \in P^w}\left(f_i^w + \overrightarrow{f}_i^w\right) - q^w \geq 0, \forall w. \tag{4}$$

Then the CP can be formulated in vector form as follows:

$$x = \begin{pmatrix} f \\ \overline{f} \\ \pi \end{pmatrix} \geq 0, F(x) = \begin{pmatrix} C - \sigma\pi \\ \overline{C} - \sigma\pi \\ \sigma^T(f + \overline{f}) - q \end{pmatrix} \geq 0, x^T F(x) = 0. \tag{5}$$

Note that if both C_i^w and $\overline{C}_i^w$ are linear functions with respect to traffic flow, CP (5) becomes a linear complementarity problem (LCP), which can be solved using algorithms such as Lemke's method, the projected successive over relaxation iteration method, the general fixed-point iteration method, or the modulus-based matrix splitting iteration method [32–36]. If either C_i^w or $\overline{C}_i^w$ are nonlinear, CP (5) becomes a nonlinear complementarity problem (NCP), which can be solved by algorithms such as Newton methods [37–39]. In this paper, route cost functions are assumed to be "convex combinations" of route travel time and out-of-pocket costs, and thus the proposed CP (5) becomes an NCP.

Specifically, route cost functions C_i^w, $\overline{C}_i^w$ are defined as

$$C_i^w = P_i^w + I_i^w, \overline{C}_i^w = \overline{P}_i^w + \overline{I}_i^w, \tag{6}$$

where P_i^w, $\overline{P}_i^w$ denote route travel time for vehicles and E-bikes, respectively, and I_i^w, $\overline{I}_i^w$ denote the corresponding out-of-pocket costs.

The route travel time is formulated as

$$P_i^w = \sum_a \delta_{ia}^w T_a, \overline{P}_i^w = \sum_a \delta_{ia}^w \overline{T}_a. \tag{7}$$

Out-of-pocket cost relate to fuel or electricity consumption, vehicle or E-bike depreciation, insurance, security, the environment, and so on. Similar to Liu and Li [31], we assume that the out-of-pocket cost is defined as a function of both travel time and travel distance, as follows:

$$I_i^w = \lambda_m P_i^w + \varphi_m LR_i, \overline{I}_i^w = \lambda_e \overline{P}_i^w + \varphi_e LR_i, \tag{8}$$

where λ_m and λ_e denote the monetary cost per unit time for vehicles and E-bikes, respectively, and φ_m and φ_e denote the monetary cost per unit distance traveled by vehicles and E-bikes, respectively. Note that values for λ_m, φ_m, λ_e, and φ_e depend on factors such as fuel price, weather, and so on. In reality, these parameters can be calibrated by data collected by surveys of stated preference.

According to Equations (6)–(8), route costs C_i^w, $\overline{C}_i^w$ are obtained by

$$C_i^w = (1 + \lambda_m)\sum_a \delta_a^i T_a + \varphi_m LR_i, \overline{C}_i^w = (1 + \lambda_e)\sum_a \delta_a^i \overline{T}_a + \varphi_e LR_i. \tag{9}$$

Note that the linear or nonlinear characteristics of route cost function depend on the function of link travel time (T_a and $\overline{T}_a$). On some urban links, bicycle lanes are separated from vehicle lanes by physical separations, so the flows of vehicles and E-bikes involve almost no interactions. The following modified BPR functions are used to model the link travel time for links with physical separations between bicycle lanes and vehicle lanes:

$$T_a = T_a^0(1 + \alpha_m(\frac{v_a}{C_a})^{\beta_m}) \tag{10}$$

$$\overline{T}_a = \overline{T}_a^0 (1 + \alpha_e (\frac{\overline{v}_a}{\overline{C}_a})^{\beta_e}) \tag{11}$$

where $v_a = \sum_w \sum_i \delta_{ia}^w f_i^w$ and $\overline{v}_a = \sum_w \sum_i \delta_{ia}^w \overline{f}_i^w$ represent vehicle flow and E-bike flow on link a, respectively, and $\alpha_m(\alpha_e)$ and $\beta_m(\beta_e)$ are constants defining how cost increases with traffic flow for vehicles (E-bikes). Note that, in reality, E-bikes have higher flexibility than vehicles and, despite lower maximum speed, E-bikes can maintain higher speeds than vehicles in congested areas. Hence, compared to the travel time of vehicles, the travel time of E-bikes is normally not significantly affected by traffic flow. That is, values of α_e and β_e can be smaller than those of α_m and β_m, respectively. Specifically, in reality, the vehicle link capacity can usually be calibrated due to designed travel speed, number of lanes, headway, etc., and the E-bike link capacity can be calibrated by real link travel data [5].

In some urban links, no independent bicycle lanes or bicycle lanes are separated from vehicle lanes by traffic markings, meaning vehicle lanes may be occupied by E-bikes and bicycle lanes may also be occupied by vehicles frequently. In this case, the link travel time functions related to links without physical separations between bicycle lanes and vehicle lanes are formulated as follows:

$$T_a = T_a^0 (1 + \alpha_m (\frac{v_a + \gamma_m \overline{v}_a}{\theta_m C_a})^{\beta_m}) \tag{12}$$

$$\overline{T}_a = \overline{T}_a^0 (1 + \alpha_e (\frac{\overline{v}_a + \gamma_e v_a}{\theta_e \overline{C}_a})^{\beta_e}) \tag{13}$$

where $\gamma_m(\gamma_e)$ is a constant characterizing the impact of traffic flow of E-bikes (vehicles) on travel cost of vehicles (E-bikes) and $\theta_m(\theta_e)$ is a constant defining how the link capacity of vehicles (E-bikes) is influenced by the traffic flow of E-bikes (vehicles).

Despite no physical separation, vehicles and E-bikes are designed to run in separated lanes or spaces, and C_a and $\overline{C}_a$ represent the capacity of these designed lanes or spaces. However, due to no physical separation, one mode may occupy the designed lanes or spaces of other mode. Considering this phenomenon of occupation, parameters θ_m and θ_e are introduced to adjust the corresponding capacity, and γ_m and γ_e are considered to adjust the corresponding traffic flow. Since the volume of a vehicle is normally larger than that of a E-bike, γ_m is assumed to be bigger than γ_e. In fact, link time Functions (10) and (11) regarding cases of physical separation can be treated as special forms of link time Functions (12) and (13) for cases without physical separation, respectively. In this special form, $\gamma_m = \gamma_e = 0$ and $\theta_m = \theta_e = 1$.

4. Uniqueness of Equilibrium Solution

Note that link travel time Functions (10)–(13) are nonlinear and the proposed traffic assignment model is an NCP. According to the theory of VI/CP [40], since the feasible region of our problem is convex and route cost Function (9) is continuous, if the Jacobian matrix J of route cost Function (9) is definitely positive, the solution of the proposed NCP is unique.

The corresponding Jacobian matrix J is:

$$J = \begin{bmatrix} \frac{\partial C_i^w}{\partial f_i^w} & \frac{\partial C_i^w}{\partial \overline{f}_i^w} \\ \frac{\partial \overline{C}_i^w}{\partial f_i^w} & \frac{\partial \overline{C}_i^w}{\partial \overline{f}_i^w} \end{bmatrix} = \begin{bmatrix} (1+\lambda_m) \sum_a \delta_a^i \dot{T}_a & (1+\lambda_m) \sum_a \delta_a^i \ddot{T}_a \\ (1+\lambda_e) \sum_a \delta_a^i \dot{\overline{T}}_a & (1+\lambda_e) \sum_a \delta_a^i \ddot{\overline{T}}_a \end{bmatrix} \tag{14}$$

where $\dot{T}_a = \frac{\partial T_a}{\partial v_a}$, $\ddot{T}_a = \frac{\partial T_a}{\partial \overline{v}_a}$, $\dot{\overline{T}}_a = \frac{\partial \overline{T}_a}{\partial v_a}$, and $\ddot{\overline{T}}_a = \frac{\partial \overline{T}_a}{\partial \overline{v}_a}$.

Theorem 1. *According to Equation (10) and Equation (11), the solution to the proposed NCP is unique in cases of physical separation.*

Proof. For cases of physical separation between vehicle lanes and bicycle lanes, $\ddot{T}_a = \dot{\bar{T}}_a = 0$. Then, J becomes:

$$J = \begin{bmatrix} (1+\lambda_m)\sum_a \delta_a^i \dot{T}_a & 0 \\ 0 & (1+\lambda_e)\sum_a \delta_a^i \ddot{\bar{T}}_a \end{bmatrix} \quad (15)$$

which is a standard diagonal matrix with positive diagonal elements. Obviously, in this case J is definitely positive. The uniqueness of the solution to the NCP under cases of physical separation is therefore proven. □

Next, we discuss the case of no physical separation between vehicle lanes and bicycle lanes on links of the transportation network.

Theorem 2. *Given link time Functions (12) and (13), if $1 - \gamma_m \gamma_e > 0$, the solution to the proposed NCP is unique for cases without physical separation.*

Proof. For cases of no physical separation between vehicle lanes and bicycle lanes, according to Equation (14), the first-order leading principal minor of J is $(1+\lambda_m)\sum_a \delta_a^i \dot{T}_a$, which is positive. Then we discuss the second-order leading principal minor, i.e., $D\prime_2$:

$$D\prime_2 = \begin{vmatrix} (1+\lambda_m)\sum_a \delta_a^i \dot{T}_a & (1+\lambda_m)\sum_a \delta_a^i \ddot{T}_a \\ (1+\lambda_e)\sum_a \delta_a^i \dot{\bar{T}}_a & (1+\lambda_e)\sum_a \delta_a^i \ddot{\bar{T}}_a \end{vmatrix}$$

$$= (1+\lambda_m)(1+\lambda_e)(\sum_a \delta_a^i \dot{T}_a \sum_a \delta_a^i \ddot{\bar{T}}_a - \sum_a \delta_a^i \ddot{T}_a \sum_a \delta_a^i \dot{\bar{T}}_a)$$

Thus, $D\prime_2 > 0$ if, and only if,

$$\sum_a \delta_a^i \dot{T}_a \sum_a \delta_a^i \ddot{\bar{T}}_a - \sum_a \delta_a^i \ddot{T}_a \sum_a \delta_a^i \dot{\bar{T}}_a > 0 \quad (16)$$

In Equation (16), $\dot{T}_a = \frac{\alpha_m \beta_m T_a^0}{\theta_m C_a}\left(\frac{v_a + \gamma_m \bar{v}_a}{\theta_m C_a}\right)^{\beta_m - 1}$, $\dot{\bar{T}}_a = \frac{\alpha_e \beta_e \bar{T}_a^0}{\theta_e \bar{C}_a}\left(\frac{\bar{v}_a + \gamma_e v_a}{\theta_e \bar{C}_a}\right)^{\beta_e - 1}$, $\ddot{T}_a = \frac{\alpha_m \beta_m \gamma_m T_a^0}{\theta_m C_a}\left(\frac{v_a + \gamma_m \bar{v}_a}{\theta_m C_a}\right)^{\beta_m - 1}$,

and $\ddot{\bar{T}}_a = \frac{\alpha_e \beta_e \gamma_e \bar{T}_a^0}{\theta_e \bar{C}_a}\left(\frac{\bar{v}_a + \gamma_e v_a}{\theta_e \bar{C}_a}\right)^{\beta_e - 1}$. Denote $A^1 = \frac{\alpha_m \beta_m T_a^0}{\theta_m C_a}\left(\frac{v_a + \gamma_m \bar{v}_a}{\theta_m C_a}\right)^{\beta_m - 1}$ and $A^2 = \frac{\alpha_e \beta_e \bar{T}_a^0}{\theta_e \bar{C}_a}\left(\frac{\bar{v}_a + \gamma_e v_a}{\theta_e \bar{C}_a}\right)^{\beta_e - 1}$, then:

$$\sum_a \delta_a^i \dot{T}_a \sum_a \delta_a^i \ddot{\bar{T}}_a - \sum_a \delta_a^i \ddot{T}_a \sum_a \delta_a^i \dot{\bar{T}}_a = (1 - \gamma_m \gamma_e) A^1 A^2 \quad (17)$$

Thus, if $1 - \gamma_m \gamma_e > 0$, $D\prime_2 > 0$. □

In summary, if $1 - \gamma_m \gamma_e > 0$, all order leading principal minors of J are positive, then the solution to the proposed NCP is unique for cases of no physical separation.

Note that values of γ_m and γ_e can impact the corresponding traffic flows of each mode due to interactions between flows of vehicles and E-bikes. In the most extreme case, vehicle lanes are occupied by all vehicles and E-bikes, and bicycle lanes are also occupied by all vehicles and E-bikes. In this case, γ_m can be treated as the vehicle equivalent of an E-bike (denoted as VE) and γ_e can be treated as the E-bike equivalent of a vehicle (denoted as EE). According to the conversion relationship, VE × EE = 1. In reality, despite no physical separation between vehicle lanes and bicycle lanes, some vehicles and E-bikes still run in the corresponding designed lanes, with not all vehicles (E-bikes) occupying the bicycle (vehicle) lane. Thus, $\gamma_m <$ VE and $\gamma_e <$ EE. Therefore, $1 - \gamma_m \gamma_e > 1 -$ VE $*$ EE $= 0$, that is, the condition $1 - \gamma_m \gamma_e > 0$ in Theorem 2 is satisfied. In summary, the unique solution to the proposed NCP can be guaranteed in reality.

5. Solution Algorithm

Several algorithms were proposed in the literature to solve the traffic assignment problem formulated as an NCP. Among these algorithms, the nonsmooth and semismooth Newton methods were widely used, the basic idea being to convert the complementarity problem into an equal system of equations so as to solve them using the general Newton method.

First, we give the following definition.

Definition 1. *A function* $\phi : R^2 \to R$ *is called an NCP function if*

$$\phi(a,b) \Leftrightarrow ab = 0, a \geq 0, b \geq 0 \tag{18}$$

According to Definition 1, the NCP function related to NCP (5) can be defined as

$$\Phi(x) = \begin{pmatrix} \phi(x_1, F_1(x)) \\ \vdots \\ \phi(x_n, F_n(x)) \end{pmatrix} \tag{19}$$

Then, the solution to NCP (5) can be obtained by solving $\Phi(x) = 0$.

Note that the NCP function significantly impacts the effective solution algorithm. The following Fischer–Burmeister (FB) function [38] is frequently used as the NCP function.

$$\phi_{FB}(a,b) = a + b - \sqrt{a^2 + b^2} \tag{20}$$

The FB Function (20) has many interesting properties, however, it is too flat in the positive orthant (the main region of interest for a complementarity problem) when dealing with a monotone complementarity problem. Chen et al. [37] introduced another NCP function, i.e.,

$$\phi_\lambda(a,b) = \lambda \phi_{FB}(a,b) + (1-\lambda)a_+ b_+ \tag{21}$$

where $\lambda \in (0,1]$ is an arbitrary parameter and $a_+ b_+$ are penalties for violating the complementarity conditions, in which, for example, z_+ is a nonnegative operator $z_+ = max(0,z)$ for $\forall z \in R$.

Based on the NCP Function (21), the equal system of equation related to NCP Function (5) is defined as

$$\Phi_\lambda(x) = \begin{pmatrix} \phi_\lambda(x_1, F_1(x)) \\ \vdots \\ \phi_\lambda(x_n, F_n(x)) \end{pmatrix} \tag{22}$$

Further, we define

$$\varphi_\lambda(a,b) = \frac{1}{2}\phi_\lambda(a,b)^2 \tag{23}$$

Then, a natural merit function $\psi_\lambda(x)$ of $\Phi_\lambda(x)$ is given by

$$\psi_\lambda(x) = \frac{1}{2}\|\Phi_\lambda(x)\|^2 = \sum_{i=1}^{n} \varphi_\lambda(x_i, F_i(x)) \tag{24}$$

where $\|\cdot\|$ is the Euclidean norm.

The NCP Function (21) and the merit Function (24) were proven by Chen et al. [37] and Xu et al. [39] to possess all the positive features of the FB Function (20) and its corresponding merit function.

Thus, the Newton method introduced by Du Luca et al. [41] to solve the proposed NCP Function (5) with NCP Function (21) and merit Function (24) is given as follows.

Algorithm 1. Global algorithm.

Step 1.1. Initialize parameters $\mu \in (0,1)$, $\omega \in \left(0, \frac{1}{2}\right)$, $\rho > 0$, $p > 2$, tolerance error $\varepsilon > 0$ to check convergence, iteration counter $k = 0$.

Step 1.2. Initialize solution vector $x^0 = \begin{pmatrix} f^0 \\ \overline{f}^0 \\ \pi^0 \end{pmatrix}$.

Step 1.3. If $\|\nabla \psi_\lambda(x^k)\| \leq \varepsilon$, then terminate. Otherwise, go to the next step.

Step 1.4. Choose V_k from the C-subdifferential $\partial_C \Phi_\lambda(x^k)^T$ of $\Phi_\lambda(x^k)$ and let $d_k \in R^{2n_1+n_2}$ be a solution of the following linear system of equations:

$$V_k d = -\Phi_\lambda(x^k). \quad (25)$$

If solution d_k cannot be found or if the descent test

$$\nabla \psi_\lambda(x^k)^T d_k \leq -\rho \|d_k\|^p \quad (26)$$

does not satisfy, set $d_k = -\nabla \psi_\lambda(x^k)^T$.

Step 1.5. Linear search. Find the smallest nonnegative integer l^k such that

$$\psi_\lambda(x^k + \mu^{l^k}) \leq \psi_\lambda(x^k) + \omega \mu^{l^k} \nabla \psi_\lambda(x^k)^T d_k \quad (27)$$

Step 1.6. Set $x^{k+1} = x^k + \mu^{l^k} d_k$, $k = k+1$ and go to Step 1.3.

Step 1.2 is for the initialization of the solution vector x^0. Although we can set the arbitrary vector as the initial solution vector, to make the global algorithm more efficient in solving the proposed NCP Function (5), the following procedure (Algorithm 2) is used to initialize the solution vector.

Algorithm 2. Initialize the solution vector.

Step 2.1. Read in a predefined route set P^w. Choose any initial vehicle demand q_v^w and E-bike demand q_e^w, $q_v^w + q_e^w = q^w$.

Step 2.2. Load demand q_v^w to route set P^w using the all-or-nothing method to obtain an initial vehicle route flow vector f^0.

Step 2.3. Update the link time and route cost C_i^w according to Equations (9)–(13).

Step 2.4. Load demand q_e^w to route set P^w using the all-or-nothing method to obtain an initial E-bike route flow vector $\overline{f}^0$.

Step 2.5. Update the route cost $\overline{C}_i^w$.

Step 2.6. Select the initial min-route cost $\pi^{w,0} = min\{C_i^w, i \in \mathbf{R}^w\}$ and set $\pi^0 = [\ldots, \pi^{w,0}, \ldots]^T$.

Step 2.7. Set the initial solution vector $x^0 = \begin{pmatrix} f^0 \\ \overline{f}^0 \\ \pi^0 \end{pmatrix}$.

Further, in Step 1.4 of the global algorithm (Algorithm 1), we first need to choose V_k from the C-subdifferential $\partial_C \Phi_\lambda(x^k)^T$ (see [37,39] for definition). Similar to Chen et al. [37], we use the following Algorithm 3 to choose V_k.

Algorithm 3. Choose $V_k \in \partial_C \phi_\lambda(x^k)^T$

Step 3.1. Let $x \in R^{2n_1+n_2}$ be given and V_i denote the ith row of a matrix $V \in R^{(2n_1+n_2)\times(2n_1+n_2)}$.
Step 3.2. Set index set $S_1 = \{i | x_i = F_i(x) = 0\}$ and $S_2 = \{i | x_i > 0, F_i(x) > 0\}$.
Step 3.3. Set $z \in R^{2n_1+n_2}$ such that $z_i = 0$ for $i \notin S_1$ and $z_i = 1$ for $i \in S_1$.
Step 3.4. Set V_i as follows:
If $i \in S_1$, set

$$V_i = \lambda\left(1 - \frac{z_i}{\|(z_i, \nabla F_i(x)^T z)\|}\right)e_i^T + \lambda\left(1 - \frac{\nabla F_i(x)^T z}{\|(z_i, \nabla F_i(x)^T z)\|}\right)\nabla F_i(x)^T. \quad (28)$$

If $i \in S_2$, set

$$V_i = \left[\lambda\left(1 - \frac{x_i}{\|(x_i, F_i(x))\|}\right) + (1-\lambda)F_i(x)\right]e_i^T + \left[\lambda\left(1 - \frac{F_i(x)}{\|(x_i, F_i(x))\|}\right) + (1-\lambda)x_i\right]\nabla F_i(x)^T \quad (29)$$

If $i \notin S_1 \cup S_2$, set

$$V_i = \lambda\left(1 - \frac{x_i}{\|(x_i, F_i(x))\|}\right)e_i^T + \lambda\left(1 - \frac{F_i(x)}{\|(x_i, F_i(x))\|}\right)\nabla F_i(x)^T \quad (30)$$

6. Numerical Examples

In this section, we present numerical examples to verify the proposed model and analyze the users' mode (vehicle and E-bike) choice behavior.

6.1. A Simple Example

First, we apply the proposed NCP to a simple network as shown in Figure 1. The network has five nodes, five links, and two OD pairs (1-5 and 2-5). Link parameters are shown in Table 1. Demands of OD pairs 1-5 and 2-5 are set to be 300 and 200, respectively. Parameters in link time Functions (10)–(13) are set to be $\alpha_m = 0.15$, $\beta_m = 4$, $\alpha_e = 0.1$, $\beta_e = 2$, $\gamma_m = 0.3$, and $\gamma_e = 3$, for any link, and parameters in route cost Function (9) are set to be $\lambda_m = 0.1$, $\varphi_m = 0.2$, $\lambda_e = 0.2$, $\varphi_e = 0.4$, and $\theta_m = \theta_e = 1.1$ for any route.

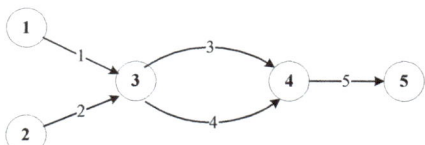

Figure 1. A simple network.

Table 1. Link parameters of network in Figure 1.

Link	1	2	3	4	5
T_a^0	10	10	20	15	10
$\overline{T}_a^0$	20	20	40	30	20
C_a	40	50	30	60	80
$\overline{C}_a$	60	80	50	100	120
LL_a	10	10	15	10	10

Table 2 shows the results of link flows for two cases. The first case demonstrates no physical separation between the vehicle lane and the bicycle lane for any link in the network. The second case regards all links in the network having physical separations between vehicle lanes and bicycle lanes. As can be seen from Table 2, the link flow patterns are quite different for the two cases, indicating that physical separation between the vehicle lane and the bicycle lane has dramatic effects on the equilibrium flow pattern. Table 3 shows the route flow and route cost of both vehicles and E-bikes, denoting that (a) the sum of route flows of vehicles and E-bikes for each OD pair is equal to the total demand of that OD pair, and (b) for any OD pair, the cost of each used route (including vehicles and E-bikes) is equal to its minimum travel cost (in bold) and the unused routes have higher costs than the minimum OD travel cost.

Table 2. Link flows of the nonlinear complementarity problem (NCP) for cases with and without physical separation.

Link	Mode	1	2	3	4	5
Without physical separation	v_a	43.69	109.46	81.006	72.156	153.15
	$\overline{v}_a$	256.31	90.54	0	346.85	346.85
With physical separation	v_a	90.18	88.55	55.36	123.37	178.73
	$\overline{v}_a$	209.82	111.45	71.03	250.24	321.27

Table 3. Route flows of the NCP for cases with and without physical separation.

Case	OD	Route	Route Flow of Vehicles	Route Flow of E-Bikes	Route Cost of Vehicles	Route Cost of E-Bikes
Without physical separation	1-5	1-3-5	12.70	0	**415.08**	429.25
		1-4-5	31.00	256.31	**415.08**	**415.08**
	2-5	2-3-5	68.30	0	**382.08**	396.24
		2-4-5	41.16	90.54	**382.08**	**382.08**
With physical separation	1-5	1-3-5	22.87	11.33	**184.61**	**184.61**
		1-4-5	67.31	198.48	**184.61**	**184.61**
	2-5	2-3-5	32.49	59.70	**155.81**	**155.81**
		2-4-5	56.05	51.76	**155.81**	**155.81**

Numbers in bold means the cost of each used route (including vehicles and E-bikes) is equal to its minimum travel cost.

Table 4 further compares some indicators of the flow patterns for cases with and without physical separation, including demand of vehicles, demand of E-bikes, and total travel time of the system. It can be seen from Table 4 that mode choice proportions are significantly influenced by physical separation between vehicle lanes and bicycle lanes. The total system travel time for cases with physical separation is much smaller than in cases without physical separation. This is because physical separation decreases the interference between vehicles and E-bikes, thereby reducing travel costs for both traffic modes.

Table 4. Indicators of the NCP for cases with and without physical separation.

Index	Demand of Vehicles ($\sum_w \sum_{i \in R^w} \sigma_i^w f_i^w$)	Demand of E-Bikes ($\sum_w \sum_{i \in R^w} \sigma_i^w \overline{f}_i^w$)	System Total Travel Time ($\sum_{a \in A}(v_a T_a + \overline{v}_a \overline{T}_a)$)
Without physical separation	153.15	346.85	148,760.5
With physical separation	178.73	321.27	63,544.0

6.2. Sensitivity Analysis

Figure 2 shows how mode choice proportions vary from the total demand. In this experiment, demands of OD pairs 1-5 and 2-5 are set to grow at the same rate. It can be seen from Figure 2 that proportion of vehicle demand decreases with increasing total demand, while the proportion of E-bike demand changes conversely. If the total demand is larger, the network tends to be more congested. As discussed before, E-bikes have higher flexibility than vehicles and can maintain higher speeds than vehicles in congested areas despite their lower maximum speeds. Hence, when the network is more congested, users of the network prefer to choose E-bikes rather than vehicles.

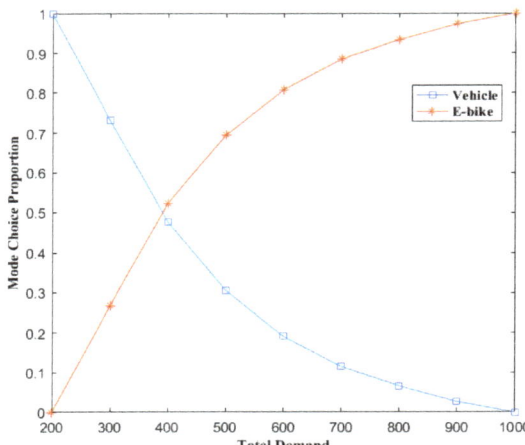

Figure 2. Mode choice proportions change with total demand for the example network.

Figure 3 shows how proportions of vehicle and E-bike demand vary by changes in values of out-of-pocket-related parameters φ_m, λ_m, φ_e, and λ_e. As shown in Equation (8), φ_m and φ_e denote the monetary cost per unit of distance traveled by vehicles and E-bikes, respectively, and λ_m and λ_e denote the monetary cost per unit of time for vehicles and E-bikes, respectively. Figure 3 shows that the proportion of vehicle (E-bikes) demand decreases with the growth of the corresponding parameters λ_m and φ_m (λ_e and φ_e). As mentioned before, out-of-pocket cost is impacted by fuel or electricity consumption, vehicle or E-bike depreciation, insurance, the environment, and so on. For example, when the price of fuel increases (values of φ_m and λ_m increase in this case), users tend to reduce vehicle use. Similarly, when the weather conditions are poor (such as raining) or the road safety conditions for nonmotor vehicles are low (values of φ_e and λ_e increase in these cases), out-of-pocket costs related to E-bikes increase, thus the choice proportion of E-bikes becomes smaller.

Table 5 shows the sensitivity analysis results of parameters related to interactions between vehicles and E-bikes (γ_m and γ_e in Equations (12) and (13)). In reality, the influence between flows of vehicles and E-bikes is mutual, that is, when the impact on vehicles from E-bikes becomes greater, the impact on E-bikes from vehicles also becomes greater simultaneously. Hence, in Table 5, the corresponding parameters γ_m and γ_e are shown to increase equidistantly. The results show that the total system total travel time increases with the degree of interaction between vehicles and E-bikes. The total travel time of each mode also tends to increase with the degree of interaction. Combined with results of Table 4, flow of vehicles and E-bikes should be physically separated as much as possible, and interference between vehicles and E-bikes should also be reduced as much as possible in links without physical separation between vehicle lanes and bicycle lanes, such as by regulating traffic.

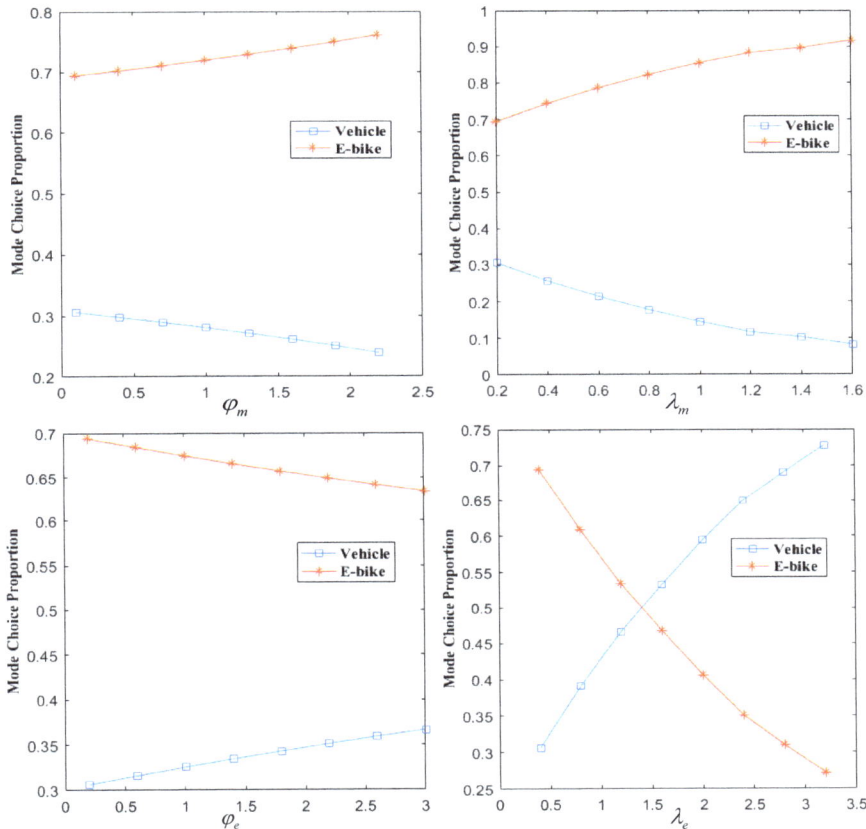

Figure 3. Sensitivity analysis regarding parameters related to out-of-pocket cost.

Table 5. Sensitivity analysis regarding parameters related to interactions between vehicles and E-bikes.

γ_m	γ_e	Total Travel Time of Vehicles ($\sum_{a \in A} v_a T_a$)	Total Travel Time of E-Bikes ($\sum_{a \in A} \overline{v}_a \overline{T}_a$)	System Total Travel Time ($\sum_{a \in A} (v_a T_a + \overline{v}_a \overline{T}_a)$)
0.05	0.5	28,934.3	41,812.6	70,746.9
0.1	1	34,368.3	51,494.2	85,862.6
0.15	1.5	40,223.1	62,836.3	103,059.4
0.2	2	45,795.2	75,477.3	121,272.5
0.25	2.5	49,974.9	88,623.3	138,598.3
0.3	3	49,546.9	99,213.6	148,760.5

6.3. A Larger Network

The proposed model is further tested using the well-known Nguyen–Dupuis network shown in Figure 4. It consists of 13 nodes, 38 bidirectional links, and 18 OD pairs (all possible combinations between the three left nodes {12, 1, 4} and the three right nodes {8, 2, 3}). Fifty routes considered by Zhu et al. [42] are used. The length of each link is set to be $LL_a = 10$, and other link characteristic parameters are shown in Table 6. Parameters in link time Functions (12) and (13) are set to be $\gamma_m = 0.2$ and $\gamma_e = 2$ for any link, and other parameters in link time Functions (10)–(13) and route cost Function (9) are set to be the same as those of the simple example. The travel demands of 18 OD pairs are shown in Table 7.

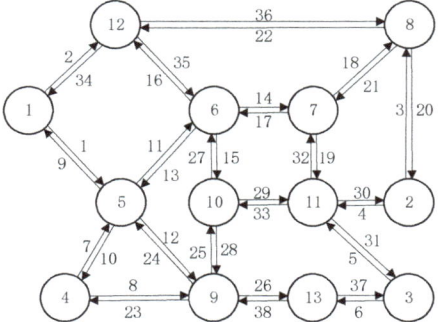

Figure 4. The Nguyen–Dupuis network.

Table 6. Link parameters of the Nguyen–Dupuis network.

Link	T_a^0	C_a	$\overline{T}_a^0$	$\overline{C}_a$	Link	T_a^0	C_a	$\overline{T}_a^0$	$\overline{C}_a$	Link	T_a^0	C_a	$\overline{T}_a^0$	$\overline{C}_a$
1	7	70	14	140	14	5	70	10	140	27	4	28	8	56
2	9	56	18	112	15	4	28	8	56	28	4	28	8	56
3	9	70	18	140	16	6	14	12	28	29	4	70	8	140
4	9	28	18	56	17	5	70	10	140	30	9	28	18	56
5	9	56	18	112	18	9	70	18	140	31	8	56	16	112
6	11	56	22	112	19	4	70	8	140	32	4	70	8	140
7	12	56	24	112	20	9	70	18	140	33	4	70	8	140
8	5	37	10	74	21	9	70	18	140	34	9	56	18	112
9	7	70	14	140	22	14	56	28	112	35	7	14	14	28
10	12	56	24	112	23	5	37	10	74	36	14	56	28	112
11	12	42	24	84	24	9	42	18	84	37	11	56	22	112
12	9	42	18	84	25	5	28	10	56	38	9	28	18	56
13	12	42	24	84	26	9	28	18	56					

Table 7. Origin–Destination (OD) pairs and the corresponding demand.

OD No.	O	D	Demand	OD No.	O	D	Demand
1	1	2	210.00	10	4	2	320.00
2	1	3	430.00	11	4	3	110.00
3	1	8	320.00	12	4	8	210.00
4	2	1	210.00	13	8	1	320.00
5	2	4	320.00	14	8	4	210.00
6	2	12	50.00	15	8	12	60.00
7	3	1	430.00	16	12	2	50.00
8	3	4	110.00	17	12	3	40.00
9	3	12	40.00	18	12	8	60.00

As discussed before, cases of physical separation are special cases of those without physical separation, with the proposed model only tested for cases of no physical separation between vehicle lanes and bicycle lanes for any link in the network. Table 8 shows the resulting link flow pattern, where, for any link, the link flow of the E-bike is larger than that of vehicle. Hence, given the OD demand shown in Table 7, the proportion of E-bike demand is larger than that of vehicle demand. The simple example proves that the proportion of vehicle demand decreases with increasing total demand, while the proportion of E-bike demand increases with the total demand. Similarly, when we reduce the total travel demand of the Nguyen–Dupuis network, vehicle choice proportion increases and E-bike choice proportion decreases.

Table 8. Link flows of the NCP for the Nguyen–Dupuis network.

Link	v_a	$\bar{v}_a$	Link	v_a	$\bar{v}_a$	Link	v_a	$\bar{v}_a$
1	83.84	335.47	14	75.87	332.90	27	26.34	60.69
2	66.79	473.90	15	24.98	74.76	28	34.38	390.82
3	109.29	175.43	16	25.79	112.23	29	61.04	434.67
4	15.97	279.31	17	77.65	332.82	30	16.56	277.95
5	51.53	249.78	18	74.01	239.21	31	46.34	250.42
6	47.25	231.44	19	3.22	226.62	32	8.14	210.53
7	56.63	115.54	20	111.05	174.44	33	60.72	451.50
8	17.06	450.78	21	70.88	255.23	34	67.33	469.30
9	86.63	336.73	22	70.93	477.68	35	26.24	102.18
10	56.37	107.38	23	16.83	459.42	36	68.68	493.60
11	74.61	305.48	24	64.80	162.84	37	46.86	236.39
12	65.86	145.52	25	36.06	359.91	38	47.25	231.44
13	78.20	281.28	26	46.86	236.39			

To check the correctness of the solutions when applying the proposed NCP model to a larger network, Table 9 shows the resulting route flows and route costs. Without loss of generality, Table 9 only shows the results for OD pairs 1-3 and 4-2. First, the sum of route flows of vehicles and E-bikes for each OD pair should equal the total demand of that OD pair. In detail, for OD pair 1-3, the total vehicle route flow is 2.36 + 19.00 + 46.86 = 68.22 and the total E-bike route flow is 129.01 + 19.13 + 126.39 + 12.39 + 74.76 = 361.78. Hence, the total flow is 68.22 + 361.78 = 430, which equals the travel demand of OD pair 1-3. Thus, the sum of vehicle and E-bike route flows for each OD pair should equal to the total demand of the OD pair, which is satisfied for OD pair 1-3. Similarly, OD pair 4-2 is also verified. Second, for any OD pair, the cost of each used route (including vehicles and E-bikes) should equal its minimum travel cost, with the unused routes having higher costs than the minimum OD travel cost. Table 9 clearly shows that the resulting route flows and costs of vehicles and E-bikes satisfy the Wardrop UEprinciple.

Table 9. Route flows of the NCP for the Nguyen–Dupuis network.

OD	OD Demand	Route	Route Flow of Vehicles	Route Flow of E-Bikes	Route Cost of Vehicles	Route Cost of E-Bikes
1-3	430.00	1-11-14-19-31	2.36	129.10	246.89	246.89
		1-11-15-29-31	0	0	246.89	246.89
		1-12-25-29-31	19.00	19.13	246.89	246.89
		1-12-26-37	46.86	126.39	246.89	246.89
		2-35-14-19-31	0	12.39	246.89	246.89
		2-35-15-29-31	0	74.76	246.89	246.89
4-2	320	7-11-14-18-20	25.49	0	269.85	281.06
		8-25-29-30	16.56	277.95	269.85	269.85
		8-25-29-32-18-20	0	0	269.85	281.06

7. Conclusions

To consider the mode choice behavior between vehicles and E-bikes, this paper presented a multimode traffic assignment model formulated as a CP. In this model, the route cost was assumed to consist of route travel time and out-of-pocket cost. Then, the BPR link travel time function was extended for cases with and without physical separation between vehicle lanes and bicycle lanes, respectively. Given the modified link travel time functions, the proposed multimode traffic assignment model became an NCP. Further, the uniqueness of the equilibrium solution to the proposed NCP was proven and a solution algorithm based on the Newton method was developed.

Numerical examples were conducted on two different size networks, with the results showing that the solution to the proposed NCP was correct, that is, the solution satisfied the Wardrop UE principle and flow conservation law. Sensitivity analysis showed that since E-bikes are more flexible than vehicles, especially in congested areas, E-bike choice proportion increased with total travel demand and vehicle choice proportion decreased accordingly. Increased in out-of-pocket costs led to a reduction of the corresponding mode choice.

Through the comparison of cases with and without physical separations, it was found that reducing the inference between vehicles and E-bikes could significantly reduce total system travel time, indicating that traffic engineers and planners should try to physically separate the flow of vehicles and E-bikes as much as possible.

In reality, due to factors such as resource constraints, it is impossible for all links to be physically separated between vehicle lanes and bicycle lanes. Hence, in future research, it would be worthwhile to optimize which links should set up physical separations and extend the proposed CP model to the network design problem. Meanwhile, the application of the proposed model should be tested on real networks, and the modified link travel time function should be verified and calibrated by real link travel data. In addition, some travelers are accustomed to certain traffic modes and do not consider other modes in reality, and some travelers may have more alternatives besides vehicles and E-bikes, such as public transportation. Hence, extending the proposed CP model to consider more types of travelers in the future would be worthwhile.

Author Contributions: Conceptualization, S.Z. and J.M.; methodology, S.Z. and J.M.; validation, S.Z. and T.T.; formal analysis, Q.S.; investigation, T.T.; resources, Q.S.; writing—original draft preparation, S.Z. and J.M.; writing—review and editing, T.T., Q.S.; supervision, Q.S.; funding acquisition, S.Z. and Q.S. All authors have read and agreed to the published version of the manuscript.

Funding: This research was funded by the Humanities and Social Science Foundation of the Ministry of Education in China, grant numbers 18YJCZH274, the Science and Technology Project of Jiangsu Province, China, grant numbers BK20190926, the National Natural Science Foundation of China, grant numbers 61771265, the Natural Science Foundation of the Jiangsu Higher Education Institutions of China, grant numbers 19KJB580003, and the Science and Technology Project of Nantong City, grant numbers JC2019062.

Acknowledgments: The authors are grateful for comments made by anonymous referees.

Conflicts of Interest: The authors declare no conflict of interest.

Appendix A Proof of the Equivalent Equations (3) and (4)

Proof. Equations (3) and (4) are equivalent if π^w has a strictly positive value. If π^w is positive, the equality $\sum_{i \in P^w} \left(f_i^w + \overline{f}_i^w \right) = q^w$ in Equation (3) must be satisfied. Therefore, to show the equivalence, it is sufficient to show that π^w cannot equal 0.

Assume π^w equals 0. Since π^w represents the minimum travel cost of OD pair w, $\pi^w = 0$ means the route flow of any route between OD pair w for both vehicles and E-bikes is 0. Thus, the demand q^w of OD pair w is zero. Note $q^w > 0$. Therefore π^w cannot be 0, thereby proving that Equations (3) and (4) are equivalent. □

References

1. Rose, G. Electric bicycles and urban transportation: Emerging issues and unresolved questions. *Transportation* **2012**, *39*, 81–96. [CrossRef]
2. Weinert, J.X.; Burke, A.F.; Wei, X. Lead-acid and lithium-ion batteries for the Chinese electric bike market and implications on future technology advancement. *J. Power Sources* **2007**, *172*, 938–945. [CrossRef]

3. Weinert, J.X.; Ma, C.; Yang, X.; Cherry, C.R. Electric two-wheelers in China: Effect on travel behavior, mode shift, and user safety perceptions in a medium-sized city. *Transp. Res. Rec. J. Transp. Res. Board* **2007**, *2038*, 62–68. [CrossRef]
4. Lin, X.; Wells, P.; Sovacool, B.K. Benign mobility? Electric bicycles, sustainable transport consumption behaviour and socio-technical transitions in Nanjing, China. *Transp. Res. Part A Policy Pract.* **2017**, *103*, 223–234. [CrossRef]
5. Jin, S.; Qu, X.; Zhou, D.; Xu, C.; Ma, D.; Wang, D. Estimating cycleway capacity and bicycle equivalent unit for electric bicycles. *Transp. Res. Part A Policy Pract.* **2015**, *77*, 225–248. [CrossRef]
6. Petzoldt, T.; Schleinitz, K.; Heilmann, S.; Gehlert, T. Traffic conflicts and their contextual factors when riding conventional vs. electric bicycles. *Transp. Res. Part F Traffic Psychol. Behav.* **2017**, *46*, 477–490. [CrossRef]
7. Wells, P.; Lin, X. Spontaneous emergence versus technology management in sustainable mobility transitions: Electric bicycles in China. *Transp. Res. Part A Policy Pract.* **2015**, *78*, 371–383. [CrossRef]
8. Di, X.; He, X.; Guo, X.; Liu, H.X. Braess paradox under the boundedly rational user equilibria. *Transp. Res. Part B Methodol.* **2014**, *67*, 86–108. [CrossRef]
9. National Research Council. *Highway Capacity Manual*; TRB, National Research Council: Washington, DC, USA, 2010.
10. Di, Z.; Yang, L.; Jianguo, Q.; Gao, Z. Transportation network design for maximizing flow-based accessibility. *Transp. Res. Part B Methodol.* **2018**, *110*, 209–238. [CrossRef]
11. Yang, H.; Bell, M.G.H. Transport bilevel programming problems: Recent methodological advances. *Transp. Res. Part B Methodol.* **2001**, *35*, 1–4. [CrossRef]
12. Cao, Z.; Ceder, A. Autonomous Shuttle Bus Service Timetabling and Vehicle Scheduling Using Skip-Stop Tactic. *Transp. Res. Part C Emerg. Technol.* **2019**, *109*, 60–78. [CrossRef]
13. Cao, Z.; Ceder, A.; Zhang, S. Real-Time Schedule Adjustments for Autonomous Public Transport Vehicles. *Transp. Res. Part C Emerg. Technol.* **2019**, *102*, 370–395. [CrossRef]
14. Chiou, S.W. An efficient algorithm for computing traffic equilibria using TRANSYT model. *Appl. Math. Model.* **2010**, *34*, 3390–3399. [CrossRef]
15. Clegg, J.; Smith, M.; Xiang, Y.; Yarrow, R. Bilevel programming applied to optimizing urban transport. *Transp. Res. Part B Methodol.* **2001**, *35*, 41–70. [CrossRef]
16. Bar-Gera, H. Origin-based algorithm for the traffic assignment problem. *Transp. Sci.* **2002**, *36*, 398–417. [CrossRef]
17. Daganzo, C.; Sheffi, Y. On stochastic models of traffic assignment. *Transp. Sci.* **1977**, *11*, 253–274. [CrossRef]
18. Bouscasse, H.; Joly, I.; Peyhardi, J. A new family of qualitative choice models: An application of reference models to travel mode choice. *Transp. Res. Part B Methodol.* **2019**, *121*, 74–91. [CrossRef]
19. Liu, Y.; Cirillo, C. A generalized dynamic discrete choice model for green vehicle adoption. *Transp. Res. Part A Policy Pract.* **2018**, *114*, 288–302. [CrossRef]
20. Bagloee, S.A.; Sarvi, M.; Wallace, M. Bicycle lane priority: Promoting bicycle as a green mode even in congested urban area. *Transp. Res. Part A Policy Pract.* **2016**, *87*, 102–121. [CrossRef]
21. Wu, J.; Florian, M.; He, S. An algorithm for multiclass network equilibrium problem in PCE of trucks: Application to the SCAG travel demand model. *Transportmetrica* **2006**, *2*, 1–9. [CrossRef]
22. García, R.; Marín, A. Network equilibrium with combined modes: Models and solution algorithms. *Transp. Res. Part B Methodol.* **2005**, *39*, 223–254. [CrossRef]
23. Kitthamkesorn, S.; Chen, A. Alternate weibit-based model for assessing green transport systems with combined mode and route travel choices. *Transp. Res. Part B Methodol.* **2018**, *103*, 291–310. [CrossRef]
24. Jie, M.; Min, X.; Qiang, M.; Lin, C. Ridesharing user equilibrium problem under OD-based surge pricing strategy. *Transp. Res. Part B Methodol.* **2020**, *134*, 1–24.
25. Bar-Gera, H.; Boyce, D.; Nie, Y. User-equilibrium route flows and the condition of proportionality. *Transp. Res. Part B Methodol.* **2012**, *46*, 440–462. [CrossRef]
26. Chen, B.Y.; Lam, W.H.K.; Sumalee, A.; Shao, H. An efficient solution algorithm for solving multiclass reliability-based traffic assignment problem. *Math. Comput. Model.* **2011**, *54*, 1428–1439. [CrossRef]
27. Dafermos, S.C. The traffic assignment problem for multiclass-user transportation networks. *Transp. Sci.* **1972**, *6*, 73–87. [CrossRef]

28. Florian, M.; Morosan, C.D. On uniqueness and proportionality in multiclass equilibrium assignment. *Transp. Res. Part B Methodol.* **2014**, *70*, 173–185. [CrossRef]
29. Nagurney, A. A multiclass, multicriteria traffic network equilibrium model. *Math. Comput. Model.* **2000**, *32*, 393–411. [CrossRef]
30. Nagurney, A.; Dong, J. A multiclass, multicriteria traffic network equilibrium model with elastic demand. *Transp. Res. Part B Methodol.* **2002**, *36*, 445–469. [CrossRef]
31. Liu, Y.; Li, Y. Pricing scheme design of ridesharing program in morning commute problem. *Transp. Res. Part C Emerg. Technol.* **2017**, *79*, 156–177. [CrossRef]
32. Cottle, R.; Pang, J.-S.; Stone, R. *The Linear Complementarity Problem*; Academic Press: San Diego, CA, USA, 1992.
33. Dong, J.-L.; Jiang, M.-Q. A modified modulus method for symmetric positive-definite linear complementarity problems. *Numer. Linear Algebra Appl.* **2009**, *16*, 129–143. [CrossRef]
34. Lemke, C.E. Bimatrix equilibrium points and mathematical programming. *Manag. Sci.* **1965**, *11*, 681–689. [CrossRef]
35. Schäfer, U. A linear complementarity problem with a P-matrix. *SIAM Rev.* **2004**, *46*, 189–201. [CrossRef]
36. Schäfer, U. On the modulus algorithm for the linear complementarity problem. *Oper. Res. Lett.* **2004**, *32*, 350–354. [CrossRef]
37. Chen, B.; Chen, X.; Kanzow, C. A penalized Fischer–Burmeister NCP-function. *Math. Program.* **2000**, *88*, 211–216. [CrossRef]
38. Fischer, A. A special Newton-type optimization method. *Optimization* **1992**, *24*, 269–284. [CrossRef]
39. Xu, M.; Chen, A.; Qu, Y.; Gao, Z. A semismooth Newton method for traffic equilibrium problem with a general nonadditive route cost. *Appl. Math. Model.* **2011**, *35*, 3048–3062. [CrossRef]
40. Nagurney, A. *Network Economics: A Variational Inequality Approach*; Springer Science & Business Media: Berlin, Germany, 2013.
41. Du Luca, T.; Facchinei, F.; Kanzou, C. A semismooth equation approach to the solution of nonlinear complementarity problems. *Math. Program.* **1996**, *75*, 407–439. [CrossRef]
42. Zhu, S.; Cheng, L.; Chu, Z.; Chen, A.; Chen, J. Identification of Network Sensor Locations for Estimation of Traffic Flow. *Transp. Res. Rec. J. Transp. Res. Board* **2014**, *2443*, 32–39. [CrossRef]

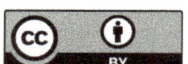

© 2020 by the authors. Licensee MDPI, Basel, Switzerland. This article is an open access article distributed under the terms and conditions of the Creative Commons Attribution (CC BY) license (http://creativecommons.org/licenses/by/4.0/).

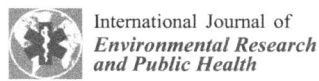

Article

Active School Transport among Children from Canada, Colombia, Finland, South Africa, and the United States: A Tale of Two Journeys

Silvia A. González [1,2,3,*], Olga L. Sarmiento [1], Pablo D. Lemoine [4], Richard Larouche [2,5], Jose D. Meisel [6], Mark S. Tremblay [2,3], Melisa Naranjo [1], Stephanie T. Broyles [7], Mikael Fogelholm [8], Gustavo A. Holguin [1], Estelle V. Lambert [9] and Peter T. Katzmarzyk [7]

[1] School of Medicine, Universidad de los Andes, Bogota 111711, Colombia; osarmien@uniandes.edu.co (O.L.S.); ms.naranjo10@uniandes.edu.co (M.N.); ga.holguin@uniandes.edu.co (G.A.H.)
[2] Healthy Active Living and Obesity Research Group, Children's Hospital of Eastern Ontario Research Institute, Ottawa, ON K1H 8L1, Canada; richard.larouche@uleth.ca (R.L.); mtremblay@cheo.on.ca (M.S.T.)
[3] School of Epidemiology and Public Health, Faculty of Medicine, University of Ottawa, Ottawa, ON, K1G 5Z3, Canada
[4] Centro Nacional de Consultoría, Bogota 110221, Colombia; plemoine@cnccol.com
[5] Faculty of Health Sciences, University of Lethbridge, 4401 University Drive, Lethbridge, AB, T1K 3M4, Canada
[6] Facultad de Ingeniería, Universidad de Ibagué, Ibagué 730001, Colombia; jd.meisel28@uniandes.edu.co
[7] Pennington Biomedical Research Center, Baton Rouge, LA 70808, USA; stephanie.broyles@pbrc.edu (S.T.B.); peter.katzmarzyk@pbrc.edu (P.T.K.)
[8] Department of Food and Nutrition, University of Helsinki, 00100 Helsinki, Finland; mikael.fogelholm@helsinki.fi
[9] Research Centre for Health through Physical Activity, Lifestyle and Sport, Division of Exercise Science and Sports Medicine, Faculty of Health Sciences, University of Cape Town, Rondebosch, Cape Town 7700, South Africa; vicki.lambert@uct.ac.za
* Correspondence: sa.gonzalez68@uniandes.edu.co; Tel.: +1-613-981-8332

Received: 6 May 2020; Accepted: 25 May 2020; Published: 28 May 2020

Abstract: Walking and biking to school represent a source of regular daily physical activity (PA). The objectives of this paper are to determine the associations of distance to school, crime safety, and socioeconomic variables with active school transport (AST) among children from five culturally and socioeconomically different country sites and to describe the main policies related to AST in those country sites. The analytical sample included 2845 children aged 9–11 years from the International Study of Childhood Obesity, Lifestyle and the Environment. Multilevel generalized linear mixed models were used to estimate the associations between distance, safety and socioeconomic variables, and the odds of engaging in AST. Greater distance to school and vehicle ownership were associated with a lower likelihood of engaging in AST in sites in upper-middle- and high-income countries. Crime perception was negatively associated to AST only in sites in high-income countries. Our results suggest that distance to school is a consistent correlate of AST in different contexts. Our findings regarding crime perception support a need vs. choice framework, indicating that AST may be the only commuting choice for many children from the study sites in upper-middle-income countries, despite the high perception of crime.

Keywords: active school transport; distance; safety; Canada; Colombia; Finland; South Africa; United States

1. Introduction

In the context of a global crisis of physical inactivity, walking and biking to and from school represent an opportunity for children to engage in regular physical activity (PA) on a daily basis [1]. Children who walk or bike to school have higher levels of PA [2] and lower measures of adiposity [3,4]. Moreover, cycling to/from school is associated with higher cardiorespiratory fitness [3] and lower cardiovascular disease risk factors [5]. In addition to the health benefits, active school transport (AST) contributes to the development of children's independent mobility [6], provides opportunities for children to interact with their local environments [7], and has the potential to mitigate the adverse environmental effects of the use of motorized vehicles around schools by reducing emissions of greenhouse gases and other pollutants [8,9]. Despite these benefits, time trends show that the prevalence of AST in low, middle- [10–13], and high-income countries (HIC) [14–22] is declining.

A multicountry study indicated that more than 50% of children reported AST in cities from upper-middle-income countries (UMIC) like Bogota in Colombia and Cape Town in South Africa and in cities from HIC like Helsinki in Finland and Bath in the UK [2]. These findings can be understood, in part, within a "need vs. choice" framework, where the drivers to engage in AST differ according to the context [23]. This framework proposes that for low and middle-income countries (LMIC), the involvement in AST may be a result of a need given the limited car availability [4,23]. In contrast, for HIC, AST could be a choice driven by the availability of policies and infrastructure that support AST [4,24]. This framework suggests that the drivers for AST may differ according to the context and taking those differences into account is essential for policymaking processes.

Although previous studies have shown associations between AST and several correlates, including distance, motor vehicle ownership, perceived safety, land use mix, walking and cycling infrastructure, walkability, urban form, and social interactions [25–29], there is evidence that shows that associations and the direction of association may differ across countries [25]. Furthermore, distance between home and school has been described as the most consistent correlate of AST [26,27,30], and together with safety perceptions and resources availability, such as car ownership, are among the main factors that influence AST and can guide public policy design [31]. However, the studies that have objectively measured the distance to school have been conducted only in HIC [30]. Therefore, the generalizability of these results to UMIC and the relevance of these factors in the design of AST policies is unclear.

In this context, international studies using comparable methods and including sites that differ on sociodemographic characteristics can help to elucidate the association between AST with potential correlates such as distance and crime safety. Furthermore, a review of the policy environment in these contexts is crucial to determine the relevance of environmental variables like distance and safety in the practice to promote AST. Therefore, the objectives of this study are twofold: (1) to determine the associations between AST and measures of distance between home and school and crime safety among children from study sites located in five culturally and socioeconomic different countries and (2) to describe the main policies related to AST in the research sites included in this study.

2. Materials and Methods

The International Study of Childhood Obesity, Lifestyle and the Environment (ISCOLE) is a multinational, cross-sectional study conducted among 9–11-year-old children from study sites in 12 countries. More details on the study design and methods can be found elsewhere [32]. Analyses reported in the present study include data from five ISCOLE sites: Ottawa (Canada), Bogota (Colombia), Helsinki, Espoo, and Vantaa; onwards, we will use Helsinki as a collective term for the three cities (Finland), Cape Town (South Africa), and Baton Rouge (United States). Data were collected in 111 schools (Ottawa = 26, Bogota = 20, Helsinki = 25, Cape Town = 19 and Baton Rouge = 21). These sites were included in the present analyses because they provided objective data on distance between home and school measured using geographic information systems (GIS).

The institutional review board at the Pennington Biomedical Research Center (coordinating center) approved the overarching protocol, and the institutional/ethical review boards at each participating institution approved local protocols. Written informed consent was obtained from parents or legal guardians, and child assent was obtained for all participants. The data were collected from September 2011 through December 2013.

2.1. Study Setting

Our study included sites in the countries with the most unequal (South Africa) and the least unequal (Finland) distribution of income in ISCOLE, according to the Gini index [33]. The population at the city levels varied from 812,129 inhabitants in Ottawa to 7,674,366 inhabitants in Bogota [34]. Some variability was also observed in contextual variables at the national level that may be relevant to engagement in AST. The number of motor vehicles per capita ranged from 89 per 1000 inhabitants in Colombia, to 809 per 1000 inhabitants in the United States [35]. The road traffic death rate ranged from 5.1 to 31.9 deaths per 100,000 inhabitants, in Finland and South Africa, respectively [36], and robbery rate varied from 30.8 to 197.5 per 100,000 inhabitants, in Finland and Colombia, respectively [37] (Table 1).

Table 1. Sociodemographic characteristics of five country sites in the International Study of Childhood Obesity, Lifestyle and the Environment (ISCOLE).

Socio-Demographic Characteristics	Ottawa (Canada)	Bogota (Colombia)	Helsinki, Espoo & Vantaa (Finland)	Cape Town (South Africa)	Baton Rouge (US)
World bank classification [a]	High income	Upper-middle income	High income	Upper-middle income	High income
Gini index (year) [a]	34.0 (2013)	50.8 (2016)	27.1 (2017)	63.0 (2014)	41.5 (2016)
Total population at the city level	812,129	7,674,366	1,005,275	3,433,441	228,590
Population density (inhabitants per km^2)	317	4310	2739	1530	2960
Motor vehicles per 1000 inhabitants [b]	605	58	534	159	809
Estimated road traffic death rate per 100,000 population [c]	6.8	15.6	5.1	31.9	11.4
Crime rate Robbery rate per 100,000 population [d]	58.8	197.5	30.8	101.4	102

[a] World Bank Data at country level [33]; [b] World Bank Data at country level: Motor vehicles (per 1000 people) include cars, buses, and freight vehicles but not two-wheelers [35]; [c] World Health Organization data at country level: Global status report on road safety 2013 [36]; [d] Robbery at the national level, number of police-recorded offences. Definitions: "Robbery" means the theft of property from a person, overcoming resistance by force or threat of force. Where possible, the category "Robbery" should include muggings (bag-snatching) and theft with violence but should exclude pick pocketing and extortion [37].

2.2. Participants

The overall response rate for ISCOLE study was 60% [38]. The present analysis included 2960 children from the selected study sites, and 2845 remained in the analytical data set after excluding participants for whom data on AST (n = 22), parental education (n = 17), motor-vehicle availability (n = 9), and parental crime perception (n = 67) were not available. The inclusion rate per study site was 95.4% for Ottawa, 99.2% for Bogota, 90.8% for Helsinki, 56.7% for Cape Town, and 91% for Baton Rouge. The participants who were excluded from the present analysis were more likely to be overweight or obese ($p < 0.001$) and were less likely to report meeting PA guidelines (p = 0.001), compared with the included sample. In addition, their parents were more likely to report that they did not complete high school ($p < 0.001$). The five study sites were specifically selected from the 12 country sites for the ISCOLE study on the basis of the availability of geo-coded data.

2.3. Measurements

2.3.1. Active School Transport

AST was self-reported by participants, who responded to a diet and lifestyle questionnaire [32]. The questions used to assess AST were adapted for each country from the Canadian component of the 2009–2010 Health Behavior in School-aged Children Study [39]. Travel mode was assessed with the question "In the last week you were in school, the main part of your journey to school was by". The response options included active modes such as walking, bicycle, roller blades, and scooter and motorized modes such as car, motorcycle, moped (motor scooters), bus, train, tram, underground or boat, and others according to country-specific modes of transport. Other modes of transportation included active modes such as running and jogging; motorized modes such as the school van, bus feeder; and inactive nonmotorized modes such as pedicab (tricycle with a passenger compartment), and riding on the top tube of the bike's frame [4]. For this analysis, responses were collapsed into a binary variable indicating AST or nonactive travel.

2.3.2. Distance to School

Distance to school was estimated using ArcGIS 10.2 (ESRI Inc., Redlands, CA). Children's home address information was reported by the parents who responded to a demographic questionnaire. Home and school addresses were geo-coded using specific layers for each city. If parents did not provide a complete address, the closest street intersection was used. To estimate the distance between home and school, it was assumed that children took the shortest route via the street network. For the present analysis, distance was used both as a continuous and as a categorical variable using 4 levels: (1) <1000 m; (2) 1000 m–1499 m; (3) 1500 m–1999 m; and (4) ≥2000 m. The categories of distance to school were determined by previous studies and examining the continuous measurement of distance to school using smoothed locally estimated scatterplot smoothing (LOESS) curves [40].

2.3.3. Parental Perception of Crime

We included a crime perception scale adapted from the Neighborhood Environment Walkability Scale for Youth (NEWS-Y) [41], created based on five crime safety items and assessed on a 4-point Likert scale (from strongly disagree to strongly agree): "I am afraid of my child being taken or hurt by a stranger on local streets", "I am afraid of my child being taken or hurt by a stranger in my yard, driveway or common area", "I am afraid of my child being taken or hurt by a stranger in a local park", "I am afraid of my child being taken or hurt by a known 'bad' person (adult or child) in my neighborhood", and "there is a high crime rate". The crime perception variable was scored (score range 1–4) as the average of the five crime safety items (Cronbach $\alpha = 0.86$) [25], where high scores represent greater safety concerns.

2.3.4. Correlates

Sociodemographic variables were reported by the parents in response to the demographic and family health questionnaire from ISCOLE [32]. For this analysis we included age, gender, parental education, and vehicle ownership. The highest parental education variable was created based on the highest education level attained by the mother or the father (less than high school, complete high school or some college, and university degree or postgraduate degree). Vehicle ownership was reported as the number of motorized vehicles (cars, motorcycles, mopeds, and/or trucks) available for use in the household and was recoded as 0 vs.1 vs. ≥ 2 for the analyses.

2.4. Statistical Analysis

The descriptive characteristics included the means and standard deviations (SD) for continuous variables and the frequencies of categorical variables stratified by study site. Associations between distance to school and the likelihood of engaging in AST were estimated using generalized linear mixed models (SAS PROC GLIMMIX), stratifying by the World Bank country classification by income level of the countries where the study sites were located at, which grouped Bogota and Cape Town as belonging to UMIC and Ottawa, Helsinki, and Baton Rouge as belonging to HIC. The statistical models included age, gender, parental education, motorized vehicle ownership, and crime perception as potential correlates. To account for the clustering effects of schools and study sites, the multilevel models included three levels: the child, school, and study site. Study sites and schools nested within study sites were considered as having fixed effects. The denominator degrees of freedom for statistical tests pertaining to fixed effects were calculated using the Kenward and Roger approximation. These analyses were conducted using SAS version 9.3 (SAS Institute, Cary, NC, USA).

Curvilinear relationships of AST with distance to school and parent's perception of crime were estimated using smooth terms in generalized additive models (GAMs) (in GAMs the linear predictor is specified in terms of a sum of smooth functions of covariates) [42]. We employed a GAM function of mgcv package in R with binomial variance with logit link function and used thin-plate regression splines to estimate the smooth function of the covariates distance to school and parent's perception of crime. Separate GAMs were run to estimate the association of AST with distance to school and parent's perception of crime by income level of the country that the study site belonged to. We used GAM to study the association of AST with distance to school and parent's perception of crime because these models can estimate complex curvilinear relationships of unknown form among a dependent variable and smooth functions of a set of covariates and/or a set of covariates [42]. A detailed description of GAM is available elsewhere [42]. These analyses were conducted using R version 3.4.0 (The R Foundation for Statistical Computing, Vienna, Austria).

The generalized linear mixed models and the GAMS were also conducted excluding the active commuters living at 5km or more from school as sensitivity analyses.

A distance decay parameter was estimated to compare the distribution of walking distances among study sites. A specific distance decay function fitted to a real data set presents a precise description of the distribution of walking trips over distances [43]. The exponential function is used because the distances involved are relatively short [44–47]. The function used is:

$$P(d) = e^{-\beta d} \tag{1}$$

where $P(d)$ denotes the cumulative percentage of walking trips with distance equal or longer than d and β is the parameter estimated using empirical data. The parameter β was estimated by least-squares fit (FindFit in Mathematica 11.1). The resulting distance decay functions can be used to compare the distribution of walking distances among different groups [43].

2.5. AST Policies

To contextualize the policy environment of the study sites included in this analysis, we reviewed specific AST-policy documents at the city/state level. A policy search plan was developed to incorporate two different searching strategies: (1) academic databases and (2) customized Google search engines. The search strategy comprised four concepts: age group, active transport, interventions, and location of the interventions. These concepts were translated into keywords (adolescent, child, children, students, pupils, bicycling, transportation, walking, cyclists, cycling, bike, travel, intervention, implement, evaluate, change, pilot, project, environment, planning, impact, policy, project, politics, program, guidelines, methods, health impact assessment and planning techniques, Ottawa, Bogota, Helsinki, Cape Town, Baton Rouge, and Louisiana). For the customized Google search, we used the terms "Active school transportation policy + City/state" OR "City + school transport guide", OR "City + school transport guidelines"; for Bogota, the search also included the Spanish terms: *"Bogotá guías de transporte escolar"*. The eligibility criteria included: impact evaluation of programs, case studies, policy documents, official guidelines, nongovernmental information, and news. The documents selected were screened for information on regulation of AST in each city (Supplementary file 1). Finally, we extracted information from all of the documents regarding security, infrastructure, and the specific policy actions at each city. This information was complemented and validated by coauthors from each country site.

3. Results

A total sample of 2845 children from Ottawa (n = 541), Bogota (n = 912), Helsinki (n = 487), Cape Town (n = 312), and Baton Rouge (n = 593) was included in the present analysis (Table 2). The average age of participants was 10.3 ± 0.6 years, and 54% were girls. Parental education level differed between sites, reflecting the variability in socioeconomic status. Cape Town had the highest percentage of parents with less than high school as their highest education level (37.7%), while Ottawa had the lowest percentage in this category (2.0%). Overall, 67.6% of the households had access to at least one vehicle. Ottawa had the lowest percentage of households with no access to motor vehicles (3.8%), while Bogotá had the highest percentage in this category (75.8%). Finally, the average score for crime perception was 2.6 ± 1.0, ranging from 1.6 in Helsinki to 3.4 in Bogota (Table 2).

Table 2. Descriptive Characteristics of Participants Stratified by Study Site (n = 2845) in the International Study of Childhood Obesity, Lifestyle and the Environment (ISCOLE).

Socio-Demographic Variables of the Sample	Ottawa (Canada)	Bogota (Colombia)	Helsinki, Espoo & Vantaa (Finland)	Cape Town (South Africa)	Baton Rouge (US)	Total
	n = 541	n = 912	n = 487	n = 312	n = 593	n = 2845
Age [a]	10.5 (0.4)	10.5 (0.6)	10.5 (0.4)	10.2 (0.7)	10.0 (0.6)	10.3 (0.6)
Sex						
Male (%)	42.7	49.6	47.5	44.3	43.2	46.0
Female (%)	57.4	50.4	52.5	55.7	56.8	54.0
Highest parent education						
<High School (%)	2.0	31.8	2.9	37.7	8.6	17.0
Complete high-school or some college (%)	27.8	50.8	54.9	45.9	43.2	45.0
≥Bachelor degree (%)	70.2	17.4	42.2	16.4	48.2	38.0
Number of motorized vehicles in the household						
None (%)	3.8	75.8	9.4	37.5	8.3	32.5
One (%)	38.3	21.5	45.2	32.4	30.5	31.8
Two or more (%)	57.9	2.7	45.4	30.1	61.2	35.7
Crime perception score [a]	2.0 (0.7)	3.4 (0.7)	1.6 (0.6)	3.1 (0.8)	2.4 (0.8)	2.6 (1.0)
School transport characteristics						
Mode of transport to school						
Walking (%)	34.9	71.6	54.7	49.4	10.1	46.3
Bicycle, roller-blade, skateboard, scooter (%)	0.6	1.8	24.4	0.9	0.7	5.1
Bus, train, tram, underground, or boat (%)	38.1	18.7	13.3	5.4	34.5	23.3
Car, motorcycle, or moped (%)	26.5	7.3	7.6	44.3	54.3	25.0
Other [b] (%)	0.0	0.7	0.0	0.0	0.5	0.3
Distance-related variables						
Average distance to school (km) [a]	2.8 (4.2)	2.4 (3.7)	1.5 (1.7)	2.9 (3.9)	4.6 (5.1)	2.8 (4.0)

Table 2. Cont.

Socio-Demographic Variables of the Sample	Ottawa (Canada)	Bogota (Colombia)	Helsinki, Espoo & Vantaa (Finland)	Cape Town (South Africa)	Baton Rouge (US)	Total
Median of the distance to school (km)	1.5	0.8	1.0	1.5	3.3	1.3
Distance distribution among active and nonactive travelers						
<1 km (%)	36.8	56.6	50.0	38.1	19.1	41.7
1 km ≤ Distance < 1.5 Km (%)	13.2	10.6	20.9	12.0	11.6	13.2
1.5 Km ≤ Distance < 2 Km (%)	10.9	5.5	12.3	11.3	7.9	8.8
≥2 km (%)	39.2	27.4	16.8	38.7	61.4	36.2
Distance distribution among active travelers						
<1 km (%)	70.0	73.0	60.6	64.4	80.0	68.7
1 km ≤ Distance < 1.5 Km (%)	17.1	10.6	21.8	12.5	4.6	14.3
1.5 Km ≤ Distance < 2 Km (%)	4.2	4.9	12.2	11.3	3.1	7.3
≥2 km (%)	8.8	11.5	5.4	11.9	12.3	9.6
Average distance to school among active travelers (km) [a]	1.3 (2.9)	1.4 (2.7)	1.0 (0.8)	1.7 (3.2)	1.0 (1.6)	1.3 (2.4)
Active travel among children living at <1 km (%)	67.2	94.6	95.9	84.9	44.8	84.5

[a] Mean and Standard Deviation; [b] Other includes school van, bus feeder, riding on the top tube of the bike's frame, pedicab, and wheelchair.

3.1. School Transport

The overall prevalence of AST was 51.4%, ranging from 10.7% in Baton Rouge to 79.1% in Helsinki. Among all children, the average distance between home and school was 2.8 ± 4.0 km, ranging from 1.5 km in Helsinki to 4.6 km in Baton Rouge. Among children who engaged in AST, the average distance between home and school was 1.3 ± 2.4 km, ranging from 1.0 km in Helsinki and Baton Rouge, to 1.7 km in Cape Town. In the group of active travelers, 68.7% of the children lived within 1 km of the school, while 9.6% lived further than 2 km away (Table 2).

3.2. Factors Associated with AST by Income Level of the Country

Multivariable models stratified by income level of the country that the study sites belonged to showed common and differing factors associated to AST (Table 3). Number of vehicles and greater distance between home and school were negatively associated with AST in sites from both UMIC and HIC. In addition, children whose parents had a lower education level were more likely to engage in AST, only in sites from UMIC. Regarding crime perception, each unit increase in the crime perception scale was associated with 33% higher odds of AST among children from sites in UMIC (OR = 1.33 CI [1.06–1.66], $p = 0.014$), whereas an opposite association was observed among children from sites in HIC (OR= 0.37 CI [0.31–0.45], $p < 0.001$). Gender was not associated with AST and age was positively associated only among children from sites in HIC. The direction and significance of these associations remained in the sensitivity analysis excluding the children who lived at 5km or more and used AST (results not shown).

Table 3. Factors associated to active school transport in 2845 9–11-year-old children, by income level of the country.

Covariates	Sites in Upper-Middle-Income Countries [a]			Sites in High-Income Countries [b]		
	OR	95% CI	p-Value	OR	95% CI	p-Value
Highest parent education						
<High School	4.83	(2.84–8.21)	<0.001	0.89	(0.45–1.78)	0.741
Complete high-school or some college	4.21	(2.58–6.85)	<0.001	1.35	(1.01–1.81)	0.040
≥Bachelor degree	Ref.			Ref.		
Age	0.80	(0.61–1.06)	0.126	1.96	(1.49–2.58)	<0.001
Gender (ref. male)	1.27	(0.89–1.79)	0.176	0.97	(0.74–1.28)	0.838
Crime perception	1.33	(1.06–1.66)	0.014	0.37	(0.31–0.45)	<0.001
Number of motorized vehicles (ref. none)						
None	Ref.			Ref.		
One	0.24	(0.16–0.35)	<0.001	0.42	(0.24–0.72)	0.002
Two or more	0.14	(0.08–0.26)	<0.001	0.38	(0.22–0.65)	0.001
Distance to school						
<1 km	Ref.			Ref.		
1 km ≤ Distance < 1.5 Km (%)	0.12	(0.07–0.20)	<0.001	0.29	(0.21–0.42)	<0.001
1.5 Km ≤ Distance < 2 Km (%)	0.13	(0.07–0.23)	<0.001	0.15	(0.10–0.22)	<0.001
≥2 km	0.03	(0.02–0.05)	<0.001	0.02	(0.02–0.03)	<0.001

[a] Sites in upper-middle-income countries comprised Bogota and Cape Town according to the World Bank classification [35]; [b] Sites in high-income countries comprised Ottawa, Helsinki and Baton Rouge according to the World Bank classification [35].

Figure 1 shows the curvilinear relationship of AST with distance to school and parent's perception of crime by groups according to the income level of the countries. The negative association between distance and the probability of engaging in AST was stronger in sites in HIC (Chi.sq (6.7, 8.4) = 423.5, $p < 0.0001$) compared to the sites in UMIC (Chi.sq (13.1, 16.2) = 332.6, $p < 0.0001$). In HIC-sites, the results of the GAM show that the probability of engaging in AST decreased with an increase of the distance to school from 0 to 5 km. However, for UMIC-sites, the probability of engaging in AST decreased but not uniformly when the distance increased. The probability for sites in UMIC increased again when the distance took the values of 5, 12, and 15 km approximately. It is important to note that the latter estimates had a high level of uncertainty (imprecise confidence intervals) due to the small number of participants living more than 15 km away from school. However, the analysis excluding the AST users living at 5km or more, showed similar patterns (results not shown).

Moreover, for sites in HIC, the results of the GAM show that the probability of engaging in AST decreased with an increase in the parent's perception of crime from 1 to 3 (Chi.sq (3.9, 4.8) = 124.3, $p < 0.0001$). However, for sites in UMIC, the probability of AST increased with parent's perception of crime (Chi.sq (3.3, 4.1) = 99.6, $p < 0.0001$).

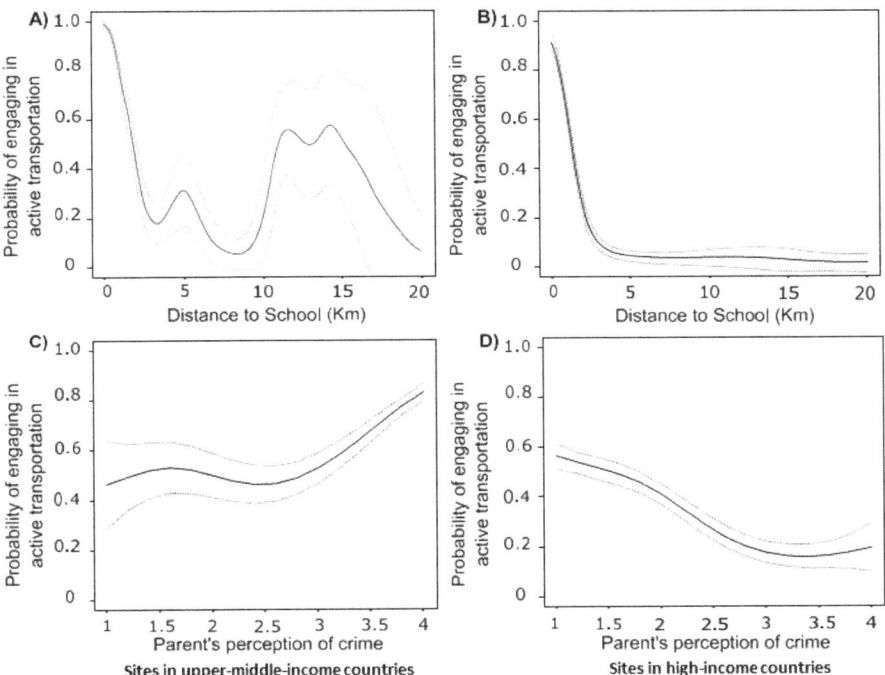

Figure 1. Associations of active transport to school with distance and crime perception by income level of the country. (**A**) Association of active transportation to school with distance between home and school among children from sites in upper middle-income countries. (**B**) Association of active transportation to school with distance between home and school among children from sites in high-income countries. (**C**) Association of active transportation to school with parental perception of crime in sites in upper middle-income countries. (**D**) Association of active transportation to school with parental perception of crime in sites in high-income countries.

Figure 2 shows the distance decay functions for each study site. This figure shows the lowest β-parameter for children from Cape Town (β = 0.87), followed by Ottawa (β = 1.05), Bogota (β = 1.15),

Finland (β = 1.16), and the highest in Baton Rouge (β = 1.54). A higher β means a steeper decline in the probability of walking as distance increases.

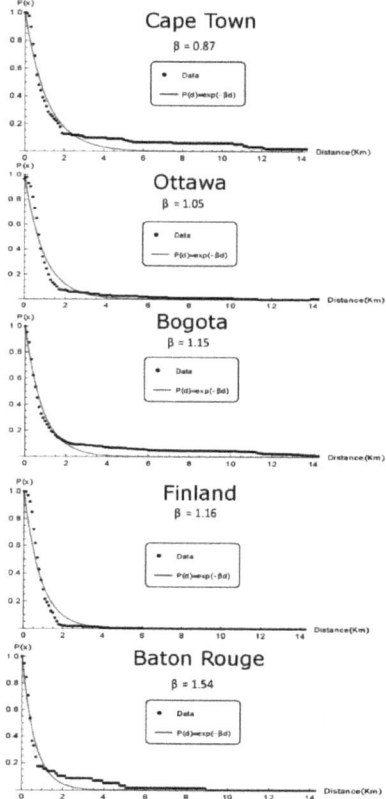

Figure 2. Distance decay curves by study site.

3.3. AST Policies

Table 4 describes AST policies in the five cities included in this analysis. All the cities had AST-related policies, and all of them proposed actions aiming to change travel behavior and to create AST supporting environments. Transport and education sectors were the main leaders and implementers of these policies, but most of them also engaged other sectors like public health, urban planning, and security. A common characteristic of the policies was the inclusion of school travel initiatives such as Safe Routes to School (Ottawa and Baton Rouge), Al colegio en bici (Bogota), and walking school buses and bicycle trains initiatives (Helsinki and Cape Town). Reflecting the importance of distance as a determinant in the mode of transport selection, all the cities had programs or initiatives that enhanced public transportation or school buses for children living at a certain distance from the school. However, the eligibility criteria to access these programs differed by city. The minimum distance between home and school to be eligible for transport support varied from 0.8 km for kindergarten children in Ottawa to 5 km for children in Cape Town.

Table 4. Description of policies that support active school transport in Ottawa, Bogota, Helsinki, Cape Town, and Baton Rouge.

Location	Description	Target	Sectors Involved	Impact Evaluation
Ottawa, Canada	The Ottawa Student Transportation Authority (OSTA) is responsible for all school transport initiatives and policies at the city. Regarding active school transportation (AST), OSTA provides services that support and promote the core principles of the School Active Transportation Charter. Specific actions include: (1) Assisting schools in providing safety conditions for students through management of vehicle, pedestrian, and bike traffic around schools. (2) Assessing potential hazards in all walk zones and assigning transportation services to those children who walk and face a very high risk to their safety. (3) Recommending the best routes for AST, through maps that identify unsafe intersections to avoid. (4) Submitting infrastructure improvement needs or service requirements to the appropriate departments at the city. (5) Coordinating School Travel Planning initiatives, like Active and Safe Routes to School program, that involve school communities engaged in the development of action plans for removing barriers to AST. (6) Coordinating Walking School Bus initiatives, in which children are encouraged to walk to school accompanied by a paid leader of the program. AST programs and policies are also supported by the Ottawa School Active Transportation Network, which involves OSTA, School Boards planning, Ottawa Police Services, City By-Law, Ottawa Public Health, Ottawa Public Works, Green Communities Canada, and Ottawa Safety Council [48]. School board policies determine the eligibility for bus services based on the distance between home and school as follows: kindergarten students located at ≥0.8 km, grades 1 to 8 located at ≥1.6 km, and grades 9 to 12 located at ≥3.2 km or more from their home school [48].	Parents or guardians, students, school communities	OSTA, School Boards planning, Ottawa Police Services, City By-Law, Ottawa Public Health, Ottawa Public Works, Green Communities Canada, and Ottawa Safety Council	School Travel Planning initiatives have been evaluated in Canada. Mammen et al. reported pooled data from several cities across Canada, but no specific data was provided for Ottawa. This evaluation found that after 1 year of implementation, there was no increase in AST. However, given the school-specific nature of the program, this approach may not be appropriate to evaluate its impact [49,50].

Table 4. Cont.

Location	Description	Target	Sectors Involved	Impact Evaluation
Bogotá, Colombia	The main AST policy in Bogotá is the School Mobility Plan, which was designed and enforced by the School Board and the District Department of Transport. This plan comprises guidelines for motorized and nonmotorized school transport. Each school must design its own Mobility Plan and propose strategies to promote active and sustainable mobility. The specific actions of this policy regarding AST include: (1) Assigning children to the closest schools to their homes, in order to promote active commuting. (2) Improving infrastructure prioritizing safety conditions for pedestrians and cyclists. (3) Implementing programs to promote safe walks to school among students living at 2 km or closer. (4) Implementing the program "Al Colegio en Bici", a comprehensive program to promote biking in public schools that includes a bicycle loan system, supervision, and education strategies. The education strategies comprise training in road safety, cycling skills, traffic rules, and a participatory design of safe routes [51]. Based on the distance between home and school, and considering vulnerability of children, bus services, or transport subsidies (money transfers or bus card) can be provided. Eligibility for motorized transportation benefits is defined as follows: ≥ 1 km for kindergarten children and ≥2 km for children from 1st to 11th grade.	Parents, community, students	Education, planning, mobility, sport and recreation, urban development, security road and maintenance and security department [51].	No impact evaluation

Table 4. *Cont.*

Location	Description	Target	Sectors Involved	Impact Evaluation
Helsinki, Finland	Helsinki Region Transportation (HRT) is the main authority in charge of the transport policy and mobility plans. The main policy document to guide specific actions to promote AST in Helsinki is the School Mobility Plan [52]. Each school is independent in the design and development of their mobility plan. However, the common purpose is to increase the use of walking, cycling, or public transport and make commitments in sustainable practices. Mobility plans also aim to increase the independent mobility among schoolchildren, as well as the safety in walking and cycling trails. Overall, the plan should include (1) identifying mobility problems or characteristics of the environment that make active commuting to the school difficult. (2) Assigning responsible persons for the implementation, including the school principal. (3) Formulating a mobility study at the school level. (4) Establishing objectives and achievable goals for the plan. And (5) Proposing an action plan, with specific initiatives like walking or cycling school buses, mobility lessons, or bicycle service days at school. Public transportation is encouraged through the entitlement of a Helsinki Region Transport travel card for children living at further distances based on the following criteria: children from 1st to 6th grades with journeys ≥2 km or adolescents from 7th to 9th grade with journeys ≥ 3km. For shorter distances, the use of the journey planner for cycling and walking is encouraged [52,53].	Parents or guardians, students, school communities	Transport and education	No impact evaluation

Table 4. *Cont.*

Location	Description	Target	Sectors Involved	Impact Evaluation
Cape Town, South Africa	Cape Town's Transport and Urban Development Authority (TDA) is responsible for the local transport policies. The main policy to promote AST in the city is the Non-Motorized Transport (NMT) Policy and Strategy. This document aims to create safe environments for pedestrian and cyclists in order to increase AST as a desirable and acceptable mode of transport. Specific actions related to schools and learners in this policy include: (1) promoting scholar patrols, (2) implementing bicycle/pedestrian paths and other NMT infrastructure in school priority zones, (3) introducing walking and cycling bus programs and (4) including learner safety programs as part of the school curriculum [54]. However, is important to highlight that the school transport policies are focused on the provision of motorized school transportation based on the extreme distances that most of the children walk to school and challenges that children face on their way to and from school [55,56]. Specific criteria for Western Cape province establishes that children who live at 5km or further from their school are eligible for school transport provision [55].	Community, Students	Transport, education, and urban development	No impact evaluation

Table 4. *Cont.*

Location	Description	Target	Sectors Involved	Impact Evaluation
Baton Rouge, U.S.A	The Louisiana Department of Education regulates the School Transportation for Louisiana. The main guidelines for school transportation are provided on the Louisiana School Transportation Specifications and Procedures Bulletin. However, this document is focused in motorized transportation to school and specifies that children whose home is located further than 1 mile from the school should be provided with free transportation, and children living within 1 mile can also be eligible for bus transportation in case of hazardous walking situations [57]. A more supportive policy for AST is the Complete Streets policy at the state level in Louisiana, led by the Louisiana Department of Transportation and Development (DOTD). This policy aims to create an integrated transportation network that provides access, mobility, and safety to the users of different transport modes, including active modes, in Louisiana [58]. One of the expected benefits of the implementation of this policy is increased road safety and active transportation among children. In partnership with the DOTD, school travel initiatives like Safe Routes to School (SRTS) are funded with the objective to improve the health of kids and the community by making walking and bicycling to school safer, easier, and more enjoyable. SRTS programs comprise five components: education, encouragement, enforcement, engineering and evaluation, and include specific actions, such as: (1) Teaching safety skills, (2) Creating awareness among students, pedestrians, and bicyclists, (3) Helping children to follow transit rules and (4) Improving driver behaviors [59].	Parents, Students, Schools	Transport, education, and planning	Safe Routes to School impact has been evaluated but not in Louisiana

4. Discussion

The results of this study show a tale of two journeys, one in cities from UMIC and a different one in cities from HIC. In the study sites in UMIC, higher scores on crime perception were associated with higher odds of AST and there was a curvilinear relationship between distance and the likelihood of AST. Conversely, in the study sites in HIC, children were less likely to engage in AST as distance and crime perception increased. The fact that children from sites in UMIC are engaging in AST even with high perceptions of vulnerability to crime supports the previously proposed need-based framework for physical activity. This framework suggests that for some populations AST may be the result of a need in absence of other options for transportation [4,23]. By contrast, in high-income settings AST may be a socially desirable activity [60] in a supportive context [24], which supports a choice-based framework [4,23]. These differences in AST patterns should be considered for evaluating existing policy approaches and to support the development of new policy, regulation, design, and program interventions for children.

Safety concerns are one of the main barriers to AST reported by parents [22,61,62]. Our results for the sites in HIC are consistent with previous and recent evidence [63,64]. However, our findings indicate a counter-intuitive association among children from sites in UMIC. These results indicate that for many children, safety concerns are not a barrier for AST and suggest that these children could be engaging in AST due to a necessity. Our results contribute to fill the gap identified by recent studies in LMIC that make a call for the collection and report on cross-country differences in the drivers of AST that can be related to socioeconomic status, such as distance, car ownership, and safety [65]. Despite the fact that supporting evidence from other UMIC is scarce, similar associations have been reported in disadvantaged populations from HIC as observed in children from urban-dwellings in Baltimore [66]. Similarly, a longitudinal study on younger children in Quebec, Canada reported that those living in poverty were more likely to engage in AST during the first school years, despite being exposed to unsafe environments, which has been defined by the authors as environmental injustice [18]. These results add to the concept that in low income communities AST is a need instead of a choice. In addition, previous research in low income groups of adults [67] and children [68,69] has yielded conflicting findings regarding the relationship between crime and different measures of AST and PA. Our policy review evidenced that safety is mentioned as a priority in the agenda of AST promotion in our study sites. Interventions like Safe Routes to School, the Walking School Bus, or Al colegio en bici could serve as examples from cities in HIC and UMIC to improve safety and reinforce AST where it is already prevalent. These strategies highlight the importance of parents, school, and community involvement, as well as interaction between these groups. However, more evidence and impact evaluation of the different outcomes of these strategies are needed. Recent systematic reviews have reported the effectiveness of Safe Routes to School and Walking School Bus initiatives in other HIC contexts, but few interventions have been implemented in UMIC [50,70]. Future studies comparing multiple programs of UMIC and HIC settings should also be conducted.

The negative association with access to motorized vehicles observed in this study is consistent with previous literature showing that children from households with at least one motorized vehicle available for use are less likely to engage in AST [25,71,72]. However, when examining ISCOLE country sites individually, this relationship was not significant in many country sites [25]. Presumably, vehicle ownership may favor motorized travel to a greater extent when parents perceive that it is more convenient to drive their children to school [73,74]. In North America, AST has declined considerably over the last 50 years [17,21,22]. For example, in the United States, 49% of children 5–14 years engaged in AST in 1969, but only 13% engaged in AST in 2009 [22]. These trends and our findings suggest that in HIC settings, interventions should focus on children from households that own a car and live at a walkable distance from school, which could potentially shift from motorized to active modes of transport. Our study shows that 73.3% of children in Bogota, 79.1% in Helsinki, and 50.3% in Cape Town engage in AST, which reflect even higher AST patterns than those observed in the 1960s in the United States. Future studies should assess the factors associated with AST in a HIC setting like

Finland and in UMIC like Colombia and South Africa. To our knowledge, no previous study in LMICs examined perceived convenience of driving among parents or to what extent the (re)development of built environments designed to prioritize cars could or has affected AST, as it has been observed in HIC [61]. Such research may be particularly important in the context of the PA transition [75], which is characterized among other things by a shift from active to motorized transportation.

The negative association observed between distance to school and AST in HIC and in UMIC is consistent with previous studies that have reported that distance is one of the main correlates of AST [26,27,30,64,71,76,77]. However, our results show different parameters and inflection points by study site and by income level of the country, respectively. Specifically, the distance decay parameters indicate that children from Cape Town and Ottawa are willing to actively travel for longer distances. Nonetheless it is in Cape Town and Bogota where the percentage of children have the highest likelihood of walking more than 5 km. These results align with the proposed need vs. choice framework [4,23]. Similarly, the curvilinear relationship between AST and distance observed for sites in UMIC suggests an increased probability of engaging in AST among children living 5 km or further from the school. Considering that previous studies in HIC have proposed distances between 1.4 and 1.6 km as thresholds for socially normative walking distances for children [78], we hypothesize that our results for sites in UMIC could be related to poverty conditions. Children who are walking those extreme distances because they have no other choice, usually face risks and challenges that eventually would lead them to give up active commuting [60]. For this reason, these groups should be the target for cycling or multimodal transportation initiatives that improve their quality of life while at the same time allowing them to maintain active behaviors for an acceptable part of their journey. Initiatives that provide the bicycles to children through a loan system, like Al colegio en bici in Bogota and Qubeka in Cape Town could be scalable to cities in LMIC to provide access to the required equipment for cycling to school. The policy review indicated that all the study sites are committed to provide school bus services or subsidies for children living at certain distances from school; however, our results could suggest a limited implementation of these initiatives in the sites in UMIC. The findings from this study could contribute to understand the role of urban planning and safety promotion at the local level in the engagement on AST. These associations are relevant for the promotion of health in urban contexts, and increasingly car-dependent societies, taking into account the multiple health and environmental benefits of active transportation [79].

Strengths of the present study include the implementation of a standardized protocol across countries which facilitated comparisons, the objective measurement of distance between households and schools and the use of a crime subscale with a satisfactory internal consistency, and the systematic search of local policies. However, our findings should be interpreted cautiously considering the following limitations. First, the cross-sectional design of the study does not allow the inference of causality. For instance, we cannot rule out the possibility that the observed relationship between perceived crime and AST might be attributable to reverse causality (i.e., parents may be more concerned about crime because their child engages in AST). Second, AST was assessed only for the journey "to school", which may be a potential source of bias, considering that some children may engage in AST only on the journey "to home". Third, the distance estimations assumed that children took the shortest route via the street network to go to school, which may not represent the actual route travelled [26,80]. However, a previous study that compared routes measured by global positioning systems and estimated by GIS found similar travel distances, despite the route discordance [81]. Fourth, correlates of walking and cycling may differ but the low prevalence of cycling in all the countries, except for Finland, did not allow for the assessment of these relationships separately. Fifth, there could be a risk of recall bias and social desirability bias in the AST and parental perception of crime variables, due to the self-reported nature of these variables. Finally, sixth, regarding the results for UMIC, it is important to note the lower inclusion rate of participants from Cape Town, which led to having an overrepresentation of children from Bogotá in the UMIC subsample.

Policy Implications

Our results can be of interest for policy-makers from multiple sectors in high-income countries and UMIC. Ideally, these findings should be taken into account in conjunction, as evidence suggests that the most promising policies are those that address distance concerns and safety perceptions improvements [82]. The following points summarize the relevance of our findings for policy-design in different contexts:

- Distance: Distance is a key determinant for school-siting policies that aim to create dense school networks and encourage active transportation by the location of schools at reasonable distances from residential neighborhoods. Through the design of school-siting and land use policies, policy-makers can manage the strong influence that distance can have on the engagement in AST. This could be a relevant strategy for settings that are experiencing urbanization and growing processes. Extreme distances can be addressed by multimodal transportation strategies that combine motorized travel and AST, such as bike-friendly features in public transportation infrastructure or safe routes for walking from bus stops to schools.
- Safety: policy-makers can contribute to address the parents' concerns about crime perceptions through the identification of potential risks and the design of safe routes for children living at walkable distances from the schools. Strategies that involve adult accompaniment along the trip to school can encourage the involvement in AST. These strategies are pertinent for HIC settings where safety is inversely related to AST and for UMIC settings where an inverse association was not observed, but safety improvement can contribute to making AST a sustainable behavior.
- Car-ownership: policy-makers cannot restrict car-ownership, however, motorized transportation can be made less convenient for short trips through policy. Initiatives such as parking restrictions around schools and traffic management strategies can discourage the use of motorized modes and replace those trips with active options.

5. Conclusions

Distance to school is a consistent correlate of AST in differing contexts. Our findings regarding crime perception support the need vs. choice framework, indicating that AST may be the only travel mode available for many children from UMIC settings, despite the high perception of crime. These findings could contribute to the design of policies and programs intended to promote active commuting among children. The observed differences in the correlates of AST by country-income level further substantiate our previous recommendation for context-specific evidence to guide local interventions [25]. Future studies to address models of transportation to school behaviors should be conducted taking into account the local context of the studied area and the potential differences within and between regions. Policies and programs should be implemented to promote AST and ensure that safe routes are available with the goal of reversing the declining trend of AST in HIC and to maintain and increase prevalence of AST in UMIC settings, before unintended consequences of development change these patterns.

Supplementary Materials: The following are available online at http://www.mdpi.com/1660-4601/17/11/3847/s1, Figure S1 Policy search flow chart.

Author Contributions: Conceptualization, S.A.G., O.L.S., S.T.B., and P.T.K.; Data curation, S.A.G. and P.D.L.; Formal analysis, S.A.G., O.L.S., P.D.L., J.D.M. and S.T.B. Funding acquisition, O.L.S., and P.T.K.; Investigation, S.A.G., O.L.S., M.S.T., M.N., S.T.B., M.F., G.A.H., E.V.L., and P.T.K.; Methodology, S.A.G., O.L.S., P.D.L., J.D.M., S.T.B. and P.T.K.; Supervision, O.L.S.; Visualization, P.D.L., and J.D.M.; Writing—original draft, S.A.G.; Writing—review and editing, O.L.S., P.D.L., R.L., J.D.M., M.S.T., M.N., S.T.B., M.F., G.A.H., E.V.L., and P.T.K. All authors have read and agreed to the published version of the manuscript.

Funding: ISCOLE was funded by The Coca-Cola Company. With the exception of requiring that the study be global in nature, the study sponsor had no role in study design, data collection and analysis, decision to publish, or preparation of manuscripts. GH was funded by Colciencias (Grant number FP44842-080). SG and OS were funded by the Research Office at the Universidad de los Andes.

Acknowledgments: We thank the ISCOLE External Advisory Board, the ISCOLE participants, and their families who made this study possible.

Conflicts of Interest: The authors declare no conflicts of interest. ISCOLE was funded by The Coca-Cola Company. With the exception of requiring that the study be global in nature, the study sponsor had no role in study design, data collection and analysis, decision to publish, or preparation of manuscripts.

References

1. Stanley, R.M.; Maher, C.; Dollman, J. Modelling the contribution of walking between home and school to daily physical activity in primary age children. *BMC Public Health* **2015**, *15*, 445. [CrossRef] [PubMed]
2. Denstel, K.D.; Broyles, S.T.; Larouche, R.; Sarmiento, O.L.; Barreira, T.V.; Chaput, J.-P.; Church, T.S.; Fogelholm, M.; Hu, G.; Kuriyan, R.; et al. Active school transport and weekday physical activity in 9–11-year-old children from 12 countries. *Int. J. Obes. Suppl.* **2015**, *5*, S100–S106. [CrossRef] [PubMed]
3. Larouche, R.; Saunders, T.J.; Faulkner, G.E.J.; Colley, R.; Tremblay, M. Associations between active school transport and physical activity, body composition, and cardiovascular fitness: A systematic review of 68 studies. *J. Phys. Act. Health* **2014**, *11*, 206–227. [CrossRef] [PubMed]
4. Sarmiento, O.; Lemoine, P.; Gonzalez, S.; Broyles, S.; Denstel, K.; Larouche, R.; Onywera, V.; Barreira, T.; Chaput, J.-P.; Fogelholm, M.; et al. Relationships between active school transport and adiposity indicators in school-age children from low-, middle- and high-income countries. *Int. J. Obes. Suppl.* **2015**, *5*, 107–114. [CrossRef]
5. Andersen, L.B.; Wedderkopp, N.; Kristensen, P.; Moller, N.C.; Froberg, K.; Cooper, A.R. Cycling to school and cardiovascular risk factors: A longitudinal study. *J. Phys. Act. Health* **2011**, *8*, 1025–1033. [CrossRef]
6. Tranter, P.; Pawson, E. Children's Access to Local Environments: A case-study of Christchurch, New Zealand. *Local Environ.* **2001**, *6*, 27–48. [CrossRef]
7. Fusco, C.; Moola, F.; Richichi, V. Toward an understanding of children's perceptions of their transport geographies: (Non)active school travel and visual representations of the built environment. *J. Transp. Geogr.* **2012**, *20*, 62–70. [CrossRef]
8. Marshall, J.D.; Wilson, R.D.; Meyer, K.L.; Rajangam, S.K.; McDonald, N.C.; Wilson, E.J. Vehicle Emissions during Children's School Commuting: Impacts of Education Policy. *Environ. Sci. Technol.* **2010**, *44*, 1537–1543. [CrossRef]
9. Maibach, E.; Steg, L.; Anable, J. Promoting physical activity and reducing climate change: Opportunities to replace short car trips with active transportation. *Prev. Med.* **2009**, *49*, 326–327. [CrossRef]
10. Costa, F.F.; Silva, K.S.; Schmoelz, C.P.; Campos, V.C.; de Assis, M.A.A. Longitudinal and cross-sectional changes in active commuting to school among Brazilian schoolchildren. *Prev. Med.* **2012**, *55*, 212–214. [CrossRef]
11. Yang, Y.; Hong, X.; Gurney, J.G.; Wang, Y. Active Travel to and from School Among School Age Children During 1997–2011 and Associated Factors in China. *J. Phys. Act. Health* **2017**, *14*, 1–25. [CrossRef]
12. Onywera, V.O.; Adamo, K.B.; Sheel, A.W.; Waudo, J.N.; Boit, M.K.; Tremblay, M. Emerging evidence of the physical activity transition in Kenya. *J. Phys. Act. Health* **2012**, *9*, 554–562. [CrossRef] [PubMed]
13. Trang, N.H.H.D.; Hong, T.K.; Dibley, M.J. Active commuting to school among adolescents in Ho Chi Minh City, Vietnam: Change and predictors in a longitudinal study, 2004 to 2009. *Am. J. Prev. Med.* **2012**, *42*, 120–128. [CrossRef] [PubMed]
14. Meron, D.; Rissel, C.; Reinten-Reynolds, T.; Hardy, L.L. Changes in active travel of school children from 2004 to 2010 in New South Wales, Australia. *Prev. Med.* **2011**, *53*, 408–410. [CrossRef]
15. van der Ploeg, H.P.; Merom, D.; Corpuz, G.; Bauman, A.E. Trends in Australian children traveling to school 1971–2003: Burning petrol or carbohydrates? *Prev. Med.* **2008**, *46*, 60–62. [CrossRef]
16. Lewis, N.; Dollman, J.; Dale, M. Trends in physical activity behaviours and attitudes among South Australian youth between 1985 and 2004. *J. Sci. Med. Sport* **2007**, *10*, 418–427. [CrossRef]
17. Gray, C.E.; Larouche, R.; Barnes, J.D.; Colley, R.C.; Bonne, J.C.; Arthur, M.; Cameron, C.; Chaput, J.-P.; Faulkner, G.; Janssen, I.; et al. Are we driving our kids to unhealthy habits? Results of the active healthy kids Canada 2013 report card on physical activity for children and youth. *Int. J. Environ. Res. Public Health* **2014**, *11*, 6009–6020. [CrossRef]

18. Pabayo, R.; Gauvin, L.; Barnett, T.A. Longitudinal Changes in Active Transportation to School in Canadian Youth Aged 6 Through 16 Years. *Pediatrics* **2011**, *128*, e404–e413. [CrossRef]
19. Pavelka, J.; Sigmundová, D.; Hamřík, Z.; Kalman, M.; Sigmund, E.; Mathisen, F. Trends in Active Commuting to School among Czech Schoolchildren from 2006 to 2014. *Cent. Eur. J. Public Health* **2017**, *25* (Suppl. 1), S21–S25. [CrossRef]
20. Grize, L.; Bringolf-Isler, B.; Martin, E.; Braun-Fahrländer, C. Trend in active transportation to school among Swiss school children and its associated factors: Three cross-sectional surveys 1994, 2000 and 2005. *Int. J. Behav. Nutr. Phys. Act.* **2010**, *7*, 28. [CrossRef]
21. McDonald, N.C. Active transportation to school: trends among U.S. schoolchildren, 1969–2001. *Am. J. Prev. Med.* **2007**, *32*, 509–516. [PubMed]
22. McDonald, N.C.; Brown, A.L.; Marchetti, L.M.; Pedroso, M.S. U.S. School Travel, 2009 an assessment of trends. *Am. J. Prev. Med.* **2011**, *41*, 146–151. [CrossRef] [PubMed]
23. Salvo, D.; Reis, R.S.; Sarmiento, O.L.; Pratt, M. Overcoming the challenges of conducting physical activity and built environment research in Latin America: IPEN Latin America. *Prev. Med.* **2014**, *69*, S86–S92. [CrossRef] [PubMed]
24. Tremblay, M.S.; Barnes, J.D.; González, S.A.; Katzmarzyk, P.T.; Onywera, V.O.; Reilly, J.J.; Tomkinson, G.R. Global Matrix 2.0 Research Team Global Matrix 2.0: Report Card Grades on the Physical Activity of Children and Youth Comparing 38 Countries. *J. Phys. Act. Health* **2016**, *13*, S343–S366. [CrossRef]
25. Larouche, R.; Sarmiento, O.L.; Broyles, S.T.; Denstel, K.D.; Church, T.S.; Barreira, T.V.; Chaput, J.-P.; Fogelholm, M.; Hu, G.; Kuriyan, R.; et al. Are the correlates of active school transport context-specific? *Int. J. Obes. Suppl.* **2015**, *5*, S89–S99. [CrossRef]
26. Panter, J.R.; Jones, A.P.; van Sluijs, E.M. Environmental determinants of active travel in youth: A review and framework for future research. *Int. J. Behav. Nutr. Phys. Act.* **2008**, *5*, 34. [CrossRef]
27. Pont, K.; Ziviani, J.; Wadley, D.; Bennett, S.; Abbott, R. Environmental correlates of children's active transportation: A systematic literature review. *Health Place* **2009**, *15*, 849–862. [CrossRef]
28. Kerr, J.; Rosenberg, D.; Sallis, J.F.; Saelens, B.E.; Frank, L.D.; Conway, T.L. Active commuting to school: Associations with environment and parental concerns. *Med. Sci. Sports Exerc.* **2006**, *38*, 787–794. [CrossRef]
29. Molina-García, J.; Queralt, A. Neighborhood Built Environment and Socioeconomic Status in Relation to Active Commuting to School in Children. *J. Phys. Act. Health* **2017**, *14*, 761–765. [CrossRef]
30. Wong, B.Y.-M.; Faulkner, G.; Buliung, R. GIS measured environmental correlates of active school transport: A systematic review of 14 studies. *Int. J. Behav. Nutr. Phys. Act.* **2011**, *8*, 39. [CrossRef]
31. Stewarta, O.; Moudon, A.V.; Claybrooke, C. Common ground: Eight factors that influence walking and biking to school. *Transp. Policy* **2012**, *24*, 240–248. [CrossRef]
32. Katzmarzyk, P.T.; Barreira, T.V.; Broyles, S.T.; Champagne, C.M.; Chaput, J.-P.; Fogelholm, M.; Hu, G.; Johnson, W.D.; Kuriyan, R.; Kurpad, A.; et al. The International Study of Childhood Obesity, Lifestyle and the Environment (ISCOLE): Design and methods. *BMC Public Health* **2013**, *13*, 900. [CrossRef] [PubMed]
33. World Bank Gini Index (World Bank Estimates). Available online: https://data.worldbank.org/indicator/SI.POV.GINI?locations=ZA (accessed on 31 October 2017).
34. World Population Review World Population. Available online: https://worldpopulationreview.com/world-cities/ (accessed on 1 January 2018).
35. The World Bank. *World Development Indicators*; The World Bank: Washington, DC, USA, 2011. Available online: http://documents.worldbank.org/curated/en/245401468331253857/World-development-indicators-2011 (accessed on 31 October 2017).
36. World Health Organization. In *Global Status Report on Road Safety*; World Health Organization: Luxembourg, 2013. Available online: https://www.who.int/violence_injury_prevention/road_safety_status/2013/en/ (accessed on 31 October 2017).
37. United Nations Office on Drugs and Crime Robbery Statistics. Available online: https://data.unodc.org/#state:0 (accessed on 15 July 2018).
38. Katzmarzyk, P.T.; Barreira, T.V.; Broyles, S.T.; Champagne, C.M.; Chaput, J.-P.; Fogelholm, M.; Hu, G.; Johnson, W.D.; Kuriyan, R.; Kurpad, A.; et al. Relationship between lifestyle behaviors and obesity in children ages 9-11: Results from a 12-country study. *Obesity* **2015**, *23*, 1696–1702. [CrossRef] [PubMed]
39. Gropp, K.; Janssen, I.; Pickett, W. Active transportation to school in Canadian youth: should injury be a concern? *Inj. Prev.* **2013**, *19*, 64–67. [CrossRef]

40. Cleveland, W.S.; Devlin, S.J.; Grosse, E. Regression by local fitting: Methods, properties, and computational algorithms. *J. Econom.* **1988**, *37*, 87–114. [CrossRef]
41. Rosenberg, D.; Ding, D.; Sallis, J.F.; Kerr, J.; Norman, G.J.; Durant, N.; Harris, S.K.; Saelens, B.E. Neighborhood Environment Walkability Scale for Youth (NEWS-Y): Reliability and relationship with physical activity. *Prev. Med.* **2009**, *49*, 213–218. [CrossRef]
42. Wood, S. *Generalized Additive Models: An Introduction with R*, 2nd ed.; Taylor & Francis Group: Boca Raton, FL, USA, 2017.
43. Yang, Y.; Diez-Roux, A.V. Walking Distance by Trip Purpose and Population Subgroups. *Am. J. Prev. Med.* **2012**, *43*, 11–19. [CrossRef]
44. Iacono, M.; Krizek, K.J.; El-Geneidy, A. Measuring non-motorized accessibility: Issues, alternatives, and execution. *J. Transp. Geogr.* **2010**, *18*, 133–140. [CrossRef]
45. Fotheringham, A.S.; O'Kelly, M.E. *Spatial Interaction Models: Formulations and Applications*; Kluwer Academic Publishers: Dordrecht, The Netherlands, 1989.
46. de Vries, J.J.; Nijkamp, P.; Rietveld, P. Exponential or Power Distance-Decay for Commuting? An Alternative Specification. *Environ. Plan. A* **2009**, *41*, 461–480. [CrossRef]
47. Signorino, G.; Pasetto, R.; Gatto, E.; Mucciardi, M.; La Rocca, M.; Mudu, P. Gravity models to classify commuting vs. resident workers. An application to the analysis of residential risk in a contaminated area. *Int. J. Health Geogr.* **2011**, *10*, 11. [CrossRef]
48. Ottawa Student Transportation Authority School Active Transportation Policy. 2016. Available online: http://www.ottawaschoolbus.ca/wp-content/uploads/2016/06/T23_-_V1_Student_Active_Transportation.pdf (accessed on 17 July 2018).
49. Mammen, G.; Stone, M.R.; Faulkner, G.; Ramanathan, S.; Buliung, R.; O'Brien, C.; Kennedy, J. Active school travel: An evaluation of the Canadian school travel planning intervention. *Prev. Med.* **2014**, *60*, 55–59. [CrossRef] [PubMed]
50. Larouche, R.; Mammen, G.; Rowe, D.A.; Faulkner, G. Effectiveness of active school transport interventions: a systematic review and update. *BMC Public Health* **2018**, *18*, 206. [CrossRef] [PubMed]
51. Secretaria de Educación del Distrito Movilidad Escolar. Available online: http://www.educacionbogota.edu.co/es/temas-estrategicos/movilidad-escolar (accessed on 15 March 2018).
52. City of Helsinki School Transport. Available online: https://www.hel.fi/helsinki/en/childhood-and-education/comprehensive/student-assistance/school-transport/ (accessed on 18 March 2018).
53. Toiskallio, K.; Wood, M. Mobility Management Guidance for Primary Schools in the Helsinki Metropolitan area. Available online: https://julkaisut.valtioneuvosto.fi/handle/10024/78070 (accessed on 4 May 2018).
54. City of Cape Town's Transport and Urban Development Authority NMT Policy And Strategy Volume 2: Policy Framework. 2015. Available online: https://tdacontenthubstore.blob.core.windows.net/resources/b4bb0a1e-e7f0-42ce-9071-bca907515f7e.pdf (accessed on 10 May 2018).
55. Western Cape Government Western Cape Education Department Policy on Learner Transport Schemes. 2013. Available online: https://wcedonline.westerncape.gov.za/circulars/circulars13/e25_13_A.pdf (accessed on 10 May 2018).
56. Department of Transport National Learner Transport Policy. 2015. Available online: https://www.gov.za/sites/www.gov.za/files/39314_gon997.pdf (accessed on 10 May 2018).
57. Division of Administration State of Louisiana Part CXIII. Bulletin 119—Louisiana School Transportation Specifications and Procedures. In *Louisiana Administrative Code*; Division of Administration State of Louisiana Part CXIII: Baton Rouge, LA, USA, 2016; p. 26. Available online: http://www.doa.la.gov/Pages/osr/lac/LAC-28.aspx (accessed on 10 May 2018).
58. The Louisiana Department of Transportation and Development Complete Streets Policy. 2010. Available online: http://wwwsp.dotd.la.gov/Inside_LaDOTD/Divisions/Multimodal/Highway_Safety/Complete_Streets/Complete%20Streets%20Legislative%20Reports/Complete%20Streets%20Legislative%20Update%20Final.pdf (accessed on 10 May 2018).
59. Safe Routes to School. Louisiana Safe Routes to School. Available online: https://www.ltrc.lsu.edu/ltc_11/pdf/LouisianaSafeRoutestoSchool.pdf (accessed on 10 May 2018).
60. Goenka, S.; Andersen, L.B. Urban design and transport to promote healthy lives. *Lancet* **2016**, *388*, 2851–2853. [CrossRef]

61. Mitra, R. Independent Mobility and Mode Choice for School Transportation: A Review and Framework for Future Research Independent Mobility and Mode Choice for School Transportation: A Review and Framework for. *Transp. Rev.* **2013**, *33*, 21–43. [CrossRef]
62. Zhu, X.; Lee, C. Correlates of Walking to School and Implications for Public Policies: Survey Results from Parents of Elementary School Children in Austin, Texas. *J. Public Health Policy* **2009**, *30*, S177–S202. [CrossRef]
63. Aranda-Balboa, M.J.; Huertas-Delgado, F.J.; Herrador-Colmenero, M.; Cardon, G.; Chillón, P. Parental barriers to active transport to school: A systematic review. *Int. J. Public Health* **2020**, *65*, 87–98. [CrossRef]
64. Rothman, L.; Macpherson, A.K.; Ross, T.; Buliung, R.N. The decline in active school transportation (AST): A systematic review of the factors related to AST and changes in school transport over time in North America. *Prev. Med.* **2018**, *111*, 314–322. [CrossRef]
65. Uddin, R.; Mandic, S.; Khan, A. Active commuting to and from school among 106,605 adolescents in 27 Asia-Pacific countries. *J. Transp. Heal* **2019**, *15*, 100637. [CrossRef]
66. Rossen, L.M.; Pollack, K.M.; Curriero, F.C.; Shields, T.M.; Smart, M.J.; Furr-Holden C, D.M.; Cooley-Strickland, M. Neighborhood incivilities, perceived neighborhood safety, and walking to school among urban-dwelling children. *J. Phys. Act. Health* **2011**, *8*, 262–271.
67. Foster, S.; Giles-Corti, B. The built environment, neighborhood crime and constrained physical activity: An exploration of inconsistent findings. *Prev. Med.* **2008**, *47*, 241–251. [CrossRef]
68. Durand, C.P.; Dunton, G.F.; Spruijt-Metz, D.; Pentz, M.A. Does community type moderate the relationship between parent perceptions of the neighborhood and physical activity in children? *Am. J. Heal. Promot.* **2012**, *26*, 371–380. [CrossRef] [PubMed]
69. DeWeese, R.S.; Yedidia, M.J.; Tulloch, D.L.; Ohri-Vachaspati, P. Neighborhood perceptions and active school commuting in low-income cities. *Am. J. Prev. Med.* **2013**, *45*, 393–400. [CrossRef] [PubMed]
70. Jones, R.A.; Blackburn, N.E.; Woods, C.; Byrne, M.; van Nassau, F.; Tully, M.A. Interventions promoting active transport to school in children: A systematic review and meta-analysis. *Prev. Med.* **2019**, *123*, 232–241. [CrossRef] [PubMed]
71. Mitra, R.; Buliung, R.N. Built environment correlates of active school transportation: Neighborhood and the modifiable areal unit problem. *J. Transp. Geogr.* **2012**, *20*, 51–61. [CrossRef]
72. Zhang, R.; Yao, E.; Liu, Z. School travel mode choice in Beijing, China. *J. Transp. Geogr.* **2017**, *62*, 98–110. [CrossRef]
73. Faulkner, G.E.; Richichi, V.; Buliung, R.N.; Fusco, C.; Moola, F. What's "quickest and easiest?": Parental decision making about school trip mode. *Int. J. Behav. Nutr. Phys. Act.* **2010**, *7*, 62. [CrossRef]
74. McDonald, N.C.; Aalborg, A.E. Why Parents Drive Children to School: Implications for Safe Routes to School Programs. *J. Am. Plan. Assoc.* **2009**, *75*, 331–342. [CrossRef]
75. Katzmarzyk, P.T.; Mason, C. The physical activity transition. *J. Phys. Act. Health* **2009**, *6*, 269–280. [CrossRef]
76. Larouche, R. Built Environment Features that Promote Cycling in School-Aged Children. *Curr. Obes. Rep.* **2015**, *4*, 494–503. [CrossRef]
77. Rodríguez-López, C.; Salas-Fariña, Z.M.; Villa-González, E.; Borges-Cosic, M.; Herrador-Colmenero, M.; Medina-Casaubón, J.; Ortega, F.B.; Chillón, P. The Threshold Distance Associated With Walking From Home to School. *Heal Educ. Behav.* **2017**, *44*, 857–866. [CrossRef]
78. Chillón, P.; Panter, J.; Corder, K.; Jones, A.P.; Van Sluijs, E.M.F. A longitudinal study of the distance that young people walk to school. *Health Place* **2015**, *31*, 133–137. [CrossRef] [PubMed]
79. Pucher, J.; Buehler, R. Walking and Cycling for Healthy Cities. *Built Environ.* **2010**, *36*, 391–414. [CrossRef]
80. Buliung, R.N.; Larsen, K.; Faulkner, G.E.J.; Stone, M.R. The "path" not taken: Exploring structural differences in mapped-versus shortest-network-path school travel routes. *Am. J. Public Health* **2013**, *103*, 1589–1596. [CrossRef]
81. Duncan, M.J.; Mummery, W.K. GIS or GPS? A Comparison of Two Methods For Assessing Route Taken During Active Transport. *Am. J. Prev. Med.* **2007**, *33*, 51–53. [CrossRef] [PubMed]
82. Larouche, R.; Saidla, K. Public Policy and Active Transportation. In *Children's Active Transportation*, 1st ed.; Larouche, R., Ed.; Elsevier: Amsterdam, The Netherlands, 2018; pp. 155–172.

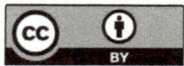

© 2020 by the authors. Licensee MDPI, Basel, Switzerland. This article is an open access article distributed under the terms and conditions of the Creative Commons Attribution (CC BY) license (http://creativecommons.org/licenses/by/4.0/).

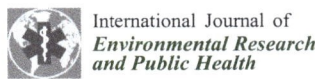

Article

How Does Commute Time Affect Labor Supply in Urban China? Implications for Active Commuting

Xiaoyu Wang [1], Jinquan Gong [1] and Chunan Wang [2,*]

[1] National School of Development, Peking University, Beijing 100871, China; xiaoyuwangecon@pku.edu.cn (X.W.); jinquang@pku.edu.cn (J.G.)
[2] School of Economics and Management, Beihang University, Beijing 100191, China
* Correspondence: chnwang@buaa.edu.cn

Received: 25 May 2020; Accepted: 24 June 2020; Published: 27 June 2020

Abstract: This paper identifies the causal effect of commute time on labor supply in urban China and provides implications for the development of active commuting. Labor supply is measured by daily workhours, workdays per week and weekly workhours, and city average commute time is adopted as an instrumental variable to correct the endogenous problem of individual commute time. We find that in urban China, commute time does not have effect on daily labor supply but has negative effects on workdays per week and weekly labor supply. These results are different from those found in Germany and Spain, and are potentially related to the intense competition among workers in the labor market of China. Moreover, the effect of commute time on workdays per week is stronger for job changed workers. In addition, the effects of commute time on labor supply are not different between males and females. Finally, policy implications for active commuting are discussed.

Keywords: commute time; labor supply; endogeneity; active commuting; China

1. Introduction

Active transportation and commuting are efficient ways to improve individuals' physical activities, ameliorate individuals' health status, and reduce air pollution. In recent years, many big cities in China, such as Beijing, have built a large number of exclusive bike lanes and encourage people to go to work using this healthy and green method. In fact, active commuting does not merely relate to health and the environment, but might also have a close relationship with economic activities. Compared with traditional urban transportation modes, such as the subway, buses, and cars, active commuting will inevitably increase individuals' commute time. It has been shown that commute time might significantly affect labor supply [1–3]. Accordingly, if commute time is proved to have negative effects on labor supply, a potential conflict between active commuting and economic development may arise, which might threaten the development of active commuting to some extent. In this case, in order to better benefit from the functions of active commuting and transportation, remedies should be considered to mitigate the negative effects.

In this paper, we aim to identify the causal effect of commute time on labor supply in urban China, and provide policy implications for the promotions of active commuting.

There are divergent theoretical views on how to model the relationship between commuting and labor supply in the literature. Some studies assume that the number of workdays is fixed and that the number of workhours per day can be chosen [4], while other studies make the opposite assumption [5]. Therefore, valid empirical evidence of the causal effect of commuting on labor supply will shed some lights on this theoretical debate. Previous research has found that, in Germany, commute distance has a positive effect on daily and weekly labor supply but no effect on the number of workdays [1]. It has also been found that commute distance has a negative effect on productivity measured by worker's absenteeism in Germany [2]. In Spain, it was found that longer commute time results in workers providing more daily labor supply [3]. It has been shown that when workers are free to make decisions on their daily labor supply but subject to daily exogenous variation in commute time, commute time has a negative effect on job-offer acceptance decisions of substitute teachers in Michigan [6].

In our study, labor supply is measured by daily workhours, workdays per week, and weekly workhours. These three measurements of labor supply are necessary since they capture different relationships between commute time and labor supply. Specifically, for a large proportion of workers, commute time is the fixed cost for daily workhours, while it is the variable cost for weekly workhours because workers can choose the number of workdays [4,5,7]. Using the China Health and Nutrition Survey (CHNS), and combining the fixed effect model and instrumental variable method, we find that commute time does not have a significant effect on daily workhours in China, which is in contrast with the findings in Germany and Spain [1,3]. On the other hand, commute time significantly decreases the number of workdays per week and weekly workhours. In addition, heterogeneous effects of commute time are found between job changed and job unchanged workers. Finally, policy implications for the development of active commuting are discussed.

This paper contributes to the literature by comparing the heterogeneous impacts of commute time on labor supply in China and other countries (i.e., Germany and Spain). The patterns observed in urban China, namely, that longer commute time does not significantly affect daily workhours but significantly decreases the number of workdays per week and weekly workhours, might closely relate to the intense competition among workers in the labor market of China. Such a particularity of China's labor market implies that in order to better promote active commuting, the Chinese government should pay more attention to the amelioration of transportation infrastructure.

The remainder of this paper is organized as follows. The next section discusses the theoretical model established in this study, provides detailed information on the data employed, and introduces the identification strategy and the specification of the model. Section 3 presents empirical results and additional results. Section 4 discusses the reasons for different results across countries and policy implications for the development of active commuting. The final section concludes.

2. Methods

2.1. The Theoretical Model

Previous theoretical research presents a model of monocentric cities with decentralized employment [8]. This model proposes if the work location is assumed to be fixed, longer commuting will be compensated by lower house prices, or by higher wages when residential location is assumed to be fixed. Although the effect of commuting on labor supply can be analyzed based on White's model, a large amount of the literature casts doubt on the ability of the monocentric model to explain actual commuting behavior in the US [9–12].

The model we set up in this paper does not assume that the city is monocentric and that work places are located in the center of city. On the contrary, work locations can be altered if workers change their jobs. Since the data we use is longitudinal, in which people surveyed stay in the same residential location, we assume that people do not change their residential locations. Hourly wage is a function of distance from residential location to work location, that is, $w(d)$, in which w is the hourly wage and d is the round-trip commute distance.

Assume that the individual utility function is given by $U(x,l)$, and that a worker wants to maximize utility subjected to their budget constraint:

$$\max_{x,l} U(x,l) \\ s.t. \: x + w(d)l = I_0 + w(d) - (tw(d) + m)d, \tag{1}$$

in which x is consumption; l is leisure, I_0 is non-labor income; t is the commute time for each unit of commute distance; td is the round trip commute time; and m the is the monetary cost of each unit of commute distance. The budget constraint can be rewritten as:

$$x = I_0 + w(d) - (tw(d) + m)d - w(d)l. \tag{2}$$

Putting the above specification into the utility function and maximizing the utility function:

$$U_l - U_x w = 0. \tag{3}$$

The optimal values of x and l are then as follows:

$$x^* = x(w(d), I_0 + w(d) - (tw(d) + m)d), \tag{4}$$

$$l^* = l(w(d), I_0 + w(d) - (tw(d) + m)d). \tag{5}$$

We assume that all workers have the same utility level; differentiate with respect to distance (d) and apply the envelope theorem:

$$w_d = \frac{tw + m}{1 - td - l} = \frac{tw + m}{n}, \tag{6}$$

in which $n = 1 - td - l$ is the labor supply. $w_d > 0$ implies that higher wage compensates longer commute distance or commute time.

First, the marginal effect of commute distance on labor supply is:

$$\frac{\partial n}{\partial d} = -t - \frac{\partial l}{\partial d}, \tag{7}$$

in which:

$$\begin{aligned}
\frac{\partial l}{\partial d} &= \left(\frac{\partial l^h}{\partial w} - \frac{\partial l}{\partial m}l\right)w_d + \frac{\partial l}{\partial m}(w_d - (tw + m) - tdw_d) \\
&= \frac{\partial l^h}{\partial w}w_d + (1 - td - l)\frac{\partial l}{\partial m}w_d - \frac{\partial l}{\partial m}(tw + m) \\
&= \frac{\partial l^h}{\partial w}w_d + \frac{\partial l}{\partial m}(nw_d - (tw + m)) \\
&= \frac{\partial l^h}{\partial w}w_d.
\end{aligned} \tag{8}$$

Note that the superscript "h" denotes Hicksian. Combining the two equations above, the marginal effect of commute distance on labor supply will be:

$$\frac{\partial n}{\partial d} = -t - \frac{\partial l^h}{\partial w}w_d. \tag{9}$$

According to economic theory, given the individual's utility is unchanged, the increase of hourly wage will substitute leisure time, that is, $\frac{\partial l^h}{\partial w} < 0$. Considering also $w_d > 0$, if the absolute value of $\frac{\partial l^h}{\partial w}$ or w_d is large enough, the commute distance will have a positive effect on labor supply, that is, $\frac{\partial n}{\partial d} > 0$. Furthermore, given constant commute time per unit of commute distance, commute time increases labor supply. However, if the absolute value of the product is not large enough, the commute distance will decrease labor supply, that is, $\frac{\partial n}{\partial d} < 0$.

In addition, the change of commute time per unit of commute distance t can be understood as the variation of transport condition in an urban area. Then, the marginal effect of transportation condition on labor supply is given by:

$$\frac{\partial n}{\partial t} = -d - \frac{\partial l}{\partial t} = -d + \frac{\partial l}{\partial I}dw = d\left(-1 + \frac{\partial l}{\partial I}w\right), \tag{10}$$

in which I is used to denote the total income of a worker, that is, $I_0 + w(d) - (tw(d) + m)d \equiv I$. Due to the positive income effect, the increase of total income will increase the leisure time, that is, $\frac{\partial l}{\partial I} > 0$. Under this specification, when $\frac{\partial l}{\partial I}$ or w is large enough, the commute time per unit of commute distance or the deterioration of transportation condition will have a positive effect on labor supply, that is, $\frac{\partial n}{\partial t} > 0$. Therefore, commute time will have a positive effect on working hours given that commute distance is held constant. Nevertheless, when the product of $\frac{\partial l}{\partial I}$ and w is small, the deterioration of transportation condition will then decrease labor supply.

To summarize, the derivation of theoretical model leads to the following propositions.

Proposition 1. *The change of commute distance, such as induced by job change, has a positive effect on the wage, but its effect on labor supply is uncertain.*

Proposition 2. *Better transportation conditions do not affect the wage, and its effect on labor supply is uncertain.*

2.2. Data and Descriptive Statistics

The dataset adopted in this study was drawn from the China Health and Nutrition Survey (CHNS) provided by the Chinese Center for Disease Control and Prevention and the Population Research Center of the University of North Carolina in the USA. The first round was in 1989. The next eight waves followed in 1991, 1993, 1997, 2000, 2004, 2006, 2009, and 2011. The study population is composed of respondents from the provinces of Guangxi, Guizhou, Heilongjiang, Henan, Hubei, Hunan, Jiangsu, Liaoning, and Shandong in China. This sample is diverse, with variation found in a wide-ranging set of socioeconomic factors, which include income, employment, education, and modernization and other related health, nutritional and demographic measures. The detailed information on commute time and other data at both individual and household levels make it ideal for examining the effect of commute time on labor supply.

To take advantage of controlling individual-specific, time-invariant effects, attention was restricted to a longitudinal subsample in the dataset. We further limited the sample to workers aged between 16 and 60 years who were surveyed in the urban areas. Note that urban areas in this paper include all urban, suburban, and town communities in the CHNS. For the purpose of this study, we also limited the sample to surveys after 2004 since CHNS only included questions on commute time for workers from 2004. We defined three variables relating to labor supply in this study, that is, workhours per day, workdays per week, and weekly workhours.

In line with the previous studies on labor supply, some variables reflecting socioeconomic and demographic characteristics of the respondents were specified. As illustrated in numerous economics studies, an individual's status relating to smoking and chronic conditions is a signal of health and affects that individual's labor supply decision, and was thus included in the labor supply function. In addition to health status, other demographic characteristics involved in the empirical analysis included age, the number of children less than or equal to 6 years old, and the number of family members in the household. In order to capture the wealth effect on labor supply, we also controlled for family wealth in the regression. Family wealth included house value and values of appliances, vehicles, machines, and equipment owned. Family income affects individual labor supply and thus was also controlled in our analysis. Family income, in this study, was defined as household non-labor income, other family members' labor income, and housing subsidy, in which housing subsidy was calculated by subtracting the annual rent the family pays from the annual fair market rent.

To correct the endogenous problem of individual commute time, we used the average commute time in the city, which was constructed as the average of individual workers' commute times in the city, as the instrumental variable for individual commute time. To avoid the problem that city characteristics may be potentially correlated with city average commute time and individual labor supply, we controlled for city-level human capital, measured by city average education level, and the ratio of employment from the non-public sector, as a variable from the labor demand side. We further controlled the fraction of workers changing job in the city to reflect the city labor market condition.

Finally, after excluding those observations with relevant missing information, a total sample of 1077 individuals and 2727 observations was retained. The descriptive statistics of commute time, labor supply variables, and other important variables in 2004, 2006, 2009 and 2011 are presented in Table 1.

Table 1. Descriptive statistics.

	2004		2006	
	Mean	S.D.	Mean	S.D.
Daily workhours	8.05	1.37	7.93	1.24
Workdays per week	5.51	0.82	5.43	0.85
Weekly workhours	44.56	11.75	43.30	10.93
Hourly wage	8.42	7.28	11.16	15.91
Commute time	29.17	25.00	34.04	25.86
Family wealth	85,218.59	223,544.99	68,030.82	179,556.20
Other family members' income	67,335.48	51,489.82	71,479.22	57,398.39
Age	39.86	9.38	41.05	9.47
Cigarette	0.32	0.47	0.33	0.47
Number of children less than 6 years old	0.17	0.38	0.15	0.37
Number of family members	3.22	1.15	3.10	1.09
City job change rate	0.16	0.09	0.11	0.07
City average education	11.07	0.96	11.45	1.13
City non-public employment rate	0.29	0.15	0.37	0.13
City average commute time	29.17	6.15	34.04	7.29
N	604		693	
	2009		2011	
	Mean	S.D.	Mean	S.D.
Daily workhours	8.02	1.47	8.11	1.37
Workdays per week	5.44	0.84	5.54	0.89
Weekly workhours	43.71	11.19	45.10	11.59
Hourly wage	13.90	13.75	15.54	17.93
Commute time	36.09	26.11	34.68	25.84
Family wealth	298,918.15	325,010.84	941,293.65	1,665,275.68
Other family members' income	93,313.23	70,074.26	110,297.02	98,893.49
Age	41.86	9.53	42.74	9.10
Cigarette	0.34	0.47	0.34	0.47
Number of children less than 6 years old	0.16	0.40	0.14	0.37
Number of family members	3.21	1.23	3.27	1.27
City job change rate	0.15	0.08	0.14	0.08
City average education	11.29	1.24	11.24	1.22
City non-public employment rate	0.43	0.18	0.44	0.17
City average commute time	36.09	5.82	34.68	6.50
N	775		655	

On average, round trip commute time increased from 29.17 min in 2004 to 36.09 min in 2009 and then decreased to 34.68 min in 2011. All three labor supply variables decreased in 2006 first and then increased. For example, typical workers worked 8.05 h per day, 5.51 days per week, and 44.56 h per week in 2004. In 2006, daily working hours decreased to 7.93, working days decreased to 5.43, and weekly working hours also decreased. However, from 2009 to 2011, people worked longer per day, more days per week, and also had higher weekly working hours.

Family wealth and family income had a similar increasing trend. The proportion of smoking people was consistently around 33% across different years. The number of children aged less than 6 years in the household was around 0.14–0.17 and the number of family members in the household was around 3.2. The percentage of job changing workers ranged from 11% to 16%. Average years of education in the city was around 11 years. The ratio of non-public employment increased from 29% in 2004 to 44% in 2011.

2.3. Empirical Methodology

In this paper, we aim to investigate the causal effect of commute time on labor supply, measured by working hours per day, number of workdays per week, and weekly workhours. However, following the standard labor supply literature, controlling commute time, hourly wage, and other variables in regressions cannot provide a consistent estimator for such a causal effect, due to the following two reasons.

First, commute time is endogenous, especially when residential location and work location can be chosen by individual workers and such a decision is made based on the working hours. For example, long workhours may cause workers to move to places closer to the work places. In this research, worker's residential location is assumed to be fixed in the longitudinal data. However, there are still two factors accounting for the change of commute time, that is, the changes of work location and transportation conditions in the city. As a result, the reverse causal effect of labor supply on work location decision cannot be ruled out, resulting in the endogeneity problem. Nevertheless, since city transportation conditions provide a good instrumental variable for commute time, we adopted the average commute time in the city to measure the city transportation conditions. Note that as the city average commute time is an aggregate variable, it can at least partially correct the endogeneity of individual commute time. From this perspective, although the city average commute time is not flawless, it might work as a valid instrumental variable to some extent.

Second, wages may also be endogenous. Given the residence location, workers can find jobs based on job characteristics, such as daily workhours, number of workdays per week, total weekly workhours, hourly wage, and commute time. Labor supply, wage, and commute time are simultaneously chosen. In this research, as hourly wage was not the variable of interest, in order to avoid the endogeneity problems, a totally reduced form was adopted first, and hourly wage was not included in the regression. Hourly wage was included in a subsequent regression to perform a robustness check.

The basic regression form is:

$$\log(Y_{it}) = \beta_0 + \beta_1 \log(T_{it}) + \beta_2 X_{it} + v_i + \mu_t + u_{it}, \tag{11}$$

in which Y_{it} measures labor supply variables, that is, daily workhours, working days per week, and weekly workhours; T_{it} is the round trip commute time; X_{it} are other time-varying independent variables, controlling for individual, household, demographic, and city characteristics; v_i is the individual time-invariant unobserved heterogeneity; μ_t captures the year fixed effect; and u_{it} is the error term. β_1 is the elasticity of labor supply with respect to commute time. The fixed effect is the model that fit using the above equation.

The first-stage regression for commute time is:

$$\log(T_{it}) = \alpha_0 + \alpha_1 \log(\overline{T}_j) + \alpha_2 X_{it} + v_i + \mu_t + \varepsilon_{it}, \tag{12}$$

in which $\overline{T}_j$ is the average commute time in city j where individual i lives, and ε_{it} is the error term. We also applied a fixed effect model to the above equation.

Note that by using the modified Wald test and the Cumby–Huizinga test, we found that the problems of heteroscedasticity and autocorrelation in the error terms exist. Therefore, in all regressions, we adjusted standard errors by clustering around individuals.

3. Results

3.1. First-Stage Results for Individual Commute Time

To validate the use of city average commute time as a good instrumental variable for individual commute time, two conditions need to be checked. First, the city average commute time should have a strong correlation with individual commute time. Second, the city average commute time should not correlate with the error term in Equation (11).

Table 2 presents regression results when the dependent variable is individual commute time, and independent variables are city average commute time and those which we controlled in the labor supply regression. Column (1) of Table 2 shows that city average commute time, that is, city transportation conditions, has a strong relationship with individual commute time. The elasticity is 0.875, which means that a 1% increase in city average commute time will enhance individual commute time by 0.875%. Controlling city level characteristics additionally, the correlation is still significant at the 1% level, which is shown in column (2) of Table 2. In labor supply regressions in the second stage, hourly wage was controlled. Thus, in order to show that city average commute time is still a good instrumental variable, we controlled the hourly wage in the first stage and present results in column (3) of Table 2. We find that there still exists a strong correlation between individual commute time and city average commute time, given other independent variables and hourly wage.

Table 2. Effect of city average commute time on individual commute time.

VARIABLES	(1)	(2)	(3)
	Dependent Variable: Log (Individual Commute Time)		
Log (City average commute time)	0.875 ***	0.920 ***	0.920 ***
	(0.131)	(0.133)	(0.133)
Log (Hourly wage)			−0.0101
			(0.0365)
Cigarette	−0.0638	−0.0625	−0.0637
	(0.0638)	(0.0640)	(0.0644)
Age	0.00844	0.0141	0.0148
	(0.00920)	(0.0107)	(0.0109)
Number of children less than 6 years old	0.0864	0.0917	0.0924
	(0.0626)	(0.0626)	(0.0627)
Number of family members	0.00289	0.00184	0.000963
	(0.0291)	(0.0291)	(0.0295)
Log (Asset)	−0.0126	−0.0121	−0.0120
	(0.0123)	(0.0123)	(0.0123)
Log (Other family members' income)	0.0553 **	0.0550 **	0.0580 **
	(0.0272)	(0.0273)	(0.0289)
Stroke	−0.864 *	−0.859 *	−0.856 *
	(0.497)	(0.499)	(0.500)
Fracture	−0.00158	−0.00491	−0.00422
	(0.0771)	(0.0768)	(0.0769)
Blood pressure	0.153 *	0.152 *	0.150 *
	(0.0860)	(0.0867)	(0.0863)
Diabetes	0.0934	0.0969	0.101
	(0.165)	(0.163)	(0.163)
Myocardial infarction	0.713	0.672	0.670
	(0.577)	(0.600)	(0.601)
City job change rate		−0.107	−0.107
		(0.238)	(0.239)
City average education		−0.00749	−0.00743
		(0.0359)	(0.0359)
City non-public employment rate		−0.324	−0.324

Table 2. Cont.

VARIABLES	(1)	(2)	(3)
	\multicolumn{3}{c}{Dependent Variable: Log (Individual Commute Time)}		
		(0.204)	(0.204)
Constant	−0.686	−0.854	−0.893
	(0.471)	(0.580)	(0.592)
Observations	2727	2727	2727
R-squared	0.652	0.653	0.653
Number of id	1077	1077	1077
Year FE	YES	YES	YES
F value	44.907	47.978	47.923
Under-identification test	45.164	48.306	48.268
Partial R-squared between IV and dependent variable	0.017	0.017	0.017

Note: Coefficients of year fixed effect are not reported; Standard errors adjusted for clustering around individuals are in parentheses; *** $p < 0.01$, ** $p < 0.05$, * $p < 0.1$.

Results in Table 2 support that there is a significantly positive correlation between city average commute time and individual commute time. City average commute time reflects the transportation conditions in the city. Individual commute time is the time workers spend between residential location and work location, which should be affected by the city transportation conditions. A city with high average commute time has poor transportation conditions, which increase the commute time for commuters.

In addition, city average commute time is a macro condition in the city. Thus, it does not correlate with the factors that affect an individual's labor supply and appears in the error term in Equation (11).

Finally, in the last three rows of Table 2, we calculate the F value of the first-stage regression; conduct the under-identification test; and calculate the partial R-squared between the instrumental variable and the dependent variable. These tests can support the validity of city average commute time as the instrumental variable.

3.2. Hourly Wage and Commute Time

Table 3 presents estimated results for the effect of commute time on hourly wage. The result of the fixed effect model, shown in column (1) of Table 3, demonstrates that commute time does not have a significant effect on wage. According to column (2) of Table 3, even when city average commute time is adopted to correct the endogeneity problem of individual commute time, such an effect is still insignificant. Because health status may have an effect on the worker's productivity, in column (3) we include several health conditions, including stroke, fracture, high blood pressure, diabetes, and myocardial infarction. However, estimation results do not show a significant effect of commute time on hourly wage, which is different from the findings in theoretical derivations.

In addition, cigarette smoking has a negative effect on hourly wage since smoking can impact health and then reduce labor productivity. Even when more health variables are included in the regression, the cigarette variable still has a significant and large negative effect on wage. The labor market demand side variable measured by the ratio of non-public employment in the city, city human capital level, and labor market conditions measured by job changed ratio in the city do not have a significant effect on hourly wage.

Table 3. Hourly wage regression results.

VARIABLES	(1) FE	(2) FE + 2SLS	(3) FE + 2SLS
	Dependent Variable: Log (Hourly Wage)		
Log (Commute time)	0.00423	−0.0475	−0.0544
	(0.0193)	(0.109)	(0.109)
Cigarette	−0.116 *	−0.118 *	−0.118 *
	(0.0629)	(0.0632)	(0.0623)
Experience	0.00596	0.00471	0.00550
	(0.0143)	(0.0145)	(0.0144)
Experience square	−0.000398 *	−0.000377	−0.000389 *
	(0.000226)	(0.000231)	(0.000231)
City job change rate	0.0612	0.0779	0.0737
	(0.169)	(0.170)	(0.171)
City average education	0.00455	0.00438	0.00613
	(0.0271)	(0.0272)	(0.0274)
City non-public employment rate	−0.0609	−0.0733	−0.0794
	(0.160)	(0.162)	(0.159)
Stroke			0.280
			(0.383)
Fracture			0.0449
			(0.0424)
Blood pressure			−0.179 **
			(0.0761)
Diabetes			0.393 ***
			(0.112)
Myocardial infarction			−0.184 *
			(0.109)
Constant	1.924 ***	2.101 ***	2.095 ***
	(0.406)	(0.577)	(0.573)
Observations	2727	2727	2727
R-squared	0.766	0.766	0.769
Number of id	1077	1077	1077
Year FE	YES	YES	YES

Note: Coefficients of year fixed effect are not reported; Standard errors adjusted for clustering around individuals are in parentheses; *** $p < 0.01$, ** $p < 0.05$, * $p < 0.1$.

3.3. Second-Stage Results for Daily Labor Supply

In the second stage, we studied how commute time affects labor supply, in which three variables were used to measure labor supply, that is, daily workhours, workdays per week, and weekly workhours.

The fixed effect model in column (1) of Table 4 shows that commute time has a positive relationship with working hours per day. As commute time may be endogenous, in column (2) of Table 4, we adopt city average commute time as an instrumental variable to correct the endogeneity problem. Result shows that commute time insignificantly decreases daily workhours. The family income and asset variables may be endogenous. Compared with column (2), we control the asset and other family members' income variables additionally in column (2). We find that the effect of commute time on daily labor supply, that is, the coefficient of interest, changes little when we control these two variables. Based on this result, although there might exist an endogeneity problem of the family income and asset variables, given the very limited impacts on the magnitude and significance of the coefficient of interest, the inclusion of asset and other family members' income variables as control variables might not be an important issue.

Because commute time does not have any significant relationship with hourly wage, as shown in Section 3.2, we can infer that in labor supply regressions controlling wage additionally will not change the value and significance level of commute time. The regression result in column (4) supports this claim. Since wage and labor supply are simultaneously determined in labor market, the endogeneity problem in terms of hourly wage is still an issue. Column (5) in Table 4, in which the interaction term of experience and age is adopted as an instrumental variable for hourly wage, shows that commute time still has insignificant effect on daily workhours. An interesting result is the positive effect of the number of cigarettes on daily labor supply. One possible explanation is that the cigarette variable represents the workers' occupations. For example, blue collar workers work more hours and are also more likely to smoke. However, this explanation is rejected by the result that controlling occupations additionally does not alter the value and significance level of the cigarette variable. A second explanation is that the cigarette variable represents ambition and a smoking person has strong incentive to work.

Table 4. Effect of commute time on labor supply—daily workhours.

	(1)	(2)	(3)	(4)	(5)
	\multicolumn{5}{c}{Dependent Variable: Log (Daily Workhours)}				
VARIABLES	FE	FE + 2SLS	FE + 2SLS	FE + 2SLS	FE + 2SLS
Log (Commute time)	0.00259	−0.0306	−0.0332	−0.0332	−0.0333
	(0.00675)	(0.0377)	(0.0377)	(0.0364)	(0.0418)
Log (Hourly wage)				−0.138 ***	0.107
				(0.0179)	(0.194)
Cigarette	0.0555 **	0.0538 **	0.0529 **	0.0366 *	0.0656 *
	(0.0228)	(0.0228)	(0.0226)	(0.0190)	(0.0375)
Age	−0.00118	-4.23×10^{-6}	0.000773	0.0105 ***	−0.00670
	(0.00211)	(0.00258)	(0.00270)	(0.00289)	(0.0139)
Number of children less than 6 years old	−0.0441 ***	−0.0419 **	−0.0408 **	−0.0312 *	−0.0481 *
	(0.0166)	(0.0167)	(0.0171)	(0.0159)	(0.0252)
Number of family members	−0.00443	−0.00383	−0.00479	−0.0168 **	0.00448
	(0.00748)	(0.00756)	(0.00761)	(0.00745)	(0.0186)
City job change rate	0.0330	0.0441	0.0452	0.0460	0.0445
	(0.0618)	(0.0630)	(0.0629)	(0.0602)	(0.0695)
City average education	0.00170	0.00159	0.00114	0.00199	0.000485
	(0.00997)	(0.0100)	(0.0101)	(0.00971)	(0.0112)
City non-public employment rate	−0.0271	−0.0346	−0.0354	−0.0443	−0.0286
	(0.0597)	(0.0624)	(0.0625)	(0.0573)	(0.0716)
Log (Asset)			−0.00276	−0.00119	−0.00397
			(0.00328)	(0.00309)	(0.00447)
Log (Other family members' income)			0.00415	0.0443 ***	−0.0268
			(0.00919)	(0.0111)	(0.0581)
Constant	2.105 ***	2.162 ***	2.132 ***	1.609 ***	2.535 ***
	(0.110)	(0.129)	(0.140)	(0.154)	(0.748)
Observations	2727	2727	2727	2727	2727
R-squared	0.563	0.563	0.563	0.615	0.563
Number of id	1077	1077	1077	1077	1077
Health conditions	YES	YES	YES	YES	YES
Year FE	YES	YES	YES	YES	YES

Note: Columns (2), (3), (4), and (5) adopt city average commute time as instrumental variable for individual commute time; Column (5) additionally adopts the interaction term of experience and age as instrumental variable for hourly wage; Coefficients of year fixed effect and health conditions are not reported; Standard errors adjusted for clustering around individuals are in parentheses; *** $p < 0.01$, ** $p < 0.05$, * $p < 0.1$.

3.4. Second-Stage Results for Workdays per Week

The second measurement for labor supply is workdays per week. For workers' daily labor supply, commute time is fixed cost. However, for weekly labor supply, commute time is a variable cost. Given total weekly workhours, workers can reduce workdays per week and increase daily labor supply to minimize cost. Even when we relax the assumption that total weekly workhours are constant, workers can still reduce cost by decreasing workdays.

Table 5 displays regression results for workdays per week. When city average commute time is used as an instrumental variable to correct individual commute time's endogeneity problem, the coefficient of individual commute time changes from an insignificant positive effect to a significant negative effect. Even when we control the family income and asset variables, such a result is still valid. Controlling hourly wage additionally, the coefficient of commute time does not change. Adopting the interaction term of experience and age to correct bias caused by the endogeneity of hourly wage, the coefficient of commute time is still unchanged. To summarize, a 1% increase in commute time will significantly decrease workdays per week by 0.0735%.

Table 5. Effect of commute time on labor supply—workdays per week.

	(1)	(2)	(3)	(4)	(5)
	Dependent Variable: Log (Workdays per Week)				
VARIABLES	FE	FE + 2SLS	FE + 2SLS	FE + 2SLS	FE + 2SLS
Log (Commute time)	0.00316	−0.0702 *	−0.0735 *	−0.0735 *	−0.0735 *
	(0.00606)	(0.0407)	(0.0416)	(0.0395)	(0.0410)
Log (Hourly wage)				−0.123 ***	−0.0208
				(0.0162)	(0.132)
Cigarette	0.0315 *	0.0277	0.0264	0.0118	0.0240
	(0.0185)	(0.0190)	(0.0192)	(0.0172)	(0.0263)
Age	−0.00210	0.000482	0.00132	0.00994 ***	0.00278
	(0.00166)	(0.00225)	(0.00268)	(0.00301)	(0.0100)
Number of children less than 6 years old	0.00778	0.0127	0.0146	0.0231	0.0161
	(0.0151)	(0.0165)	(0.0170)	(0.0166)	(0.0189)
Number of family members	−0.00475	−0.00343	−0.00536	−0.0161 **	−0.00717
	(0.00694)	(0.00721)	(0.00749)	(0.00762)	(0.0135)
City job change rate	−0.00852	0.0161	0.0172	0.0180	0.0173
	(0.0562)	(0.0597)	(0.0602)	(0.0563)	(0.0591)
City average education	−0.00858	−0.00882	−0.00951	−0.00875	−0.00938
	(0.0101)	(0.0106)	(0.0106)	(0.00993)	(0.0106)
City non-public employment rate	0.0670	0.0503	0.0494	0.0415	0.0480
	(0.0517)	(0.0536)	(0.0539)	(0.0499)	(0.0533)
Log (Asset)			−0.00379	−0.00239	−0.00355
			(0.00301)	(0.00279)	(0.00319)
Log (Other family members' income)			0.00818	0.0439 ***	0.0142
			(0.00799)	(0.00987)	(0.0401)
Constant	1.844 ***	1.970 ***	1.912 ***	1.447 ***	1.833 ***
	(0.117)	(0.141)	(0.141)	(0.132)	(0.528)
Observations	2727	2727	2727	2727	2727
R-squared	0.563	0.568	0.568	0.625	0.568
Number of id	1077	1077	1077	1077	1077
Health conditions	YES	YES	YES	YES	YES
Year FE	YES	YES	YES	YES	YES

Note: Columns (2), (3), (4), and (5) adopt city average commute time as an instrumental variable for individual commute time; Column (5) additionally adopts the interaction term of experience and age as an instrumental variable for hourly wage; Coefficients of year fixed effect and health conditions are not reported; Standard errors adjusted for clustering around individuals are in parentheses; *** $p < 0.01$, ** $p < 0.05$, * $p < 0.1$.

3.5. Second-Stage Results for Weekly Workhours

Weekly workhours are defined as the product of daily workhours and workdays per week. As we took the logarithm in three dependent variables in terms of labor supply, the coefficients in weekly workhours regression are equal to the sum of coefficients in the daily workhours and workdays per week regressions.

According to Table 6, the elasticity of weekly workhours with respect to commute time is −0.107. This means that when individual commute time increases 1%, workers will work 0.107% less hours in a week. The cigarette variable has a positive effect on weekly workhours. Family income and asset variables have insignificant effects on weekly workhours. Controlling these two variables additionally does not alter the value and significance level of individual commute time. City characteristics, that is, city average education attainment, employment change ratio, and non-public employment rate, do not have effects on individual weekly workhours. Even by adopting the interaction term of experience and age as an instrumental variable to correct the hourly wage's endogeneity problem, such a causal effect does not change.

Table 6. Effect of commute time on labor supply—weekly workhours.

	(1)	(2)	(3)	(4)	(5)
	Dependent Variable: Log (Weekly Workhours)				
VARIABLES	FE	FE+2SLS	FE+2SLS	FE+2SLS	FE+2SLS
Log (Commute time)	0.00575	−0.101 *	−0.107 *	−0.107 **	−0.107 *
	(0.00937)	(0.0574)	(0.0585)	(0.0537)	(0.0624)
Log (Hourly wage)				−0.261 ***	0.0858
				(0.0243)	(0.249)
Cigarette	0.0871 ***	0.0815 ***	0.0794 **	0.0484 **	0.0896 *
	(0.0307)	(0.0310)	(0.0309)	(0.0237)	(0.0475)
Age	−0.00328	0.000477	0.00209	0.0204 ***	−0.00392
	(0.00273)	(0.00348)	(0.00399)	(0.00418)	(0.0181)
Number of children less than 6 years old	−0.0363 *	−0.0291	−0.0261	−0.00802	−0.0321
	(0.0217)	(0.0233)	(0.0239)	(0.0215)	(0.0320)
Number of family members	−0.00918	−0.00725	−0.0101	−0.0329 ***	−0.00269
	(0.0108)	(0.0113)	(0.0114)	(0.0107)	(0.0246)
City job change rate	0.0245	0.0602	0.0623	0.0640	0.0618
	(0.0873)	(0.0903)	(0.0908)	(0.0818)	(0.0973)
City average education	−0.00688	−0.00723	−0.00837	−0.00677	−0.00890
	(0.0146)	(0.0152)	(0.0153)	(0.0138)	(0.0166)
City non-public employment rate	0.0399	0.0157	0.0140	−0.00286	0.0195
	(0.0807)	(0.0867)	(0.0870)	(0.0740)	(0.0957)
Log (Asset)			−0.00655	−0.00358	−0.00753
			(0.00474)	(0.00421)	(0.00583)
Log (Other family members' income)			0.0123	0.0882***	−0.0126
			(0.0125)	(0.0148)	(0.0741)
Constant	3.950 ***	4.132 ***	4.043 ***	3.056 ***	4.368 ***
	(0.167)	(0.201)	(0.212)	(0.210)	(0.977)
Observations	2727	2727	2727	2727	2727
R-squared	0.568	0.577	0.578	0.676	0.578
Number of id	1077	1077	1077	1077	1077
Health conditions	YES	YES	YES	YES	YES
Year FE	YES	YES	YES	YES	YES

Note: Columns (2), (3), (4), and (5) adopt city average commute time as an instrumental variable for individual commute time; Column (5) additionally adopts the interaction term of experience and age as an instrumental variable for hourly wage; Coefficients of year fixed effect and health conditions are not reported; Standard errors adjusted for clustering around individuals are in parentheses; *** $p < 0.01$, ** $p < 0.05$, * $p < 0.1$.

3.6. Additional Results: Job Changed and Unchanged Workers

There are three possibilities that can explain workers reporting a change in commute time. The first possibility is the change of residential or work locations. In the CHNS subsample we selected, residential location was fixed. Therefore, a change of work location will alter commute time. The second is the change of transportation conditions in the city. Better transportation conditions reduce individual commute time. Third, commute time is self-reported and may thus vary due to measurement errors.

We separated the data based on whether respondents changed their jobs since the previous survey. When individuals find new jobs, they can simultaneously choose their work location, wage, and commute time to maximize their utility. Proposition 1 proposes theoretically that, for individuals who change jobs, longer commute time will be compensated by a higher wage. For individuals who do not change jobs, there is no causal relationship between wage and commute time. In both cases, commute time can have positive or negative effects on labor supply.

Table 7 shows the labor supply and wage regression results for the subsample of job changed workers. Table 8 presents results for job unchanged workers.

Table 7. Labor supply and wage for job changed workers.

VARIABLES	(1) Log (Daily Workhours)	(2) Log (Workdays per Week)	(3) Log (Weekly Workhours)	(4) Log (Hourly Wage)
Log (Commute time)	−0.0544	−0.243 *	−0.298	0.234
	(0.160)	(0.127)	(0.242)	(0.328)
Cigarette	0.0119	−0.0625	−0.0506	−0.0442
	(0.0863)	(0.0891)	(0.156)	(0.250)
Age	−0.00751	−0.00560	−0.0131	
	(0.00875)	(0.0107)	(0.0165)	
Number of children less than 6 years old	−0.0771	−0.0758	−0.153	
	(0.0853)	(0.0601)	(0.117)	
Number of family members	−0.0336	0.0412	0.00756	
	(0.0310)	(0.0341)	(0.0501)	
Log (Asset)	0.00228	−0.000458	0.00183	
	(0.0160)	(0.0140)	(0.0234)	
Log (Other family members' incomes)	−0.0459	0.0395	−0.00635	
	(0.0391)	(0.0379)	(0.0629)	
City job change rate	−0.172	−0.145	−0.317	0.949
	(0.313)	(0.354)	(0.529)	(0.820)
City average education	−0.0153	−0.0677	−0.0830	0.0627
	(0.0414)	(0.0486)	(0.0728)	(0.128)
City non-public employment rate	0.163	0.399	0.562	−0.394
	(0.256)	(0.261)	(0.453)	(0.497)
Experience				0.0790
				(0.0569)
Experience square				−0.00127
				(0.000825)
Constant	3.288 ***	2.776 ***	6.065 ***	−0.664
	(0.765)	(0.871)	(1.284)	(2.562)
Observations	296	296	296	296
R-squared	0.695	0.607	0.643	0.761
Number of id	139	139	139	139
Health conditions	YES	YES	YES	YES
Year FE	YES	YES	YES	YES

Note: Columns (1), (2), (3), and (4) adopt city average commute time as an instrumental variable for individual commute time; Column (4) additionally adopts the interaction term of experience and age as an instrumental variable for hourly wage; Coefficients of year fixed effect and health conditions are not reported; Standard errors adjusted for clustering around individuals are in parentheses; *** $p < 0.01$, ** $p < 0.05$, * $p < 0.1$.

Commute time has a positive effect on hourly wage for job changed workers. However, this effect is insignificant. In contrast, commute time has an insignificant negative effect on the hourly wage for job unchanged workers.

For individuals who change jobs, commute time decreases daily workhours and weekly workhours insignificantly, while it significantly decreases workdays per week. Furthermore, the effects are larger than those in the full sample. For example, in the full sample, the elasticity for workdays per week is −0.0735, while it is −0.243 for the job changed subsample.

For individuals who do not change job, individual commute time is insignificant in four regressions and the absolute values are also less than those in the subsample of job changed workers.

Table 8. Labor supply and wage for job unchanged workers.

VARIABLES	(1) Log (Daily Workhours)	(2) Log (Workdays Per Week)	(3) Log (Weekly Workhours)	(4) Log (Hourly Wage)
Log (Commute time)	−0.0140	−0.0465	−0.0605	−0.0713
	(0.0352)	(0.0444)	(0.0564)	(0.112)
Cigarette	0.0620 ***	0.0340 *	0.0960 ***	−0.122 *
	(0.0238)	(0.0183)	(0.0290)	(0.0648)
Age	0.000842	−9.73 × 10^{-5}	0.000745	
	(0.00283)	(0.00294)	(0.00405)	
Number of children less than 6 years old	−0.0334 **	0.0187	−0.0147	
	(0.0148)	(0.0183)	(0.0218)	
Number of family members	−0.00210	−0.0131 *	−0.0152	
	(0.00740)	(0.00697)	(0.0107)	
Log (Asset)	−0.00175	−0.00330	−0.00505	
	(0.00326)	(0.00308)	(0.00468)	
Log (Other family members' incomes)	0.00751	0.00588	0.0134	
	(0.00959)	(0.00787)	(0.0125)	
City job change rate	0.0721	0.00565	0.0778	0.0573
	(0.0624)	(0.0604)	(0.0893)	(0.175)
City average education	0.000592	−0.00572	−0.00513	0.00260
	(0.0100)	(0.0109)	(0.0151)	(0.0288)
City non-public employment rate	−0.0681	0.0374	−0.0307	−0.0813
	(0.0640)	(0.0548)	(0.0868)	(0.170)
Experience				0.00261
				(0.0153)
Experience square				−0.000370
				(0.000249)
Constant	2.017 ***	1.884 ***	3.901 ***	2.275 ***
	(0.130)	(0.139)	(0.196)	(0.578)
Observations	2492	2492	2492	2492
R-squared	0.570	0.578	0.591	0.773
Number of id	990	990	990	990
Health conditions	YES	YES	YES	YES
Year FE	YES	YES	YES	YES

Note: Columns (1), (2), (3), and (4) adopt city average commute time as an instrumental variable for individual commute time; Column (4) additionally adopts the interaction term of experience and age as an instrumental variable for hourly wage; Coefficients of year fixed effect and health conditions are not reported; Standard errors adjusted for clustering around individuals are in parentheses; *** $p < 0.01$, ** $p < 0.05$, * $p < 0.1$.

3.7. Additional Results: Male and Female Workers

Since females do more household work than males in China, commute time may have heterogeneous effects on labor supply for males and females. Tables 9 and 10 show results for job changed and unchanged workers, respectively, in which the interaction term of commute time and female dummy is controlled. Since this interaction term has an endogeneity problem, the interaction term of city average commute time and female dummy is used as an instrumental variable. Both tables show that gender does not play a role in the effect of commute time on labor supply.

Table 9. Labor supply and wage for job changed workers based on gender.

VARIABLES	(1) Log (Daily Workhours)	(2) Log (Workdays per Week)	(3) Log (Weekly Workhours)	(4) Log (Hourly Wage)
Log (Commute time) × Female dummy	0.00278	0.0183	0.0210	0.138
	(0.170)	(0.179)	(0.293)	(0.381)
Log (Commute time)	−0.0559	−0.253	−0.309	0.158
	(0.202)	(0.169)	(0.320)	(0.435)
Cigarette	0.0113	−0.0666	−0.0553	−0.0713
	(0.103)	(0.103)	(0.182)	(0.269)
Age	−0.00756	−0.00591	−0.0135	
	(0.00922)	(0.0113)	(0.0178)	
Number of children less than 6 years old	−0.0769	−0.0745	−0.151	
	(0.0829)	(0.0621)	(0.118)	
Number of family members	−0.0337	0.0410	0.00728	
	(0.0314)	(0.0338)	(0.0506)	
Log (Asset)	0.00233	−0.000140	0.00219	
	(0.0167)	(0.0152)	(0.0246)	
Log (Other family members' incomes)	−0.0455	0.0421	−0.00336	
	(0.0450)	(0.0465)	(0.0751)	
City job change rate	−0.172	−0.141	−0.313	0.979
	(0.308)	(0.353)	(0.523)	(0.823)
City average education	−0.0153	−0.0678	−0.0831	0.0628
	(0.0415)	(0.0489)	(0.0731)	(0.127)
City non-public employment rate	0.163	0.399	0.562	−0.388
	(0.257)	(0.261)	(0.453)	(0.500)
Experience				0.0708
				(0.0657)
Experience square				−0.00117
				(0.000921)
Constant	3.286 ***	2.760 ***	6.046 ***	−0.530
	(0.752)	(0.870)	(1.259)	(2.707)
Observations	296	296	296	296
R-squared	0.695	0.607	0.643	0.761
Number of id	139	139	139	139
Health conditions	YES	YES	YES	YES
Year FE	YES	YES	YES	YES

Note: Columns (1), (2), (3), and (4) adopt city average commute time as an instrumental variable for individual commute time; Column (4) additionally adopts the interaction term of experience and age as an instrumental variable for hourly wage; Coefficients of year fixed effect and health conditions are not reported; Standard errors adjusted for clustering around individuals are in parentheses; *** $p < 0.01$, ** $p < 0.05$, * $p < 0.1$.

Table 10. Labor supply and wage for job unchanged workers based on gender.

VARIABLES	(1) Log (Daily Workhours)	(2) Log (Workdays per Week)	(3) Log (Weekly Workhours)	(4) Log (Hourly Wage)
Log (Commute time) × Female dummy	−0.0396	0.0175	−0.0220	0.0187
	(0.0563)	(0.0511)	(0.0803)	(0.164)
Log (Commute time)	0.00438	−0.0547	−0.0503	−0.0799
	(0.0462)	(0.0590)	(0.0730)	(0.144)
Cigarette	0.0617 ***	0.0341 *	0.0958 ***	−0.122 *
	(0.0238)	(0.0183)	(0.0290)	(0.0648)
Age	0.000704	−3.61 × 10^{-5}	0.000668	
	(0.00289)	(0.00299)	(0.00413)	
Number of children less than 6 years old	−0.0347 **	0.0193	−0.0154	
	(0.0150)	(0.0187)	(0.0222)	
Number of family members	−0.00285	−0.0128 *	−0.0156	
	(0.00752)	(0.00706)	(0.0109)	
Log (Asset)	−0.00167	−0.00334	−0.00500	
	(0.00329)	(0.00310)	(0.00472)	
Log (Other family members' incomes)	0.00763	0.00583	0.0135	
	(0.00960)	(0.00783)	(0.0125)	
City job change rate	0.0654	0.00865	0.0740	0.0604
	(0.0647)	(0.0608)	(0.0906)	(0.178)
City average education	0.000185	−0.00554	−0.00535	0.00274
	(0.00999)	(0.0110)	(0.0151)	(0.0289)
City non-public employment rate	−0.0679	0.0373	−0.0306	−0.0812
	(0.0643)	(0.0549)	(0.0869)	(0.170)
Experience				0.00239
				(0.0154)
Experience square				−0.000369
				(0.000249)
Constant	2.023 ***	1.881 ***	3.905 ***	2.279 ***
	(0.130)	(0.139)	(0.196)	(0.580)
Observations	2492	2492	2492	2492
R-squared	0.570	0.578	0.591	0.773
Number of id	990	990	990	990
Health conditions	YES	YES	YES	YES
Year FE	YES	YES	YES	YES

Note: Columns (1), (2), (3), and (4) adopt city average commute time as an instrumental variable for individual commute time; Column (4) additionally adopts the interaction term of experience and age as an instrumental variable for hourly wage; Coefficients of year fixed effect and health conditions are not reported; Standard errors adjusted for clustering around individuals are in parentheses; *** $p < 0.01$, ** $p < 0.05$, * $p < 0.1$.

4. Discussions

One of the main findings of this paper is that commute time does not have significant effect on daily workhours but significantly reduces workdays per week and weekly workhours. This result is different from findings in Germany and Spain, in which commute time significantly increases daily workhours. In addition, our results also differ from the findings in Germany that show commute time slightly increases weekly workhours but does not affect the number of workdays.

One reason for the different patterns might relate to the methodology. The study for Germany considers an employer-induced change in workplace location and thus uses an exogenous individual commute time. In the study for Spain, the endogeneity of individual commute time is corrected by using the prices of an individual's house. Given the availability of the data, in this paper, we use the city average commute time as the instrumental variable to correct the endogeneity. Although we employ a distinct methodology compared with the studies for Germany and Spain, given the discussion on the instrumental variable in this paper, our methodology is valid and effective for the understanding of the causal effect of commute time. Consequently, the different methodologies might not be the main reason for the heterogeneous effects of commute time on daily labor supply found in Germany, Spain, and China.

Another reason might be the different degrees of competition intensity among workers in the labor market. In Germany and Spain, the competition intensity among workers is relatively low compared to China. In such circumstances, workers might have stronger bargaining power and accordingly have the possibility to discuss the number of working hours when they sign a working contract with employers. If workers have to suffer a longer commute time, they may choose to work longer in a working day and work fewer days in a week in order to lower the total cost of the commute time in a week. In this scenario, the longer commute time may increase the daily workhours, which is the case in Germany and Spain. However, the competition among workers is more intense in China than Germany and Spain. Workers in China have very limited bargaining power and have to follow job requirements strictly according to the willingness of employers. Thus, we may observe in China that a longer commute time of workers does not significantly affect the daily workhours. In addition, as workers have more flexibility in choosing a job with the desired number of working days in China, a longer commute time may decrease the number of working days in a week and hence the number of weekly workhours.

According to our preliminary insights about how commute time affects labor supply in urban China, we can identify the following policy implications for the promotion of active commuting. In Germany and Spain, as an increase in commute time has positive effects on labor supply, the economic consequences of active commuting will not be a big issue. However, as the weekly labor supply will be reduced by a longer commute time in urban China, the promotion of active commuting might be detrimental to the economic development to some extent. Therefore, local governments in China should invest more in transportation infrastructure, for instance, building more exclusive bike lanes and sidewalks. In this way, better infrastructure can not only encourage people to choose active commuting, but also shorten the commute time effectively and mitigate the potential adverse effects of active commuting.

Further, because we observe that the negative effect of commute time is particularly strong and significant for job changed workers, it might be more efficient to give priority to the infrastructure investments mentioned above in urban areas where house rental is more active.

5. Conclusions

This paper investigates the impact of commute time on labor supply in urban China and discusses the implications for the promotion of active commuting. Based on the CHNS panel data, we measure labor supply by daily workhours, workdays per week, and weekly workhours, using the analytical framework of combining a fixed effect model and instrumental variables. The main findings can be summarized as follows.

First, in contrast with existing empirical evidence from Germany and Spain, the effect of commute time on daily labor supply is insignificant in urban China. Furthermore, commute time decreases workdays per week and weekly workhours. These distinct patterns might closely relate to the different degrees of competition intensity among workers in labor markets. Second, commute time does not have a significant effect on labor supply for job unchanged workers, while the effect of commute time on workdays per week is large and statistically significant for job changed workers. Since job changed workers can choose a new job with different job characteristics, commute time will have a strong effect. Third, there is no statistically significant difference in the effects of commute time on labor supply between males and females. In addition, smoking is found to have a negative effect on hourly wage and positive effects on daily and weekly workhours. The former may relate to the fact that smoking can impact health and then reduce labor productivity, while the latter may relate to the possibility that smoking represents ambition and a smoking person has a strong incentive to work. Finally, policy implications for promoting active commuting are discussed.

Author Contributions: J.G. designed the empirical study; X.W., J.G. and C.W. performed the empirical study; X.W., J.G. and C.W. wrote the paper. All authors have read and agreed to the published version of the manuscript.

Funding: This research was funded by School of Economics and Management, Beihang University.

Conflicts of Interest: The authors declare no conflict of interest.

References

1. Gutiérrez-i-Puigarnau, E.; van Ommeren, J.N. Labor supply and commuting. *J. Urban Econ.* **2010**, *68*, 82–89. [CrossRef]
2. Van Ommeren, J.N.; Gutiérrez-i-Puigarnau, E. Are workers with a long commute less productive? An empirical analysis of absenteeism. *Reg. Sci. Urban Econ.* **2011**, *41*, 1–8. [CrossRef]
3. Commuting Time and Labor Supply: A Causal Effect? IZA Discussion Paper No. 5529. 2011. Available online: https://www.iza.org/publications/dp/5529/commuting-time-and-labour-supply-a-causal-effect (accessed on 19 December 2019).
4. Cogan, J.F. Fixed costs and labor supply. *Econometrica* **1981**, *49*, 945–963. [CrossRef]
5. Parry, I.W.H.; Bento, A. Revenue recycling and the welfare effects of road pricing. *Scand. J. Econ.* **2001**, *103*, 645–671. [CrossRef]
6. Gershenson, S. The causal effect of commute time on labor supply: Evidence from a natural experieenceeriment involving substitute teachers. *Transp. Res. Part A Policy Pract.* **2013**, *54*, 127–140. [CrossRef]
7. Black, D.A.; Kolesnikova, N.; Taylor, L.J. Why do so few women work in New York (and so many in Minneapolis)? Labor supply of married women across US cities. *J. Urban Econ.* **2014**, *79*, 59–71. [CrossRef]
8. White, M.J. Location choice and commuting behavior in cities with decentralized employment. *J. Urban Econ.* **1988**, *24*, 129–152. [CrossRef]
9. Hamilton, B.W. Wasteful commuting again. *J. Political Econ.* **1989**, *97*, 1497–1504. [CrossRef]
10. Hamilton, B.W.; Röell, A. Wasteful commuting. *J. Political Econ.* **1982**, *90*, 1035–1053. [CrossRef]
11. Small, K.A.; Song, S. "Wasteful" commuting: A resolution. *J. Political Econ.* **1992**, *100*, 888–898. [CrossRef]
12. White, M.J. Urban commuting journeys are not "wasteful". *J. Political Econ.* **1988**, *96*, 1097–1110. [CrossRef]

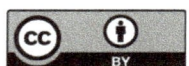

© 2020 by the authors. Licensee MDPI, Basel, Switzerland. This article is an open access article distributed under the terms and conditions of the Creative Commons Attribution (CC BY) license (http://creativecommons.org/licenses/by/4.0/).

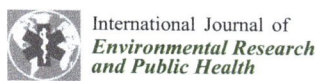

Article

Everyday Pedelec Use and Its Effect on Meeting Physical Activity Guidelines

Hedwig T. Stenner *, Johanna Boyen, Markus Hein, Gudrun Protte, Momme Kück, Armin Finkel, Alexander A. Hanke and Uwe Tegtbur

Institute of Sports Medicine, Hannover Medical School, 30625 Hanover, Germany;
boyen.johanna@mh-hannover.de (J.B.); 1.markushein@gmail.com (M.H.); gudrun.protte@gawnet.ch (G.P.);
kueck.momme@mh-hannover.de (M.K.); armin.finkel@gmx.de (A.F.);
Hanke.Alexander@mh-hannover.de (A.A.H.); tegtbur.uwe@mh-hannover.de (U.T.)
* Correspondence: stenner.hedwig@mh-hannover.de; Tel.: +49-511-532-5499

Received: 15 May 2020; Accepted: 30 June 2020; Published: 3 July 2020

Abstract: Pedelecs (e-bikes with electrical support up to 25 km·h^{-1}) are important in active transportation. Yet, little is known about physiological responses during their everyday use. We compared daily pedelec (P) and bicycle (B) use to determine if pedelecs are a suitable tool to enhance physical activity. In 101 employees, cycling duration and intensity, heart rate (HR) during P and B were recorded via a smartphone app. Each recording period was a randomized crossover design and lasted two weeks. The ride quantity was higher in P compared to B (5.3 ± 4.3 vs. 3.2 ± 4.0 rides·wk^{-1}; $p < 0.001$) resulting in a higher total cycling time per week for P (174 ± 146 min·wk^{-1}) compared to B (99 ± 109 min·wk^{-1}; $p < 0.001$). The mean HR during P was lower than B (109 ± 14 vs. 118 ± 17 bpm; $p < 0.001$). The perceived exertion was lower in P (11.7 ± 1.8 vs. 12.8 ± 2.1 in B; $p < 0.001$). The weekly energy expenditure was higher during P than B (717 ± 652 vs. 486 ± 557 metabolic equivalents of the task [MET]·min·wk^{-1}; $p < 0.01$). Due to a sufficient HR increase in P, pedelecs offer a more active form of transportation to enhance physical activity.

Keywords: active transportation; heart rate; pedelec; e-bike; cycling

1. Introduction

Insufficient physical activity and sedentary behavior are major risk factors for death from cardiovascular diseases, cancer, and diabetes worldwide [1]. The positive effects of physical activity have prompted leading health organizations to create activity guidelines to benefit health. However, globally, 25% of adults do not meet recommendations for physical activity [1]. Physical activity is important for all ages and should be integrated into daily life; for example, the workplace is a key setting where sedentary behavior can be reduced [2]. As active forms of transportation and commuting become more popular, a trip to and from the workplace offers the potential for increased productivity and a reduction in injuries and absenteeism [3,4]. The American College of Sports Medicine (ACSM) guidelines include cardiorespiratory exercise training of ≥150 min·wk^{-1} moderate-intensity (64–76% of maximum heart rate (HR$_{max}$), or 3–5.9 MET) or ≥75 min·wk^{-1} vigorous-intensity (77–95% HR$_{max}$ or 6–8.7 MET), or a combination of both, respectively [5].

In the course last decade, there has been a great deal of technological progress in the bicycle market with an increased number of pedelecs [6]. The number of pedelecs sold in Germany has steadily increased in recent years. In 2017, there were 720,000; in 2018, that number reached 980,000, which is an increase of 36% compared to the previous year [7]. Pedelecs are bicycles with electrical motor supports that can be gradually added. The motor is only active as long as the rider pedals, supporting a speed up to 25 km/h^{-1}. At higher speeds, the work has to be done by the rider alone. The assumed advantages of a pedelec vs. a normal bicycle are shorter travel times, longer travel distances, and a higher number of trips. For longer commuting distances, challenging weather conditions, or the transportation of heavy loads, pedelecs are becoming increasingly popular [8,9].

However, current knowledge about the positive health effects of pedelecs usage remains sparse. Questionnaire studies show that pedelec trip distances were significantly longer compared with bicycles, but that physical activity levels were similar. This suggests that pedelec users may compensate for the lower exertion per kilometer by traveling for longer distances [10,11].

The physiological response of pedelec use in experimental studies shows increasing physical fitness, meeting physical activity recommendations determined by questionnaires, and in a laboratory setting for pedelec use [12]. Our goal is, however, to measure the physiological adjustments in everyday use.

We hypothesize that pedelec usage produces similar health-promoting effects compared with adult employees' bicycle usage. Therefore, pedelecs are a suitable tool to enhance physical activity. Thus, the primary outcome was the total pedelec ride time minutes per week and the achieved heart rate, compared to bicycle rides.

Furthermore, we aimed to compare the results to ACSM guidelines for physical activities [5].

2. Materials and Methods

2.1. Study Design

The study was planned as an observational crossover study. To address the two different workplace settings of blue and white-collar workers, four different companies from Hanover, Germany, were chosen for the study. The employees were informed about the study via intranet, mail, and posters. Informative registration events were organized in the companies for interested employees. One hundred and nineteen volunteers were recruited. 101 (47 females, 54 males, age 43 ± 11 years, weight 82 ± 17 kg, for further details, see Table 1) were included in the study and met the following inclusion criteria: male and female workers between the ages of 18 and 65. Eighteen subjects were disqualified based on our exclusion criteria: diabetes, tumor diseases, coronary heart disease or arterial occlusive disease, unadjusted hypertension, an operation in the last eight weeks, a joint replacement six months prior to the study or suffering from other severe conditions counter indicating physical exercise. All participants were informed of the risks involved in this study and gave written informed consent prior to participation. The study protocol was approved by the ethics committee of Hannover Medical School (No. 6901-2015). The study was conducted in accordance with the Declaration of Helsinki.

Table 1. General subject information ($n = 101$). S1 and S2 display sequence association of S1: bicycle first vs. S2: pedelec first.

	All Mean ± SD	S1 Bicycle First Mean ± SD	S2 Pedelec First Mean ± SD	S1 vs. S2 p-Value
Gender (men/female)	54/47	27/24	27/23	0.915
Age (years)	43 ± 11	44 ± 12	42 ± 11	0.369
Height (cm)	174 ± 9	173 ± 9	175 ± 10	0.370
Bodyweight (kg)	82 ± 17	84 ± 19	81 ± 15	0.469
Body mass index (kg·m^{-2})	27.0 ± 4.8	27.6 ± 5.0	26.5 ± 4.4	0.218
Fat mass (%)	27 ± 9	28 ± 9	26 ± 9	0.381
Maximum Power output (W·kg^{-1})	2.6 ± 0.6	2.6 ± 0.7	2.6 ± 0.6	0.618
VO$_2$ peak (mL·kg^{-1}·min^{-1})	32 ± 8	32 ± 8	33 ± 8	0.674

VO$_2$ peak = Peak oxygen consumption.

2.2. Preliminary Physiological Testing

Before starting the study, all subjects visited the laboratory to undergo a brief physical examination by a physician. Additionally, body weight and body fat were determined using a direct-segmental multi-frequency bio-impedance scale (Inbody720, Biospace, Seoul, Korea). Height was measured using a stadiometer, and body weight was determined using a calibrated scale (Seca 764, seca GmbH & Co.

KG, Hamburg, Germany). Body Mass Index (BMI) was calculated as the ratio of weight (in kg)/squared standing height (m^2). Participants performed a graded exercise test on a cycle ergometer (Ergoselect 200, ergoline, Bitz, Germany). The test started at a workload of 20 W (for women) or 50 W (for men) for one minute and increased by 16.6 W every minute. Participants cycled until volitional exhaustion. Throughout the test, heart rate (HR) was recorded using a 12-channel-electrocardiogram (CardioSoft, GE Healthcare, Boston, USA) and respiratory gas exchange was measured breath-by-breath using an indirect calorimetry system (Masterscreen CPX, Becton Dickinson, Franklin Lakes, USA) HR and respiratory exchange values were averaged every 30 s. Peak oxygen consumption and maximum heart rate (HR$_{max}$) was determined as the highest 30 s average during the exercise test.

2.3. Flow Protocol and Randomization

The observational flow protocol is displayed in Figure 1. All subjects were randomly assigned to two-week pedelec or bicycle use in a randomized crossover design. Participants were randomized in every company 1:1 into the two groups (sequence 1 or sequence 2) using a previously computer-based list of random numbers generated by a collaborator. Detailed information on the sequences pictured in Figure 1. The participants were informed about the group assignment, due to the nature of the used hardware (especially the pedelec motor) blinding was impossible.

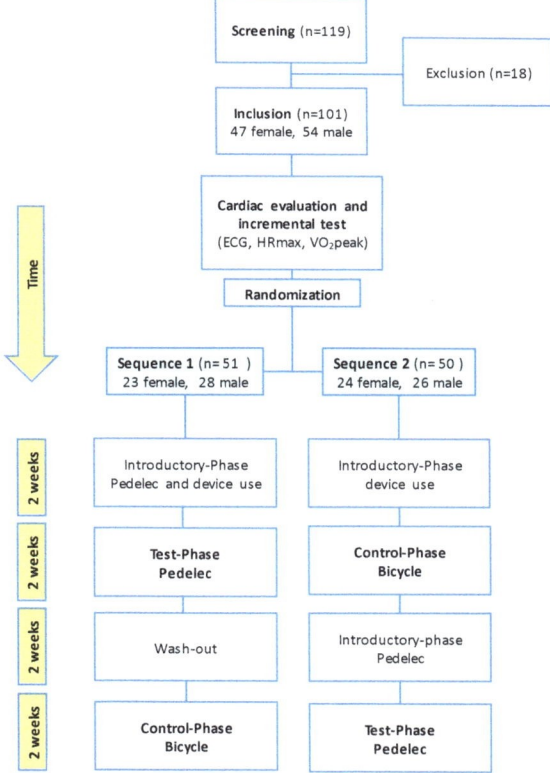

Figure 1. Flow chart of the study. Note the crossover design of sequences enabling each participant to be included in both groups, pedelec test group (P) and bicycle control group (B).

According to the participants' preferences, subjects were equipped with different pedelec models (city, trekking, mountain, carrier bikes). To eliminate the effect of curiosity, a two-week familiarization period with pedelecs was conducted before the recording period with the pedelec. To ensure that pedelec use did not have any effects on bicycle use, all subjects who started with the pedelec had a two weeks washout phase without pedelec before activities with the bicycle were recorded (Figure 1).

2.4. Trip Documentation via Monitoring Tools

Subjects recorded HR, duration, and perceived exertion of cycling digitally and in paper form during both observation periods. HR and Borg-scale were recorded via a smartphone app and a chest strap (Polar H7 Bluetooth smart, Polar, Kempele, Finland). The app was exclusively developed for this study (Inside m2m GmbH, Garbsen, Germany). Furthermore, an activity monitor (ActiGraph GT9X Link, Actigraph, Pensacola, FL, USA) was worn for assessing daily activity. The data were recorded via the app and transferred directly to an MHH database and saved on an internal university server. To detect changes in daily physical activity, participants were instructed to wear an activity monitor for the whole day during both periods. Activity monitor data were recorded in 1-min epochs. A wear time validation algorithm was used [13] and physical activity intensity was divided into two categories by a cut-off value of 1951 counts: sedentary to light ($\leq$1951 counts) and moderate to very vigorous ($\geq$1952 counts) [14]. The activity monitor had to be worn for $\geq$10 h day^{-1} to be considered a valid wear day [15]. Only subjects with $\geq$7 valid wear days in both observation periods were included in activity monitor analysis.

2.5. Measured Parameters

The duration of physical activity was recorded in one-minute intervals. Rating of perceived exertion (RPE) was given on the basis of the Borg-scale [16]. HR for a trip was calculated as average (without zeroes) over the duration of the trip. If more than 50% of the HR data were missing for a single trip, the trip was not taken into account for HR analysis. In 88 pedelec users (87%) and 62 bicycle users (61%), data sets were fully received.

2.6. Intensity Calculation

Regularly, MET calculation is based on oxygen consumption (VO_2) during individuals' exercise testing. During daily biking, we were not able to directly measure VO_2. Thus, we calculated MET based on HR and VO_2 derived from data of the graded exercise test. To estimate VO_2 (mL/min/kg) for a given heart rate, the following equation was calculated using linear regression:

$$VO2 = 0.23 \times HR - 1.72(\text{sex}) + 0.05(\text{age}) - 8.63 \qquad (1)$$

with the factor 1 for men (sex = 1) and factor 2 for women (sex = 2). Therefrom exercise intensity in MET was calculated by dividing VO_2 with 3.5 mL/min/kg (equals 1 MET).

2.7. Statistical Analysis

Following a Kolmogorov–Smirnov test to verify normal distribution of the data, a student's paired *t*-test was performed to analyze differences between P and B. The differences in intensity for all rides classified by %HR$_{max}$ were analyzed with an unpaired student's *t*-test. Values are presented as mean ± standard deviation (SD). An alpha of $p < 0.05$ was considered to be statistically significant. All analyses were carried out with the SPSS software package for Windows® (Version 24, IBM Corp., Armonk, NY, USA).

3. Results

3.1. Trip Documentation/Monitoring

Randomized sequencing did not affect ride time. Pedelec ride time, as well as bicycle ride time, did not show significant differences Pedelec time Sequence (S1 vs. S2: $p = 0.26$, bicycle time S1 vs. S2:

$p = 0.31$). Total ride time was 35 ± 61% lower in B than in P ($p > 0.001$; Figure 2, Table 2). The number of trips was higher with P than B (5.3 ± 4.3 to 3.2 ± 4.0 trips·wk^{-1}) ($p < 0.001$). Average trip duration did not differ between P and B (37.5 ± 23.5 to 40.3 ± 27.8 min/trip) ($p = 0.45$). During the two-week observation periods, 91% of the subjects used the provided pedelec and 69% used their own bicycle.

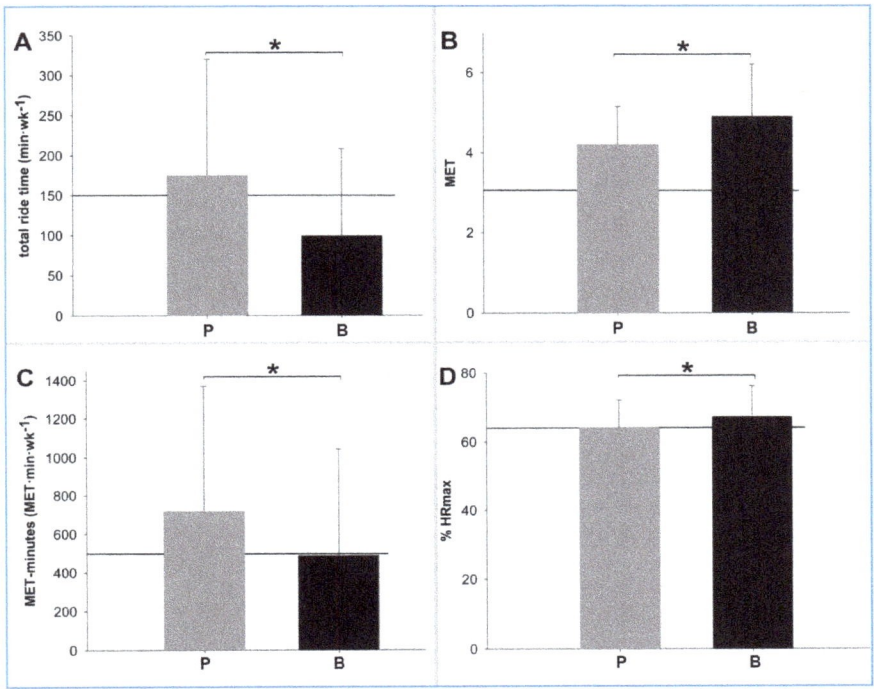

Figure 2. (**A**) Total ride time; (**B**) single trip intensity; (**C**) weekly metabolic rate; (**D**) mean intensity classified by %HR$_{max}$; P—light grey: During pedelec use; B—dark grey: Bicycle use; The solid line shows the minimum requirements for moderate-intensity exercise as recommended by the ACSM; Significant differences between activity types ($p < 0.05$) are marked with a *.

Table 2. Further results.

	P Mean ± SD	B Mean ± SD	*p*-Value
Number of trips (wk^{-1})	5.3 ± 4.3	3.2 ± 4.0	$p < 0.001$
Trip duration (min)	37.5 ± 23.5	40.3 ± 27.8	$p = 0.45$
Total ride time (min·wk^{-1})	174 ± 146	99 ± 109	$p < 0.001$

The distance from the participant's home to their work was divided as follows: 1–3 km 7%, >3–5 km 13%, >5–10 km 15%, >10 km 18%, >20 km 31%, >50 km 16%.

Daily activity monitor wear time did not differ between the two observation periods (P 856 ± 72 min, B 864 ± 62 min, $p = 0.28$).

3.2. Measured Parameters

Daily activity time in the category sedentary to light did not show significant differences between the observation periods (P 805 ± 79 min, B 810 ± 77 min, $p = 0.63$) nor did moderate to vigorous activity (P 50.9 ± 35.0 min, B 54.3 ± 47.7 min, $p = 0.50$).

Mean HR was 8 ± 13% lower during P than B (109 ± 14 vs., $p < 0.001$) 118 ± 17 bpm. In both groups, %HR_{max} was in the range of ACSM recommendations [9] for both (Figure 2, Table 2).

Subjects perceived exertion was lower during P than during B (Borg-scale: 11.7 ± 1.8 to 12.8 ± 2.1, $n = 70$) ($p < 0.001$).

3.3. Calculated Intensity

Metabolic rate calculated from absolute HR during rides was lower in P than B, but sufficient to meet ACSM recommendations [9] for moderate-intensity in both (Figure 2). Energy expenditure expressed as the weekly metabolic rate was higher during P than during B ($p < 0.01$), meeting ACSM recommendations [9] in P but not in B (Figure 2, Table 2).

4. Discussion

Pedelec use requires similar physical effort as bicycle use, and therefore it is a suitable tool to enhance health-promoting physical activity. B achieved 35% less total time than P with 99 ± 109 min·wk^{-1}. When riding P, the HF was only 8% lower than during B at 109 ± 14 bpm.

While both groups met ACSM criteria for moderate activity with respect to mean HR, total ride time was significantly less in B without achieving the recommended activity time of 150 min·wk^{-1}.

However, taking MET and MET- min·wk^{-1} into account, our data clearly support that even though P usage is less exhausting than B (as described by lower MET) in our population, the total MET minutes per week were even higher in P as compared to B.

The results of our study suggest that pedelecs are used more often than normal bicycles in everyday use when no usage specifications are made. Similar observations have been made by Fyhri and Fearnley, who showed an increase of trips with the pedelec compared to the bicycle [17]. However, while more trips were executed, the average duration per trip showed no significant difference. We, therefore, assume that the participants mainly used the pedelecs for the same routes as the bicycles, but more often. This finding indicates that commuting and day-to-day tasks (e.g., grocery shopping), rather than additional recreational trips, were the main usage purpose.

Volume and intensity are the two parameters to evaluate if physical activity is sufficient to expect health promotion effects. Several other studies already showed that the heart rate during single trips with the pedelec can be classified as moderate by ACSM standards [17,18], and the pedelec was therefore assumed to be a promising mode meeting physical activity guidelines [18]. Our study is one of the first where no minimum riding requirements were made, and cardiorespiratory intensity during real-world pedelec usage patterns was analyzed in a large cohort.

In accordance with previous studies, our data confirm that the average heart rate during everyday pedelec use was significantly lower than during cycling, but was still high enough to be classified as moderate by ACSM standards [5]. This was supported by the calculation of the metabolic costs of P which also classify it as moderate intensity, but significantly less intense than B. The lower intensity was also perceived by the subjects, resulting in the reporting of lower exertion during P. This has been observed in other studies as well [18–20]. Lower perceived exertion has been reported to be a motivation to replace other modes of transportation (e.g., car or public transport) by the pedelec [21] and might, therefore, be the main reasons for the higher usage pattern we observed with the pedelec [17].

Importantly the weekly metabolic rate was significantly higher during P than B, showing higher energy expenditure while pedelecs were used. This shows that the volume compensates for the lower intensity observed during P. We can, therefore, assume that pedelecs may have beneficial health effects as reported previously [4,22] and we can confirm previous assumptions that the pedelec is an alternative to the bicycle for fulfilling health care guidelines [19].

The absence of differences in general activity between the two observation periods can be explained by the fact that cycling activity is not accurately recorded by the Actigraph activity monitor [23,24]. Therefore, neither pedelec use nor cycling affects the recorded total daily activity. The participants still wore the device all day to make sure every activity was recorded. The absence of changes in general activity indicates that using the pedelec did not influence other physical activities as observed in other activity promoting interventions [25]. Our findings are in accordance with other studies, which showed that the additional activity with the pedelec did not reduce other physical activities [22]. Our participants were very active in addition to the pedelec/bicycle use as activity counts for moderate to very vigorous activity were higher than the activities observed in other studies [22]. Hence, even in generally active people, the pedelec can be a health-promoting active transportation mode.

Pedelec use can help to meet the recommendations for physical activity, despite motor support. This shows that the integration of pedelecs in the form of active transportation to work is an important resource and should be supported by employers.

Limitations

Although our study design included an introduction period where the participants got used to the pedelec, two weeks might have been not enough time to eliminate the effect of curiosity. Equipping the participants with GPS devices would have given our study further benefits in making pedelec and bicycle trips more comparable regarding speed, distance, and altitude. Recording the support level during the pedelec rides would have given further inside into the actual usage behavior as well. A further limitation is the relatively high number of participants who did not record heart rate during the trips due to technical limitations and based on measurements throughout the year with corresponding seasonal weather differences. For further studies, we, therefore, recommend easier to handle and more accepted options of heart rate recording, e.g., photoplethysmographic measurement on the wrist. As we only examined a two-week period, further research is necessary to clarify if the observed effects endure over longer time periods and a larger study population.

The examined population showed BMI and fat values slightly above desirable normal range but within average ranges in Germany, and thus, effects should be comparable to the general population.

5. Conclusions

On the basis of a real-world setting, our study showed that pedelecs could be a suitable method to enhance health-promoting physical activity in healthy adults. While the average physiological response is high enough to achieve beneficial adaptions, individual preconditions need to be taken into account for every pedelec user. As we only examined a two-week period, further research is necessary to clarify if the observed effects endure over longer time periods.

Author Contributions: Data curation, H.T.S. and A.F.; formal analysis, M.K. and M.H.; funding acquisition, U.T.; investigation, H.T.S., J.B., M.H., G.P. and A.F.; methodology, U.T.; project administration, U.T.; resources, U.T.; software, M.K.; validation, M.K.; visualization, A.A.H.; writing—original draft, H.T.S. and M.H.; writing—review and editing, H.T.S., J.B., M.H., G.P., A.A.H. and U.T. All authors have read and agreed to the published version of the manuscript.

Funding: Funding for the study was provided by the Bundesministerium für Bildung und Forschung Grant 16SNI012D. The results of the study are presented clearly, honestly, and without fabrication, falsification, or inappropriate data manipulation. The authors thank the participants for dedicating their time. Furthermore, we acknowledge support by the Open Access Publication Fund of Hannover Medical School (MHH) to cover publication fees.

Acknowledgments: The authors thank the participants for dedicating their time.

Conflicts of Interest: The authors declare no conflict of interest.

References

1. World Health Organization (WHO) Physical Activity. Available online: http://www.who.int/mediacentre/factsheets/fs385/en/ (accessed on 15 May 2020).
2. WHO. *Global Action Plan on Physical Activity 2018–2030: More Active People for a Healthier World*; World Health Organization: New York, NY, USA, 2018; ISBN 978-92-4-151418-7.
3. van Dongen, J.M.; Proper, K.I.; van Wier, M.F.; van der Beek, A.J.; Bongers, P.M.; van Mechelen, W.; van Tulder, M.W. Systematic review on the financial return of worksite health promotion programmes aimed at improving nutrition and/or increasing physical activity. *Obes. Rev. Off. J. Int. Assoc. Study Obes.* **2011**, *12*, 1031–1049. [CrossRef]
4. de Geus, B.; De Smet, S.; Nijs, J.; Meeusen, R. Determining the intensity and energy expenditure during commuter cycling. *Br. J. Sports Med.* **2007**, *41*, 8–12. [CrossRef]
5. Garber, C.E.; Blissmer, B.; Deschenes, M.R.; Franklin, B.A.; Lamonte, M.J.; Lee, I.-M.; Nieman, D.C.; Swain, D.P. American College of Sports Medicine position stand. Quantity and quality of exercise for developing and maintaining cardiorespiratory, musculoskeletal, and neuromotor fitness in apparently healthy adults: Guidance for prescribing exercise. *Med. Sci. Sports Exerc.* **2011**, *43*, 1334–1359. [CrossRef] [PubMed]
6. Rose, G. E-bikes and urban transportation: Emerging issues and unresolved questions. *Transportation* **2012**, *39*, 81–96. [CrossRef]
7. Zweirad-Industrie-Verband, E.V. Zahlen–Daten–Fakten zum Deutschen E-Bike-Markt 2018–2019. Available online: https://www.ziv-zweirad.de/fileadmin/redakteure/Downloads/PDFs/PM_2020_11.03._Fahrrad-_und_E-Bike_Markt_2019.pdf (accessed on 1 June 2020).
8. MacArthur, J.; Dill, J.; Person, M. Electric Bikes in North America: Results of an Online Survey. *Transp. Res. Rec. J. Transp. Res. Board* **2014**, *2468*, 123–130. [CrossRef]
9. Haustein, S.; Møller, M. Age and attitude: Changes in cycling patterns of different e-bike user segments. *Int. J. Sustain. Transp.* **2016**, *10*, 836–846. [CrossRef]
10. Castro, A.; Gaupp-Berghausen, M.; Dons, E.; Standaert, A.; Laeremans, M.; Clark, A.; Anaya-Boig, E.; Cole-Hunter, T.; Avila-Palencia, I.; Rojas-Rueda, D.; et al. Physical activity of electric bicycle users compared to conventional bicycle users and non-cyclists: Insights based on health and transport data from an online survey in seven European cities. *Transp. Res. Interdiscip. Perspect.* **2019**, *1*, 100017. [CrossRef]
11. Nordengen, S.; Ruther, D.C.; Riiser, A.; Andersen, L.B.; Solbraa, A. Correlates of Commuter Cycling in Three Norwegian Counties. *Int. J. Environ. Res. Public. Health* **2019**, *16*, 4372. [CrossRef] [PubMed]
12. Bourne, J.E.; Sauchelli, S.; Perry, R.; Page, A.; Leary, S.; England, C.; Cooper, A.R. Health benefits of electrically-assisted cycling: A systematic review. *Int. J. Behav. Nutr. Phys. Act.* **2018**, *15*, 116. [CrossRef]
13. Choi, L.; Liu, Z.; Matthews, C.E.; Buchowski, M.S. Validation of accelerometer wear and nonwear time classification algorithm. *Med. Sci. Sports Exerc.* **2011**, *43*, 357–364. [CrossRef] [PubMed]
14. Freedson, P.S.; Melanson, E.; Sirard, J. Calibration of the Computer Science and Applications, Inc. accelerometer. *Med. Sci. Sports Exerc.* **1998**, *30*, 777–781. [CrossRef] [PubMed]
15. Troiano, R.P.; McClain, J.J.; Brychta, R.J.; Chen, K.Y. Evolution of accelerometer methods for physical activity research. *Br. J. Sports Med.* **2014**, *48*, 1019–1023. [CrossRef] [PubMed]
16. Borg, G. Psychophysical scaling with applications in physical work and the perception of exertion. *Scand. J. Work. Environ. Health* **1990**, *16*, 55–58. [CrossRef] [PubMed]
17. Fyhri, A.; Fearnley, N. Effects of e-bikes on bicycle use and mode share. *Transp. Res. Part Transp. Environ.* **2015**, *36*, 45–52. [CrossRef]
18. Gojanovic, B.; Welker, J.; Iglesias, K.; Daucourt, C.; Gremion, G. Electric bicycles as a new active transportation modality to promote health. *Med. Sci. Sports Exerc.* **2011**, *43*, 2204–2210. [CrossRef]
19. Simons, M.; Van Es, E.; Hendriksen, I. Electrically assisted cycling: A new mode for meeting physical activity guidelines? *Med. Sci. Sports Exerc.* **2009**, *41*, 2097–2102. [CrossRef]
20. Sperlich, B.; Zinner, C.; Hébert-Losier, K.; Born, D.-P.; Holmberg, H.-C. Biomechanical, cardiorespiratory, metabolic and perceived responses to electrically assisted cycling. *Eur. J. Appl. Physiol.* **2012**, *112*, 4015–4025. [CrossRef]
21. Paul, F.; Bogenberger, K. Evaluation-method for a Station Based Urban-pedelec Sharing System. *Transp. Res. Procedia* **2014**, *4*, 482–493. [CrossRef]

22. Peterman, J.E.; Morris, K.L.; Kram, R.; Byrnes, W.C. Pedelecs as a physically active transportation mode. *Eur. J. Appl. Physiol.* **2016**, *116*, 1565–1573. [CrossRef]
23. Herman Hansen, B.; Børtnes, I.; Hildebrand, M.; Holme, I.; Kolle, E.; Anderssen, S.A. Validity of the ActiGraph GT1M during walking and cycling. *J. Sports Sci.* **2014**, *32*, 510–516. [CrossRef]
24. Steeves, J.A.; Bowles, H.R.; McClain, J.J.; Dodd, K.W.; Brychta, R.J.; Wang, J.; Chen, K.Y. Ability of thigh-worn ActiGraph and activPAL monitors to classify posture and motion. *Med. Sci. Sports Exerc.* **2015**, *47*, 952–959. [CrossRef] [PubMed]
25. Mansoubi, M.; Pearson, N.; Biddle, S.J.H.; Clemes, S.A. Using Sit-to-Stand Workstations in Offices: Is There a Compensation Effect? *Med. Sci. Sports Exerc.* **2016**, *48*, 720–725. [CrossRef] [PubMed]

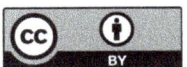

© 2020 by the authors. Licensee MDPI, Basel, Switzerland. This article is an open access article distributed under the terms and conditions of the Creative Commons Attribution (CC BY) license (http://creativecommons.org/licenses/by/4.0/).

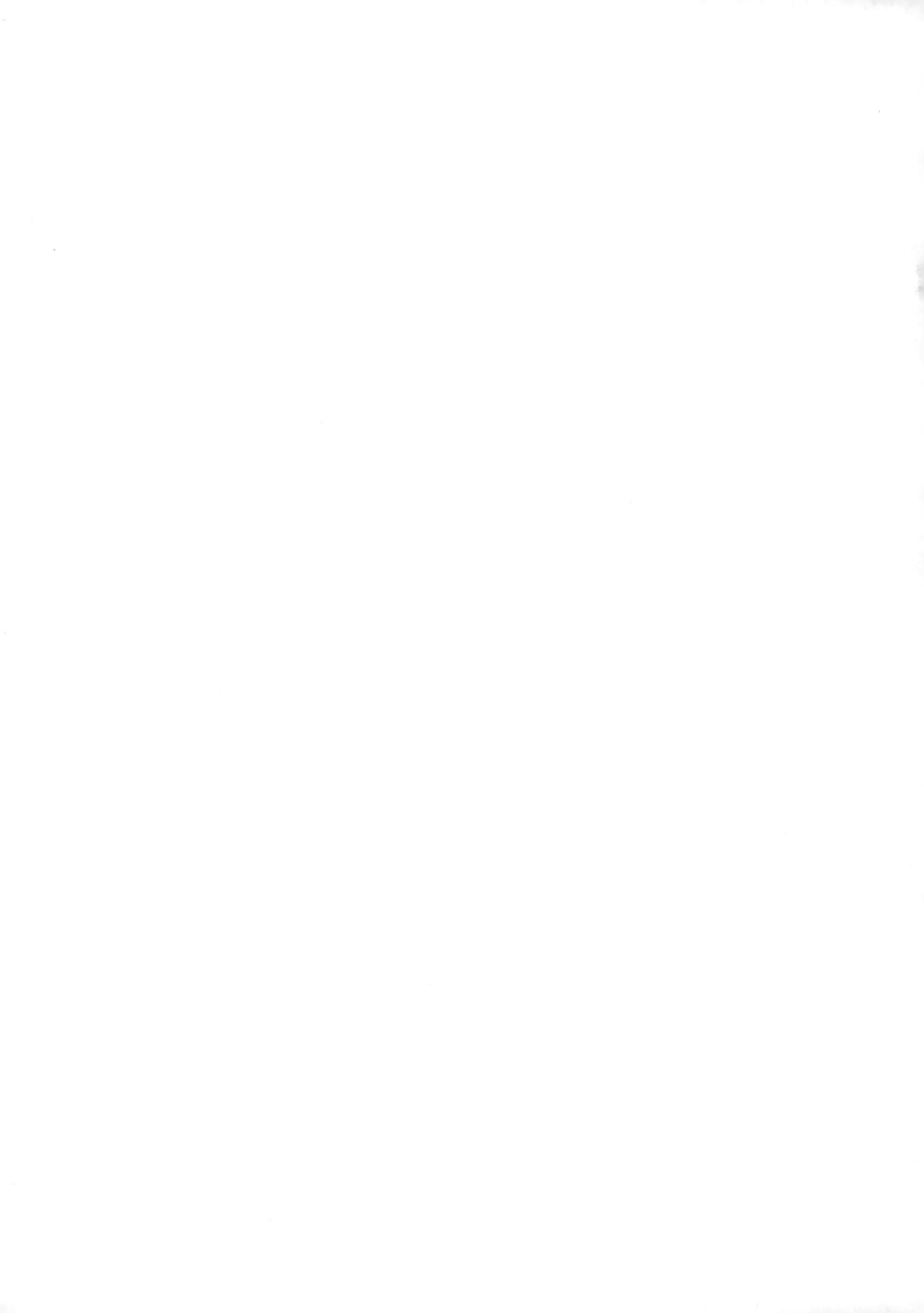

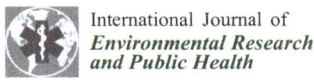 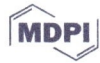

Article

Profiles of Active Transportation among Children and Adolescents in the Global Matrix 3.0 Initiative: A 49-Country Comparison

Silvia A. González [1,2,*], Salomé Aubert [1], Joel D. Barnes [1], Richard Larouche [1,3] and Mark S. Tremblay [1,2]

1. Healthy Active Living and Obesity Research Group, Children's Hospital of Eastern Ontario Research Institute, Ottawa, ON K1H 8L1, Canada; saubert@cheo.on.ca (S.A.); j@barnzilla.ca (J.D.B.); richard.larouche@uleth.ca (R.L.); mtremblay@cheo.on.ca (M.S.T.)
2. School of Epidemiology and Public Health, Faculty of Medicine, University of Ottawa, Ottawa, ON K1G 5Z3, Canada
3. Faculty of Health Sciences, University of Lethbridge, 4401 University Drive, Lethbridge, AB T1K 3M4, Canada
* Correspondence: sa.gonzalez68@uniandes.edu.co; Tel.: +1-613-9818332

Received: 27 June 2020; Accepted: 14 August 2020; Published: 18 August 2020

Abstract: This article aims to compare the prevalence of active transportation among children and adolescents from 49 countries at different levels of development. The data was extracted from the Report Cards on Physical Activity for Children and Youth from the 49 countries that participated in the Global Matrix 3.0 initiative. Descriptive statistics and a latent profile analysis with active transportation, Human Development Index and Gini index as latent variables were conducted. The global average grade was a "C", indicating that countries are succeeding with about half of children and youth (47–53%). There is wide variability in the prevalence and in the definition of active transportation globally. Three different profiles of countries were identified based on active transportation grades, Human Development Index (HDI) and income inequalities. The first profile grouped very high HDI countries with low prevalence of active transport and low inequalities. The second profile grouped low and middle HDI countries with high prevalence of active transportation and higher inequalities. And the third profile was characterized by the relatively high prevalence of active transportation and more variability in the socioeconomic variables. Promising policies from countries under each profile were identified. A unified definition of active transportation and contextualized methods for its assessment are needed to advance in surveillance and practice.

Keywords: cycling; walking; health promotion; policy; latent profile analysis; surveillance

1. Introduction

The world is experiencing a crisis of physical inactivity with almost 80% of adolescents not achieving the recommended 60 min of daily moderate to vigorous physical activity for health [1]. In this context, transportation, as a daily necessity to move from one place to another, represents a promising domain to promote the accumulation of physical activity in children and adolescents in a convenient and habitual manner [2]. Specifically, active transportation to/from school is an opportunity to integrate physical activity into children's and adolescent's routines [3].

Active transportation comprises non-motorized travel modes like walking, cycling or riding a scooter, among others [4]. The use of these active modes leads not only to health benefits such as greater levels of cardiorespiratory fitness [3,5] and better cardiometabolic health indicators [6] among children who actively commute, but also to other co-benefits, such as better mental health outcomes [7,8], greater interaction with their environment [9], and reduced transportation-related emissions and pollution [10]. Despite these benefits, current evidence suggests that this behaviour is declining in many countries [11].

In the same way that physical inactivity prevalence varies widely across countries [1], a wide variation in active transportation could be expected. These variations represent an opportunity to identify those countries that are succeeding with active transportation behaviours, and those that require action to increase active transportation or prevent a decline in this behaviour. However, to the best of our knowledge, the few international comparisons of data on active transportation among children and adolescents include mostly small groups of countries or the availability of national representative data is limited [11–13]. Therefore, the Global Matrix 3.0 of Report Card grades on physical activity among children and youth provides an opportunity to describe and examine the global situation of active transportation. For the first time, 49 countries from all continents reported data on an active transportation indicator at the national level [14]. The aims of this study were to compare the prevalence of active transportation among children and adolescents from 49 countries participating in the Global Matrix 3.0, to identify a set of profiles to group the countries according to their prevalence of active transport and sociodemographic variables, and to discuss policies and practices implemented across different countries to increase active transportation.

2. Materials and Methods

The Global Matrix 3.0 was an international initiative released in 2018 and led by the Active Healthy Kids Global Alliance (AHKGA). This project brought together 513 researchers and physical activity leaders from 49 countries around the world [15]. All the participating countries followed a harmonized process to develop Report Cards on the physical activity of children and youth. A detailed description of the countries' involvement and the process to develop the Report Cards has been published elsewhere and is briefly described here [14].

In each country, National Report Card Committees gathered the best and most recent national surveillance data available up to 2018 to inform and grade ten specific indicators related to physical activity among children and adolescents: Overall Physical Activity, Organized Sport and Physical Activity, Active Play, Active Transportation, Sedentary Behaviours, Physical Fitness, Family and Peers, School, Community and Environment, and Government [14]. The analyses presented in this paper are focused on the Active Transportation indicator.

According to the benchmarks proposed by AHKGA to harmonize and guide the development of the Report Cards, the Active Transportation indicator was described as the "percentage of children and youth who use active transportation to get to and from places (e.g., school, park, mall, friend's house)" [14]. Report card leaders were instructed to inform this indicator by the best, preferably nationally representative, data available for children and adolescents between five and 17 years, and a grade was assigned according to the prevalence following a common rubric established by the AHKGA (Table 1).

The prevalence of active transportation reported by each country and the related details presented in each Report Card, including policies, practices, strategies to improve the grade and research gaps, were extracted from the Report Cards and from related publications in English, Spanish or French, including brief reports, posters and peer-reviewed articles. These publications were reviewed, and relevant information was summarized by two of the authors of this manuscript. Based on the grades provided, numerical equivalents were assigned (Table 1), and average estimates of the grades for active transportation were calculated at the global level and by groups of countries according to their level of development determined by the Human Development Index (HDI). The HDI is a composite index created by the United Nations Development Programme (New York, NY, USA) to rank countries based on key dimensions of human development such as education, life expectancy and gross national income per capita [16]. HDI ranges from 0 to 1 and for the present analysis we used the continuous index and a categorical variable that classified countries in three categories: low and medium (HDI < 0.70), high (HDI ≥ 0.70 to <0.80) and very high (HDI ≥ 0.80) [16]. It was included as a variable of interest in this analysis based on the variability in active transportation observed across HDI clusters in previous analysis of the Global Matrix [14]. Also, the Gini index for each country was retrieved from the World Bank estimates. The Gini index provides a measure of inequality in income distribution. It ranges from 0 (perfect equality) to 100 (perfect inequality) [17]. The Gini index was included in this analysis considering previous international evidence that has shown that income inequality is a relevant variable related to physical activity levels and taking into account the importance of socioeconomic inequalities in transport as an essential activity for economic and social development [18,19].

Table 1. Global Matrix 3.0 grading rubric.

Grade	Interpretation [a]	Numerical Equivalents [b]
A+	94–100%	15
A	We are succeeding with a large majority of children and youth (87–93%)	14
A−	80–86%	13
B+	74–79%	12
B	We are succeeding with well over half of children and youth (67–73%)	11
B−	60–66%	10
C+	54–59%	9
C	We are succeeding with about half of children and youth (47–53%)	8
C−	40–46%	7
D+	34–39%	6
D	We are succeeding with less than half but some children and youth (27–33%)	5
D−	20–26%	4
F	We are succeeding with very few children and youth (<20%)	2
INC [c]	Incomplete—insufficient or inadequate information to assign a grade	

[a] For this article, the interpretation corresponds to the percentage of children and youth who use active transportation to get to and from places (e.g., school, park, mall, friend's house). [b] Letter grades were converted to numerical equivalents for analyses purposes. [c] INC: incomplete

A latent profile analysis (LPA) was conducted to identify groups or profiles of countries based on the numerical grades for active transportation and the two sociodemographic variables at the country level, the HDI and the Gini index. LPA is a probability-based statistical procedure that allows to identify classes or profiles that group observations sharing similar patterns of the variables of interest [20]. The analysis was performed to look for the best model solution for one to five possible profiles. Models were compared to choose the solution with the best fit based on the Akaike information criterion (AIC), sample-adjusted Bayesian information criterion (SABIC) and the bootstrapped likelihood ratio test (BLRT) as indicators of model fit. All statistical analyses were performed using SAS 9.4 (SAS Institute, Cary, NC, USA) and R (version 3.4.1, The R Foundation for Statistical Computing, Vienna, Austria). The tidyLPA package [21] was used for the LPA.

3. Results

A total of 47 countries (96%) in the Global Matrix 3.0 had sufficient evidence (determined by each country's National Report Card Committee) on active transportation to assign a grade. The grades ranged from "A−" in Japan, Nepal and Zimbabwe to "F" in Chile (Table 2). The global average for active transportation was "C". The average grade by HDI was "C+" for low to medium HDI countries, "C" for high HDI countries and "C−" for very high HDI countries, as previously reported by Aubert et al. [14]. The HDI of the included countries varied from 0.448 in Ethiopia to 0.985 in Jersey. According to the Gini index, the country with the most unequal distribution of income was South Africa with a Gini index of 63, while Slovenia had the lowest inequality score, with a Gini of 25.4 (Table 2).

Table 2. Active transportation grades and sociodemographic variables of the 49 countries participating in the Global Matrix 3.0.

Country	Active Transport Grade	Active Transport Numerical Grade	Human Development Index (HDI) [a]	HDI Classification	Gini Index [b]
Australia	D+	6	0.939	Very high	34.7
Bangladesh	C−	7	0.579	Low to medium	32.4
Belgium (Flanders)	C+	9	0.896	Very high	27.7
Botswana	C	8	0.698	Low to medium	60.5
Brazil	C	8	0.754	High	51.3
Bulgaria	B−	10	0.794	High	37.4
Canada	D−	4	0.920	Very high	34.0
Chile	F	2	0.847	Very high	47.7
China	C+	9	0.738	High	42.2
Colombia	B	11	0.727	High	50.8
Czech Republic	C+	9	0.878	Very high	25.9
Denmark	B+	12	0.925	Very high	28.2
Ecuador	C−	7	0.739	High	45.0
England	C−	7	0.909	Very high	33.2
Estonia	D	5	0.865	Very high	32.7
Ethiopia	C	8	0.448	Low to medium	39.1
Finland	B+	12	0.895	Very high	27.1
France	C−	7	0.897	Very high	32.7
Germany	C−	7	0.926	Very high	31.7
Ghana	C+	9	0.579	Low to medium	42.4
Guernsey Channel Islands	D	5	0.975	Very high	40.0
Hong Kong	B+	12	0.917	Very high	N/A
India	B−	10	0.624	Low to medium	35.1
Japan	A−	13	0.903	Very high	32.1
Jersey	D+	6	0.985	Very high	41.0
Lebanon	D	5	0.763	High	31.8
Lithuania	C−	7	0.848	Very high	37.4
Mexico	C+	9	0.762	High	43.4
Nepal	A−	13	0.558	Low to medium	32.8
Netherlands	B−	10	0.924	Very high	29.3
New Zealand	C−	7	0.915	Very high	N/A
Nigeria	B	11	0.527	Low to medium	43.0
Poland	C	8	0.855	Very high	31.8
Portugal	C−	7	0.843	Very high	35.5
Qatar	N/A	N/A	0.856	Very high	N/A
Scotland	C	8	0.909	Very high	33.2
Slovenia	C	8	0.890	Very high	25.4
South Africa	C	8	0.666	Low to medium	63.0
South Korea	B+	12	0.901	Very high	31.6
Spain	B−	10	0.884	Very high	36.2
Sweden	C	8	0.913	Very high	29.2
Taiwan	C−	7	0.885	Very high	33.6
Thailand	C	8	0.740	High	37.8
United Arab Emirates	INC	N/A	0.840	Very high	N/A
United States	D−	4	0.920	Very high	41.5

Table 2. *Cont.*

Country	Active Transport Grade	Active Transport Numerical Grade	Human Development Index (HDI) [a]	HDI Classification	Gini Index [b]
Uruguay	C	8	0.795	High	39.7
Venezuela	B−	10	0.767	High	46.9
Wales	D+	6	0.909	Very high	33.2
Zimbabwe	A−	13	0.516	Low to medium	43.2
Global average	C	8.29	NA	NA	NA
Low to medium HDI countries	C+	9.67	NA	NA	NA
High HDI countries	C	8.5	NA	NA	NA
Very high HDI counties	C−	7.78	NA	NA	NA

[a] Data at the national level from the United Nations Development Programme [16]. [b] Data at the national level from the World Bank [17]. Abbreviations: HDI, Human Development Index; INC, Incomplete, N/A, Not available; NA, Not Applicable.

Table 3 presents the prevalence and rationales behind the grades for each country, as well as the sources and characteristics of the information reported. Active transportation among children and adolescents varied between 15% in Chile and 86% in Japan and Nepal. Among the countries that assigned a grade for active transportation, 83% ($n = 39$) did not provide details of the prevalence stratified by sex. In the majority (62%) of countries that reported data by sex, the prevalence of active transportation was slightly higher for males. More than half of the countries (65%) reported data for both children and adolescents, however, the age groups included varied from one country to another. Most countries (87%) only included data on school trips, and only two countries (Ecuador and the United States) clearly reported active transportation to other destinations. Regarding the direction of the trips, about half of the countries (49%) reported active transportation to and from school or other destinations. In more than half of the countries (65%), the frequency of active transportation reported was not clear. The most common frequencies reported were "daily" ($n = 3$), "typically" or "usually" ($n = 3$) and "on a regular basis" ($n = 2$). Regarding the source of information, 64% ($n = 30$) of the countries used data from surveys and studies with national representativeness, 8.5% ($n = 4$) used local studies, and 19% ($n = 9$) used both local and national studies. International surveys such as the Global School-Based Student Health Survey (GSHS) [22] and the Health Behaviour of School-aged Children (HBSC) [23] were among the sources of information in seven countries.

The best LPA model grouped the Global Matrix 3.0 countries into three profiles according to the grades for active transportation, the HDI and the Gini index. The three-profile model had the best fit statistics according to the criteria proposed by Nylund et al. for model selection [24]. The preferred model showed the lowest values for the AIC (359.8), SABIC (331.1) and the BLRT (24.8), and a significant p value for the BLRT ($p = 0.041$). Table 4 shows the descriptive statistics for the latent variables among the three profiles identified. In profile 1 ($n = 25$) 72% of the countries had active transportation grades below "C", 96% of the countries had a very high HDI, and 72% had relatively low Gini indices (below 40). In profile 2 ($n = 7$), 85% of the countries had active transportation grades equal to or greater than "C", all of them had a low to medium HDI and 43% had Gini indices above 40. In profile 3 ($n = 17$), 94% of the countries had active transportation grades equal to or greater than "C", 53% had a high HDI and 35% had a very high HDI, and 47% had Gini indices above 40. For countries with missing values in any of the variables of interest, the LPA assigned a profile based on the values available for the remaining variables. Figure 1 presents a plot of the scaled data for the three profiles.

Table 3. Rationale for grades and information reported on active transportation by 49 countries involved in the Global Matrix 3.0.

Grade	Country	Rationale	Gender	Age	Destination and Direction	Frequency	Source of Information and Year	Profile
A−	Japan	86% of students used active transportation to school from home.	Not reported	6–17 years	To school	On a regular basis	The National Sports-Life Survey of Young People (SSF), 2015 [25]	3
A−	Nepal	86% of children and youth of 15–20 years used active transportation to get to and from places.	Not reported	15–20 years	Not specified	Not clear	Physical Activity Level and Associated Factors Among Higher Secondary School Students in Banke, Nepal: A Cross-Sectional Study, 2013 [26]	2
A−	Zimbabwe	Over 80% of children and adolescents used active transport to and from school, with variation between provinces as well as between rural and urban areas.	82% of girls and 79% of boys engaged in active transport to and from school	8–16 years	To and from School	Not clear	The Zimbabwe Baseline [27] and Global school-based health survey (GSHS) Zimbabwe 2003 [28]	2
B+	Denmark	78% of children and adolescents reported cycling, walking, or using children's scooters as transport (e.g., to school) at least two times per week.	Not reported	7–15 years	To school	At least two times per week	Danish Sports Habits Study 2016 [29]	3
B+	Finland	77% of children and adolescents actively commuted to school, on foot or by bike.	9 years old 79% of boys, 81% of girls 11 years old 85% of boys, 81% of girls 13 years old 80% of boys, 77% of girls 15 years old 59% of boys, 63% of girls	9–15 years	To school	Not clear	National Physical Activity Behaviour Study for Children and Adolescents 2016 (LIITU) [30]	3
B+	Hong Kong	80% of the adolescent males and 77% of the adolescent females actively travelled to school at least once per week. 52% of primary school children used active travel to/from school at least 5 times per week.	80% adolescent males and 77% adolescent females	Primary and secondary	To and from school	At least 5 times per week and at least once per week	Understanding Children's Activity and Nutrition (UCAN) study, 2011–2012 [31]	3
B+	South Korea	79.4% of children and adolescents reported walking or cycling to/from places, with an average duration of 39 min per day.	84.3% of boys and 73.8% of girls took active modes of transport	12–17 years	Not specified	Not clear	Korea National Health and Nutrition Examination Survey, 2016 [32]	3
B	Colombia	71.7% of children and adolescents in Colombia reported walking or biking as their main mode of transport to or from school in the previous week.	Not reported	6–17 years	To and from school	Main mode during the last 7 days	National Survey of Nutrition (ENSIN) 2015 [33]	3
B	Nigeria	The majority (61% to 80%) of Nigerian children and adolescents engage in some form of active transportation, mostly walking to and from school.	Not reported	5–13 years	To and from school	Not clear	2 different studies on rural and urban populations in Nigeria, conducted in 2011 [34] and 2013 [35]	2

Table 3. *Cont.*

Grade	Country	Rationale	Gender	Age	Destination and Direction	Frequency	Source of Information and Year	Profile
B−	Bulgaria	64% of children and youth reported walking, biking, or skating, etc. to go to school and back.	Not reported	Not specified	To and from school	Not clear	Bulgarian Active Kids survey, 2016 [36]	3
B−	India	Approximately 65% of children/adolescents (weighted average) reported walking or cycling to school on a regular basis.	Not reported	5–17 years	To school	On a regular basis	7 different studies at the national and local level conducted between 2005 and 2018 [12,13,37–41]	2
B−	Netherlands	90% of the adolescents commute actively to school. 36% of the children commute actively to school	Not reported	Not specified	To school	At least three days per week	Lifestyle monitor National Survey, 2017 [42]	1
B−	Spain	55% and 56.9% of children between 6 and 9 years old walked to and from school, respectively. In Catalonia, 61.3% of children between 3 to 14 years old walked to and from school.	Not reported	3–14 years	To and from school	Not clear	Food, Physical Activity, Child developmentand Obesity study (ALADINO) 2011 [43], and the Catalan Health Survey (ESCA) 2016 [44]	3
B−	Venezuela	63% of adolescents might walk at least 10 min to move from one place to another.	Not reported	Not specified	Not specified	Not clear	Venezuelan Study of Nutrition and Health [45]	3
C+	Belgium (Flanders)	55.5% of parents of 6-9-year old children reported that their child uses active transportation, and 58.9% of 10- to 17-year-olds adolescents reported to mainly use active transportation to travel to school.	Not reported	6 to 9 and 10 to 17	To school	Not clear	Belgian National Food Consumption Survey 2014 [46]	1
C+	China	56.3% of Chinese children (aged 6–18 years) reported going to and from school by walk or bicycle.	Not reported	9 to 17 years	To and from school	Daily	Physical Activity and Fitness in China—The Youth Study (PAFCTYS), 2016 [47]	3
C+	Czech Republic	On average, 57% (weighted mean: 59%) of children and adolescents reported using active transport to get to and from school.	Not reported	9–17 years	To and from school	Not clear	Health Behaviour in School-aged Children Study (HBSC)2006, 2010, and 2014 [48] and International Physical Activity and Environment Network Study (IPEN), 2013–2015 [49]	1
C+	Ghana	About 54% of children and youth especially those in the rural areas walk to school and back home covering about 2 km.	Not reported	Not specified	To and from school	Not clear	Not specified	2
C+	Mexico	54.8% of children 3 years and older walked to school and 1.5% rode bicycles. 69% of 10–14-year-olds walked or rode a bicycle to school.	Not reported	3 years and older	To school	Not clear	Intercensal Survey of the National Institute of Statistics and Geography (INEGI), 2015 [50] and the National Health and Nutrition Survey 2016 (ENSANUT) [51]	3

177

Table 3. Cont.

Grade	Country	Rationale	Gender	Age	Destination and Direction	Frequency	Source of Information and Year	Profile
C	Botswana	49% of 13-15-year-olds walked or rode a bike to and from school at least one day during the past 7 days.	Not reported	13–15	To and from school	At least one of the last 7 days	2005 Botswana School-based Student Health Survey (GSHS) [13]	3
C	Brazil	55.0% of children and youth in Brazil used active transportation to get to and from school.	Not reported	6 to 21	To and from school	Not clear	18 different national and regional studies conducted between 2008 and 2017 [52]	3
C	Ethiopia	Approximately 48% of children and youth (31% in urban and 65% rural) walked to and from school.	Not reported	Not specified	To and from school	Not clear	Experts' opinion	2
C	Poland	47.4% of 10- to 17-year-olds reported walking to school and 52.3% walking from school. 5.5% and 5.2% travel to and from school by bicycle, respectively. 41% and 5% of lower-secondary students walk and cycle to school, respectively. While 36% and 3% of upper-secondary school students walk and cycle to school, respectively.	Not reported	10–19 years	To and from school	Not clear	Study of Physical Activity of School Children Aged 9–17 by the Institute of Mother and Child, 2013 [53] and the All-Poland survey of physical activity and sedentary lifestyles for middle school, high school and university students, 2011 [54]	1
C	Scotland	51% and 52% of school age children and adolescents, respectively, actively commuted to school (walking, cycling, skating or using scooter).	Not reported	4–18 years	To school	Not clear	Hands up Scotland Survey (HUS) 2016 [55], Transport and Travel in Scotland (TATIS) 2016 [56]	1
C	Slovenia	Almost 49% of children commute actively to and from school and additional 12% commute actively from school only.	52% of boys and 50% of girls commute actively to school	5–15 years	To and from school	Not clear	Analysis of Children's Development in Slovenia study (ACDSi) 2013–16 [57,58]	1
C	South Africa	63% of school-aged children walk to school. 81% of children and adolescents in Cape Town walk to school without adult supervision in low-income settings, and 61% of parents reported concerns about their children safety.	Not reported	6–15 years	To school	Not clear	General Household Survey, 2013 [59] and two local studies conducted in Cape Town, 2016 [60,61]	3
C	Sweden	48% and 57% of children and adolescents used active transportation to and from school in the winter and summer months, respectively.	Not reported	6–15 years	To and from school	Not clear	Children's Routes to School Survey 2015–16 [62]	1
C	Thailand	53.4% children and adolescents used active transportation (walking, cycling, using a wheelchair, in-line skating or skateboarding) to get to and from places.	54.7% of girls and 52.4% of boys used active transportation	6–17 years	Not specified	Not clear	Thailand Physical Activity ChildrenSurvey (TPACS) 2015 [63]	3
C	Uruguay	51.2% of adolescents between 13 and 15 years old went to the school walking or bicycling 4 or more days per week.	Not reported	13–15 years	To school	4 or more days per week	Global School-Based Student Health Survey (GSHS) 2012 [64]	3

Table 3. Cont.

Grade	Country	Rationale	Gender	Age	Destination and Direction	Frequency	Source of Information and Year	Profile
C−	Bangladesh	41.1% students aged 13–17 years used active transport to commute to or from school at all seven days prior to the survey.	Not reported	13–17 years	To and from school	Last 7 days	Bangladesh School-based Student Health Survey (GSHS), 2014 [65]	2
C−	Ecuador	42.7% of 5–17 years-old children reported going to school or work by foot or bike.	Boys: 42%; Girls: 41%	5–17 years	To school, work or other destinations	Not clear	Not specified	3
C−	England	On average, 42.5% of children and adolescents used active modes of transport to school everyday.	Not reported	5–16 years	To school	Every day	National Travel Survey 2016 [66], Health Survey for England 2015 [67] and Walking and Cycling Statistics 2016 [68]	1
C−	France	44% of the 3–10 years old and 43% of the 11–14 years old used active transportation to go to school according to the National Study of Individual Nutritional Consumption 2014–2015. And 41% of the 6–10-year-olds reported using active transportation to school according to the Health Study of the Environment, Biosurveillance, Physical Activity, and Nutrition 2015.	Not reported	3–14 years	To school	Not clear	National Study of Individual Nutritional Consumption (INCA) 2014–2015 [69] and the Health Study of the Environment, Biosurveillance, Physical Activity and Nutrition (ESTEBAN) 2015 [70]	1
C−	Germany	Approximately 40% of the children and adolescents commute actively to school.	Not reported	Not specified	To school	Not clear	Not specified	1
C−	Lithuania	45% of 7–8 aged children used active transport to school and 57.9% used active transport from school to home. 84% of children and adolescents (11–13 year) walked to/from school. 12% of youths and adolescents (15–24 year) reported to engage regularly in cycling from one point to another.	Not reported	7–24 years	To and from school	Not clear	4 different studies and one special report Eurobarometer on Sport and Physical Activity, between 2012 and 2017 [71–75]	1
C−	New Zealand	45% of children and adolescents aged 5–14 years usually used active transport to school according to the NZ Health Survey, 43% of children and youth aged 5–17-year-olds usually used active transport to and from school according to the Active NZ Survey. 30% of children aged 5–12 years and 31% of adolescents aged 13–17 years used active transport to school according to the Health and Lifestyles Survey and the NZ Household Travel Survey, respectively. 24% of 6-year-olds in a longitudinal cohort study usually used active transport to get to and from school.	Not reported	5–17 years	To and from school	Not clear	New Zealand Health Survey 2016/2017 [76], Active NZ Survey 2018 [77], Health and Lifestyles Survey 2016 [78], NZ Household Travel Survey 2015–2018 [79], and the Growing Up in New Zealand study 2010 [80]	1

Table 3. Cont.

Grade	Country	Rationale	Gender	Age	Destination and Direction	Frequency	Source of Information and Year	Profile
C−	Portugal	A study with urban school-aged children showed that 45% of participants commuted actively to and from school. Another study in the countryside region found that 30% of the participants (aged 7 to 8 years) commuted either by foot or cycling on a regular basis during school days (ARSA 2012).	Not reported	7–8 years and 15–24 years	To and from school	Not clear	A study in public schools from the Porto area [81] and the Health Study of the Child Population of the Alentejo Region, 2012 [82]	1
C−	Taiwan	33–46% of children and adolescents reported walking or cycling to school most of the days.	Not reported	7–18 years	To school	Most of the days	Student Participation in Physical Activity Survey, 2015 [83] and Health Behaviour Survey in Junior High School Students, 2016 [84]	1
D+	Australia	National data shows that 43% of 12–17 year-olds usually travel to/from school using active transport, other state and regional studies shows that 37% of primary students and 36% of secondary students use active transport as their usual mode to get to school.	Not reported	12–17 years	To school	Usual mode—each week (Usual defined as at least 5 trips out of 10 or on at least 2.5 school days)	National Secondary Students Diet and Activity Survey 2012–2013 [85], ACT Year 6 Physical Activity and Nutrition Survey 2015 [86], Child Population Health Survey [87], Queensland Child Preventive Health Survey 2018 [88], NSW School Physical Activity and Nutrition Survey 2015 [89], Victorian Child Health and Wellbeing survey 2016 [90]	1
D+	Jersey	37% of 10–15-year-olds traveled to school by active modes.	Not reported	10–15 years	To school	Not clear	Health Related Behaviour Questionnaire 2014 [91]	1
D+	Wales	44% primary school children and 34% secondary school pupils traveled actively to school. In another survey, 33.8% and 36.1% of children and young people aged 11–16 years walked/cycled to and from school, respectively.	Not reported	11–16 years	To and from school	Not clear	National Survey for Wales (2016–17) [92] and The Health Behaviour of School-aged Children (HBSC)/School Health Research Network (SHRN) Survey 2017 [93]	1
D	Estonia	The percentage of use of active transport varied between 36–56%. Specifically, 35% of children walked to school and back home, while 14% of children rode a bike to go to school. The grading process took into account the number of subjects, age range and used methodology of different studies.	Not reported	7–17 years	To and from school	Not clear	Children's Physical Activity Study 2015 and Schools in Motion Survey 2018 [94]	1
D	Guernsey Channel Islands	On average, 31% of children and adolescents reported active travel (walking, bicycle or scooter) to school on the day of the survey (43% of primary school pupils and 25% of secondary pupils.	Not reported	Primary and secondary (grades 6, 8 and 10)	To school	On the day of the survey	Guernsey Young People Survey 2016–2017 [95]	1

Table 3. *Cont.*

Grade	Country	Rationale	Gender	Age	Destination and Direction	Frequency	Source of Information and Year	Profile
D	Lebanon	36.8% of Lebanese adolescents between the ages of 13 and 18 reported walking or biking to school.	Not reported	13–17 years	To school	Not clear	Global School-Based Student Health Survey 2016 (GSHS) [96]	1
D–	Canada	21% of 5- to 19-year-olds in Canada typically use active modes of transportation (e.g., walk, bike), and 16% use a combination of active and inactive modes of transportation to travel to and from school (2014–16 CANPLAY, CFLRI).	Not reported	5 to 19	To and from school	Typical use	Kids CANPLAY 2014–2016 [97]	1
D–	United States	38% of adolescents walked or used a bicycle for at least 10 min continuously once or more in a typical week to get to and from places, and 23% of youth actively commuted 5–7 days per week.	45% of boys and 32% of girls reported any active transportation in a typical week	12–19 years	To and from multiple places	5 to 7 days on a typical week	National Health and Nutrition Examination Survey (NHANES 2015–16) [98]	1
F	Chile	15% of children and youth (weighted average) rode a bike or walked to and from school (ranging from 0.29% to 32.2% in different samples and regions).	Not reported	Not specified	To and from school	Not clear	National Survey of Quality of life 2015–2016 (ENCAVI) [99], Survey of Urban Quality of Life Perception 2015 (EPCVU) [100], a cross-sectional study of seventh grade students in the Maule region 2014 [101], and a cross-sectional study in Valparaíso 2017 [102]	1
INC	United Arab Emirates	There was no current data available to grade this indicator.	NA	NA	NA	NA	NA	1
N/A	Qatar	Active transportation indicator is excluded from the report according to stakeholders' group recommendation. This indicator is still not applicable in Qatar due to unsafe roads and the hot climate during most times of the year.	N/A	N/A	N/A	N/A	N/A	1

Abbreviations: INC, incomplete; NA, not applicable.

Table 4. Descriptive statistics of the latent variables by country profile.

Profile (% of Countries)	Active Transportation Grade				Human Development Index				Gini Index			
	Mean	SD	Min	Max	Mean	SD	Min	Max	Mean	SD	Min	Max
1 n = 25 (51%)	6.08	2.55	0.00	10.00	0.89	0.05	0.763	0.985	33.78	5.29	25.44	47.70
2 n = 7 (14.3%)	10.14	2.34	7.00	13.00	0.55	0.06	0.448	0.624	38.29	4.81	32.40	43.20
3 n = 17 (34.7%)	9.82	1.88	7.00	13.00	0.80	0.09	0.666	0.925	42.08	10.58	27.10	63.0

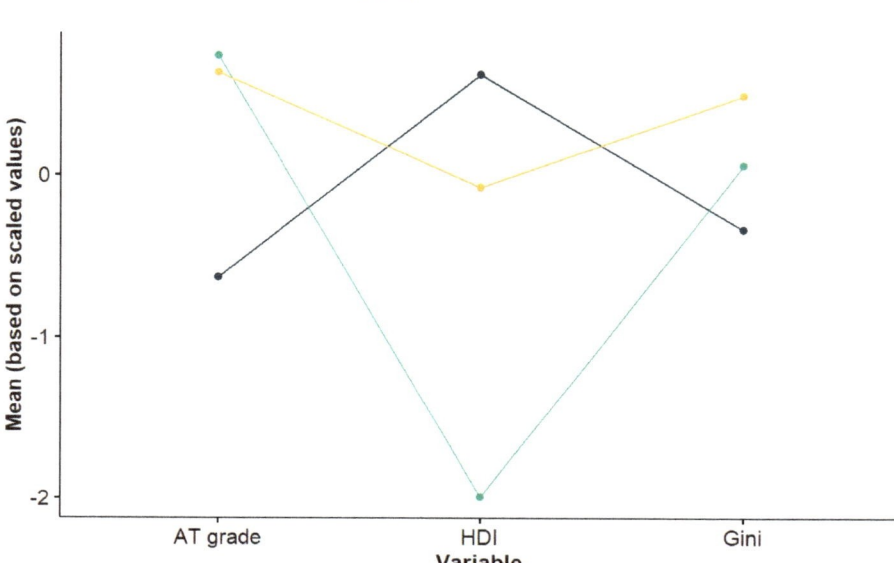

Figure 1. Country profiles for active transportation and sociodemographic variables of countries in the Global Matrix 3.0. The range of values for the active transportation grade, Human Development Index and the Gini index varied notably between variables, therefore they were converted to z-scores to be expressed in the same range of values and to ease their graphic depiction.

The availability of details related to active transportation in the report cards, beyond the reported prevalence, varied across countries. Table 5 summarizes the information provided by countries in terms of practices and policies, strategies proposed to improve the grades and research gaps identified by expert groups in each country. Twenty-four countries provided at least one of these details. The policies and practices identified by the expert groups included school siting policies, transport policies that prioritize active modes of commuting, walking challenges and special events, and multi-component programs that comprise educational strategies, enforcement of regulation to improve traffic safety, and providing infrastructure and resources at several levels (children, teachers, schools and communities). The most common topics in the strategies proposed to improve the grades were improving safety conditions, providing supportive infrastructure, developing informational and education strategies, and involving parents, schools and communities in the promotion of active transportation. Several research gaps were identified, but the most frequent across countries was the need to study active transportation to destinations other than school (Table 5).

Table 5. Policies and practices, strategies to improve the grade and research gaps in active transportation identified in the Global Matrix 3.0.

Grade	Country	Profile	Policies/Practices	How to Improve the Grade	Gaps
A−	Japan	3	Since 1953 Japan has a "walking to school practice" resulting from the implementation of the article 49 of the School Education Act, which regulates the siting of public schools in urban areas of Japan. This article establishes that the commuting distances are 4 km for elementary schools and 6 km for junior high schools. Based on these, the boards of education must ensure that children attend to schools located within those distances to allow children to walk to school [14,103,104].	Not reported	Research on active transportation to destinations other than schools (e.g., going shopping, going to the park, sports clubs or cram schools) [104].
A−	Zimbabwe	2	Not reported	1. Through public health messages to highlight the benefits of active transportation and reduce the prestige/status symbol associated with motorized transportation. 2. Implementing policies that encourage and provide safe and walkable neighborhoods and bike lanes, etc. [105].	There is a need of data reporting the time invested in active transportation and distance to and from school, as well as research data on the correlates of active transportation, and more recent data is required [105].
B+	Finland	3	Not reported	Not reported	There is no comparable published data available about active school commutes for upper secondary students when the distance between home and school is less than 5 km. More information is needed about active transportation to other destinations [106].
B+	Hong Kong	3	The high density of Hong Kong could be one of the factors facilitating active transportation to school. Since most districts in Hong Kong are highly self-contained, children can attend schools located at walkable distance from their home [107,108].	1. Encouraging active travel to destinations other than school may provide additional health benefits for children and adolescents. 2. Promoting cycling to and from school and other destinations in districts with a bicycle track [107,108].	Data about active transportation to destinations other than school, as well as the relationship between active transportation, physical activity and health-related outcomes. Also, data on the duration of active travel trips is required [107,108].
B	Colombia	3	In Bogota, the capital city of Colombia, the program "Bike to school" is implemented in public schools to promote cycling as a sustainable mode of transportation to school and other destinations in the city. The program was created in order to address the barriers to access to education and to decrease the dropout rates. Bike to school program includes the following strategies: (a) bicycle loan, (b) workshops on skills and abilities to ride a bicycle, (c) basic mechanics and road safety education, (d) participatory mapping of safe routes, (e) daily trips from a meeting point to school with adult supervision, and (f) extracurricular activities to develop responsible behaviours in the roads and to visit other destinations of interest in the city [109,110]. Another promising practice to encourage walking and cycling, but with recreational purposes, are the Open Streets programs, or Ciclovias. Colombia currently has 67 of these programs that close main roads to motorized vehicles and open them for leisure activities on Sundays and holidays [109,111]. Walking and cycling are the main activities performed by children who attend Ciclovia in Bogota [112]. Also, Colombia has a specific law to support the use of bicycles as the main mode of transport at the national level (Law 1811 of 2016). This law establishes the responsibility of public transportation systems to allow multi-modal trips through the provision of bike-supporting infrastructure, and encourages schools to implement programs to promote cycling [111].	1. Improving safety conditions and infrastructure to keep promoting and maintaining active transportation as a desirable behaviour since early ages [109].	Not reported

Table 5. Cont.

Grade	Country	Profile	Policies/Practices	How to Improve the Grade	Gaps
B	Nigeria	2	The National Transport Policy in Nigeria is under review with the aim to strengthen the inclusion of non-motorized transport infrastructure and to create better non-motorized transport options for urban residents. This review is the result of a workshop on streets design led by the Federal Ministry of Transport in 2017 and is a good example of the concerted efforts to improve the conditions for active transportation in Nigeria [114,115]. Another example is the Non-Motorized Transport Policy developed in Lagos, which aims to prioritize walking, cycling and public transportation as the main modes of transport [114]. This policy specifically addresses active transportation to school through two strategies: (a) public awareness through the creation of a curriculum about road safety and benefits of active transportation for primary and secondary school students. And (b) regulations that include the creation of route plans for students to go to school, and the implementation of access and safety measures such as speed limits, traffic calming infrastructure and school zone signaling [116].	Not reported	Not reported
C+	Ghana	2	The Community Day Senior High Schools, built in various districts in Ghana, seem to be encouraging active transportation to school. The students who attend to this schools usually walk to and from school every day, some of them covering more than two kilometers [117].	Not reported	Not reported
C+	Mexico	3	Not reported	1. Promoting active transportation among Mexican children and adolescents. 2. Communities and governments should provide appropriate safety conditions on streets, sidewalks and neighborhoods to promote walking and cycling among children and adolescents [18].	Data on all age groups and stratified by age group and sex is desirable for future surveys [18].
C	Brazil	3	Not reported	Local authorities should be encouraged to create a monitoring system to generate standardized and detailed reports on active transportation to school to support planning and evaluation of public policies [19].	Data on time invested in active transportation, the distance to the school and other environmental and mobility-related factors such as bike paths, traffic and conditions of the city is lacking [52].
C	Ethiopia	2	Not reported	1. Building sidewalks to encourage active transportation in all cities in Ethiopia. 2. Encouraging and supporting children and adolescents to travel to and from school through active transportation [120].	Active transportation specific studies in Ethiopia are required [120].
C	Scotland	1	Not reported	Not reported	No data available on active commuting to and from places other than school [121].
C	Sweden	1	A national cycling strategy has been adopted in Sweden to improve safety and increase cycling [122]. The strategy aims to increase cycling through five action lines: (a) creating more bicycle-friendly municipalities, (b) focusing on various types of cyclists (where children are highlighted as a population of interest), (c) giving higher priority to bicycle traffic in community planning, (d) building more functional and user-friendly cycling infrastructure and (e) strengthening research an innovation on cycling [123].	Not reported	Not reported

Table 5. *Cont.*

Grade	Country	Profile	Policies/Practices	How to Improve the Grade	Gaps
C	Uruguay	3	Not reported	Creating policies to encourage the creation of cycle lanes and safe sidewalks.	Data on active transportation in a wider age range and to locations other than school.
C−	Ecuador	3	Not reported	Reinforcing programs aiming to promote active transportation [124].	Not reported
C−	France	1	Not reported	Not reported	Research is needed on the characteristics of active transportation of children and adolescents (frequency, mode, distance covered) and on the potential barriers to this in order to develop effective promotion program [125].
C−	Lithuania	1	Not reported	1. Promoting and facilitating safe active transport to get to school and other destinations. 2. Prioritizing active transportation promotion as a key factor at schools and communities. 3. Involving parents, schools, community and policy makers in the promotion of active transportation [7].	1. Research on the prevalence and trends of active transport in Lithuania, considering the most popular modes of active transportation used to get to/from different points or destinations (e.g., parks, shops, sport fields) among children and adolescents as well as studying the role of active transport in achieving recommended levels of physical activity. 2. Research on health and social benefits of active transportation is needed. 3. Evaluating the impact of the cycling paths and interventions at the school, community and municipality levels. 4. Examining the potential moderators and mediators of active transport behaviour change to help refine interventions [7].
C−	New Zealand	1	Not reported.	Strategies to encourage active travel to school are needed, especially for girls, younger children, and older adolescents [126]. This strategies should have a multi-sectoral y culturally appropriate approach, including urban planning, initiatives a the school and community level, social marketing campaigns and family support [127].	Nationally representative data on active transportation to school and other destinations that is comparable between countries and across time is desirable [127].
C−	Taiwan	1	Not reported	Local governments and schools should work together to create a safe and convenient environment for active transportation [128].	Research on the contribution of active transportation to overall physical activity in children and adolescents, and about motivations and barriers for active transportation is needed [128].

Table 5. *Cont.*

Grade	Country	Profile	Policies/Practices	How to Improve the Grade	Gaps
D+	Australia	1	The Australian Capital Territory has implemented the Ride or Walk to School program since 2012 aiming to build the capacity of primary schools to support and promote active travel to and from school. The program was designed with a participatory approach including students and different stakeholders. The strategies of the program include: (a) resources for teachers and students, (b) provision of bikes and helmets, (c) safe routes maps, (d) workshops to increase skills, and (e) four annual active travel events. This program was expanded to high schools since 2016 [129]. In Western Australia, the Department of Transport implemented the program "Your Move Schools". This is a community-focused program that promotes active and sustainable transportation providing: (a) teaching resources, (b) expert advice and (c) access to funding (up to $5000 AUD) to promote active transportation through bike education workshops, wayfinding, bike supporting infrastructure like bike shelters, bike repair stations, bike skills tracks and bicycle parkings [129]. In the Northern Territory, the Nightcliff Walk and Wheel initiative is aimed at encouraging students to walk and cycle to school. This is a local project in two dense suburbs lead by principals and parents from four schools. The project has a focus on roads safety for children and has implemented activities such as the Ride2School days, increasing cycling to school [129].	1. Encouraging families to active commute at least part of the way, promoting the use of park and walk/ride/scoot zones away from school grounds to reduce traffic. 2. Creating and promoting safe routes to schools and engage schools to promote their use. 3. Creating greater awareness of actual distances between home and school and the travel time for active modes. 4. Highlighting the benefit of students travelling to school carrying their school bags as an opportunity to be active while carrying a load, which could contribute to improve their muscular fitness [129].	1. Nationally representative data for primary and secondary students. 2. Data on the use of active transportation to other destinations. 3. Data on the use of multi-modal transport combining active transport with public transport. 4. Research about how far families and children are willing to travel using active transportation [129].
D+	Wales	1	The report card mentioned the following initiatives led by charities to promote active travel to school: 1. Active Journeys—Sustrans School active travel program promotes active transportation through different actions like: (a) providing support to schools to develop active travel plans, (b) delivering activities and lessons, (c) offering free incentives to promote active travel, (d) providing resources and online travel challenges for the school community, and (e) rewarding schools with the School Mark award for achieving excellence in active and sustainable travel [130]. 2. Living Streets Walking initiatives: This charity has two main strategies for schools, the WOW Year-Round Walk to School challenge and the Five-Days Walking challenge. Both of these aim to engage primary and secondary students to walk to school encouraging them with an interactive travel tracker and the provision of incentives at the end of the challenge. This charity also encourages the celebration of the Walk to School Week in May every year [131].	Not reported	More research is needed on how children and young people travel to other places including shops, parks and friends' or relatives' houses [132].
D	Guernsey Channel Islands		Guernsey has an integrated transport strategy in place that promotes active travel with the aim of having a positive impact on the environment and the population's health [133]. The On-island Integrated Transport Strategy aims to encourage active travel, followed by the use of public transport and to reduce the use of private motor vehicles. This strategy was initially planned to progressively advance to a taxation policy for high emission vehicles to support the promotion of active travel. However, there are other actions in this strategy aimed at increasing active travel to school, such as: (a) Bikeability training at primary schools, (b) increasing the investments in walking and cycling infrastructure to improve safety for active commuters, (c) revising the speed limits to enhance the safety of vulnerable populations using active travel, and (d) developing and implementing travel plans for schools [134].	Through the implementation of the integrated transport initiative that supports active travel [133].	Not reported

Table 5. Cont.

Grade	Country	Profile	Policies/Practices	How to Improve the Grade	Gaps
D	Lebanon	1	Not reported	Not reported	Nationally representative samples for children and adolescents and on all active transportation means are required to gain a better understanding of this indicator [135,36].
D−	Canada	1	In Ontario, the Minister of Education expanded the funding for initiatives that improve the cognitive, physical, social and emotional well-being of students. Specifically walking school buses and biking-to-school programs have benefited from this increase in the funding [137]. These initiatives are part of the Ontario Active School Travel program (formerly Active & Safe Routes to School) which comprise five components: (a) education activities to foster the skills, confidence, and awareness such as workshops and route mapping. (b) Encouragement activities to inspire students, parents and school staff to try active travel modes. For example, walk and wheel seasonal events or walking school buses. (c) Engineering actions to create safe and accessible school sites, neighbourhoods and routes to school, such as school siting, signaling, parking restrictions, crosswalk improvements or crossing guards. (d) Enforcement of traffic policies to improve safety around schools. (e) Evaluations to measure the measure success, and demonstrate impact of the actions [138]. In 2017, three organizations in Canada (Canada Bikes, Green Communities Canada and the National Active and Safe Routes to School Working Group) created an active transportation alliance to advocate for the adoption and funding of a national active transportation strategy [137]. However, this strategy is not yet in place.	1. Creating a culture of active transportation, to make active transportation the norm. 2. Establishing lower speed limits in school areas. 3. Implementing traffic-calming devices (e.g., speed bumps/humps, chicanes, narrower intersections) to enhance compliance with speed limits, mainly in low-income areas, where more children engage in active transportation. 4. Hiring more crossing guards at busy intersections near schools. 5. Considering more progressive policies for low-income areas, to access to funding for active transportation interventions. 6. Considering children's active transportation when planning schools and recreation facilities. 7. Encouraging schools to implement "drop-off spots" from which driven children could safely walk to school in groups [137].	1. Research on active transportation to destinations such as parks, stores, recreation facilities and other places. 2. Studies on children's preferences for cycling and how to harness them in interventions. 3. More research is needed on how to facilitate children's independent mobility. 4. More research is needed on the use of mixed modes of transportation to and from destinations [137].
D−	United States	1	Safe Routes to School is a movement to promote walking and bicycling to school, improving safety, health and physical activity levels. Actions at the local level incorporate the six E's integrated approach: (a) education through the provision of training in skills and knowledge to walk and bicycle safely and teaching the benefits of active transportation. (b) Encouragement to motivate children to travel actively through events and activities. (c) Engineering to improve streets and neighborhoods in order to make them more convenient for walking and bicycling. (d) Enforcement of safety regulation. (e) Evaluation of the success and opportunities to improve the initiatives in place. And (f) equity to ensure that the program benefits all demographic groups. Actions at the regional and state level are focused on finding funding and ensuring the proper use of the resources invested in the program. At the federal level, the Safe Routes Partnership advocates for policy and funding support and provides expert help, ideas and resources for the leaders at all levels [139].	1. Investing in infrastructure, programs, and policies that promote active transportation to and from school. 2. Allocating funding to provide and improve infrastructure to encourage active transportation (e.g., sidewalks, crosswalks, bike lanes, trails, etc.). 3. Encouraging children at home to use active transportation to school and other neighborhood locations. 4. Investing in infrastructure and policies such as Safe Routes to School and walking school buses. 5. Informing parents (at all income levels) about the benefits of active transportation [140].	1. The study of locations where children and adolescents walk and bike, duration and distance of trips as well as the main reasons for not engaging in active transportation. 2. Surveillance systems should include children under 12 years old [140].

187

4. Discussion

Our results suggest that about half of children and adolescents use active modes of transportation to get to and from places, mainly to and/or from school. However, a pooled estimate of the global prevalence of active transportation cannot be calculated from the Global Matrix 3.0 data for reasons that will be discussed below. Despite the clear gradient in average grades according to HDI that has been discussed in previous publications [141–143], our results show variability within HDI groups and the LPA allowed us to examine the clustering of this sample of countries according to three variables of interest (active transportation grades, level of development and income inequality).

4.1. Comparability of Data

There was wide variability between countries in the prevalence of active transportation, and high involvement in this behaviour was reported across countries with very different socioeconomic contexts (e.g., Japan, Zimbabwe, Nepal, Denmark and Finland). However, the data reported by the countries presented in Table 3 show important methodological differences that should be accounted for when comparing the prevalence of active transportation between countries. One of the issues that can affect the comparability of data is the difference in the frequency of use of active transportation reported by the countries. Depending on the cut-point used to define children as active travelers, the prevalence will vary widely, and the use of active transportation can be overestimated or underestimated. Similarly, the prevalence may vary depending on the direction of active transportation assessed since different modes can be used to go to and from school. As observed in previous comparisons of surveillance systems measuring active transportation, the prevalence of active transportation varies greatly according to the construct assessed [144]. In the group of countries included in this analysis, the frequencies reported varied from daily to at least twice per week. Even when the source of information was the same survey (e.g., the GSHS across countries), different frequencies were reported [136,145–147]. Regarding the construct assessed, the destination for active transportation is also relevant. Despite the broad definition of active transportation in the Global Matrix 3.0 benchmarks [14], most of the evidence available on active transportation in children is focused on the journeys to and from school, as observed in this analysis and in previous literature [148]. Only Ecuador and the United States reported the use of active transportation to other destinations, which could suggest an underestimation of the involvement in active transportation in other countries since trips to places such as parks and other people's homes are also relevant opportunities to engage in this behaviour [149]. These findings point to a need for the development of harmonized and contextualized measurements. Our results are consistent with the findings reported by Herrador-Colmenero et al. in a systematic review, in which the formulation of a standardized question is proposed to overcome the heterogeneity in measures to assess active transportation [150]. Based on these insights, initiatives like the Global Matrix and organizations like the AHKGA can contribute to the improvement of surveillance systems for the evaluation of active transportation among children.

The Global Matrix initiative aims to better understand the global variation of certain physical activity indicators [14]. Specifically, active transportation is one of the most strategic indicators in the Global Matrix 3.0 to contribute to this aim, due to the low amount of INC grades, and the good dispersion of grades across countries [14]. However, the availability of transportation-relevant contextual variables at the country level to understand these variations was limited. Therefore, the LPA provides an exploratory approach to identify subgroups that share similar patterns of variables [20,151], and provides a unique opportunity to identify the ways in which countries in the Global Matrix 3.0 cluster, according to the grades for active transportation and contextual variables. The identified profiles can be useful for the discussion of the different contexts in which active transportation needs to be maintained or increased. A description of the three profiles is provided below.

4.2. Country Profiles for Active Transportation and Sociodemographic Variables

Profile 1 included mainly countries with a very high HDI and low income inequality, mostly with a reported prevalence of active transportation under 50%. Mainly, countries from North America, Europe and Oceania were grouped in this profile. While the countries with the lowest prevalence of active transportation were classified in this group (Chile, the United States and Canada), it also included some countries with non-negligible prevalence of active transportation such as the Netherlands, Belgium and the Czech Republic. This means that although all of these countries have a similar development level, there are other relevant factors influencing active travel among children. First, some of these are countries where long distances between destinations and the perceived convenience of driving may undermine opportunities for active travel [102,152–154]. Second, urban planning and policies that have prioritized people instead of cars, as well as supportive infrastructure have made active modes a convenient and safe alternative to commute [155,156]. Interventions in countries under this profile should aim to increase active transportation addressing the issues of distance and convenience, attempting to discourage the use of motorized vehicles for short trips, and trying to shift the social norms to consider active modes the default option for commuting as it occurs in many European countries. A useful example among the policies reported in the Report Cards is the National Cycling Policy from Sweden, which aims to prioritize cycling in the community and municipalities planning [123].

Profile 2 grouped mostly countries with high prevalence of active transportation, low to medium HDI and higher income inequalities. In most of these countries, access to motorized vehicles is limited, and active travel is happening despite multiple safety concerns [157,158] and the lack of supportive infrastructure [143]. Therefore, for many families, active transportation is likely to reflect necessity rather than choice [159]. Also, many of the countries in this group report important differences between children from rural and urban areas [117,120,145]. As suggested by a previous systematic review on active transportation in Africa, these differences could be indicative of the physical activity transition that these countries are experiencing [157,160]. In this context, for the countries classified in this profile, preserving active travel while providing improved safety and infrastructure conditions should be a priority. It is important to design strategies to avoid the unintended consequences that economic growth can have on the mode of transport for children and adolescents. A good example of the approaches needed in countries under this profile is the Non-Motorized Transport Policy from Lagos, Nigeria. This policy aims to prioritize active modes of transportation over motorized options, communicating the benefits and importance of active transportation, as well as improving safety conditions for students using active modes to go to school [116].

Profile 3 had more variability in terms of HDI and income inequality, however, the relatively high prevalence of active transportation was a main feature in common between this group of countries. Some of the most successful countries in active transportation are grouped under this profile. However, the conditions in which it is happening are very different. There are countries such as Finland, Denmark, Japan, South Korea and Hong Kong where the use of active modes is supported by the design of compact cities, school siting policies that ensure that children attend to schools located at a walkable distance from home, and supportive infrastructure and regulations [103,104,108,141,155,161]. These factors have made walking and cycling safe options for the daily commuting. Conversely, there are countries like Colombia, Brazil, Mexico, Venezuela and South Africa, where active transportation is prevalent despite safety concerns, the lack of supportive infrastructure and regulations and is likely to be a necessity-driven behaviour [52,60,61,162–165]. Similarly to profile 2, almost half of the countries in this profile have a relatively high Gini coefficient. However, this profile also includes countries with very low inequality, such as Finland and Denmark. Income inequality has been previously documented as a negative correlate of physical activity and organized sports involvement [14,19]. Notwithstanding, the high prevalence of active transportation in both equal and unequal societies are consistent with literature that suggest that active transportation modes could be an opportunity to bridge the inequities in transportation [18] as well as in other domains of physical activity. Due to the diversity of contexts found in this profile, different approaches are needed to promote or maintain active travel. School siting policies that take into account the proximity between schools and children's homes, like those implemented in Japan and Hong Kong [103,104,107], can be useful for growing cities. Also, multi-component strategies, such as the Bike to school program in Colombia are a good reference for countries that aim to provide access, skills, and support to bike to school in safe conditions [110]. Furthermore, Ciclovias or Open Streets programs are a good model for countries where active transportation to school is already prevalent and aim to increase walking and cycling to other destinations in the leisure time [112,166].

Regarding the strategies to improve active transportation, it is concerning to find that major correlates of active transportation such as distance and the perceived convenience of driving are not mentioned among the strategies proposed by the Report Card teams. Future versions of the Report Cards, as tools to communicate evidence to stakeholders, should take these important factors into consideration in order to advocate for active transportation addressing its most important drivers.

Our results can contribute to the call for measures of conditions related to all children wellbeing made by a recent commission sponsored by the WHO, UNICEF and The Lancet. This commission identified that inequities and climate change are undermining children's right to a healthy environment in both, the poorest and wealthiest countries [167]. Given that the transportation sector accounts for almost 25% of global greenhouse gas emissions [168], local, regional, and national policymakers and practitioners should implement interventions that support children's active transportation in all socioeconomic contexts.

4.3. Strengths and Limitations of the Study

Strengths of this study include the availability of active transportation data from 47 countries from all continents, and the harmonized selection of the best available evidence in each country. Our analyses contributed with a diverse context perspective to the emerging evidence on international comparisons of active transportation, which has focused on specific groups of countries in previous studies [169,170]. Although most countries reported nationally representative data on active transportation, in some countries, the best available evidence consisted of local data. The main limitations of the study were the diversity in the quality of the data reported, and the broad benchmark proposed for active transportation in the Global Matrix 3.0, which led to variations in the definition of active transportation across countries. The important amount of missing data in the Community and Environment indicator (26%) and the heterogeneity of the data reported across countries did not allow to include it as a variable of interest in the LPA, despite its relevance for active transportation. For example, including data on average distances for active transportation by country in future studies could strengthen the model and enrich the profiling of countries as distance is one of the most consistent predictors of active transportation. Also, since we analyzed aggregated data at the country level, a sample size of 47 is small and has limited power for the LPA. This could partly explain the heterogeneity observed in the profiles, mainly in profile 1. Regarding the policies and practices reviewed, there was also heterogeneity in the information reported across countries. Future versions of the Global Matrix can strengthen the guidance on desirable information to report in this regard, such as the inclusion of active transportation to school in National Education Acts or their equivalents in each country. The sample included in this study represents approximately 25% of the total countries in the world. The inclusion of a larger sample of countries in future studies could provide a clearer picture of profiles according to active transportation and sociodemographic variables.

5. Conclusions

This work allowed for a deeper exploration of the active transportation information reported by all the countries participating in the Global Matrix 3.0. Based on our findings, we identified the need to standardize definitions of active transportation to be able to make more meaningful comparisons. The LPA conducted allows for the inference that countries belonging to a specific profile have a greater probability of sharing certain characteristics among them compared to the countries belonging to other profiles. Given the variation by geographic region and even HDI, this approach is useful for identification of more meaningful groupings that can facilitate the cross-fertilization of efforts to promote active transportation, and therefore, to "power the movement to get kids moving", as is intended by the Global Matrix initiative [171]. The Active Healthy Kids Global Alliance can contribute to improving active travel surveillance providing guidance to countries involved in future versions of the Global Matrix. A more comprehensive approach to active transportation surveillance that considers duration, distance, frequency, direction, other destinations than school and the contribution of active transportation to school to overall active transportation, could improve the understanding of this behaviour and its potential to increase overall physical activity.

Author Contributions: Conceptualization, S.A.G. and S.A.; methodology, S.A.G. and J.D.B.; software, J.D.B.; formal analysis, S.A.G. and J.D.B.; investigation, S.A.G., S.A., J.D.B. and M.S.T.; resources, M.S.T.; data curation, S.A.G., S.A. and J.D.B.; writing—original draft preparation, S.A.G.; writing—review and editing, S.A., J.D.B., R.L. and M.S.T.; visualization, J.D.B.; supervision, M.S.T.; project administration, S.A.; funding acquisition, M.S.T. All authors have read and agreed to the published version of the manuscript.

Funding: S.A.G. was supported by the Government of Ontario and the University of Ottawa through the Ontario Trillium Scholarship for doctoral studies.

Acknowledgments: The authors would like to acknowledge the then Active Healthy Kids Global Alliance Executive Committee for modifying and standardizing the benchmarks and grading rubric and leading this international initiative. We are grateful for all the hard work by each participating country's Report Card Work Group and Leaders and all other members of their Report Card Committees. We also want to thank Megan Forse for her work compiling the data from the report cards.

Conflicts of Interest: The authors declare no conflict of interest.

References

1. Sallis, J.F.; Bull, F.; Guthold, R.; Heath, G.W.; Inoue, S.; Kelly, P.; Oyeyemi, A.L.; Perez, L.G.; Richards, J.; Hallal, P.C. Progress in physical activity over the Olympic quadrennium. *Lancet* **2016**, *388*, 1325–1336. [CrossRef]
2. Ikeda, E.; Hinckson, E.; Witten, K.; Smith, M. Assessment of direct and indirect associations between children active school travel and environmental, household and child factors using structural equation modelling. *Int. J. Behav. Nutr. Phys. Act.* **2019**, *16*, 1–17. [CrossRef] [PubMed]
3. Larouche, R.; Saunders, T.J.; Faulkner, G.E.J.; Colley, R.; Tremblay, M. Associations between active school transport and physical activity, body composition, and cardiovascular fitness: A systematic review of 68 studies. *J. Phys. Act. Health* **2014**, *11*, 206–227. [CrossRef]
4. Centers for Disease Control and Prevention (CDC) Transportation Health Impact Assessment Toolkit. Available online: https://www.cdc.gov/healthyplaces/transportation/promote_strategy.htm (accessed on 20 August 2019).
5. Lubans, D.R.; Boreham, C.A.; Kelly, P.; Foster, C.E. The relationship between active travel to school and health-related fitness in children and adolescents: A systematic review. *Int. J. Behav. Nutr. Phys. Act.* **2011**, *8*, 5. [CrossRef] [PubMed]
6. Andersen, L.B.; Wedderkopp, N.; Kristensen, P.; Moller, N.C.; Froberg, K.; Cooper, A.R. Cycling to school and cardiovascular risk factors: A longitudinal study. *J. Phys. Act. Health* **2011**, *8*, 1025–1033. [CrossRef]
7. Sun, Y.; Liu, Y.; Tao, F.B. Associations between active commuting to school, body fat, and mental well-being: Population-based, cross-sectional study in China. *J. Adolesc. Health* **2015**, *57*, 679–685. [CrossRef]
8. Ruiz-Ariza, A.; de la Torre-Cruz, M.J.; Redecillas-Peiró, M.T.; Martínez-López, E.J. Influencia del desplazamiento activo sobre la felicidad, el bienestar, la angustia psicológica y la imagen corporal en adolescentes. *Gac. Sanit.* **2015**, *29*, 454–457. [CrossRef]
9. Fusco, C.; Moola, F.; Richichi, V. Toward an understanding of children's perceptions of their transport geographies: (non)active school travel and visual representations of the built environment. *J. Transp. Geogr.* **2012**, *20*, 62–70. [CrossRef]
10. Marshall, J.D.; Wilson, R.D.; Meyer, K.L.; Rajangam, S.K.; McDonald, N.C.; Wilson, E.J. Vehicle Emissions during Children's School Commuting: Impacts of Education Policy. *Environ. Sci. Technol.* **2010**, *44*, 1537–1543. [CrossRef]

11. Larouche, R. Last Child Walking?-Prevalence and Trends in Active Transportation. In *Children's Active Transportation*; Larouche, R., Ed.; Elsevier Inc.: Cambridge, UK, 2018; pp. 53–71. ISBN 978-0-12-811931-0.
12. Larouche, R.; Sarmiento, O.L.; Broyles, S.T.; Denstel, K.D.; Church, T.S.; Barreira, T.V.; Chaput, J.-P.; Fogelholm, M.; Hu, G.; Kuriyan, R.; et al. Are the correlates of active school transport context-specific? *Int. J. Obes. Suppl.* **2015**, *5*, S89–S99. [CrossRef]
13. Guthold, R.; Cowan, M.J.; Autenrieth, C.S.; Kann, L.; Riley, L.M. Physical activity and sedentary behavior among schoolchildren: A 34-country comparison. *J. Pediatr.* **2010**, *157*, 43–49.e1. [CrossRef] [PubMed]
14. Aubert, S.; Barnes, J.D.; Abdeta, C.; Abi Nader, P.; Adeniyi, A.F.; Aguilar-Farias, N.; Andrade Tenesaca, D.S.; Bhawra, J.; Brazo-Sayavera, J.; Cardon, G.; et al. Global Matrix 3.0 Physical Activity Report Card Grades for Children and Youth: Results and Analysis From 49 Countries. *J. Phys. Act. Health* **2018**, *15*, S251–S273. [CrossRef] [PubMed]
15. Aubert, S.; Barnes, J.D.; Forse, M.L.; Turner, E.; González, S.A.; Kalinowski, J.; Katzmarzyk, P.T.; Lee, E.Y.; Ocansey, R.; Reilly, J.J.; et al. The international impact of the active healthy kids global alliance physical activity report cards for children and youth. *J. Phys. Act. Health* **2019**, *16*, 679–697. [CrossRef] [PubMed]
16. United Nations Development Programme. *Human Development Report 2016 "Human Development for Everyone"*; United Nations Development Programme: New York, NY, USA, 2016.
17. The World Bank Gini index (World Bank Estimate). Available online: https://datacatalog.worldbank.org/gini-index-world-bank-estimate-1 (accessed on 25 December 2019).
18. Lee, R.J.; Sener, I.N.; Jones, S.N. Understanding the role of equity in active transportation planning in the United States. *Transp. Rev.* **2017**, *37*, 211–226. [CrossRef]
19. Elgar, F.J.; Pförtner, T.K.; Moor, I.; De Clercq, B.; Stevens, G.W.J.M.; Currie, C. Socioeconomic inequalities in adolescent health 2002–2010: A time-series analysis of 34 countries participating in the Health Behaviour in School-aged Children study. *Lancet* **2015**, *385*, 2088–2095. [CrossRef]
20. Stanley, L.; Kellermanns, F.W.; Zellweger, T.M. Latent Profile Analysis: Understanding Family Firm Profiles. *Fam. Bus. Rev.* **2017**, *30*, 84–102. [CrossRef]
21. Rosenberg, J.M.; Beymer, P.N.; Anderson, D.J.; Schmidt, J.A. tidyLPA: An R Package to Easily Carry Out Latent Profile Analysis (LPA) Using Open-Source or Commercial Software. *J. Open Source Softw.* **2018**, *3*, 978. [CrossRef]
22. World Health Organization Global School-Based Student Health Survey (GSHS). Available online: https://www.who.int/ncds/surveillance/gshs/en/ (accessed on 15 August 2020).
23. Roberts, C.; Freeman, J.; Samdal, O.; Schnohr, C.W.; de Looze, M.E.; Nic Gabhainn, S.; Iannotti, R.; Rasmussen, M. International HBSC Study Group The Health Behaviour in School-aged Children (HBSC) study: Methodological developments and current tensions. *Int. J. Public Health* **2009**, *54* (Suppl. 2), 140–150. [CrossRef]
24. Nylund, K.L.; Asparouhov, T.; Muthén, B.O. Deciding on the number of classes in latent class analysis and growth mixture modeling: A Monte Carlo simulation study. *Struct. Equ. Model.* **2007**, *14*, 535–569. [CrossRef]
25. Sasakawa Sports Foundation. *The 2015 SSF National Sports-Life Survey of Children and Young People. Executive Summary*; Sasakawa Sports Foundation: Tokyo, Japan, 2015.
26. Paudel, S.; Subedi, N.; Mehata, S. Physical activity level and associated factors among higher secondary school students in banke, Nepal: A cross-sectional study. *J. Phys. Act. Health* **2016**, *13*, 168–176. [CrossRef]
27. Makaza, D.; Khumalo, B.; Makoni, P.; Mazulu, M.; Dlamini, K.; Tapera, E.; Banda, M.; Mlalazi, T.; Gundani, P.; Chaibva, C. Nutritional Status and Physical Fitness Profiles, Knowledge, Attitudes, Nutritional and Physical Activity Practices of Zimbabwean Primary School Children: The Zimbabwe Baseline Study. Unpublished manuscript. National University of Science and Technology: Bulawayo, Zimbabwe, 2015.
28. Sithole, E. *Global School-Based Health Survey Zimbabwe*, Unpublished Report; Harare, Zimbabwe, 2003.
29. Pilgaard, M.; Rask, S. Danskernes Motions- og Sportsvaner. 2016. Available online: https://www.idan.dk/vidensbank/downloads/danskernes-motions-og-sportsvaner-2016/9a94e44b-4cf5-4fbe-ac89-a696011583d5 (accessed on 15 August 2020).
30. Kokko, S.; Mehtälä, A.; Villberg, J.; Ng, K.; Hämylä, R. *The Physical Activity Behaviours of Children and Adolescents in Finland. Results of the LIITU Study*; Kokko, S., Mehtäla, A., Eds.; National Sports Council: Helsinki, Finland, 2016.
31. Huang, W.Y.; Wong, S.H.; He, G. Is a change to active travel to school an important source of physical activity for Chinese children? *Pediatr. Exerc. Sci.* **2017**, *29*, 161–168. [CrossRef] [PubMed]

32. Korea Centers for Disease Control and Prevention. *The Seventh Korea National Health and Nutrition Examination Survey (KNHANES VII-1). User Guide*; Korea Centers for Disease Control and Prevention: Chung-cheonbuk-do, Korea, 2018.
33. Instituto Colombiano del Bienestar Familiar; Instituto Nacional de Salud; Ministerio de la Protección Social. *Encuesta Nacional de la Situación Nutricional en Colombia 2015 ENSIN*; Instituto Colombiano de Bienestar Familiar: Bogotá, Colombia, 2018.
34. Usman Ahmadu, B.; Maigana Usiju, N.; Ibrahim, A.; Adamu Adiel, A.; Tumba, D.; Rimamchika, M.; Solomon, J.D. Lingering hunger among primary school pupils residing in rural areas of Borno State, North-Eastern Nigeria: Implication for education and food supplementation programs. *Glob. Adv. Res. J. Food Sci. Technol.* **2012**, *1*, 093–097.
35. Adeomi, A.A.; Adeoye, O.A.; Bamidele, J.O.; Abodunrin, O.L.; Odu, O.; Adeomi, O.A. Pattern and determinants of the weight status of school-age children from rural and urban communities of Osun state, Nigeria: A comparative study. *J. Med. Nutr. Nutraceuticals* **2015**, *4*, 107. [CrossRef]
36. BG Be Active. *First Bulgarian Report Card 2018 Active Healthy Kids*; BG Be Active: Plovdiv, Bulgaria, 2018.
37. Mohan, A.; Harish, R. Be Activ Chennai Study. Madras Diabetes Research Foundation, Chennai, India. Unpublished Work. 2018.
38. Ghattu, K.; Kalyanaraman, K. Mysuru Study. CSI Holdsworth Memorial Hospital, Mysuru, India. Unpublished Work, 2018.
39. Tetali, S.; Edwards, P.; Roberts, G.V.S.M.I. How do children travel to school in urban India? A cross-sectional study of 5842 children in Hyderabad. *BMC Public Health* **2016**, *16*, 1–7. [CrossRef] [PubMed]
40. Dandona, R.; Anil Kumar, G.; Ameratunga, S.; Dandona, L. Road use pattern and risk factors for non-fatal road traffic injuries among children in urban India. *Injury* **2011**, *42*, 97–103. [CrossRef] [PubMed]
41. Anitha Rani, M.; Sathiyasekaran, B.W.C. Behavioural determinants for obesity: A cross-sectional study among urban adolescents in India. *J. Prev. Med. Public Health* **2013**, *46*, 192–200. [CrossRef]
42. Dutch National Institute for Public Health and the Environment (RIVM) Leefstijlmonitor. Available online: https://www.rivm.nl/leefstijlmonitor (accessed on 15 August 2020).
43. *Ministerio de Sanidad Servicios Sociales e Igualdad Estudio ALADINO 2015: Estudio de Vigilancia del Crecimiento, Alimentación, Actividad Física, Desarrollo Infantil y Obesidad en España 2015*; Agencia Española de Consumo, Seguridad Alimentaria y Nutrición: Madrid, Spain, 2016.
44. Direcció General de Planificació en Salut; Departament de Salut; Institut d'Estadística de Catalunya Enquesta de Salut de la Població, Estadística Oficial Prevista al Pla estadístic de Catalunya Vigent. Available online: https://salutweb.gencat.cat/ca/el_departament/estadistiques_sanitaries/enquestes/esca/ (accessed on 15 August 2020).
45. Méndez-pérez, B.; Martín-rojo, J.; Castro, V.; Herrera-cuenca, M.; Landaeta-jiménez, M.; Ramírez, G.; Vásquez, M.; Rivas, P.H.; Rosalía, C. Estudio Venezolano de Nutrición y Salud : Perfil antropométrico y patrón de actividad física. Grupo del Estudio Latinoamericano de Nutrición y Salud. The Venezuelan Study of Nutrition and Health : Anthropometric profile and pattern of physical activity. *Venez Nutr.* **2017**, *30*, 53–67.
46. Bel, S.; Van den Abeele, S.; Lebacq, T.; Ost, C.; Brocatus, L.; Stiévenart, C.; Teppers, E.; Tafforeau, J.; Cuypers, K. Protocol of the Belgian food consumption survey 2014: Objectives, design and methods. *Arch. Public Health* **2016**, *74*, 1–11. [CrossRef]
47. Chen, P. Physical activity, physical fitness, and body mass index in the Chinese child and adolescent populations: An update from the 2016 Physical Activity and Fitness in China—The Youth Study. *J. Sport Health Sci.* **2017**, *6*, 381–383. [CrossRef]
48. Pavelka, J.; Sigmundová, D.; Hamřík, Z.; Kalman, M.; Sigmund, E.; Mathisen, F. Trends in Active Commuting to School among Czech Schoolchildren from 2006 to 2014. *Cent. Eur. J. Public Health* **2017**, *25* (Suppl. 1), S21–S25. [CrossRef]
49. Vorlíček, M.; Rubín, L.; Dygrýn, J.; Mitáš, J. Pomáhá aktivní docházka/dojížďka českým adolescentům plnit zdravotní doporučení pro pohybovou aktivitu? *Tělesná Kult.* **2018**, *40*, 112–116. [CrossRef]
50. Instituto Nacional de Estadística y Geografía-INEGI Encuesta Intercensal. Available online: http://www.inegi.org.mx/est/contenidos/Proyectos/encuestas/hogares/especiales/ei2015/ (accessed on 28 March 2020).
51. Romero-Martínez, M.; Shamah-Levy, T.; Cuevas-Nasu, L.; Gómez-Humarán, I.M.; Gaona-Pineda, E.B.; Gómez-Acosta, L.M.; Rivera-Dommarco, J.Á.; Hernández-ávila, M. Diseño metodológico de la encuesta nacional de salud y nutrición de medio camino 2016. *Salud Publica Mex.* **2017**, *59*, 299–305. [CrossRef] [PubMed]

52. Ferrari, G.L.D.M.; De Victo, E.R.; Ferrari, T.K.; Solé, D. Active transportation to school for children and adolescents from Brazil: A systematic review. *Rev. Bras. Cineantropometria Desempenho Hum.* **2018**, *20*, 406–414. [CrossRef]
53. Mazur, J.; Oblacińska, A.; Jodkowska, M. *Physical Activity of School Children Aged 9–17*; Institute of Mother and Child: Warsaw, Poland, 2013.
54. Wojtyła-Buciora, P.; Bołdowski, T.; Wojtyła, C.; Żukiewicz-Sobczak, W.; Juszczak, K.; Łabędzka-Gardy, M.; Wojtyła, A.; Krauss, H. An all-Poland survey of physical activity and sedentary lifestyles for middle school, high school and university students. *J. Health Inequalities* **2017**, *1*, 70–77. [CrossRef]
55. Riley, R.; Mohun, R. *Travel to School in Scotland. Hands Up Scotland Survey 2016: National Summary Report*; Sustrans: Bristol, England, 2017.
56. Transport Scotland. *Transport and Travel in Scotland 2016*; National Statistics: Edinburgh, Scotland, 2017.
57. Jurak, G.; Kovač, M.; Starc, G. The ACDSi 2013-the analysis of children's development in slovenia 2013: Study protocol. *Anthropol. Noteb.* **2013**, *19*, 123–143.
58. Starc, G.; Kovač, M.; Strel, J.; Pajek, M.B.; Golja, P.; Robič, T.; Kotnik, K.Z.; Grum, D.K.; Filipčič, T.; Sorí, M.; et al. The ACDSi 2014—A decennial study on adolescents' somatic, motor, psychosocial development and healthy lifestyle: Study protocol. *Anthropol. Noteb.* **2015**, *21*, 107–123.
59. *Statistics South Africa General Household Survey 2013*; Statistics South Africa: Pretoria, South Africa, 2015.
60. Simons, A.; Koekemoer, K.; van Niekerk, A.; Govender, R. Parental supervision and discomfort with children walking to school in low-income communities in Cape Town, South Africa. *Traffic Inj. Prev.* **2018**, *19*, 391–398. [CrossRef]
61. Koekemoer, K.; Van Gesselleen, M.; Van Niekerk, A.; Govender, R.; Van As, A.B. Child pedestrian safety knowledge, behaviour and road injury in Cape Town, South Africa. *Accid. Anal. Prev.* **2017**, *99*, 202–209. [CrossRef]
62. *Swedish Transport Administration Children's Routes to School, TRV 2013/54076*; Swedish Transport Administration: Borlänge, Sweden, 2015.
63. Amornsriwatanakul, A.; Bull, F.; Rosenberg, M. *Thailand Physical Activity Children Survey*; Thailand Physical Activity Research Centre and University of Western Australia: Perth, Australia, 2015.
64. World Health Organization Global School-Based Student Health Survey (GSHS)-Datasets. Available online: https://www.who.int/ncds/surveillance/gshs/datasets/en/ (accessed on 15 August 2020).
65. World Health Organization 2014 Global School-based Student Health Survey (GSHS) results: Bangladesh Survey. 2014. Available online: https://www.who.int/ncds/surveillance/gshs/BDH2014_public_use_codebook.pdf?ua=1 (accessed on 16 August 2020).
66. Department of Transport National Travel Survey: England 2016. Statistical Release. 2016. Available online: https://assets.publishing.service.gov.uk/government/uploads/system/uploads/attachment_data/file/633077/national-travel-survey-2016.pdf (accessed on 16 August 2020).
67. NatCen Social Research; University College London. *Department of Epidemiology and Public Health Health Survey for England, 2015*; UK Data Service: Colchester, England, 2017.
68. Department for Transport Walking and Cycling Statistics, England. 2016. Available online: https://assets.publishing.service.gov.uk/government/uploads/system/uploads/attachment_data/file/674503/walking-and-cycling-statistics-england-2016.pdf (accessed on 16 August 2020).
69. Agence Nationale de Sécurité Sanitaire ANSES. Étude Individuelle Nationale des Consommations Alimentaires 3. 2017. Available online: https://www.anses.fr/fr/system/files/NUT2014SA0234Ra.pdf (accessed on 16 August 2020).
70. *Équipe de Surveillance et D'épidémiologie Nutritionnelle (Esen) Étude de Santé sur L'environnement, la Biosurveillance, L'activité Physique et la Nutrition (Esteban) 2014–2016*; Volet Nutrition, Chapitre Activité Physique et Sédentarité; Santé Publique France: Saint Maurice, Switzerland, 2017.
71. Emeljanovas, A.; Gruodyte–Raciene, R.; Sukys, S.; Mieziene, B.; Rutkauskaite, R.; Trinkuniene, L.; Fatkulina, N.; Gerulskiene, I.; Balsyte, V.; Zabolotnaja, T.; et al. *The Lithuanian Physical Activity Report Card for Children and Youth*; Lithuanian Sports University: Kaunas, Lithuania, 2018.
72. Wijnhoven, T.M.A.; Van Raaij, J.M.A.; Yngve, A.; Sjöberg, A.; Kunešová, M.; Duleva, V.; Petrauskiene, A.; Rito, A.I.; Breda, J. WHO European childhood obesity surveillance initiative: Health-risk behaviours on nutrition and physical activity in 6-9-year-old schoolchildren. *Public Health Nutr.* **2015**, *18*, 3108–3124. [CrossRef]

73. Meškaitė, A.; Dadelienė, R.; Kowalski, I.M.; Burokienė, S.; Doveikienė, J.; Juocevičius, A.; Raistenskis, J. 11-15 Metų Mokinių Fizinio Aktyvumo Ir. *Sveik. Moksl.* **2012**, *22*, 49–53.
74. Žaltauskė, V. Lietuvos 7–8 metų Vaikų Fizinis Aktyvumas ir jo Sąsajos su Individualiais, Šeimos ir Mokyklos Aplinkos Veiksniais. 2017. Available online: https://193.219.163.160/cris/handle/20.500.12512/95687 (accessed on 16 August 2020).
75. European Comission Special Eurobarometer 472. Report Sport and Physical Activity; European Union. 2018. Available online: https://ec.europa.eu/commfrontoffice/publicopinion/index.cfm/ResultDoc/download/DocumentKy/82432 (accessed on 16 August 2020).
76. Ministry of Health Annual Update of Key Results 2016/17: New Zealand Health Survey 2017. Available online: https://www.health.govt.nz/publication/annual-update-key-results-2016-17-new-zealand-health-survey (accessed on 16 August 2020).
77. *Sport New Zealand Active NZ and Active NZ Young People*; Sport New Zealand: Wellington, New Zealand, 2018.
78. Health Promotion Agency. *2016 Health and Lifestyles Survey: Methodology Report*; Health Promotion Agency: Wellington, New Zealand, 2017.
79. Ministry of Transport. *Household Travel Survey*; Ministry of Transport: Wellington, New Zealand, 2018.
80. Morton, S.M.B.; Carr, P.E.A.; Bandara, D.K. *Growing Up in New Zealand: A Longitudinal Study of New Zealand Children and Their Families*; Report 1: Before We Are Born; University of Auckland: Auckland, New Zealand, 2010.
81. Pizarro, A.N.; Santos, M.P.; Ribeiro, J.C.; Mota, J. Physical activity and active transport are predicted by adolescents' different built environment perceptions. *J. Public Health* **2012**, *20*, 5–10. [CrossRef]
82. *Administração Regional de Saúde do Alentejo (ARSA) Estudo de Saúde da População Infantil da Região Alentejo–Relatório*; Núcleo Regional do Alentejo da Plataforma Contra a Obesidade da ARSA: Évora, Portugal, 2012.
83. Ministry of Education. *Report of Student Participation in Physical Activity School Year 2015–2016*; Sports Administration, Ministry of Education: Taipei City, Taiwan, 2017.
84. Health Promotion Administration. *Report of Health Behavior Survey in Junior High School Students 2016*; Ministry of Health and Welfare: Taipei City, Taiwan, 2017.
85. Cancer Council Victoria National Secondary Students' Diet and Activity (NaSSDA) survey 2012–2013. Available online: http://www.cancer.org.au/news/media-releases/increase-in-teenagers-screen-use-a-new-threat-to-long-term-health.html (accessed on 6 March 2020).
86. *Epidemiology Section ACT Health Year 6 ACT Physical Activity and Nutrition Survey*; ACTdata Collection; Epidemiology Section: Canberra, Australia, 2015.
87. Centre for Epidemiology and Evidence NSW Ministry of Health. *Child Population Health Survey*; Centre for Epidemiology and Evidence: New South Wales, Australia, 2015.
88. Queensland Health. *Queensland Child Preventive Health Survey 2018*, Report of the Chief Health Officer Queensland; Brisbane, QLD, Australia, 2018.
89. Hardy, L.; Mihrshahi, S.; Drayton, B.; Bauman, A. *NSW Schools Physical Activity and Nutrition Survey (SPANS) 2015*; Full Report; NSW Department of Health: Sydney, NSW, Australia, 2016.
90. Department of Education and Early Childhood Development. *Victorian Child Health and Wellbeing Survey (VCHWS)*; Department of Education and Early Childhood Development: Victoria, Australia, 2013.
91. Scriven, J.; Morris, S.; Irving, P.; Sheehan, D. Evaluating physical literacy levels of KS1 children in Jersey, Channel Islands Poster. Presented at UKSCA National Conference, Leicester, UK, 4–6 August 2017.
92. Welsh Government National survey for Wales 2016/17 2017. Available online: https://gov.wales/national-survey-wales-april-2016-march-2017 (accessed on 16 August 2020).
93. Hewitt, G.; Anthony, R.; Moore, G.; Melendez-Torres, G.; Murphy, S. *Student Health and Wellbeing In Wales: Report of the 2017/18 Health Behaviour in School-aged Children Survey and School Health Research Network Student Health and Wellbeing Survey*; Cardiff University: Cardiff, UK, 2019.
94. *Research Group of Physical Activity for Health Children's Physical Activity Study 2015 and Schools in Motion Survey 2018*; University of Tartu, Institute of Sport Sciences and Physiotherapy: Tartu, Estonia, 2018.
95. States of Guernsey Guernsey Young People's Survey 2016/2017. 2016. Available online: https://www.gov.gg/ypsurveyarchive (accessed on 18 August 2020).
96. World Health Organization NCDs: Lebanon Global School-Based Student Health Survey (GSHS) Implementation. 2017. Available online: https://www.who.int/ncds/surveillance/gshs/lebanon/en/ (accessed on 16 August 2020).

97. *Canadian Fitness and Lifestyle Research Institute Bulletin 5: Active Transportation Among Children and Youth*; Canadian Fitness and Lifestyle Research Institute: Ottawa, ON, Canada, 2018.
98. National Center for Health Statistics. *National Health and Nutrition Examination Survey*; U.S. Department of Health and Human Services, CDC, National Center for Health Statistics: Hyattsville, MD, USA, 2016.
99. Ministerio de Salud de Chile Encuesta Nacional de Calidad de Vida 2015–2016 (ENCAVI). 2017. Available online: http://www.sochmet.cl/wp-content/uploads/2017/06/Resultados_Abril2017_ENCAVI_2015-16_Depto_Epidemiolog%C3%ADa_MINSAL.pdf (accessed on 16 August 2020).
100. Ministerio de Vivienda y Urbanismo Encuesta de Percepción de Calidad de Vida Urbana (EPCVU 2015). 2016. Available online: http://calidaddevida.colabora.minvu.cl/doc2016/Resultados%20Encuesta%20Percepci%C3%B3n%20de%20Calidad%20de%20Vida%20Urbana%202015.pdf (accessed on 16 August 2020).
101. García-Hermoso, A.; Saavedra, J.M.; Olloquequi, J.; Ramírez-Vélez, R. Associations between the duration of active commuting to school and academic achievement in rural Chilean adolescents. *Environ. Health Prev. Med.* **2017**, *22*, 31. [CrossRef] [PubMed]
102. Rodríguez-Rodríguez, F.; Cristi-Montero, C.; Celis-Morales, C.; Escobar-Gómez, D.; Chillón, P. Impact of distance on mode of active commuting in Chilean children and adolescents. *Int. J. Environ. Res. Public Health* **2017**, *14*, 1334. [CrossRef] [PubMed]
103. Mori, N.; Armada, F.; Willcox, D.C. Walking to school in Japan and childhood obesity prevention: New lessons from an old policy. *Am. J. Public Health* **2012**, *102*, 2068–2073. [CrossRef] [PubMed]
104. Tanaka, C.; Tanaka, S.; Inoue, S.; Miyachi, M.; Suzuki, K.; Abe, T.; Reilly, J.J. Results from the Japan's 2018 report card on physical activity for children and youth. *J. Exerc. Sci. Fit.* **2019**, *17*, 20–25. [CrossRef]
105. Munambah, N.; Matsungo, T.; Makaza, D.; Mahachi, C.; Mlalazi, T.; Masocha, V.; Makoni, P.; Khumalo, B.; Rutsate, S.; Mandaza, D.; et al. *Physical Activity and the Nutritional Status of School-Aged Children in Zimbabwe: Current Research Evidence and Policy Implications*; Active Health Kids Zimbabwe: Harare, Zimbabwe, 2018.
106. Tammelin, T.; Kämppi, K.; Aalto-Nevalainen, P.; Aira, A.; Halme, N.; Husu, P.; Inkinen, V.; Joensuu, L.; Kokko, S.; Korsberg, M.; et al. *Finland's Report Card 2018–Physical Activity for Children and Youth*; The LIKES Research Centre for Physical Activity and Health: Jyväskylä, Finland, 2018.
107. Wong, S.H.S.; Huang, W.Y.J.; Sit, C.H.P.; Wong, M.C.S.; Sum, R.K.M.; Wong, S.W.S. *The 2018 Active Healthy Kids Hong Kong Report Card on Physical Activity for Children and Youth*; The Chinese University of Hong Kong: Hong Kong, China, 2018.
108. Huang, W.Y.; Wong, S.H.S.; Sit, C.H.P.; Wong, M.C.S.; Sum, R.K.W.; Wong, S.W.S.; Yu, J.J. Results from the Hong Kong's 2018 report card on physical activity for children and youth. *J. Exerc. Sci. Fit.* **2019**, *17*, 14–19. [CrossRef]
109. Gonzalez, S.A.; Triana, C.A.; Garcia, J.; Sarmiento, O.L. *Report Card on Physical Activity of Children and Youth—Colombia 2018–2019*; Universidad de los Andes: Bogota, Colombia, 2018.
110. Hidalgo, D.; Miranda, L.; Lleras, N.; Ríos, J. Al Colegio en Bici: Bike-to-School Program in Bogotá, Colombia. *Transp. Res. Rec. J. Transp. Res. Board* **2016**, *2581*, 66–70. [CrossRef]
111. Sarmiento, O.; Torres, A.; Jacoby, E.; Pratt, M.; Schmid, T.L.; Stierling, G. The Ciclovía-Recreativa: A Mass-Recreational Program With Public Health Potential. *J. Phys. Act. Health* **2010**, *7*, 163–180. [CrossRef]
112. Triana, C.A.; Sarmiento, O.L.; Bravo-Balado, A.; González, S.A.; Bolívar, M.A.; Lemoine, P.; Meisel, J.D.; Grijalba, C.; Katzmarzyk, P.T. Active streets for children: The case of the Bogotá Ciclovía. *PLoS ONE* **2019**, *14*, e0207791. [CrossRef]
113. Congreso de la República de Colombia Ley 1811 de 2016 por la cual se Otorgan Incentivos Para Promover el uso de la Bicicleta en el Territorio Nacional y se Modifica el Código Nacional de Tránsito. 2016. Available online: https://dapre.presidencia.gov.co/normativa/normativa/LEY%201811%20DEL%2021%20DE%20OCTUBRE%20DE%202016.pdf (accessed on 16 August 2020).
114. Akinroye, K.K.; Adeniyi, A.F.; Odukoya, O.O.; Adedoyin, R.A.; Odior, S.; Oyeyemi, A.L.; Metseagharun, E.; Fawehinmi, O.S.; Ezeigwe, N.; Ayorinde, R.O. *2018 Nigerian Report Card on Physical Activity for Children and Youth*; Nigerian Heart Foundation: Ibadan, Nigeria, 2018.
115. FIA Foundation Walking the Talk: Supporting Nigeria to Adopt Policies for Active Mobility-FIA Foundation. Available online: https://www.fiafoundation.org/blog/2017/november/walking-the-talk-supporting-nigeria-to-adopt-policies-for-active-mobility (accessed on 10 February 2020).

116. Lagos State Ministry of Transportation; Lagos Metropolitan Area Transport Authority; United Nations Environment Programme; Institute for Transportation and Development Policy. *Lagos Non-Motorised Transport Policy Empowering Pedestrians and Cyclists for a Better City*; Institute for Transportation and Development Policy: Lagos, Nigeria, 2018.
117. Nyawornota, V.K.; Luguterah, A.; Sofo, S.; Aryeetey, R.; Badasu, M.; Nartey, J.; Assasie, E.; Donkor, S.K.; Dougblor, V.; Williams, H.; et al. Results from Ghana's 2018 Report Card on Physical Activity for Children and Youth. *J. Phys. Act. Health* **2018**, *15*, S366–S367. [CrossRef]
118. Galaviz, K.; Argumedo García, G.; Gaytán-González, A.; González-Casanova, I.; González Villalobos, M.; Jáuregui, A.; Jáuregui Ulloa, E.; Medina, C.; Pacheco Miranda, Y.; Pérez Rodríguez, M.; et al. *Mexican Report Card on Physical Activity of Children and Youth 2018*; Universidad de Guadalajara: Guadalajara, Jal, Mexico, 2018.
119. Silva, D.A.S.; Christofaro, D.G.D.; Ferrari, G.L.D.M.; da Silva, K.S.; Nardo, N., Jr.; Silva, R.J.D.S.; Fernandes, R.A.; Barbosa Filho, V.C. *Report Card Brazil 2018: It's Time to Take Care of Children and Teenagers! Report on Physical Activity in Brazilian Children and Adolescents*; Federal University of Santa Catarina: Florianopolis, Santa Catarina, Brazil, 2018.
120. Abdeta, C.; Teklemariam, Z.; Deksisa, A.; Abera, E. *Ethiopia's 2018 Report Card on Physical Activity for Children and Youth*; Active Healthy Kids Ethiopia: Harar, Ethiopia, 2018.
121. Active Healthy Kids Scotland. *Active Healthy Kids Scotland Report Card 2018*; University of Strathclyde: Glasgow, Scotland, 2018.
122. Delisle Nyström, C.; Larsson, C.; Alexandrou, C.; Ehrenblad, B.; Eriksson, U.; Friberg, M.; Hagströmer, M.; Lindroos, A.K.; Nyberg, G.; Löf, M. *Active Healthy Kids Sweden 2018*; Karolinska Insitutet: Huddinge, Sweden, 2018.
123. Ministry of Enterprise and Innovation. *A National Cycling Strategy for More and Safer Cycling*; Government Offices of Sweden: Stockholm, Sweden, 2017.
124. Andrade, S.; Ochoa-Aviles, A.; Freire, W.; Romero-Sandoval, N.; Orellana, D.; Contreras, T.; Pillco, J.L.; Sacta, J.; Andrade Muñoz, D.; Ramírez, P.; et al. Results from Ecuador's 2018 Report Card on Physical Activity for Children and Youth. *J. Phys. Act. Health* **2018**, *15*, S344–S346. [CrossRef] [PubMed]
125. Aubert, S.; Aucouturier, J.; Vanhelst, J.; Fillon, A.; Genin, P.; Ganière, C.; Praznoczy, C.; Larras, B.; Schipman, J.; Duclos, M.; et al. France's 2018 Report Card on Physical Activity for Children and Youth: Results and International Comparisons. *J. Phys. Act. Health* **2020**, 1–8. [CrossRef] [PubMed]
126. Smith, M.; Ikeda, E.; Hinckson, E.; Duncan, S.; Maddison, R.; Meredith-Jones, K.; Walker, C.; Mandic, S. *New Zealand's 2018 Report Card on Physical Activity for Children and Youth*; The University of Auckland: Auckland, New Zealand, 2018.
127. Smith, M.; Ikeda, E.; Duncan, S.; Maddison, R.; Hinckson, E.; Meredith-Jones, K.; Walker, C.; Mandic, S. Trends and measurement issues for active transportation in New Zealand's physical activity report cards for children and youth: NZ child/youth active transport trends. *J. Transp. Health* **2019**, *15*, 100789. [CrossRef]
128. Chang, C.-K.; Wu, C.-L.; Chen, L.-J.; Fang, S.-H.; Hung, C.-W.; Jiang, R.-S.; Lee, P.-C.; Wang, W.-Y.; Wu, C.-M. *The Active Healthy Kids Taiwan Report Card 2018 on Physical Activity for Children and Youth*; National Taiwan University of Sport: Taichung, Taiwan, 2018.
129. Active Healthy Kids Australia. *Muscular Fitness: It's Time for a Jump Start. The 2018 Active Healthy Kids Australia Report Card on Physical Activity for Children and Young People*; Active Healthy Kids Australia: Adelaide, Australia, 2018.
130. Sustrans Active Journeys. *Getting Young People Active on the Journey to School*; Sustrans: Bristol, England, 2019.
131. Living Streets. *Walk to School with Living Streets*; Living Streets: London, UK, 2019.
132. Stratton, G.; Edwards, L.; Tyler, R.; Blain, D.; Bryant, A. *Active Healthy Kids Wales 2018 Report Card*; Active Healthy Kids Wales: Wales, UK, 2018.
133. Williams, A.; Whitman, L.; Page, Y.L.; Page, C.L.; Chester, G.; Sebire, S.J. Results from the Bailiwick of Guernsey's 2018 Report Card on Physical Activity for Children and Youth. *J. Phys. Act. Health* **2018**, *15*, S368–S369. [CrossRef] [PubMed]
134. The States of Deliberation of the Island of Guernsey. *The On-Island Integrated Transport Strategy-First Periodic Review*; Committee for the Environment & Infrastructure: St. Martin, Guernsey, 2019.
135. Abi Nader, P.; Majed, L.; Sayegh, S.; Hadla, R.; Borgi, C.; Hawa, Z.; Mattar, L.; Fares, E.-J.; Chamieh, M.C.; Habib-Mourad, C.; et al. Results from Lebanon's 2018 Report Card on Physical Activity for Children and Youth. *J. Phys. Act. Health* **2018**, *15*. in press. [CrossRef]

136. Nader, P.A.; Majed, L.; Sayegh, S.; Mattar, L.; Hadla, R.; Chamieh, M.C.; Mourad, C.H.; Fares, E.J.; Hawa, Z.; Bélanger, M. First physical activity report card for children and youth in Lebanon. *J. Phys. Act. Health* **2019**, *16*, 385–396. [CrossRef]
137. ParticipACTION. *The Brain + Body Equation: Canadian Kids Need Active Bodies to Build Their Best Brains. The 2018 ParticipACTION Report Card on Physical Activity for Children and Youth*; ParticipACTION: Toronto, ON, Canada, 2018.
138. Ontario Active School Travel Steps to Success-Ontario Active School Travel. Available online: https://ontarioactiveschooltravel.ca/steps-to-success-the-5-es/#fivees%7C4 (accessed on 14 February 2020).
139. Safe Routes Partnership Safe Routes to School|Safe Routes Partnership. Available online: https://www.saferoutespartnership.org/safe-routes-school (accessed on 15 February 2020).
140. National Physical Activity Plan Alliance. *The 2018 United States Report Card on Physical Activity for Children and Youth*; National Physical Activity Plan Alliance: Washington, DC, USA, 2018.
141. Aubert, S.; Barnes, J.D.; Aguilar-Farias, N.; Cardon, G.; Chang, C.-K.; Delisle Nyström, C.; Demetriou, Y.; Edwards, L.; Emeljanovas, A.; Gába, A.; et al. Report Card Grades on the Physical Activity of Children and Youth Comparing 30 Very High Human Development Index Countries. *J. Phys. Act. Health* **2018**, *15*, S298–S314. [CrossRef]
142. González, S.A.; Barnes, J.D.; Abi Nader, P.; Susana Andrade Tenesaca, D.; Brazo-Sayavera, J.; Galaviz, K.I.; Herrera-Cuenca, M.; Katewongsa, P.; López-Taylor, J.; Liu, Y.; et al. Report Card Grades on the Physical Activity of Children and Youth From 10 Countries With High Human Development Index: Global Matrix 3.0. *J. Phys. Act. Health* **2018**, *15*, S284–S297. [CrossRef]
143. Manyanga, T.; Barnes, J.D.; Abdeta, C.; Adeniyi, A.F.; Bhawra, J.; Draper, C.E.; Katapally, T.R.; Khan, A.; Lambert, E.; Makaza, D.; et al. Indicators of Physical Activity Among Children and Youth in 9 Countries With Low to Medium Human Development Indices: A Global Matrix 3.0 Paper. *J. Phys. Act. Health* **2018**, *15*, S274–S283. [CrossRef]
144. Whitfield, G.P.; Paul, P.; Wendel, A.M. Active Transportation Surveillance—United States, 1999–2012. *MMWR. Surveill. Summ.* **2015**, *64*, 1–17. [CrossRef]
145. Manyanga, T.; Munambah, N.E.; Mahachi, C.B.; Makaza, D.; Mlalazi, T.F.; Masocha, V.; Makoni, P.; Sithole, F.; Khumalo, B.; Rutsate, S.H.; et al. Results from Zimbabwe's 2018 Report Card on Physical Activity for Children and Youth. *J. Phys. Act. Health* **2018**, *15*, s433–s435. [CrossRef] [PubMed]
146. Tladi, D.M.; Monnaatsie, M.; Shaibu, S.; Sinombe, G.; Mokone, G.G.; Gabaitiri, L.; Malete, L.; Omphile, H. Results from Botswana's 2018 Report Card on Physical Activity for Children and Youth. *J. Phys. Act. Health* **2018**, *15*, s320–s322. [CrossRef] [PubMed]
147. Brazo-Sayavera, J.; Del Campo, C.; Rodríguez, M.J.; da Silva, I.C.M.; Merellano-Navarro, E.; Olivares, P.R. Results from Uruguay's 2018 Report Card on Physical Activity for Children and Youth. *J. Phys. Act. Health* **2018**, *15*, s425–s426. [CrossRef] [PubMed]
148. Larouche, R.; Sarmiento, O.L.; Stewart, T. Active Transportation—Is the School Hiding the Forest. In *Children's Active Transportation*; Elsevier: Amsterdam, The Netherlands, 2018; pp. 243–258.
149. Williams, G.C.; Borghese, M.M.; Janssen, I. Objectively measured active transportation to school and other destinations among 10–13 year olds. *Int. J. Behav. Nutr. Phys. Act.* **2018**, *15*. [CrossRef] [PubMed]
150. Herrador-Colmenero, M.; Pérez-García, M.; Ruiz, J.R.; Chillón, P. Assessing modes frequency of commuting to school in youngsters: A systematic review. *Pediatr. Exerc. Sci.* **2014**, *26*, 291–341. [CrossRef]
151. Oberski, D. Mixture Models: Latent Profile and Latent Class Analysis. In *Modern Statistical Methods for HCI*; Robertson, J., Kaptein, M., Eds.; Human–Computer Interaction Series; Springer: Cham, Switzerland, 2016; pp. 275–287.
152. Lee, C.; Zhu, X.; Yoon, J.; Varni, J.W. Beyond distance: Children's school travel mode choice. *Ann. Behav. Med.* **2013**, *45*. [CrossRef]
153. McDonald, N.C.; Aalborg, A.E. Why Parents Drive Children to School: Implications for Safe Routes to School Programs. *J. Am. Plan. Assoc.* **2009**, *75*, 331–342. [CrossRef]
154. Faulkner, G.E.; Richichi, V.; Buliung, R.N.; Fusco, C.; Moola, F. What's "quickest and easiest?": Parental decision making about school trip mode. *Int. J. Behav. Nutr. Phys. Act.* **2010**, *7*, 62. [CrossRef]
155. Pucher, J.; Buehler, R. Making cycling irresistible: Lessons from the Netherlands, Denmark and Germany. *Transp. Rev.* **2008**, *28*, 495–528. [CrossRef]
156. Pucher, J.; Dijkstra, L. Making Walking and Cycling Safer: Lessons from Europe. *Transp. Q.* **2000**, *54*, 25–50.

157. Larouche, R.; Oyeyemi, A.L.; Prista, A.; Onywera, V.; Akinroye, K.K.; Tremblay, M.S. A systematic review of active transportation research in Africa and the psychometric properties of measurement tools for children and youth. *Int. J. Behav. Nutr. Phys. Act.* **2014**, *11*, 1–18. [CrossRef] [PubMed]
158. Oyeyemi, A.L.; Larouche, R. Prevalence and Correlates of Active Transportation in Developing Countries. In *Children's Active Transportation*; Elsevier: Amsterdam, The Netherlands, 2018; pp. 173–191.
159. Salvo, D.; Reis, R.S.; Sarmiento, O.L.; Pratt, M. Overcoming the challenges of conducting physical activity and built environment research in Latin America: IPEN Latin America. *Prev. Med. (Baltim.)* **2014**, *69*, S86–S92. [CrossRef] [PubMed]
160. Katzmarzyk, P.T.; Mason, C. The physical activity transition. *J. Phys. Act. Health* **2009**, *6*, 269–280. [CrossRef] [PubMed]
161. Broberg, A.; Sarjala, S. School travel mode choice and the characteristics of the urban built environment: The case of Helsinki, Finland. *Transp. Policy* **2015**, *37*, 1–10. [CrossRef]
162. Sarmiento, O.L.; Lemoine, P.; Gonzalez, S.A.; Broyles, S.T.; Denstel, K.D.; Larouche, R.; Onywera, V.; Barreira, T.V.; Chaput, J.-P.; Fogelholm, M.; et al. Relationships between active school transport and adiposity indicators in school-age children from low-, middle- and high-income countries. *Int. J. Obes. Suppl.* **2015**, *5*, S107–S114. [CrossRef] [PubMed]
163. Arango, C.M.; Parra, D.C.; Eyler, A.; Sarmiento, O.; Mantilla, S.C.; Gomez, L.F.; Lobelo, F. Walking or bicycling to school and weight status among adolescents from Montería, Colombia. *J. Phys. Act. Health* **2011**, *8* (Suppl. 2), S171–S177. [CrossRef]
164. Herrera-Cuenca, M.; Méndez-Pérez, B.; Landaeta-Jiménez, M.; Marcano, X.; Guilart, E.; Sotillé, L.; Romero, R. Results from Venezuela's 2018 Report Card on Physical Activity for Children and Youth. *J. Phys. Act. Health* **2018**, *15*, s427–s429. [CrossRef]
165. Jáuregui, A.; Medina, C.; Salvo, D.; Barquera, S.; Rivera-Dommarco, J.A. Active Commuting to School in Mexican Adolescents: Evidence From the Mexican National Nutrition and Health Survey. *J. Phys. Act. Health* **2015**, *12*, 1088–1095. [CrossRef]
166. Torres, A.; Sarmiento, O.L.; Stauber, C.; Zarama, R. The Ciclovia and Cicloruta programs: Promising interventions to promote physical activity and social capital in Bogotá, Colombia. *Am. J. Public Health* **2013**, *103*, e23–e30. [CrossRef]
167. Clark, H.; Coll-Seck, A.M.; Banerjee, A.; Peterson, S.; Dalglish, S.L.; Ameratunga, S.; Balabanova, D.; Bhan, M.K.; Bhutta, Z.A.; Borrazzo, J.; et al. A future for the world's children? A WHO–UNICEF–Lancet Commission. *Lancet* **2020**, *395*, 605–658. [CrossRef]
168. Sims, R.; Schaeffer, R.; Creutzig, F.; Cruz-Núñez, X.; D'Agosto, M.; Dimitriu, D.; Figueroa Meza, M.J.; Fulton, L.; Kobayashi, S.; Lah, O.; et al. Transport. In *Climate Change 2014: Mitigation of Climate Change. Contribution of Working Group III to the Fifth Assessment Report of the Intergovernmental Panel on Climate Change*; Edenhofer, O., Pichs-Madruga, R., Sokona, Y., Farahani, E., Kadner, S., Seyboth, K., Adler, A., Baum, I., Brunner, S., Eickemeier, P., et al., Eds.; Cambridge University Press: Cambridge, UK; New York, NY, USA, 2014; pp. 599–670.
169. Peralta, M.; Henriques-Neto, D.; Bordado, J.; Loureiro, N.; Diz, S.; Marques, A. Active Commuting to School and Physical Activity Levels among 11 to 16 Year-Old Adolescents from 63 Low- and Middle-Income Countries. *Int. J. Environ. Res. Public Health* **2020**, *17*, 1276. [CrossRef] [PubMed]
170. Aguilar-Farias, N.; Martino-Fuentealba, P.; Carcamo-Oyarzun, J.; Cortínez-O'Ryan, A.; Cristi-Montero, C.; Von Oetinger, A.; Sadarangani, K.P. A regional vision of physical activity, sedentary behaviour and physical education in adolescents from Latin America and the Caribbean: Results from 26 countries. *Int. J. Epidemiol.* **2018**, *47*, 976–986. [CrossRef] [PubMed]
171. Tremblay, M.S.; Gray, C.E.; Akinroye, K.; Harrington, D.M.; Katzmarzyk, P.T.; Lambert, E.V.; Liukkonen, J.; Maddison, R.; Ocansey, R.T.; Onywera, V.O.; et al. Physical Activity of Children: A Global Matrix of Grades Comparing 15 Countries. *J. Phys. Act. Health* **2014**, *11*, S113–S125. [CrossRef] [PubMed]

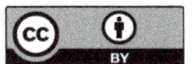

© 2020 by the authors. Licensee MDPI, Basel, Switzerland. This article is an open access article distributed under the terms and conditions of the Creative Commons Attribution (CC BY) license (http://creativecommons.org/licenses/by/4.0/).

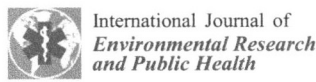 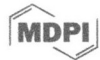

Article

Association between Perceived Neighborhood Built Environment and Walking and Cycling for Transport among Inhabitants from Latin America: The ELANS Study

Gerson Ferrari [1,*], André Oliveira Werneck [2], Danilo Rodrigues da Silva [3], Irina Kovalskys [4], Georgina Gómez [5], Attilio Rigotti [6], Lilia Yadira Cortés Sanabria [7], Martha Cecilia Yépez García [8], Rossina G. Pareja [9], Marianella Herrera-Cuenca [10], Ioná Zalcman Zimberg [11], Viviana Guajardo [12], Michael Pratt [13], Cristian Cofre Bolados [1,14], Emilio Jofré Saldía [1], Carlos Pires [15], Adilson Marques [16,17], Miguel Peralta [16,17], Eduardo Rossato de Victo [18], Mauro Fisberg [18,19] and on behalf of the ELANS Study Group [†]

1. Laboratorio de Ciencias de la Actividad Física, el Deporte y la Salud, Facultad de Ciencias Médicas, Universidad de Santiago de Chile, USACH, Santiago 7500618, Chile; cristian.cofre@usach.cl (C.C.B.); emilio.jofre.s@usach.cl (E.J.S.)
2. Department of Nutrition, School of Public Health, Universidade de São Paulo (USP), São Paulo 01246-904, Brazil; andreowerneck@gmail.com
3. Department of Physical Education, Federal University of Sergipe—UFS, São Cristóvão 49100-000, Brazil; danilorpsilva@gmail.com
4. Carrera de Nutrición, Facultad de Ciencias Médicas, Pontificia Universidad Católica Argentina, Buenos Aires C1107 AAZ, Argentina; ikovalskys@gmail.com
5. Departamento de Bioquímica, Escuela de Medicina, Universidad de Costa Rica, San José 11501-2060, Costa Rica; georgina.gomez@ucr.ac.cr
6. Centro de Nutrición Molecular y Enfermedades Crónicas, Departamento de Nutrición, Diabetes y Metabolismo, Escuela de Medicina, Pontificia Universidad Católica, Santiago 8330024, Chile; arigotti@med.puc.cl
7. Departamento de Nutrición y Bioquímica, Pontificia Universidad Javeriana, Bogotá 110231, Colombia; ycortes@javeriana.edu.co
8. Colégio de Ciencias de la Salud, Universidad San Francisco de Quito, Quito 17-1200-841, Ecuador; myepez@usfq.edu.ec
9. Instituto de Investigación Nutricional, Lima 15026, Peru; rpareja@iin.sld.pe
10. Centro de Estudios del Desarrollo, Universidad Central de Venezuela (CENDES-UCV)/Fundación Bengoa, Caracas 1053, Venezuela; manyma@gmail.com
11. Departamento de Psicobiologia, Universidade Federal de São Paulo, São Paulo 04023-062, Brazil; iona.zimberg@gmail.com
12. Nutrition, Health and Wellbeing Area, International Life Science Institute (ILSI) Argentina, Santa Fe Av. 1145, CABA C1059ABF, Argentina; viviana.guajardo@comunidad.ub.edu.ar
13. Institute for Public Health, University of California San Diego, La Jolla, CA 92093-0021, USA; mipratt@health.ucsd.edu
14. Facultad de Salud, Instituto de Ciencias del Deporte, Escuela de Ciencias del Deporte y la Actividad Física, Universidad Santo Tomas Santiago de Chile, Santiago 5520540, Chile
15. Center for Research in Neuropsychology and Cognitive and Behavioral Intervention (CINEICC), Faculty of Psychology and Educational Sciences, University of Coimbra, 3000-115 Coimbra, Portugal; carlosandrepires@gmail.com
16. CIPER, Faculdade de Motricidade Humana, Universidade de Lisboa, 1499-002 Lisbon, Portugal; adncmpt@gmail.com (A.M.); miguel.peralta14@gmail.com (M.P.)
17. ISAMB, Faculdade de Medicina, Universidade de Lisboa, 1649-028 Lisbon, Portugal
18. Departamento de Pediatria da Universidade Federal de São Paulo, São Paulo 04023-061, Brazil; eduardorossato93@gmail.com (E.R.d.V.); mauro.fisberg@gmail.com (M.F.)
19. Instituto Pensi, Fundação José Luiz Egydio Setubal, Hospital Infantil Sabará, São Paulo 01227-200, Brazil
* Correspondence: gerson.demoraes@usach.cl; Tel.: +56-9-5398-0556

† Membership of the ELANS Study Group is provided in the Acknowledgments section of the manuscript; elansstudy2014@gmail.com.

Received: 11 August 2020; Accepted: 10 September 2020; Published: 16 September 2020

Abstract: Purpose: This study aimed to examine the associations of the perceived neighborhood built environment with walking and cycling for transport in inhabitants from Latin American countries. Methods: This cross-sectional study involved 9218 participants (15–65 years) from the Latin American Study of Nutrition and Health, which included a nationally representative sample of eight countries. All participants completed the International Physical Activity Questionnaire-Long Form for measure walking and cycling for transport and the Neighborhood Environment Walkability Scale-Abbreviated. Furthermore, perceived proximity from home to public open spaces and shopping centers was assessed. Results: Perceived land use mix-access (OR: 1.32; 95%CI: 1.16,1.50) and the existence of many alternative routes in the neighbourhood (1.09 1.01,1.17) were associated with higher odds of reporting any walking for transport (≥10 min/week). Perceived slow speed of traffic (1.88 1.82,1.93) and few drivers exceeding the speed limits (1.92; 1.86,1.98) were also related to higher odds of reporting any walking for transport. The odds of reporting any cycling for transport (≥10 min/week) were higher in participants perceiving more walking/cycling facilities (1.87 1.76,1.99), and better aesthetics (1.22 1.09,1.38). Conclusions: Dissimilar perceived neighborhood built environment characteristics were associated with walking and cycling for transport among inhabitants from Latin America.

Keywords: transport physical activity; walking; cycling; neighborhood built environment; Latin America

1. Introduction

Physical activity has beneficial effects on numerous health outcomes. Higher physical activity levels decrease the risk of cardiovascular disease (CVD), including coronary heart disease, type 2 diabetes, colon cancer, and breast cancer, as well as increasing life expectancy [1]. Active transportation (i.e. walking and cycling for travel purposes) has been recommended as a practical way of incorporating more physical activity into daily life [2] and those who engage in active transportation tend to be more active in duration and frequency than those without active transportation [3]. Furthermore, a systematic review and meta-analysis of 531,333 participants reported that active transportation had a significantly reduced risk of all-cause mortality, cardiovascular disease incidence and diabetes [4].

Recently, Latin America has undergone a rapid urbanization process with demographic, epidemiological and socioeconomic changes and is currently the most urbanized region in the world (around 80% of Latin Americans live in cities) [5]. The urbanization change people's behaviour and in most cases decrease the physical activity levels. Between 2001 and 2016, the prevalence of physical inactivity (not meeting the physical activity recommendation proposed by the World Health Organization) increased by more than 5 percentage points in Latin America (from 33.4% in 2001 to 39.1% in 2016) [6]. Overall, the prevalence of physical inactivity (<150 min/week in moderate-to-vigorous physical activity) ranging from 26.9% (Chile) to 47% (Costa Rica and Venezuela). Physical inactivity (>40%) was prevalent in Brazil (43.5%), Argentina (43.7%), Venezuela (47.1%), and Costa Rica (48.0%) [7]. Furthermore, the highest mean of total sedentary behavior per day were in Costa Rica (524.6 min/day) followed by Brazil (455.1 min/day) [8]. The Latin American region is characterized by high population density, disorganized and heavy traffic, air and noise pollution, rising crime rates, high-income inequality, high levels of poverty, and population aging [9,10]. The dissimilar features of Latin American countries reduce, to translate findings from high-income countries (e.g., the United States, European countries) to this particular region. Therefore, the investigation of how the built environment can influence physical activity during transportation is warranted.

Different studies have explored associations between neighborhood built environmental (destination accessibility, street connectivity, recreational facilities, and public transport) and walking or cycling for transport [11–13] and found that characteristics related to active transport infrastructure, connectivity, walkability, safety and aesthetics were associated with higher physical activity during transportation. Nonetheless, most previous research was done in the high-income countries [14–16]. Only one of the existing Latin American studies used a representative sample of the urban population which may limit the generalizability of the observed associations, but it was related to a representative sample of only one city per country [13,17,18] and had not sufficient power and variability to assess walking and cycling separately. Therefore, the purpose of the present study was to examine the associations of the perceived neighborhood built environment with walking and cycling for transport in a representative sample of inhabitants from eight Latin America countries.

2. Material and Methods

2.1. Study Design and Sample

We use data from Estudio Latinoamericano de Nutrición y Salud (Latin American Study of Nutrition and Health, ELANS—https://es.elansstudy.com/). ELANS was an observational, cross-sectional, epidemiological multi-country (Argentina, Brazil, Chile, Colombia, Costa Rica, Ecuador, Peru, and Venezuela) study that uses a common design and comparable methods across countries. ELANS analyses a large representative sample from these eight countries and focuses on urban populations [19]. The main criteria for countries participate in ELANS were as follows: (a) data were collected from participants (15–65 years of age) selected; (b) at least the minimum number of participants per country according to the sample size; c) investigators were selected for the ELANS study based on their ability to collect the data which included investigator experience, funding availability, completed pilot work and having translated ELANS materials and diversity of their geographic location in Latin America.

Data collection dates ranged from September 2014 to February 2015. The overarching ELANS protocol was approved by the Western Institutional Review Board (#20140605) and is registered at ClinicalTrials.gov (#NCT02226627). Ethical approval was obtained from each local institutional review board (Brazil: 689.294; Chile: 14-179; Costa Rica: VI-6480-2013; Ecuador: 2014-057M; Peru: 352-2014/CIEI-IIN), and participants' informed consent was obtained before data collection.

The entire ELANS study consisted of 9218 (4809 women; aged 15–65 years) participants who were chosen using a random complex, multistage sample design, stratified by conglomerates, with all regions of each country represented, and random selection of Primary Sampling Units (PSUs) and Secondary Sampling Units (SSUs) according to probability proportional to size method. The PSUs were areas (e.g., counties, municipalities, neighborhoods, residential areas) within each selected city in each country. An "n" size proportional to the population weight was used for the range of PSUs. In this instance, a simple random sampling of "n" with replacement was achieved to adhere to the principle of statistical independence of the selection of the areas included in the PSU sample. For these random selections, the probability proportional to size (PPS) method was applied. Therefore, within each of the areas included in the PSU allocation, a representative sample of SSUs was randomly selected using the PPS method.

For the selection of households, we implemented a four-step, systematic randomization procedure by establishing a selection interval (k): a) the total urban population was used to proportionally define the main regions and to select cities representing each region, including key cities and other representative cities in the region, using a random method and sampling criteria, while attempting to cover the determined urban population; b) the sampling points (survey tracts) of each city were randomly designated, and c) clusters of households were selected from each sampling unit. Addresses were chosen systematically using standard random route techniques, beginning with an initial address designated at random. The households were designated with three regular jumps; that is, a particular household was selected by randomly picking the first home and subsequently skipping three households; d) the designated respondent within each household was selected using the birthday method (half chosen using the next birthday; the other half using the last birthday).

In total, a number of 92 cities were participants in the study and the sampling size essential for sufficient accuracy was calculated with a 95% confidence level and a maximum error of 3.5% and a survey design effect of 1.75 based on guidance from the National Center for Health Statistics [20], and calculations of the minimum sample sizes required per sex, age group and socioeconomic status were performed for each country [19,21]. The exclusion criteria adopted were: (a) pregnant and lactating women; (b) persons with physical or mental disabilities; (c) unsigned consent form; (d) individuals living in non-family residential environments; and (e) individuals who could not read. More information on the ELANS study is provided in Fisberg et al. [19].

The perceived neighborhood built environment and walking and cycling for transport procedure used in ELANS consist of self-reported data collected by questionnaires. The questionnaires (perceived neighborhood built environment and walking and cycling for transport) used in the ELANS were interviewer-administered during the home visit, and 9218 (15–65 years old) adults had complete data.

2.2. Perceived Neighborhood Built Environment

The Neighborhood Environment Walkability Scale-Abbreviated (NEWS-A) adapted for the current study was used to collect data of perceived neighborhood built environment [22]. The NEWS-A was translated from English into the language of the participanting countries (Spanish and Portuguese) and the scale adaptation also encompassed the addition of two items to the safety from crime subscale, an item measuring the proximity of shopping centers and three items gauging the proximity to three types of public open space (metropolitan parks, playgrounds and public squares). The reliability and validity survey of NEWS-A have been previously shown in several countries with all included scales having test-retest reliability intraclass correlations >0.50 [23,24].

The NEWS-A is one of several recently developed questionnaires designed to measure residents' perceptions of the environmental attributes of their local area [25]. The NEWS was designed to obtain residents' perceptions of how neighborhood characteristics found in the transportation and urban planning literature were related to a higher frequency of walking and cycling for transport [26].

The NEWS-A include items that represent seven subscales: land use mix–diversity, land use mix-access, street connectivity, walking/cycling facilities, aesthetics, safety from traffic, and safety from crime (Table 1) [22]. The land use mix-diversity scale is assessed by the perceived walking proximity from home to twenty-three different types of destinations, with responses ranging from 1–5-min walking distance (coded as 5 = high walkability) to >30-min walking distance (coded as 1 = low walkability). The remaining six scales are average ratings of items answered on a four-point Likert scale (1 = strongly disagree to 4 = strongly agree). Scales were scored in a direction consistent with higher walkability and safety, with individual items reversed when necessary. Scoring details are described elsewhere [22]. Cronbach's alpha was used to measure the internal consistency of the neighborhood environment characteristics' scales. The scales 'street connectivity' (Cronbach's alpha: 0.433) and 'safety from traffic' (Cronbach's alpha: 0.191) from NEWS-A were not included in the results due to low internal consistency. Instead, the individual items were analysed separately. On the other hand, the Cronbach's alpha was higher for 'land use mix-diversity' (Cronbach's alpha: 0.897), 'land use mix-access' (Cronbach's alpha: 0.693), 'walking/cycling facilities' (Cronbach's alpha: 0.613), 'aesthetics' (Cronbach's alpha: 0.804), 'safety from crime' (Cronbach's alpha: 0.805), 'distance to parks' (Cronbach's alpha: 0.620).

Table 1. Summary of environmental scales, NEWS-A.

Scale	Items
Land use mix-diversity	About how long would it take to get from your home to the nearest businesses or facilities listed below if you walked to them? Items: convenience/small grocery store, supermarket, blacksmith, fruit/vegetable market, laundry/dry cleaners, clothing store, post office, library, university/school, other educational centers, book store, fast food restaurant or street food, bakery/coffee shop, bank, non-fast food restaurant, video store, pharmacy/drug store, salon/barber shop, your job or school, public transport stop, park or square, gym or fitness facility
Land use mix-access	Stores are within easy walking distance of my home. It is easy to walk to a transit stop (bus, train) from my home. There are many places to go within easy walking distance of my home. The streets in my neighborhood are hilly, making my neighborhood difficult to walk in (reversed). There are major barriers to walking in my local area that make it hard to get from place to place (for example, freeways, railway lines, rivers) (reversed).
Street connectivity	The streets in my neighborhood do not have many cul-de-sacs (dead-end streets). The distance between intersections in my neighborhood is usually short (100 yards or less; the length of a football field or less). There are many alternative routes for getting from place to place in my neighborhood. (I don't have to go the same way every time).
Walking/cycling facilities	There are sidewalks on most of the streets in my neighborhood. Sidewalks are separated from the road/traffic in my neighborhood by parked cars. There is a grass/dirt strip that separates the streets from the sidewalks in my neighborhood.
Aesthetics	There are trees along the streets in my neighborhood. There are many interesting things to look at while walking in my neighborhood. There are many attractive natural sights in my neighborhood (such as landscaping, views). There are attractive buildings/homes in my neighborhood.
Safety from traffic	There is so much traffic along nearby streets that it makes it difficult or unpleasant to walk in my neighborhood (reversed). The speed of traffic on most nearby streets is usually slow (50 km/h or less) Most drivers exceed the posted speed limits while driving in my neighborhood (reversed) There are crosswalks and pedestrian signals to help walkers cross busy streets in my neighborhood.
Safety from crime	My neighborhood streets are well lit at night. Walkers and bikers on the streets in my neighborhood can be easily seen by people in their homes. There is a high crime rate in my neighborhood (reversed). The crime rate in my neighborhood makes it unsafe to go on walks during the day (reversed). The crime rate in my neighborhood makes it unsafe to go on walks at night (reversed). The parks, public squares, green areas and recreation areas in my neighborhood are unsafe during the day (reversed).* The parks, public squares, green areas and recreation areas in my neighborhood are unsafe at night (reversed).*

* items not in the NEWS-A scale.

2.3. Walking and Cycling for Transport

Participants reported their walking and cycling for tranport levels by completing the long-form of the last seven days, interview version of the International Physical Activity Questionnaire (IPAQ) in Spanish and Portuguese [27]. We used only the questions that covered the active transport-related domain [21]. The IPAQ has been validated to assess PA in individuals aged 15–69 years in several countries [28,29].

The participants were instructed to report the frequency and duration (bouts of ≥10 min) of walking and cycling for transport domain. Specifically, the following questions were asked: (a) "During the last seven days, did you walk or use a bicycle (pedal cycle) for at least 10 min continuously to get to and from places?" (Yes, No); (b) "During the last seven days, on how many days did you walk or ride a bicycle for at least 10 min at a time to go from place to place?"; (c) "How much time did you usually spend on one of those days to bicycle or walk from place to place?" These questions were asked separately for walking and cycling. IPAQ walking and cycling for transport data are reported as min/week. Time (min/week) spent in each activity (i.e., walking and cycling) was calculated and used in the analysis. In this study, we used walking and cycling for transport separately. Details on the assessment of walking and cycling for transport by IPAQ have been published elsewhere [21].

2.4. Sociodemographic Characteristics

Information about demographics including age by year (15–65 years), and sex was collected using standard questionnaires. Socioeconomic status was evaluated by questionnaire using country-specific definitions based on national norms, laws, and the questionnaires used on national surveys in each country and included equivalent characteristics for all countries. Given the variablility in categoririzing socioeconomic status, a standard three level system (low, medium, high) was developed and included equivalent characteristics for all countries [30–36]. Detailed information can be found in a previous publication [19].

2.5. Statistical Analysis

Data analyses were performed with IBM SPSS, v.22 (SPSS Inc., IBM Corp., Armonk, New York, NY, USA). Descriptive statistics included mean, standard deviations (SD), and percentages were presented. Weighting was done considering sociodemographic characteristics, sex, socioeconomic level, and country [19].

Multilevel logistic regression models, with the individual as the first level and the country as the second level, were used to estimate the overall associations of neighborhood characteristics with walking and cycling for transport (odds ratio: OR; confidence interval 95%: 95%CI) with a binary dependent variable (0 = "<10 min of walking or cycling/week", 1 = "≥10 min of walking or cycling/week"). Multilevel logistic regression modelling is a statistical method used to estimate the odds that an event will occur (yes/no outcome) while taking the dependency of data into account—participants from the same country are more likely to function in the same way than participants from different countries. This valuable information is taken into account when estimating the effects of independent variables on the outcome [37].

We present the results of walking and cycling for transport separately. Models were adjusted for sex, age, and socioeconomic level—these variables were included as independent variables in the logistic regression. We present the overall and country-specific results. A significance level of 5% was considered ($p < 0.05$).

3. Results

3.1. Descriptive Results

Table 2 describes the participants' characteristics. The total sample with all complete data included 9218 participants. Overall, 52.2% of the sample consisted of women and the mean age was 35.8 (SD: 14.0) years. The percentages reporting ≥10 min/week walking and cycling for transport were 75.2% and 9.7%. The percentages reporting ≥10 min/week walking for transport ranged between 59.9% (Venezuela) and 83.5% (Costa Rica). While cycling for transport ranged between 2.5% (Venezuela) and 15.9% (Costa Rica). The levels of ≥10 min/week cycling for transport in the last seven days were much lower in contrast to ≥10 min/week walking for transport.

The perceived neighborhood built environment varied greatly across countries. Land use mix-diversity was the highest in Colombia (mean: 3.1; SD: 0.7), and the lowest in Venezuela (mean: 2.4; SD: 0.8) assessed with a 5-point scale. The differences in means of the other environmental variables across the countries were relatively small, about 0.6, in the variables assessed with a 4-point scale. The overall mean scores of proximity of public open spaces (mean: 3.3; SD: 1.1) and of shopping centers (mean: 4.0; SD: 1.3) (5-points scales) indicated greater perceived proximity of public open spaces than to shopping centers. The mean scores of the items of street connectivity and safety from traffic were similar across all countries (differences ≤ 0.4) (Table 3).

Table 2. Demographic characteristics and walking and cycling for transport.

Variables	Overall	Argentina	Brazil	Chile	Colombia	Costa Rica	Ecuador	Peru	Venezuela
Sample size (n)	9218	1266	2000	879	1230	798	800	1113	1132
Age, mean (SD)	35.8 (14.0)	36.8 (13.9)	36.5 (13.8)	36.4 (14.2)	36.9 (14.6)	35.2 (13.9)	34.3 (14.0)	34.2 (13.6)	35.0 (13.8)
Sex (%)									
Men	47.8	45.3	47.1	48.4	49.0	49.4	49.6	47.0	48.8
Women	52.2	54.7	52.9	51.6	51.0	50.6	50.4	53.0	51.2
Socioeconomic level (%)									
Low	52.0	48.7	45.8	46.8	63.3	32.8	49.9	47.9	77.7
Medium	38.4	46.2	45.8	44.1	31.2	53.6	37.1	31.9	16.8
High	9.5	5.1	8.5	9.1	5.4	13.5	13.0	20.2	5.5
Walking for transport ≥ 10 min/week (%)	75.2	69.0	72.6	75.1	79.3	83.5	85.0	85.4	59.9
Cycling for transport ≥ 10 min/week (%)	9.7	10.7	11.3	12.9	9.9	15.9	9.3	6.6	2.5

SD: standard deviation.

Table 3. Overall and country perceived-environment scores.

	Overall	Argentina	Brazil	Chile	Colombia	Costa Rica	Ecuador	Peru	Venezuela
Land use mix-diversity (score 1–5)	2.8 (0.8)	2.9 (0.8)	2.6 (0.8)	2.6 (0.6)	3.1 (0.7)	2.8 (0.8)	3.0 (0.6)	2.7 (0.7)	2.4 (0.8)
Land use mix-access (score 1–4)	3.0 (0.4)	3.2 (0.4)	3.0 (0.4)	3.2 (0.4)	2.9 (0.4)	3.2 (0.4)	2.9 (0.4)	3.0 (0.4)	3.0 (0.4)
Walking/cycling facilities (score 1–4)	2.8 (0.6)	2.9 (0.5)	2.7 (0.6)	3.2 (0.6)	2.7 (0.5)	2.8 (0.8)	2.6 (0.4)	2.6 (0.7)	2.8 (0.6)
Aesthetics (score 1–4)	2.6 (0.7)	2.6 (0.7)	2.5 (0.7)	2.9 (0.8)	2.7 (0.6)	2.6 (0.7)	2.4 (0.6)	2.3 (0.7)	2.6 (0.7)
Safety from crime (score 1–4)	2.5 (0.6)	2.4 (0.5)	2.4 (0.6)	2.8 (0.6)	2.6 (0.5)	2.6 (0.6)	2.6 (0.5)	2.6 (0.5)	2.2 (0.6)
Proximity to public open spaces (score 1–5)	3.3 (1.1)	3.0 (1.0)	3.6 (1.0)	2.6 (0.8)	3.3 (1.0)	2.7 (0.9)	3.4 (0.9)	3.6 (1.0)	3.8 (1.1)
Proximity to shopping centres [1]	4.0 (1.3)	3.1 (1.5)	4.5 (0.9)	4.0 (1.2)	4.0 (1.2)	3.5 (1.4)	4.3 (1.0)	4.1 (1.2)	3.9 (1.4)
Street connectivity items [2]									
The streets in my neighborhood do not have many cul-de-sacs (dead-end streets).	2.5 (0.9)	2.6 (1.0)	2.7 (0.9)	2.7 (1.1)	2.5 (0.8)	2.4 (0.9)	2.3 (0.8)	2.3 (0.8)	2.5 (0.9)
The distance between intersections in my neighborhood is usually short (100 yards or less; the length of a football field or less).	2.8 (0.8)	3.0 (0.8)	2.7 (0.8)	3.0 (0.9)	2.9 (0.7)	2.9 (0.8)	2.8 (0.7)	2.9 (0.8)	2.7 (0.8)
There are many alternative routes for getting from place to place in my neighborhood. (I don't have to go the same way every time.)	3.0 (0.8)	3.1 (0.8)	3.0 (0.8)	3.2 (0.8)	3.0 (0.7)	3.1 (0.8)	3.0 (0.7)	3.0 (0.7)	3.0 (0.7)
Safety from traffic items [2]									
There is so much traffic along nearby streets that it makes it difficult or unpleasant to walk in my neighbourhood. (reversed)	2.4 (0.9)	2.3 (0.9)	2.3 (0.9)	2.4 (0.9)	2.5 (0.8)	2.3 (1.0)	2.5 (0.8)	2.6 (0.8)	2.4 (0.8)
The speed of traffic on most nearby streets is usually slow (50 km/h or less).	2.6 (0.8)	2.4 (0.8)	2.7 (0.8)	2.6 (0.9)	2.6 (0.7)	2.5 (0.9)	2.6 (0.7)	2.5 (0.7)	2.5 (0.8)
Most drivers exceed the posted speed limits while driving in my neighbourhood. (reversed)	2.3 (0.8)	2.2 (0.8)	2.1 (0.8)	2.3 (0.9)	2.4 (0.8)	2.2 (0.9)	2.3 (0.8)	2.4 (0.8)	2.4 (0.8)
There are crosswalks and pedestrian signals to help walkers cross busy streets in my neighbourhood.	2.4 (0.9)	2.4 (0.9)	2.6 (0.9)	2.8 (0.9)	2.3 (0.8)	2.3 (0.9)	2.4 (0.8)	2.2 (0.8)	2.1 (0.9)

The "street connectivity" and "safety from traffic" items were analyzed individually due to low internal consistency; Results presented as mean (standard deviation). [1] 5-point scale: 5 min (1), 6–10 min (2), 11–20 min (3), 20–30 min (4), 30+ min (5). [2] 4-point scale: strongly disagree (1), disagree (2), agree (3), strongly agree (4).

3.2. Perceived Neighborhood Built Environmental and Walking for Transport

Estimated associations of perceived neighborhood built environment subscales with walking for transport are shown in Table 4. In overall, perceived land use mix-access (OR: 1.32; 95%CI: 1.16, 1.50) and the existence of many alternative routes in the neighbourhood (OR: 1.09; 95%CI: 1.01, 1.17) were associated with higher odds of reporting any walking for transport (defined as ≥10 min/week). Perceived slow speed of traffic (OR: 1.88; 95%CI: 1.82, 1.93) and few drivers exceeding the speed limits (OR: 1.92; 95%CI: 1.86, 1.98) were also related to higher odds of reporting any walking for transport.

There were different associations among countries between walking for transport and perceived neighborhood built environment subscales. Argentina was the country with the strongest associations between perceived aspects of the neighborhood built environment (land use mix-diversity, land use mix-access, aesthetics, safety from crime, streets in neighbourhood do not have many cul-de-sacs, the existence of many alternative routes in the neighbourhood, much traffic, and most drivers exceed the posted speed limits) and walking for transport (Table 4).

3.3. Perceived Neighborhood Built Environmental and Cycling for Transport

Estimated associations of perceived neighborhood built environment subscales with cycling for transport are presented in Table 5. In the overall analyses, the odds of reporting any cycling for transport (defined as ≥10 min/week) were higher in participants perceiving more walking/cycling facilities (OR: 1.87; 95%CI: 1.76, 1.99), and better aesthetics (OR: 1.22; 95%CI: 1.09, 1.38).

Distinct associations by country were observed between perceived neighborhood built environment characteristics and cycling for transport. Brazil was the country with the strongest associations between perceived aspects of the neighborhood built environment (land use mix-diversity, and proximity of public open space, and shopping centers) and cycling for transport (Table 5).

Table 4. Multilevel logistic regression models (OR (95%CI)) for walking for transport (0: <10 min/week, 1: ≥10 min/week) by country.

Independent Variables	Overall OR (95%CI)	p	Argentina OR (95%CI)	p	Brazil OR (95%CI)	p	Chile OR (95%CI)	p	Colombia OR (95%CI)	p	Costa Rica OR (95%CI)	p	Ecuador OR (95%CI)	p	Peru OR (95%CI)	p	Venezuela OR (95%CI)	p
Land use mix-diversity (score 1-5) [1]	1.97 (1.90, 2.04)	0.430	1.62 (1.51, 1.75)	<0.001	1.18 (1.02, 1.36)	0.023	1.17 (0.85, 1.59)	0.337	1.68 (1.54, 1.85)	0.001	1.30 (0.99, 1.72)	0.062	1.22 (0.84, 1.78)	0.302	1.00 (0.74, 1.35)	1.000	0.91 (0.75, 1.10)	0.315
Land use mix-access (score 1-4) [1]	1.32 (1.16, 1.50)	<0.001	1.49 (1.07, 2.08)	0.018	1.06 (0.81, 1.40)	0.671	1.24 (0.80, 1.91)	0.334	3.07 (1.90, 4.95)	<0.001	1.03 (0.64, 1.65)	0.913	0.66 (0.35, 1.27)	0.213	1.16 (0.68, 1.96)	0.586	1.49 (1.08, 2.05)	0.016
Walking/cycling facilities (score 1-4) [1]	0.97 (0.88, 1.06)	0.454	0.90 (0.68, 1.21)	0.488	0.83 (0.68, 1.00)	0.054	1.03 (0.77, 1.39)	0.820	1.21 (0.88, 1.68)	0.243	1.15 (0.89, 1.50)	0.294	0.83 (0.51, 1.35)	0.459	0.76 (0.55, 1.04)	0.089	0.98 (0.79, 1.21)	0.830
Aesthetics (score 1-4) [1]	1.03 (0.95, 1.11)	0.517	1.36 (1.07, 1.74)	0.013	1.84 (1.72, 1.99)	0.037	1.04 (0.81, 1.33)	0.786	1.18 (0.87, 1.59)	0.297	1.07 (0.80, 1.42)	0.646	1.03 (0.72, 1.48)	0.862	1.81 (1.29, 2.55)	0.001	0.97 (0.80, 1.18)	0.766
Safety from crime (score 1-4) [1]	1.05 (0.95, 1.15)	0.344	1.51 (1.16, 1.96)	0.002	1.22 (1.00, 1.49)	0.055	0.71 (0.52, 0.96)	0.027	0.82 (0.59, 1.13)	0.225	0.88 (0.64, 1.23)	0.458	0.86 (0.57, 1.29)	0.460	0.80 (0.53, 1.21)	0.287	1.15 (0.91, 1.46)	0.249
Proximity to public open spaces (score 1-5) [2]	1.01 (0.95, 1.06)	0.811	0.88 (0.77, 1.02)	0.081	1.06 (0.95, 1.18)	0.339	1.28 (1.03, 1.59)	0.023	0.98 (0.83, 1.16)	0.834	1.05 (0.82, 1.34)	0.712	0.79 (0.61, 1.03)	0.078	1.14 (0.93, 1.39)	0.207	0.98 (0.86, 1.12)	0.777
Proximity to shopping centers [2]	1.00 (0.95, 1.04)	0.856	1.00 (0.91, 1.11)	0.955	0.99 (0.88, 1.11)	0.854	1.03 (0.89, 1.20)	0.694	0.97 (0.84, 1.13)	0.715	1.05 (0.90, 1.22)	0.567	0.92 (0.73, 1.17)	0.512	0.97 (0.82, 1.14)	0.671	1.05 (0.94, 1.16)	0.395
Street connectivity items [3]																		
The streets in my neighbourhood do not have many cul-de-sacs (dead-end streets).	0.98 (0.93, 1.04)	0.568	1.85 (1.74, 1.97)	0.016	1.05 (0.93, 1.19)	0.409	1.00 (0.85, 1.18)	0.962	1.08 (0.88, 1.32)	0.450	0.88 (0.70, 1.10)	0.251	0.97 (0.75, 1.27)	0.842	1.14 (0.91, 1.42)	0.245	1.05 (0.90, 1.21)	0.541
The distance between intersections in my neighbourhood is usually short (100 yards or less; the length of a football field or less).	1.01 (0.94, 1.08)	0.805	0.98 (0.82, 1.15)	0.770	0.98 (0.86, 1.12)	0.791	0.95 (0.77, 1.17)	0.634	1.07 (0.84, 1.35)	0.596	1.25 (0.97, 1.62)	0.079	1.29 (0.97, 1.73)	0.082	1.06 (0.83, 1.36)	0.623	1.00 (0.85, 1.18)	0.980
There are many alternative routes for getting from place to place in my neighbourhood. (I don't have to go the same way every time.)	1.09 (1.01, 1.17)	0.021	1.25 (1.05, 1.47)	0.010	0.95 (0.82, 1.10)	0.485	1.17 (0.94, 1.47)	0.167	1.29 (1.02, 1.63)	0.032	0.96 (0.74, 1.25)	0.775	1.15 (0.84, 1.57)	0.393	0.93 (0.70, 1.25)	0.644	1.15 (0.96, 1.39)	0.132

Table 4. Cont.

Independent Variables	Overall OR (95%CI)	Overall p	Argentina OR (95%CI)	Argentina p	Brazil OR (95%CI)	Brazil p	Chile OR (95%CI)	Chile p	Colombia OR (95%CI)	Colombia p	Costa Rica OR (95%CI)	Costa Rica p	Ecuador OR (95%CI)	Ecuador p	Peru OR (95%CI)	Peru p	Venezuela OR (95%CI)	Venezuela p
Safety from traffic items [3]																		
There is so much traffic along nearby streets that it makes it difficult or unpleasant to walk in my neighbourhood (reversed).	0.99 (0.93, 1.06)	0.856	1.76 (1.64, 1.90)	0.002	1.11 (0.97, 1.27)	0.136	0.94 (0.78, 1.14)	0.521	0.87 (0.71, 1.08)	0.205	1.03 (0.82, 1.29)	0.810	0.98 (0.74, 1.30)	0.900	1.10 (0.86, 1.42)	0.438	1.22 (1.02, 1.46)	0.028
The speed of traffic on most nearby streets is usually slow (50 km/h or less).	1.88 (1.82, 1.93)	<0.001	0.93 (0.79, 1.09)	0.367	0.92 (0.81, 1.04)	0.181	0.88 (0.73, 1.06)	0.188	0.88 (0.71, 1.08)	0.238	1.73 (1.57, 1.92)	0.008	1.02 (0.76, 1.36)	0.917	0.81 (0.62, 1.04)	0.103	0.86 (0.73, 1.02)	0.092
Most drivers exceed the posted speed limits while driving in my neighbourhood (reversed).	1.92 (1.86, 1.98)	0.016	1.32 (1.09, 1.60)	0.004	1.79 (1.69, 1.91)	0.001	1.01 (0.82, 1.25)	0.903	0.93 (0.75, 1.17)	0.549	1.73 (1.57, 1.93)	0.011	1.21 (0.92, 1.59)	0.177	1.00 (0.77, 1.31)	0.974	0.82 (0.69, 0.98)	0.026
There are crosswalks and pedestrian signals to help walkers cross busy streets in my neighbourhood.	0.99 (0.93, 1.05)	0.689	1.00 (0.86, 1.17)	0.968	1.01 (0.89, 1.16)	0.857	1.06 (0.88, 1.29)	0.542	1.00 (0.83, 1.22)	0.965	1.10 (0.89, 1.37)	0.360	0.80 (0.61, 1.04)	0.098	1.09 (0.87, 1.38)	0.440	0.96 (0.83, 1.13)	0.646

Overall percentage of correct prediction: null model: 75.2%; full model: 82.8%. OR: odds ratio; CI: confidence interval. Multilevel logistic regression model (country as 2nd level) with walking time (0: <10 min/week, 1: ≥10 min/week) as dependent variable, adjusted for sex, age, and socioeconomic level; [1] higher scores indicate perception of higher land use mix-diversity, higher land use mix-access, more walking/cycling facilities, better aesthetics, and more safety from crime; [2] higher scores indicate greater proximity; [3] 4-point scale: strongly disagree (1), disagree (2), agree (3), strongly agree (4).

Table 5. Multilevel logistic regression models (OR (95%CI)) for cycling for transport (0: <10 min/week, 1: ≥10 min/week) by country.

Independent Variables	Overall OR (95%CI)	p	Argentina OR (95%CI)	p	Brazil OR (95%CI)	p	Chile OR (95%CI)	p	Colombia OR (95%CI)	p	Costa Rica OR (95%CI)	p	Ecuador OR (95%CI)	p	Peru OR (95%CI)	p	Venezuela OR (95%CI)	p
Land use mix-diversity (score 1-5) [1]	1.10 (0.99, 1.23)	0.085	0.84 (0.63, 1.11)	0.214	1.42 (1.15, 1.75)	0.001	1.45 (0.95, 2.20)	0.084	0.94 (0.69, 1.27)	0.684	1.04 (0.77, 1.40)	0.787	1.48 (0.90, 2.44)	0.121	0.80 (0.53, 1.21)	0.287	0.85 (0.47, 1.53)	0.593
Land use mix-access (score 1-4) [1]	1.10 (0.91, 1.34)	0.334	1.57 (1.35, 1.91)	0.019	1.17 (0.78, 1.77)	0.446	0.85 (0.48, 1.51)	0.589	1.07 (0.57, 2.00)	0.828	1.19 (0.69, 2.05)	0.522	1.99 (0.88, 4.53)	0.100	2.30 (1.07, 4.93)	0.032	2.39 (0.84, 6.82)	0.103
Walking/cycling facilities (score 1-4) [1]	1.87 (1.76, 1.99)	0.036	0.89 (0.59, 1.32)	0.548	0.99 (0.75, 1.31)	0.937	0.78 (0.53, 1.15)	0.211	1.21 (0.78, 1.86)	0.399	0.74 (0.56, 0.98)	0.034	0.75 (0.40, 1.42)	0.382	0.83 (0.54, 1.28)	0.410	0.56 (0.27, 1.17)	0.123
Aesthetics (score 1-4) [1]	1.22 (1.09, 1.38)	0.001	1.46 (1.04, 2.05)	0.029	1.21 (0.95, 1.53)	0.115	1.43 (1.02, 2.02)	0.041	1.42 (0.95, 2.14)	0.091	1.24 (0.91, 1.69)	0.167	1.48 (1.30, 1.79)	0.004	1.10 (0.70, 1.73)	0.688	1.05 (0.57, 1.95)	0.879
Safety from crime (score 1-4) [1]	0.95 (0.82, 1.09)	0.433	0.94 (0.63, 1.38)	0.734	1.29 (0.96, 1.73)	0.092	0.85 (0.57, 1.26)	0.407	1.44 (1.28, 1.67)	<0.001	1.03 (0.72, 1.46)	0.881	0.79 (0.47, 1.32)	0.365	0.96 (0.54, 1.70)	0.882	1.23 (0.57, 2.65)	0.601
Proximity to public open spaces (score 1-5) [2]	1.03 (0.95, 1.11)	0.537	1.02 (0.83, 1.26)	0.814	1.31 (1.11, 1.55)	0.001	0.97 (0.74, 1.28)	0.838	0.96 (0.76, 1.21)	0.719	1.64 (1.48, 1.85)	0.002	1.21 (0.85, 1.73)	0.281	0.85 (0.65, 1.12)	0.247	0.92 (0.60, 1.41)	0.705
Proximity to shopping centers [2]	1.02 (0.95, 1.09)	0.589	0.90 (0.78, 1.05)	0.182	1.21 (1.00, 1.45)	0.047	1.18 (0.96, 1.45)	0.115	0.99 (0.81, 1.20)	0.910	1.21 (1.03, 1.43)	0.024	0.90 (0.69, 1.18)	0.452	0.95 (0.76, 1.19)	0.682	0.96 (0.69, 1.33)	0.799
Street connectivity items [3]																		
The streets in my neighbourhood do not have many cul-de-sacs (dead-end streets).	0.95 (0.88, 1.03)	0.240	0.91 (0.75, 1.11)	0.357	0.99 (0.82, 1.18)	0.872	0.94 (0.76, 1.16)	0.588	1.77 (1.59, 2.00)	0.032	0.99 (0.78, 1.26)	0.954	0.92 (0.65, 1.30)	0.635	1.15 (0.86, 1.54)	0.336	0.99 (0.62, 1.58)	0.971
The distance between intersections in my neighbourhood is usually short (100 yards or less; the length of a football field or less).	0.92 (0.84, 1.01)	0.078	0.95 (0.75, 1.21)	0.691	0.88 (0.72, 1.06)	0.172	1.07 (0.81, 1.40)	0.636	0.96 (0.70, 1.32)	0.795	0.87 (0.67, 1.14)	0.316	0.58 (0.40, 0.85)	0.005	1.32 (0.91, 1.91)	0.145	0.73 (0.43, 1.21)	0.224
There are many alternative routes for getting from place to place in my neighbourhood (I don't have to go the same way every time).	1.07 (0.96, 1.19)	0.224	1.06 (0.83, 1.37)	0.637	1.00 (0.81, 1.24)	0.976	1.12 (0.81, 1.55)	0.499	0.90 (0.65, 1.25)	0.526	1.62 (1.19, 2.20)	0.002	0.82 (0.55, 1.22)	0.327	0.78 (0.51, 1.20)	0.267	1.23 (0.69, 2.21)	0.485

Table 5. Cont.

Independent Variables	Overall		Argentina		Brazil		Chile		Colombia		Costa Rica		Ecuador		Peru		Venezuela	
	OR (95%CI)	p	OR (95%CI)	p	OR (95%CI)	p	OR (95%CI)	p	OR (95%CI)	p	OR (95%CI)	p	OR (95%CI)	p	OR (95%CI)	p	OR (95%CI)	p
Safety from traffic items [3]																		
There is so much traffic along nearby streets that it makes it difficult or unpleasant to walk in my neighbourhood (reversed).	1.03 (0.94, 1.13)	0.568	1.08 (0.85, 1.38)	0.523	1.03 (0.84, 1.26)	0.766	1.08 (0.85, 1.38)	0.540	0.87 (0.66, 1.14)	0.309	0.98 (0.78, 1.24)	0.893	1.16 (0.81, 1.66)	0.419	1.22 (0.87, 1.71)	0.258	0.93 (0.53, 1.65)	0.809
The speed of traffic on most nearby streets is usually slow (50 km/h or less).	1.01 (0.92, 1.10)	0.904	0.82 (0.65, 1.03)	0.091	0.96 (0.79, 1.15)	0.642	1.10 (0.86, 1.42)	0.438	1.39 (1.06, 1.74)	0.086	1.22 (0.96, 1.56)	0.100	0.77 (0.52, 1.14)	0.189	1.00 (0.70, 1.41)	0.979	0.99 (0.58, 1.68)	0.963
Most drivers exceed the posted speed limits while driving in my neighbourhood (reversed).	1.09 (0.99, 1.20)	0.089	0.99 (0.76, 1.30)	0.962	1.21 (0.98, 1.49)	0.075	0.78 (0.60, 1.03)	0.077	1.18 (0.89, 1.56)	0.259	1.61 (1.24, 2.10)	<0.001	0.93 (0.65, 1.35)	0.708	0.92 (0.64, 1.33)	0.672	1.08 (0.61, 1.91)	0.793
There are crosswalks and pedestrian signals to help walkers cross busy streets in my neighbourhood.	1.00 (0.92, 1.09)	0.965	0.92 (0.74, 1.16)	0.492	1.07 (0.88, 1.30)	0.514	1.00 (0.77, 1.29)	0.997	1.20 (0.93, 1.55)	0.163	0.82 (0.66, 1.02)	0.080	0.94 (0.65, 1.36)	0.743	1.02 (0.75, 1.39)	0.906	0.95 (0.58, 1.56)	0.842

Overall percentage of correct prediction: null model: 90.3%; full model: 94.7%. OR: odds ratio; CI: confidence interval. Multilevel logistic regression model (country as 2nd level) with cycling time (0: <10 min/week, 1: ≥10 min/week) as dependent variable, adjusted for sex, age, and socioeconomic level; [1] higher scores indicate perception of higher land use mix-diversity, higher land use mix-access, more walking/cycling facilities, better aesthetics, and more safety from crime; [2] higher scores indicate greater proximity; [3] 4-point scale: strongly disagree (1), disagree (2), agree (3), strongly agree (4).

4. Discussion

The present study aimed to investigate whether different perceived built environment characteristics are associated with walking and cycling for transportation. Our main findings were that land use mix-diversity and mix-access, the presence of different alternative routes to access the destination, lower speed limit in the roads, as well as the majority of the drivers respecting speed limit, were associated with higher walking for transportation. The presence of walking or cycling facilities and a higher aesthetics were associated with higher cycling for transportation. We also highlight some regional specific associations land use mix-diversity (Argentina, Brazil, and Colombia), aesthetics (Argentina, Brazil, and Peru), safety from crime (Argentina and Chile - inverse), proximity to public open spaces (Chile), few dead-end streets (Argentina) and low traffic along the nearby streets (Argentina and Venezuela) were associated with higher odds of walking for transport in specific countries. Similarly, land use mix-diversity (Brazil), land use mix-access (Peru), proximity to public open spaces (Brazil and Costa Rica), few dead-end streets (Colombia), the distance between intersections in the neighbourhood (Ecuador), different alternative routes to access the destination (Costa Rica) and the majority of the drivers respecting speed limit (Costa Rica) were associated with higher odds of cycling for transport in specific countries.

Our findings regarding walking for transport are in line with previous findings from economic developed countries [12,13]. In this sense, we found that factors related to walkability as connectivity as well as related to traffic safety were the most associated with higher walking for transport. These findings highlight the role of planning compact cities aiming to shift the transportation mode towards higher active transportation through increasing the land use mix-access and connectivity [38,39].

In addition, our findings support the important role of traffic safety on walking for transportation. Therefore, measures for traffic calming and safety as lowering the speed limit of the roads can increase physical activity during transportation as well as reduce road injuries [40] and consequently, impact secondary health outcomes, producing a disability-adjusted life-years gain [38].

The findings also pointed out the role of aesthetics in transportation through cycling. Even the majority of evidence found that aesthetics is important most for leisure-time activities as walking during leisure-time [12,41,42], some previous studies also found an association between aesthetics and physical activity during transport [12,13,43], therefore, a pleasant environment seems to be determinant for the choice of cycling for transportation. Another finding was related to the association of cycling facilities with the adoption of cycling for transportation, which highlightes the need for urban infrastructure supporting cyclists, as the build of bike paths as well as the expansion of integrated transportation systems with infrastructure for cyclists, including bike-sharing and parking [44,45].

Our findings showed that there were more perceived environmental correlates of walking than cycling for transportation across countries. Country-specific associations can guide specific policies for each country included in the present study. For example, different correlates related to connectivity, land use, safety from crime, aesthetics and safety from traffic were associated with walking for transportation in Argentina, while only aesthetics and land use mix-diversity were associated with walking for transportation in Brazil. Similarly, Costa Rica presented the highest number of correlates of cycling for transportation, including the distance of public open spaces, the number of alternative routes and few drivers exceeding the speed limit, while other countries presented more specific unique determinants as land usemix-access for Peru and other did not present correlates as Argentina, Chile, and Venezuela.

Our results shows positive association between walking for transport and land use mix-diversity in Argentina, Brazil and Colombia; land use mix-access was positively associated in overall, Argentina, Colombia, and Venezuela. We found an unequal association between the neighborhood built environment characteristics (e.g., aesthetics [Argentina, Brazil, and Peru], safety from crime [Argentina, and Chile], distance to public open spaces [and Chile]) and walking for transportation by country. The documentary analysis of the ten Latin American cities show several programs in Latin America that positively impact active transportation [44]. Several cities have implemented policies and programs aimed promoting walking and cycling for transport. Some of the most relevant and commonly implemented programs are the Ciclovia Recreativa Programs, and the implementation of Bus Rapid Transit systems (BRT) projects [44,46]. In Latin America, BRT systems have been implemented in Brazil, Ecuador, Peru, Mexico, and Colombia where they are considered an efficient and cost-effective solution for urban mobility [47]. Although the main objective of BRT is to increase urban mobility and reduce transport-related time, they also have the potential to stimulate the use of walking and cycling for transport and reduce car ownership use, thus promoting prysical activity [48].

Despite the health benefits of these systems implemented in Latin American countries, private car ownership in this region has been increasing steadily [49,50] such as Brazil, Argentina, Chile, and Colombia [51]. Studies show that in high-income countries, increasing car ownership does not necessarily lead to an increase in car-usage [52]. However, lower use of non-motorized modes of transport, the higher social advantage offered by owning a car, unequal public transport systems and the trend of increasing car ownership is likely to have a negative influence on walking and cycling for transport [53,54].

In our results, the odds of reporting cycling for transport was higher in respondents living in neighborhoods perceived to be more aesthetically pleasing and better walking/cycling facilities. It may be that aesthetically pleasing environments and green spaces can act as motivators for engaging in or spending more time in active transportation [55]. The way aesthetics are associated with active transportation has an important implication [13]. The aesthetics may play a different role in deciding whether or not to engage in different types of physical activity. While aesthetics may not be a relevant environmental feature for walking, it may play a more relevant role for involvement in moderate-to-vigorous physical activity [56]. Aesthetics ratings, like safety ratings, were low across all coutries, and this may be an area for improvement with less cost implications than other structural changes.

Some limitations should be considered in the interpretation of our study. These data do not include car ownership that is likely to have a negative influence on walking and cycling for transport [53,54]. We used self-reported measures of the built environment (perceived) and physical activity, which can lead to recall bias. Also, the cross-sectional design does not allow a causality interpretation, even the reverse-causality is not probable after the adjustment for sociodemographic factors as socioeconomic status. The use of self-report measures of both neighborhood environments and physical activity should be considered in the interpretation of the findings since there is evidence that items from the IPAQ—long (the measure of physical activity used in this study) may be interpreted differently across different cultures and contexts [57]. Also, the NEWS scale has been found to assess density and access to services more accurately in low-to-medium density urban environments [17]. Considering these measurement issues, some of the between-country differences in associations observed in this study might have been due to differences in the interpretation of the survey items. Furthermore, low variability within countries and the small sample sizes in some countries, especially for cycling, may lead to non significant coefficients for variable that affect walking or cycling. This study has several strengths. We presented data on the association between perceived built environment and transportation physical activity (walking and cycling) from eight different Latin-American countries, which enables a regional as well as country-specific vision with more than 9000 participants. By providing a unique Latin American dataset, the present study enabled wider cross-country comparisons and, thus, expanded the existing literature. In addition to identifying neighborhood built environment characteristcs associated with physical activity that might inform public health policies and investments, our findings should be viewed as an opportunity to inform and motivate researchers in Latin America to further examine these relationships. Prospective studies of environmental characteristics and active transportation are needed as well as evidence from intervention studies to better inform policy changes and large-scale environmental interventions.

5. Conclusions

This study showed the importance of environmental characteristics for walking and cycling for transport. In general lines, improving perceptions of neighbourhood built environment through changes in the actual neighbourhood built environment could be a target for increasing active transport among inhabitants from Latin America. Programs and policies should consider differences by country. For example, land use mix-diversity was consistently associated with higher walking and cycling for transportation in Brazil, while the respect to the speed limits by drivers was consistently associated with walking and cycling for transportation in Costa Rica. Future studies should investigate the prospective association of environmental characteristics with change in transport physical activity among Latin America countries.

Author Contributions: Conceptualization, G.F.; Formal analysis, G.F., C.P., Investigation I.K, G.G., A.R., L.Y.C.S., M.C.Y.G., R.G.P., M.H.-C., I.Z.Z., V.G., M.P. (Michael Pratt), Funding acquisition, M.F., and I.K.; Writing-review and editing: G.F., A.O.W., D.R.d.S., C.C.B., E.J.S., A.M., M.P. (Miguel Peralta), E.R.d.V. All authors have read and agreed to the published version of the manuscript.

Funding: Fieldwork and data analysis compromised in ELANS protocol was supported by a scientific grant from the Coca Cola Company, and by grant and/or support from Instituto Pensi/Hospital Infantil Sabara, International Life Science Institute of Argentina, Universidad de Costa Rica, Pontificia Universidad Católica de Chile, Pontificia Universidad Javeriana, Universidad Central de Venezuela (CENDES-UCV)/Fundación Bengoa, Universidad San Francisco de Quito, and Instituto de Investigación Nutricional de Peru. André Werneck is supported by the São Paulo Research Foundation (FAPESP) with a PhD scholarship (FAPESP process: 2019/24124-7). This paper presents independent research. The views expressed in this publication are those of the authors and not necessarily those of the acknowledged institutions. The funding sponsors had no role in study design; the collection, analyses, or interpretation of data; writing of the manuscript; or in the decision to publish the results.

Acknowledgments: The authors would like to thank the staff and participants from each of the participating sites who made substantial contributions to ELANS. The following are members of ELANS Study Group: Chairs: Mauro Fisberg and Irina Kovalskys; Co-chair: Georgina Gómez Salas; Core Group Members: Attilio Rigotti, Lilia Yadira Cortés Sanabria, Georgina Gómez Salas, Martha Cecilia Yépez García, Rossina Gabriella Pareja Torres and Marianella Herrera-Cuenca; Steering committee: Berthold Koletzko, Luis A. Moreno and Michael Pratt; Accelerometry analysis: Priscila Bezerra Gonçalves, and Claudia Alberico; Physical activity advisor: Gerson Ferrari. Nutrition Advisors: Regina Mara Fisberg and Agatha Nogueira Previdelli. Project Managers: Viviana Guajardo, and Ioná Zalcman Zimberg.

Conflicts of Interest: The authors declare no conflict of interest.

References

1. Lee, I.M.; Shiroma, E.J.; Lobelo, F.; Puska, P.; Blair, S.N.; Katzmarzyk, P.T.; Lancet Physical Activity Series Working Group. Effect of physical inactivity on major non-communicable diseases worldwide: An analysis of burden of disease and life expectancy. *Lancet* **2012**, *380*, 219–229. [CrossRef]
2. Petrunoff, N.; Wen, L.M.; Rissel, C. Effects of a workplace travel plan intervention encouraging active travel to work: Outcomes from a three-year time-series study. *Public Health* **2016**, *135*, 38–47. [CrossRef] [PubMed]
3. Rojas-Rueda, D.; de Nazelle, A.; Andersen, Z.J.; Braun-Fahrlander, C.; Bruha, J.; Bruhova-Foltynova, H.; Desqueyroux, H.; Praznoczy, C.; Ragettli, M.S.; Tainio, M.; et al. Health impacts of active transportation in europe. *PLoS ONE* **2016**, *11*, e0149990. [CrossRef] [PubMed]
4. Dinu, M.; Pagliai, G.; Macchi, C.; Sofi, F. Active commuting and multiple health outcomes: A systematic review and meta-analysis. *Sports Med.* **2019**, *49*, 437–452. [CrossRef] [PubMed]
5. United Nations. World Urbanization Prospects: The 2011 Revision. Data Tables and Highlights 2011 Revision. 2012. Available online: https://www.un.org/en/development/desa/population/publications/pdf/urbanization/WUP2011_Report.pdf (accessed on 11 September 2020).
6. Guthold, R.; Stevens, G.A.; Riley, L.M.; Bull, F.C. Worldwide trends in insufficient physical activity from 2001 to 2016: A pooled analysis of 358 population-based surveys with 1.9 million participants. *Lancet Glob. Health* **2018**, *6*, e1077–e1086. [CrossRef]
7. Ferrari, G.L.M.; Kovalskys, I.; Fisberg, M.; Gomez, G.; Rigotti, A.; Sanabria, L.Y.C.; Garcia, M.C.Y.; Torres, R.G.P.; Herrera-Cuenca, M.; Zimberg, I.Z.; et al. Socio-demographic patterning of objectively measured physical activity and sedentary behaviours in eight Latin American countries: Findings from the ELANS study. *Eur. J. Sport Sci.* **2019**, 1–12. [CrossRef]

8. Ferrari, G.L.M.; Oliveira Werneck, A.; Rodrigues da Silva, D.; Kovalskys, I.; Gomez, G.; Rigotti, A.; Yadira Cortes Sanabria, L.; Garcia, M.C.Y.; Pareja, R.G.; Herrera-Cuenca, M.; et al. Socio-demographic correlates of total and domain-specific sedentary behavior in latin america: A population-based study. *Int. J. Environ. Res. Public Health* **2020**, *17*, 5587. [CrossRef]
9. Lund, C.; De Silva, M.; Plagerson, S.; Cooper, S.; Chisholm, D.; Das, J.; Knapp, M.; Patel, V. Poverty and mental disorders: Breaking the cycle in low-income and middle-income countries. *Lancet* **2011**, *378*, 1502–1514. [CrossRef]
10. Kane, J.C.; Vinikoor, M.J.; Haroz, E.E.; Al-Yasiri, M.; Bogdanov, S.; Mayeya, J.; Simenda, F.; Murray, L.K. Mental health comorbidity in low-income and middle-income countries: A call for improved measurement and treatment. *Lancet Psychiatry* **2018**, *5*, 864–866. [CrossRef]
11. Cerin, E.; Nathan, A.; van Cauwenberg, J.; Barnett, D.W.; Barnett, A.; Council on Environment and Physical Activity (CEPA)—Older Adults working group. The neighbourhood physical environment and active travel in older adults: A systematic review and meta-analysis. *Int. J. Behav. Nutr. Phys. Act.* **2017**, *14*, 15. [CrossRef]
12. Smith, M.; Hosking, J.; Woodward, A.; Witten, K.; MacMillan, A.; Field, A.; Baas, P.; Mackie, H. Systematic literature review of built environment effects on physical activity and active transport—An update and new findings on health equity. *Int. J. Behav. Nutr. Phys. Act.* **2017**, *14*, 158. [CrossRef]
13. Kerr, J.; Emond, J.A.; Badland, H.; Reis, R.; Sarmiento, O.; Carlson, J.; Sallis, J.F.; Cerin, E.; Cain, K.; Conway, T.; et al. Perceived neighborhood environmental attributes associated with walking and cycling for transport among adult residents of 17 cities in 12 countries: The IPEN study. *Environ. Health Perspect.* **2016**, *124*, 290–298. [CrossRef] [PubMed]
14. Gao, J.; Kamphuis, C.B.M.; Dijst, M.; Helbich, M. The role of the natural and built environment in cycling duration in the Netherlands. *Int. J. Behav. Nutr. Phys. Act.* **2018**, *15*, 82. [CrossRef] [PubMed]
15. Karmeniemi, M.; Lankila, T.; Ikaheimo, T.; Puhakka, S.; Niemela, M.; Jamsa, T.; Koivumaa-Honkanen, H.; Korpelainen, R. Residential relocation trajectories and neighborhood density, mixed land use and access networks as predictors of walking and bicycling in the Northern Finland Birth Cohort 1966. *Int. J. Behav. Nutr. Phys. Act.* **2019**, *16*, 88. [CrossRef] [PubMed]
16. Nordengen, S.; Ruther, D.C.; Riiser, A.; Andersen, L.B.; Solbraa, A. Correlates of commuter cycling in three norwegian counties. *Int. J. Environ. Res. Public Health* **2019**, *16*, 4372. [CrossRef] [PubMed]
17. Cerin, E.; Conway, T.L.; Adams, M.A.; Barnett, A.; Cain, K.L.; Owen, N.; Christiansen, L.B.; van Dyck, D.; Mitas, J.; Sarmiento, O.L.; et al. Objectively-assessed neighbourhood destination accessibility and physical activity in adults from 10 countries: An analysis of moderators and perceptions as mediators. *Soc. Sci. Med.* **2018**, *211*, 282–293. [CrossRef]
18. Salvo, D.; Reis, R.S.; Stein, A.D.; Rivera, J.; Martorell, R.; Pratt, M. Characteristics of the built environment in relation to objectively measured physical activity among Mexican adults, 2011. *Prev. Chronic Dis.* **2014**, *11*, E147. [CrossRef]
19. Fisberg, M.; Kovalskys, I.; Gomez, G.; Rigotti, A.; Cortes, L.Y.; Herrera-Cuenca, M.; Yepez, M.C.; Pareja, R.G.; Guajardo, V.; Zimberg, I.Z.; et al. Latin American Study of Nutrition and Health (ELANS): Rationale and study design. *BMC Public Health* **2016**, *16*, 93. [CrossRef]
20. National Center for Health Statistics (NCHS). Analytic and Reporting Guidelines: The Third National Health and Nutrition Examination Survey, NHANES III (1988–94). Prevention, 1–47. 1996. Available online: https://wwwn.cdc.gov/nchs/data/nhanes3/3a/EXAMSE-acc.pdf (accessed on 11 September 2020).
21. Ferrari, G.L.M.; Kovalskys, I.; Fisberg, M.; Gomez, G.; Rigotti, A.; Sanabria, L.Y.C.; Garcia, M.C.Y.; Torres, R.G.P.; Herrera-Cuenca, M.; Zimberg, I.Z.; et al. Methodological design for the assessment of physical activity and sedentary time in eight Latin American countries—The ELANS study. *MethodsX* **2020**, *7*, 100843. [CrossRef]
22. Cerin, E.; Saelens, B.E.; Sallis, J.F.; Frank, L.D. Neighborhood environment walkability scale: Validity and development of a short form. *Med. Sci. Sports Exerc.* **2006**, *38*, 1682–1691. [CrossRef]
23. Cerin, E.; Sit, C.H.; Cheung, M.C.; Ho, S.Y.; Lee, L.C.; Chan, W.M. Reliable and valid NEWS for Chinese seniors: Measuring perceived neighborhood attributes related to walking. *Int. J. Behav. Nutr. Phys. Act.* **2010**, *7*, 84. [CrossRef] [PubMed]
24. Starnes, H.A.; McDonough, M.H.; Tamura, K.; James, P.; Laden, F.; Troped, P.J. Factorial validity of an abbreviated neighborhood environment walkability scale for seniors in the Nurses' Health Study. *Int. J. Behav. Nutr. Phys. Act.* **2014**, *11*, 126. [CrossRef] [PubMed]

25. Brownson, R.C.; Chang, J.J.; Eyler, A.A.; Ainsworth, B.E.; Kirtland, K.A.; Saelens, B.E.; Sallis, J.F. Measuring the environment for friendliness toward physical activity: A comparison of the reliability of 3 questionnaires. *Am. J. Public Health* **2004**, *94*, 473–483. [CrossRef] [PubMed]
26. Saelens, B.E.; Sallis, J.F.; Frank, L.D. Environmental correlates of walking and cycling: Findings from the transportation, urban design, and planning literatures. *Ann. Behav. Med.* **2003**, *25*, 80–91. [CrossRef] [PubMed]
27. Craig, C.L.; Marshall, A.L.; Sjostrom, M.; Bauman, A.E.; Booth, M.L.; Ainsworth, B.E.; Pratt, M.; Ekelund, U.; Yngve, A.; Sallis, J.F.; et al. International physical activity questionnaire: 12-country reliability and validity. *Med. Sci. Sports Exerc.* **2003**, *35*, 1381–1395. [CrossRef]
28. Kim, Y.; Park, I.; Kang, M. Convergent validity of the international physical activity questionnaire (IPAQ): Meta-analysis. *Public Health Nutr.* **2013**, *16*, 440–452. [CrossRef]
29. Ferrari, G.L.M.; Kovalskys, I.; Fisberg, M.; Gomez, G.; Rigotti, A.; Sanabria, L.Y.C.; Garcia, M.C.Y.; Torres, R.G.P.; Herrera-Cuenca, M.; Zimberg, I.Z.; et al. Anthropometry, dietary intake, physical activity and sitting time patterns in adolescents aged 15–17 years: An international comparison in eight Latin American countries. *BMC Pediatrics* **2020**, *20*, 24. [CrossRef]
30. República Bolivariana de Venezuela. *Síntesis Estadística de Pobreza e Indicadores de Desigualdad. 1er semestre 1997—2do semestre 2011*; No 2; Instituto Nacional de Estadística: Caracas, Venezuela, 2012.
31. Asociacion Investigadores de Mercado. *Grupos Socioeconómicos Chile*; Asociacion Investigadores de Mercado: Santiago, Chile, 2012.
32. IPSOS. *Estudio General de Medios*; IPSOS: Paris, France, 2012.
33. Instituto Nacional de Estadística y Censos de Ecuador. *Encuesta de Estratificación de Nivel Socioeconómico*; Instituto Nacional de Estadística y Censos de Ecuador: Quito, Ecuador, 2011.
34. Departamento Administrativo Nacional de Estadisticas de Colombia. *Proyecciones Nacionales y Departamentales de Poblacion 2005–2020, Estudios Postcensales No. 7*; Departamento Administrativo Nacional de Estadisticas de Colombia: Bogotá, Colombia, 2009.
35. Comisión de Enlace Institucional AAM-SAIMO-CEIM. *Nivel Socioeconómico. Antecedentes, Marco Conceptual, Enfoque Metodológico y Fortalezas*; Comisión de Enlace Institucional AAM-SAIMO-CEIM: Buenos Aires, Argentina, 2006.
36. Associação Brasileira de Empresas de Pesquisa (ABEP). *Critério Padrão de Classificação Econômica Brasil*; Associação Brasileira de Empresas de Pesquisa (ABEP): São Paulo, Brazil, 2013.
37. Sommet, N.; Morselli, D. Keep calm and learn multilevel logistic modeling: A simplified three-step procedure using stata, R, Mplus, and SPSS. *Int. Rev. Soc. Psychol.* **2017**, *30*, 203–218. [CrossRef]
38. Stevenson, M.; Thompson, J.; de Sa, T.H.; Ewing, R.; Mohan, D.; McClure, R.; Roberts, I.; Tiwari, G.; Giles-Corti, B.; Sun, X.; et al. Land use, transport, and population health: Estimating the health benefits of compact cities. *Lancet* **2016**, *388*, 2925–2935. [CrossRef]
39. Giles-Corti, B.; Vernez-Moudon, A.; Reis, R.; Turrell, G.; Dannenberg, A.L.; Badland, H.; Foster, S.; Lowe, M.; Sallis, J.F.; Stevenson, M.; et al. City planning and population health: A global challenge. *Lancet* **2016**, *388*, 2912–2924. [CrossRef]
40. Brown, V.; Moodie, M.; Carter, R. Evidence for associations between traffic calming and safety and active transport or obesity: A scoping review. *J. Transp. Health* **2017**, *7*, 23–37. [CrossRef]
41. Porter, A.K.; Kohl, H.W., 3rd; Perez, A.; Reininger, B.; Pettee Gabriel, K.; Salvo, D. Perceived social and built environment correlates of transportation and recreation-only bicycling among adults. *Prev. Chronic. Dis.* **2018**, *15*, E135. [CrossRef] [PubMed]
42. Heesch, K.C.; Giles-Corti, B.; Turrell, G. Cycling for transport and recreation: Associations with socio-economic position, environmental perceptions, and psychological disposition. *Prev. Med.* **2014**, *63*, 29–35. [CrossRef] [PubMed]
43. Van Dyck, D.; Cerin, E.; Conway, T.L.; De Bourdeaudhuij, I.; Owen, N.; Kerr, J.; Cardon, G.; Frank, L.D.; Saelens, B.E.; Sallis, J.F. Perceived neighborhood environmental attributes associated with adults' transport-related walking and cycling: Findings from the USA, Australia and Belgium. *Int. J. Behav. Nutr. Phys. Act.* **2012**, *9*, 70. [CrossRef]
44. Gomez, L.F.; Sarmiento, R.; Ordonez, M.F.; Pardo, C.F.; de Sa, T.H.; Mallarino, C.H.; Miranda, J.J.; Mosquera, J.; Parra, D.C.; Reis, R.; et al. Urban environment interventions linked to the promotion of physical activity: A mixed methods study applied to the urban context of Latin America. *Soc. Sci. Med.* **2015**, *131*, 18–30. [CrossRef]

45. Florindo, A.A.; Barrozo, L.V.; Turrell, G.; Barbosa, J.; Cabral-Miranda, W.; Cesar, C.L.G.; Goldbaum, M. Cycling for transportation in sao paulo city: Associations with Bike Paths, train and subway stations. *Int. J. Environ. Res. Public Health* **2018**, *15*, 562. [CrossRef]
46. Parra, D.C.; Gómez, L.F.; Pratt, M.; Samiento, O.L.; Triche, E.; Mosquera, J. Policy and built environment changes in Bogotá and their importance in health promotion. *Indoor Built Environ.* **2007**, *16*, 344–348. [CrossRef]
47. Wright, L. Bus Rapid Transit. *Sustainable Transport: A Sourcebook for Policy-Makers in Developing Cities*; Deutsche Gesellschaft für Technische Zusammenarbeit: Eschborn, Germany, 2002.
48. Sallis, J.F.; Frank, L.D.; Saelens, B.E.; Kraft, M.K. Active transportation and physical activity: Opportunities for collaboration on transportation and public health research. *Transp. Res. Part A Policy Pract.* **2004**, *38*, 249–268. [CrossRef]
49. Ureta, S. To move or not to move? Social exclusion, accessibility and daily mobility among the lowincome population in Santiago, Chile. *Mobilities* **2008**, *3*, 269–289. [CrossRef]
50. Becerra, J.M.; Reis, R.S.; Frank, L.D.; Ramirez-Marrero, F.A.; Welle, B.; Arriaga Cordero, E.; Mendez Paz, F.; Crespo, C.; Dujon, V.; Jacoby, E.; et al. Transport and health: A look at three Latin American cities. *Cad. Saúde Pública* **2013**, *29*, 654–666. [CrossRef]
51. Roberts, I.; Wentz, R.; Edwards, P. Car manufacturers and global road safety: A word frequency analysis of road safety documents. *Inj. Prev.* **2006**, *12*, 320–322. [CrossRef] [PubMed]
52. Newman, P.; Kenworthy, J. "Peak Car Use": Understanding the demise of automobile dependence. *World Transp. Policy Pract.* **2011**, *17*, 31–42.
53. Zander, A.; Rissel, C.; Rogers, K.; Bauman, A. Active travel to work in NSW: Trends over time and the effect of social advantage. *Health Promot. J. Austr.* **2014**, *25*, 167–173. [CrossRef] [PubMed]
54. Ferrari, G.; Ferrari, M.; Kovalskys, I.; Fisberg, M.; Gomez, G.; Rigotti, A.; Sanabria, L.Y.C.; Epez García, M.C.Y.; Gabriella, R.; Torres, P.; et al. Socio-demographic patterns of public, private and active travel in Latin America: Cross-sectional findings from the ELANS study. *J. Transp. Health* **2020**, *16*, 100788. [CrossRef]
55. Saelens, B.E.; Handy, S.L. Built environment correlates of walking: A review. *Med. Sci. Sports Exerc.* **2008**, *40*, S550–S566. [CrossRef]
56. Jauregui, A.; Salvo, D.; Lamadrid-Figueroa, H.; Hernandez, B.; Rivera, J.A.; Pratt, M. Perceived neighborhood environmental attributes associated with leisure-time and transport physical activity in Mexican adults. *Prev. Med.* **2017**, *103S*, S21–S26. [CrossRef]
57. Cerin, E.; Cain, K.L.; Oyeyemi, A.L.; Owen, N.; Conway, T.L.; Cochrane, T.; Van Dyck, D.; Schipperijn, J.; Mitas, J.; Toftager, M.; et al. Correlates of agreement between accelerometry and self-reported physical activity. *Med. Sci. Sports Exerc.* **2016**, *48*, 1075–1084. [CrossRef]

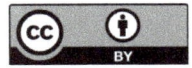

© 2020 by the authors. Licensee MDPI, Basel, Switzerland. This article is an open access article distributed under the terms and conditions of the Creative Commons Attribution (CC BY) license (http://creativecommons.org/licenses/by/4.0/).

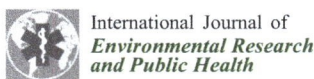 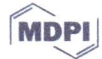

Article

Gender Influence on Students, Parents, and Teachers' Perceptions of What Children and Adolescents in Germany Need to Cycle to School: A Concept Mapping Study

Dorothea M. I. Schönbach [1,*], Catherina Vondung [2], Lisan M. Hidding [3], Teatske M. Altenburg [3], Mai J. M. Chinapaw [3] and Yolanda Demetriou [1]

1. Department of Sport and Health Sciences, Technical University of Munich, 80992 Munich, Germany; yolanda.demetriou@tum.de
2. Department of Natural and Sociological Sciences, Heidelberg University of Education, 69120 Heidelberg, Germany; vondung@ph-heidelberg.de
3. Department of Public and Occupational Health, Amsterdam Public Health Research Institute, Amsterdam UMC, Vrije Universiteit Amsterdam, 1081 BT Amsterdam, The Netherlands; l.hidding@amsterdamumc.nl (L.M.H.); t.altenburg@amsterdamumc.nl (T.M.A.); m.chinapaw@amsterdamumc.nl (M.J.M.C.)
* Correspondence: dorothea.schoenbach@tum.de; Tel.: +49-89-289-24687

Received: 13 August 2020; Accepted: 15 September 2020; Published: 20 September 2020

Abstract: Active commuting to school is highly recommended for several reasons, and in the decision-making process for doing so, a child interacts with parents and teachers. Until now, these three interactors' gender-specific perspectives on children and adolescents' need for cycling to school have been unavailable. Thus, our concept mapping study analyzed the needs of 12- to 15-year-olds in Germany for cycling to and from school daily, as perceived by students, parents, and teachers stratified by gender. From November 2019 to February 2020, 136 students, 58 parents, and 29 teachers participated. Although 87.8% of girls and 100% of boys owned a bicycle, only 44.4% of girls and 72.9% of boys cycled to school. On average, girls cycled to school on 1.6 ± 2.0 days a week and boys on 2.7 ± 2.0 days a week. A "bicycle and related equipment," the "way to school," and "personal factors" were reported needs, perceived by students and teachers of both genders and by mothers. Girls reported the additional gender-specific need for "social behavior in road traffic," mothers and female teachers reported "role of parents," and female teachers reported a "sense of safety." This study's findings could inspire the development of school-based bicycle interventions.

Keywords: childhood; adolescence; sex; active commuting to school; bicycle

1. Introduction

Only 26% of children and adolescents aged 3 to 17 in Germany achieve the physical activity (PA) as described by the guidelines of the World Health Organization (WHO) [1]. Active commuting to school (ACTS) is regarded as an additional opportunity to increase PA before and after school and is highly recommended for school-aged children and adolescents [2]. Cycling is one mode of ACTS and has additional benefits compared to walking for the following reasons: (i) Compared to 25% of walkers, 36% of children and adolescents who cycle to school meet the weekly PA recommendation [3]; (ii) ACTS by bicycle has been generally associated with higher PA intensity than walking, with positive effects on cardiovascular fitness in children and adolescents [4] leading to a risk reduction of developing cardiovascular diseases; (iii) cycling increases the mobility of students who need to manage a longer home-to-school distance when engaging in ACTS [5,6]; (iv) in cities, a bicycle is considered the fastest means of transportation for distances less than 5 km [7], which is more time-efficient (especially when car traffic is congested); and v) ACTS by bicycle is more positively associated with cycling than walking to other destinations [3], possibly establishing a potentially lifelong active travel (AT) routine by bicycle. Over time, this maintained behavior routine is useful because it predicts PA in adults [8]. Despite these well-known benefits of ACTS by bicycle and the fact that 57% to 98% of children and adolescents aged up to 17 years in Germany own a bicycle [9], why only 8% [10] to 22.2% [11] of them cycle to and from school remains as yet an unknown. Furthermore, the reasons why more boys (23.8%) than girls (20.6%) in Germany cycle to school are still unclear [11]. In a recent systematic review of school-based ACTS interventions focusing on cycling, we found that only one in seven strategies was promising and that two grade levels between 3rd and 7th grade were chosen [12]. Moreover, analysis of gender differences has been performed for only one intervention, which indicated an unexplained beneficial effect on boys but not on girls [13].

According to the Model of Children's Active Travel (M-CAT) [14], the main factors influencing children's travel behavior include "objective characteristics" of the child (e.g., age, gender, school attended), parent (e.g., social status) or family (e.g., size), and further objective elements in physical (e.g., population density), economic (e.g., costs), or political-socio-cultural environments (e.g., school). Some previous research indicates that parents' gender predicts positive associations between parental characteristics and a child's ACTS (e.g., employed mothers [15], mothers actively commuting to work [16]). Moreover, M-CAT considers parent and child's "perception elements" including attitudes (e.g., benefits or risks), the environment (e.g., favorable or unfavorable), and the child (e.g., sense of responsibility, knowledge of road safety, cycling skills) [14]. Because perception is based on "objective characteristics" [14], it can be influenced by the child or parents' gender, so perception can also impact on the child's ACTS. Previous research has reported influential factors identified by both parents of children aged 9 to 12 (e.g., perceived convenience of using the car to drive the child to school), whereas other factors were gender-specific to mothers (e.g., a child's lack of interest) [17]. In conclusion, interaction among all these factors influences the outcome, i.e., parents and children's decisions on children's engagement in ACTS, as well as events occurring during children's engagement (e.g., bullying) [14]. According to M-CAT, children make the final decision on whether they engage in a certain behavior [14], making them experts on their own behavior [18]. Their autonomy, independence, and personal responsibility increase with maturation, while the parents' role and influence as supporters or decision-makers (i.e., ultimate allowance or restriction) simultaneously decrease [14]. Besides the child and its parents, M-CAT mentions schoolteachers as important interactors in the socialization process of ACTS [14]. In addition to the teaching mission, schoolteachers also follow an educational mission according to German laws and are commonly seen as role models on who should practice whatever they emphasize in school lessons [19]. Contrary to previous research on parents, we could not find a gender-specific analysis of teachers' perspectives on ACTS.

Following this, parents at home and teachers at school educate and observe the child, making them experts on the child's behavior and needs [20]. Parents and teachers can be aware of aspects influencing their decision to support the child's ACTS [14], but the child, due to strengths, deficits, and stage of maturation, might not perceive them. This circumstance has already been confirmed in previous research, in which parents and their child had different perspectives on barriers of ACTS [15] and, conversely, needs. In addition, parents identified more barriers to ACTS than children [15]. Moreover, complementary and stimulating impulses of the child, parents, and teachers' perceptions, especially in the gender context [14], might favor a successful socialization process of ACTS [21].

Therefore, our concept mapping study analyzed how perceptions of students, parents, and teachers differed by gender about what children and adolescents aged 12 to 15 in Germany need to cycle daily to and from school. Knowledge of potential similarities and discrepancies in gender-specific perspectives of students, parents, and teachers on perceived needs is necessary to develop future gender-sensitive, school-based bicycle interventions.

2. Materials and Methods

This study used the concept mapping method, a mixed method that combines quantitative and qualitative research [22,23]. It follows a participatory approach based on group processes [22,23] and generally consists of six steps [24]. First, the study is prepared by defining the participants and developing a main question. The second step includes the generation of participants' answers to the main question. Third, participants cluster all unique answers from step two into groups of similar content and rate these answers on importance and feasibility. The fourth step includes the use of a computer program for a (hierarchical) cluster analysis and multidimensional scaling (multivariate statistical analyses). These analyses result in the representation of unique answers, obtained in the second step and structured in the third step, arranged as dots on a two-dimensional concept map. Distances between dots provide information about the frequency with which participants clustered unique answers in the same groups of similar content (i.e., the closer, the more often; the wider, the rarer). In step five, researchers interpret the concept map by identifying an adequate number of relevant clusters and, subsequently, label clusters according to their content based on participants' suggestions. The sixth step includes use of the concept map to plan or evaluate further research.

2.1. Recruitment of Participants

To address ACTS needs in both urban and suburban living areas [6,11,25] and to address the age group (older than 12 years) in which cycling-to-school rates are low [26], in October 2019, an invitation letter was sent to four secondary schools in urban or suburban areas in Germany. Three schools (one urban; two suburban), each including two classes of 7th and/or 8th graders aged 12 to 15, agreed to participate in the study. Parents and teachers were also invited to participate. Prior to the study's beginning, parents and teachers received an information letter, but only children whose parents, parents and teachers who provided signed consent forms participated. To ensure anonymity and to connect each individual's data throughout all concept mapping sessions, participants were instructed to create a five-digit ID code themselves. In all, 136 students, 58 parents, and 29 teachers participated in at least one of the sessions (drop-out rates: 26.5% for students; 79.3% for parents; 62.1% for teachers).

2.2. Concept Mapping Sessions

2.2.1. Students

All concept mapping sessions for students were conducted face-to-face at schools and were supervised by at least one trained researcher (D.M.I.S./C.V.). In each class, the sessions occurred during two regular lessons, i.e., 90 min. Based on schools' availability of sufficient computers and/or stable internet connections, sessions were conducted using either a printed or an online version. Independent of both media, sessions followed exactly the same procedure.

The first concept mapping sessions with students took place in November and December 2019. At three schools, 123 students (49 females, 72 males, 2 diverse), aged 13.1 ± 0.9 years, from six classes (22 to 32 students per class) participated. During the first session, students completed a printed or an online questionnaire via the program Survalyzer [27]. This questionnaire was structured in three sections (see Table A1): (1) personal characteristics, e.g., age and gender (see Table A2), (2) a warm-up question (why do or don't you cycle to school?), and (3) the main question (what do you need to cycle to and from school on a daily basis?). The warm-up question served as an icebreaker to introduce "cycling to school" to the students. To answer the main question, students had an individual and a group brainstorming phase. During individual brainstorming, students were stimulated to list as many answers to the main question as they could. During group brainstorming, individual students shared their written answers and checked their clarity, resulting in a list of unique answers for each class. After all classes had completed the first session, D.M.I.S. created a single list that included all unique answers from all six classes. The working process of D.M.I.S. was checked by the second researcher S.M., and any discrepancies were resolved through discussion. As a result, D.M.I.S. entered a list of 98 unique answers into the rating and clustering program Ariadne [28].

The second concept mapping sessions took place in January and February 2020; they were completed by 100 students (35 females, 64 males, 1 diverse). Here, students were asked to rate all 98 listed answers (paper/pencil with answers printed in a table or online via the program Ariadne) for both (a) importance and (b) feasibility on a five-point Likert scale (1 = very unimportant/unfeasible, 2 = unimportant/unfeasible, 3 = neutral, 4 = important/feasible, 5 = very important/feasible). Ninety-three (34 females, 59 males) and 83 students (32 females, 50 males, 1 diverse) completed the importance and feasibility ratings, respectively. Furthermore, students were asked to cluster all 98 answers (paper/pencil with answers printed on cards or online via the program Ariadne) in two to ten self-titled topic groups based on similarities between answers, with at least two answers in each; a "miscellaneous" pile was not allowed. Based on their individual ID code, each student used a personal link to access the tasks in Ariadne. Eighty-four students (30 females, 53 males, 1 diverse) completed the clustering task. Results from students who worked on the paper/pencil version were entered into Ariadne by D.M.I.S.

2.2.2. Parents and Teachers

All concept mapping sessions for parents and teachers were conducted online at home, without researchers' supervision. Prior to each session, parents and teachers received an information letter. During each working period per session, parents and teachers received a reminder asking them to participate in the study, in case they had not done so already.

The first concept mapping session with parents and teachers took place in November and December 2019. Participants included 42 parents (34 females, 8 males) aged 47.8 ± 5.5 years and 27 teachers (14 females, 13 males) aged 39.4 ± 10.9 years. During the first concept mapping session, parents and teachers completed separate online questionnaires via the program Survalyzer. Each questionnaire was structured in three sections (see Tables A3 and A4): (1) personal characteristics, e.g., age and gender (see Tables A5 and A6), (2) a warm-up question (parents: why does or doesn't your child cycle to school?; teachers: why do or don't your students cycle to school?), and (3) the main question (parents: what does your child need to cycle to and from school daily?; teachers: what do your students need to cycle to and from school daily?). The warm-up question served as an icebreaker to introduce "cycling to school" to parents and teachers. For the main question, parents and teachers listed as many answers as they could. After the first session, D.M.I.S. created lists that included all unique answers provided by parents and teachers, respectively. The working process of D.M.I.S. was checked by a second researcher (parents: P.W.; teachers: L.D.), and any discrepancies were resolved through discussion. As a result, P.W./L.D. (checked by D.M.I.S. and C.V.) entered parents' 90 and teachers' 94 unique answers into Survalyzer.

Because they completed the online questionnaire at home, parents and teachers could not participate in group brainstorming on the main question. Thus, in January 2020, an additional session was conducted in which 29 parents (10 females, 4 males, 15 unknown) and 7 teachers (1 female, 4 males, 2 unknown) checked the clarity of answers to the main question. Furthermore, parents and teachers could add new answers if inspired by other participants' answers. After the second session, D.M.I.S. revised and combined their answers where necessary, based on parents/teachers' comments, and created final lists that included all unique answers provided by parents and teachers, respectively. The working process of D.M.I.S. was checked by a second researcher (parents: P.W.; teachers: L.D.), and any discrepancies were resolved through discussion. As a result, D.M.I.S. entered revised lists of 90 parents' answers and 94 teachers' answers into Ariadne.

The third concept mapping session took place in February 2020, and was completed by 12 parents (9 females, 2 males, 1 unknown) and 11 teachers (6 females, 5 males). Here, parents and teachers rated all 90 and 94 answers listed online, via Ariadne, for both (a) importance and (b) feasibility on a five-point Likert scale (1 = very unimportant/unfeasible, 2 = unimportant/unfeasible, 3 = neutral,

4 = important/feasible, 5 = very important/feasible). Twelve parents (9 females, 2 males, 1 unknown) and 10 teachers (5 females, 5 males) completed the importance and feasibility rating. Furthermore, parents and teachers were asked to cluster all 90 and 94 answers listed online, via Ariadne, in two to ten self-titled topic groups based on similarities between answers with at least two answers in each; a "miscellaneous" pile was not allowed. Based on their individual ID code, each parent and teacher used a personal link to access the tasks in Ariadne. The clustering task was completed by 11 parents (9 females, 1 male, 1 unknown) and 10 teachers (5 females, 5 males).

2.3. Statistical Analyses and Interpretation of Concept Maps

Descriptive data from students, parents, and teachers as well as these groups' statistical gender differences (female vs. male) were analyzed using the program IBM SPSS Statistics 25 [29]. Additionally, this program was used to determine the within and between variance of days per week students cycled to the three participating schools by calculating an intraclass correlation coefficient (ICC) [30]. In the development of future intervention designs, the ICC is relevant for dealing with potential variance among participating schools.

Only students, parents, and teachers who reported their gender as female or male, and completed at least one of the two rating tasks (importance or feasibility) or the clustering task were included in analyses. The small number of fathers completing rating tasks ($n = 2$) and the clustering task ($n = 1$) did not allow for separate data analysis. Each subgroup rated and clustered the same answers, and only the analysis was stratified by gender using Ariadne. D.M.I.S. looked at all possible options of clusters, illustrated in a hierarchical cluster tree, to define an adequate number of relevant clusters for the concept map. A hierarchical cluster tree arranges all answers in one cluster at first and suggests how this cluster can be further split into two, three, four, or more clusters based on how students, mothers, or teachers clustered the answers. When considered necessary, items were reallocated into already existing clusters (indicated by arrows) or newly created clusters (indicated by circles) to ensure plausibility of answers in clusters. These procedures were checked by a second researcher (students: S.M.; parents: P.W.; teachers: L.D.). Any discrepancies were resolved through discussion. Lastly, all clusters were named according to suggestions by students, mothers, and teachers. For each cluster, average ratings of both importance and feasibility were calculated and descriptively described. These average ratings were based on the mean individual rating of all answers in each cluster. As Ariadne did not provide the participants' individual rating of all answers in each cluster, the appropriate statistical test for ordinal data (U-test) was not applicable to analyze differences in ratings [31].

3. Results

3.1. Cycling Behavior in Students

In total, 87.8% of girls and 100% of boys owned a bicycle (see Table A2). However, 44.4% of girls and 72.9% of boys cycled to school, but of these, 68.4% of girls and 62.7% of boys did not cycle to school daily. Girls cycled to school on 1.6 ± 2.0 days a week and boys on 2.7 ± 2.0 days a week.

Within and between the three participating schools, the variance of days per week students cycled to school, calculated with an ICC for 114 valid girls and boys, was 0.2 (high school in an urban area with 7th graders: 40 students; junior high school in a suburban area with 7th and 8th graders: 34 students; junior high school in a suburban area with 8th graders: 40 students).

3.2. Concept Maps and Ratings

3.2.1. Students

The concept map of the 30 girls who completed the clustering task included the following five clusters, illustrating their needs to cycle to school daily (see Figure A1): (1) "Bicycle and related equipment" (30 answers), e.g., lock, bicycle, pump, helmet, bell, reflectors, lights, bicycle basket, repair kit; (2) "Way to school" (20 answers), e.g., less traffic and roadworks, crossing guards, (wide, signposted, extra) cycle paths, (direct, shorter, simple, even) route; (3) "Requirements" (41 answers), e.g., health and environmental awareness, fun, motivation and energy, breathing fresh air, good weather conditions (no rain, warm temperatures), saving time, company of friends or classmates, later start of school lessons, liking own bicycle; (4) "Cycle training" (2 answers), e.g., cycling test, ensure cycling abilities; (5) "Social behavior in road traffic" (5 answers), e.g., more mutual respect, friendly car drivers, paying attention to avoid accidents or dangerous situations.

The concept map of the 53 boys who completed the clustering task included the following four clusters, illustrating their needs to cycle to school daily (see Figure A2): (1) "Bicycle and related equipment" (33 answers), e.g., lock, bicycle, pump, helmet, bell, reflectors, lights, bicycle basket, repair kit; (2) "Way to school" (23 answers), e.g., less traffic and roadworks, crossing guards, (wide, signposted, extra) cycle paths, (direct, shorter, simple, even) route; (3) "Requirements" (38 answers), e.g., health and environmental awareness, fun, motivation and energy, breathing fresh air, good weather conditions (no rain, warm temperatures), saving time, company of friends or classmates, later start of school lessons, liking own bicycle; (4) "Cycle training" (4 answers), e.g., cycling test, ensure cycling abilities, paying attention to avoid accidents or dangerous situations.

All four and five clusters identified in boys or girls, respectively, were rated as either unimportant/neutral or unfeasible/neutral on the Likert scale (see Table 1).

Table 1. Students' clusters and ratings of importance and feasibility by gender.

Name of Cluster	Rating of Importance		Rating of Feasibility	
	Girls ($n = 34$)	Boys ($n = 59$)	Girls ($n = 32$)	Boys ($n = 50$)
Bicycle and related equipment	3.4 ± 1.2	3.1 ± 1.3	3.5 ± 1.2	3.5 ± 1.4
Way to school	3.1 ± 1.2	2.9 ± 1.2	2.9 ± 1.3	2.8 ± 1.3
Requirements	3.0 ± 1.2	3.0 ± 1.4	2.9 ± 1.3	3.0 ± 1.4
Cycle training	3.6 ± 1.2	3.4 ± 1.3	3.7 ± 1.2	3.5 ± 1.4
Social behavior in road traffic	3.3 ± 1.2	-	3.1 ± 1.3	-

Means ± standard deviation.

3.2.2. Mothers

The concept map of the nine mothers who completed the clustering task included the following six clusters, illustrating their perceptions of what children and adolescents need to cycle to school daily (see Figure A3): (1) "Bicycle and related equipment" (26 answers), e.g., lock, (cool) bicycle, (cool) helmet, reflectors, (cool) signal clothing, (strip) lights, carrier systems, bicycle basket; (2) "Way to school" (24 answers), e.g., road lighting, (wide) cycle paths, less traffic, (uncomplicated, interesting, optimal) route, no large roadworks, crossing guards, combination of active and passive parts, speed limit; (3) "Requirements" (13 answers), e.g., health (awareness), sense of safety, self-confidence, knowledge of traffic rules, orientation skills, outdoor affinity, fitness, liking to cycle, cycling experiences; (4) "Motivation and social aspects" (12 answers), e.g., company of friends, classmates, or siblings (group trips with meeting points), sense of community, breathing fresh air; (5) "Role of the school" (7 answers), e.g., storage facilities, no vandalism, cycling projects, lighter schoolbag; (6) "Role of parents" (8 answers), e.g., trust, not taking the child to school by car, role models (obligatory helmet wearing, outdoor affinity).

All six clusters identified in mothers were rated as either unimportant/neutral or unfeasible/ neutral/feasible on the Likert scale (see Table 2).

Table 2. Mothers' clusters and ratings of importance and feasibility ($n = 9$).

Name of Cluster	Rating of Importance	Rating of Feasibility
Bicycle and related equipment	3.5 ± 1.0	4.3 ± 0.7
Way to school	3.1 ± 1.0	2.9 ± 0.9
Requirements	3.5 ± 1.0	3.8 ± 0.7
Motivation and social aspects	2.5 ± 1.0	2.9 ± 0.9
Role of the school	3.5 ± 0.9	3.6 ± 0.9
Role of parents	2.9 ± 1.0	3.7 ± 0.9

Means ± standard deviation.

3.2.3. Teachers

The concept map of the five female teachers who completed the clustering task included the following nine clusters, illustrating their perceptions of what children and adolescents need to cycle to school daily (see Figure A4): (1) "Bicycle and related equipment" (20 answers), e.g., lock, (cool) bicycle, (cool) helmet, reflectors, pump, lights; (2) "Motivation and social aspects" (15 answers), e.g., fun, incentives (scoring system, tests, class contests), rewards (certificate, price), sense of community, positive experiences in road traffic, sport interest, role models (friends, parents, teachers, siblings, classmates), good weather conditions (no rain, warm temperatures); (3) "Awareness" (5 answers), e.g., health and environmental awareness, cycling is cool (trendsetting), seeing the bicycle as sport object and means of transportation; (4) "Financial aspects" (9 answers), e.g., financial support to buy a bicycle and related equipment, appropriate clothing or a bicycle pool for cycle trainings at school; (5) "Information and services" (10 answers), e.g., information about appropriate clothing (rain jacket, pants) and carrier systems, repair service and bicycle flea market at school, information evening on advantages (environment and climate, health and fitness, saving money for fuel and public transport tickets, mobility, and independence), cycle training including traffic rules, kick-off event, school projects; (6) "Way to school" (21 answers), e.g., road lighting, cycle paths, orientation skills, less traffic around the school, cycle path guide, nice route, group trips with meeting points for friends, speed limit; (7) "Storage and changing room" (8 answers), e.g., (roofed, monitored) bicycle rack, access to changing rooms; (8) "Role of parents" (4 answers), e.g., not taking the child to school by car, support, traffic education, confidence in child; (9) "Sense of safety" (2 answers), i.e., everyone can cycle to school.

The concept map of the five male teachers who completed the clustering task included the following five clusters, illustrating their perceptions of what children and adolescents need to cycle to school daily (see Figure A5): (1) "Bicycle and related equipment" (20 answers), e.g., lock, (cool) bicycle, (cool) helmet, reflectors, pump, lights; (2) "Motivation, social aspects and awareness" (27 answers), e.g., parents not taking the child to school by car, role models (friends, parents, teachers, siblings, classmates), health and environmental awareness, cycling is cool (trendsetting), incentives (scoring system, class contests), fun, parental support, group trips with meeting points for friends, rewards (certificate, price), sense of community, positive experiences in road traffic, giving the feeling that everyone can cycle, parental confidence in child, sport interest, seeing the bicycle as sport object and means of transportation, good weather conditions (no rain, warm temperatures), saving time; (3) "Financial aspects" (10 answers), e.g., financial support to buy a bicycle and related equipment, appropriate clothing or a bicycle pool for cycle trainings at school; (4) "Information and services" (12 answers), e.g., information about appropriate clothing (rain jacket, pants) and carrier systems, repair service and bicycle flea market at school, traffic education (cycle training including traffic rules and test), information evening on advantages (environment and climate, health and fitness, saving money for fuel and public transport tickets, mobility and independence), kick-off event, school projects; (5) "Infrastructure" (25 answers) including the "way to school" and "storage and changing room," e.g., (roofed, monitored) bicycle rack, road lighting, cycle paths, speed limit, less traffic around the school, cycle path guide, access to changing rooms, nice route.

All five and nine clusters identified in male or female teachers, respectively, were rated as either neutral/important or unfeasible/neutral/feasible on the Likert scale (see Table 3).

Table 3. Teachers' clusters and ratings of importance and feasibility by gender.

Name of Cluster	Rating of Importance		Rating of Feasibility	
	Female Teachers ($n = 5$)	Male Teachers ($n = 5$)	Female Teachers ($n = 5$)	Male Teachers ($n = 5$)
Bicycle and related equipment	3.6 ± 0.8	3.7 ± 0.7	3.5 ± 0.7	3.4 ± 0.7
Motivation and social aspects	3.6 ± 1.0	3.6 ± 0.8	3.6 ± 0.9	3.5 ± 0.6
Awareness	4.0 ± 0.9		4.0 ± 0.8	
Financial aspects	3.3 ± 0.9	3.3 ± 1.0	2.8 ± 0.9	2.8 ± 1.1
Information and services	3.2 ± 1.0	3.4 ± 0.7	4.2 ± 0.8	3.7 ± 0.7
Way to school	3.6 ± 0.9	3.6 ± 0.9	3.3 ± 0.7	3.2 ± 1.0
Storage and changing room	3.3 ± 1.2		3.6 ± 1.0	
Role of parents	4.1 ± 0.7	-	3.6 ± 0.8	-
Sense of safety	4.3 ± 0.7	-	4.0 ± 0.4	-

Means ± standard deviation.

4. Discussion

Our concept mapping study analyzed factors needed by children and adolescents aged 12 to 15 in Germany to ride their bicycles to school every day based on gender perspectives of students, parents, and teachers. We found that every boy but not every girl owned a bicycle; this should be considered in future interventions (e.g., provision of bicycles) because only students who own a bicycle can actually cycle to school. Additionally, considerably more boys than girls cycled to school, in line with previous research in Germany [11]. Despite asking a similar question in this study, however, cycling rates were much higher (girls: 44.4% vs. 20.6%, boys: 72.9% vs. 23.8%) [11], suggesting that rates of cycling to school might have changed from 2003–2006 [11] and 2019. Nevertheless, cycling to school was not a daily habit in our sample, indicating room for improvement. Even though our low ICC, calculated for the within and between variance of days per week students cycled to the three participating schools, is in line with previously reported ICCs for group-randomized intervention designs (0.1 to 0.3 [32]), very low ICCs of 0.05 or 0.01 can lead to a meaningful bias in the results of significance tests [30] due to variances. Following this, researchers should keep a potential variance in mind when planning a school-based bicycle intervention (i.e., several schools per intervention condition in group-randomized designs). Contrary to our intention, we could not analyze fathers' perspectives and compare them with mothers' data due to the small number of complete data for fathers. Between girls and boys, we found one difference in clustering. Only girls clustered answers into "social behavior in road traffic." For each cluster, ratings of importance and feasibility were very similar in girls and boys. Between female and male teachers, we found differences in four clusters. Male teachers classified clusters into broader subjects, i.e., the cluster "motivation and social aspects" included "awareness" and the cluster "infrastructure" included "way to school" as well as "storage and changing room." Only female teachers clustered answers into "role of parents" and "sense of safety." For each cluster, ratings of importance and feasibility were very similar in female and male teachers.

4.1. Clusters in Concept Maps

4.1.1. Similar Clusters in Concept Maps of Mothers and Students and Teachers Independent of Gender

The need for a "bicycle and related equipment" (e.g., lock, bicycle, helmet, reflectors, lights) was stated by students, teachers, and mothers. When children and adolescents want to cycle to school, the basic necessity of bicycle ownership is indisputable. As every boy and nearly every girl in our sample owned a bicycle, providing all students in our sample with a bicycle in a future intervention does not seem necessary. Regarding bicycle-related equipment, previous research remained unclear on whether "the equipment of a child's bicycle is a potential determinant of cycling to school" [33] (p. 290). Nevertheless, the only overall effective bicycle intervention in our recent systematic review [12] was conducted in the USA and provided every child with a bicycle and related equipment (i.e., helmet, lock, lights) prior to the beginning of the intervention [34,35]. In our study, girls rated a lock and brakes as important equipment, whereas boys rated only a lock as important equipment. According to German Road Traffic Licensing Regulations, researchers might provide specific equipment (i.e., a bell, two independent brakes, two anti-slip and screwed-on pedals with two yellow reflectors shining to the front and rear, white front and red rear light, two reflectors per wheel, white front, and a red rear reflector [36]) to ensure the roadworthiness and safety of bicycles in an intervention.

Factors related to the "way to school," such as less traffic (especially around the school), (wide, signposted, extra) cycle paths, a cycle path guide, and an even route, were identified across all concept maps of students, teachers, and mothers. Traffic density and type of cycle paths (e.g., evenness) were reported as the most important factors for a cycling-friendly environment for children in previous research [37]. In addition, a cycle path guide (e.g., parental accompaniment while cycling) was positively associated with cycling behavior in children [38]. Comprehensive changes related to the way to school in school-based interventions require the involvement of municipal stakeholders.

Personal needs were represented in the cluster of students as "requirements" (e.g., motivation, company of friends or classmates), in the clusters of teachers as "motivation and social aspects" and "awareness," and in clusters of mothers as "requirements" and "motivation and social aspects." Because previous research also underlined the role of personal factors [39], it might be relevant to address the three basic psychological needs "autonomy, competence, and relatedness" of Self-Determination Theory [40] in future interventions with children and adolescents for long-term internalization of cycling-to-school behavior.

4.1.2. Unique Clusters in Concept Maps of Students (In) Dependent of Gender

"Cycle training" (e.g., cycling test, ensure cycling abilities) was identified by both girls and boys. To overcome barriers to cycle to school, cycle training is recommended by the "NZ Transport Agency" [41]. However, results from a previous study demonstrated that providing only cycle training on the school playground during physical education lessons was not effective in children's cycling-to-school behavior [42]. Following this, cycle training content should not only be chosen carefully based on needs mentioned by students but should also be implemented in the natural environment in future interventions to promote cycling to school.

The cluster "social behavior in road traffic" (e.g., more mutual respect, friendly car drivers, paying attention to avoid accidents or dangerous situations) was mentioned only by girls. Besides theoretical knowledge of traffic rules and practical cycling skills, social competences are considered essential for responsible and anticipated participation in road traffic by the "Standing Conference of the Ministers of Education and Cultural Affairs" (KMK) in Germany [43]. To acquire these competences, the KMK assigns mobility and traffic education to schools [43]. The reason boys did not mention this cluster might be explained by the observation in Germany that boys have a higher risk of injury in road traffic (accidents) due to more risky behavior than girls [44]. Therefore, the topic "social behavior in road traffic" is an important element in mobility and traffic education (especially for boys to reflect on the impact of their gender role) [44].

4.1.3. Similar and Unique Clusters in Concept Maps of Mothers, and Teachers (In) Dependent of Gender

Mothers and female teachers mentioned the "role of parents," e.g., not taking the child to school by car. Several theoretical models, for example, the M-CAT [14] or the "Social-ecological model of the correlates of active transportation" [45], consider parents' role as supporters or decision-makers. However, this role's impact decreases as the child matures [14]. Additionally, the 12- to 15-year-olds in our sample did not acknowledge their parents' role. Therefore, future interventions for this age group should empower parents to support children's need for autonomy, independence, and personal responsibility regarding mobility.

In line with theoretical models [14,45], mothers mentioned the cluster "role of the school" (e.g., storage facilities, no vandalism, cycling projects, lighter schoolbags). Additionally, the KMK has defined the teaching and educational role of mobility and traffic in schools [43], but neither students nor teachers acknowledged this. Therefore, the role of schools should be emphasized in future school-based bicycle interventions.

Mentioned by both female and male teachers, "storage and changing room" referred, for example, to a roofed and monitored bicycle rack or access to changing rooms. Even though students and mothers did not identify this cluster, the lack of or poor quality changing rooms and bicycle racks in schools have been previously reported to influence children and adolescents' PA behavior negatively [19]. Students and mothers might not have identified this need if they were satisfied by conditions at their school, but it might be relevant at schools with poor conditions.

Independent of gender, teachers identified the need for "financial aspects" (e.g., financial support to buy a bicycle and related equipment, appropriate clothing, or a bicycle pool for cycle trainings at school). In line with this, M-CAT states parents' income as a relevant factor for ACTS [14]. However, mothers and students did not mention this cluster, so financial aspects might not be a major issue for parents (who bear financial responsibility) or for students. Our assumption might be reflected in students' pervasive bicycle ownership because in our study sample, every boy owned a bicycle and only 12.2% of girls did not. This also makes it unnecessary to provide an entire bicycle pool for cycle training at the three participating schools.

Independent of gender, teachers identified the need for "information and services," e.g., information about appropriate clothing (rain jacket, pants) and carrier systems, repair service and a bicycle flea market at school, an information evening on advantages (environment and climate, health and fitness, saving money for fuel and public transport tickets, mobility and independence), cycle training including traffic rules, a kick-off event, and school projects (bicycle tour, project day). In grades 5 to 10 (students aged 10 to 15), the KMK explicitly mentions the provision of informational manuals and materials (e.g., about environment and climate), implementation of activities (e.g., ecological school trips), and cooperation with out-of-school partners (e.g., bicycle repair shops) to promote students' independent mobility [43]. However, provision of information and services might be feasible but not crucial in the development of future school-based bicycle interventions. Perhaps this is why students and mothers did not consider this need relevant.

Clusters between female and male teachers differed as only female teachers clustered answers into "sense of safety," i.e., giving the feeling that everyone can use a bicycle to engage in ACTS. As an important barrier to ACTS, children's personal safety fears were also identified in previous research [39], and this cluster might be reflected in students' identified needs for cycle training and social behavior in road traffic. Thus, future school-based bicycle interventions should attempt to establish feelings of safety among students.

4.2. Importance and Feasability

Across students, mothers, and teachers, Likert scale ratings of the degree of importance and feasibility of their provided answers showed not a single extreme response, i.e., very (un) important or (un) feasible. Participants noticeably tended to choose the unimportant/unfeasible or neutral rating categories so that ratings were very similar. Undecidedness [46], lack of motivation [47] due to the large number of participants' answers (students: 98; parents: 90; teachers: 94) that had to be rated, or a question not specific enough [48] might have led to this central tendency bias. Therefore, findings on ratings should be interpreted with caution.

4.3. Strengths and Limitations

Quantitative analysis of qualitative data in the concept mapping approach could be seen as a strength of this study. Additionally, stratified gender analyses provide a deeper understanding of different perspectives on what is needed for cycling to school. We found one and two unique gender-dependent cluster(s) in students and teachers, respectively. A limitation might be that group sessions were not conducted separately for females and males. Moreover, we could not include grades 7 and 8 in each session at every school since the schools decided the participating grades. Contrary to our previous intention, teachers did not allow us to divide classes of 22 to 32 into smaller groups of 8 to 10 students. This made conducting sessions challenging in terms of personnel, time, and resources (e.g., sufficient computers, stable internet connections) but led to a higher student recruitment rate (i.e., planned: 48; recruited: 136), which is a major strength. In general, participants were interested in the concept mapping sessions and liked getting involved by providing their opinions, which gave us an insight into their perceptions. This might explain why we also exceeded our recruitment goals for parents and teachers (58 and 29 instead of 25 each). Interestingly, more mothers than fathers contributed to the concept mapping sessions. This gender bias in our online survey's response rate aligns with previous research [49] and might be explained by differences in perceived parenting responsibilities. Due to small sample sizes as well as high drop-out rates of parents and teachers and to the few regions sampled in Germany, our findings cannot be generalized and might differ in comparison with other nations. Nevertheless, studies using the concept mapping approach in very small samples of five to eight participants are not unusual [50].

Throughout our sessions, we were confronted with several difficulties. Participants complained about the time-consuming involvement (e.g., too many answers), the type of survey (i.e., paper/pencil) and other participants' "absurd" answers (e.g., "I need training wheels"). Furthermore, non-native speakers (e.g., refugees) struggled especially with the amount of information in German. Generally, participants also found it difficult to separate ratings between importance and feasibility. In addition, participants struggled with rating tasks when answers were not applicable to their situations (e.g., students, whose parents were not worried, struggled how to rate "reduction of fear in parents"). Due to technical failures that occurred throughout the sessions with both online programs (Survalyzer, Ariadne), we could not ensure completeness of data (an inclusion criterion for Ariadne analyses). Some of these difficulties might have led to a lowered willingness and motivation to participate, thus possibly explaining the central tendency bias in importance and feasibility ratings and the relatively high drop-out rates, particularly in parents (79.3%) and teachers (62.1%), in contrast with students (26.5%).

4.4. Recommendations

Based on our experience from this study, we recommend modifying the concept mapping approach for such a complex subject and/or for its application in large groups due to school rules. To achieve participants' maximum commitment and to reduce their burden, we suggest conducting all sessions online (especially the clustering task), but in school groups supervised by researchers to ensure personal contact. Another advantage of online sessions is the immediate digital availability of collected data, which eliminates the risk of errors in transferring data manually. We further recommend removing the second online session in which participants check the clarity of answers. Instead, the first online session could be completed with a group brainstorming phase including a clarity check and a removal of duplicates. To make "ACTS by bicycle" less complex for participants (i.e., fewer answers), the main question in the first session could be specified according to factors in the "Social-ecological model of the correlates of active transportation" [45] (e.g., the needs in terms of environmental factors only). Still, to acquire a comprehensive picture of needs, the concept mapping approach could be conducted for each factor of this model based on more specific questions in different samples (e.g., different classes) in the same schools. Another possibility could be to restrict the number of answers to a more manageable number (e.g., 40 to 70) [51] by checking duplicates more strictly and combining answers after session one.

To maintain participants' motivation and to address their need for time efficiency, each provided answer could be immediately rated for importance and feasibility. In the second study session, we changed this when students received the paper/pencil version and reflected positive experiences with the procedure. Future studies could optimize rating tasks to avoid central tendency bias and inconclusive findings by replacing the five-point Likert scale with an even-point scale, i.e., a scale without a midpoint, which forces participants to choose positively or negatively. Independent of language skills, the majority of students had problems answering the question about frequency of "cycling to school (days/week)" because they cycled every day in the summer but took the bus or train in the winter. These seasonal differences align with previous Norwegian findings that reported large variations in fall (52%), winter (3%), spring (51%) [52], and in summer (22%) compared to winter (12%) [53]. Therefore, we highly recommend modifying this question to consider potential seasonal variations in surveys and to take different weather conditions into account when developing an intervention. Finally, the program Ariadne appeared to be prone to error and was perceived to be user-unfriendly, so we recommend that this program be improved for future concept mapping studies.

5. Conclusions

This study provides insight into the perceptions of girls and boys, mothers, and female and male teachers on what 12- to 15-year-old children and adolescents living in Germany need to cycle daily to school. Between genders, we found more overall similarities than differences in clusters. Students and teachers, independent of gender, and mothers mentioned the need for "bicycle and related equipment," "way to school," and "personal factors." Additionally, independent of gender, students identified "cycle training" and teachers a "storage and changing room," "financial aspects," and "information and services" as children and adolescents' needs. Furthermore, girls identified the need for "social behavior in road traffic," mothers and female teachers the "role of parents," and female teachers the "sense of safety." However, boys and male teachers did not mention these three needs. Only mothers clustered the "role of the school." Furthermore, we found bias in clusters' importance and feasibility ratings and could not draw final conclusions. Nevertheless, we hope that the combined perceptions complement each other to support the uptake and long-term maintenance of ACTS by bicycle. Our findings can be used to inform students, mothers, and teachers about their mutual perceptions and can help researchers develop school-based interventions to promote daily cycling to school.

Author Contributions: D.M.I.S. was responsible for the preparation, data collection, analyses, and interpretation of concept mapping sessions. Moreover, she drafted the manuscript. C.V. assisted in preparation and data collection. L.M.H., T.M.A. and M.J.M.C. designed the study's methodological process. Furthermore, L.M.H. advised D.M.I.S. in the methodological process and in the analyses using the program Ariadne. Y.D. acquired funding for the project and was involved in the study's preparation. C.V., L.M.H., T.M.A., M.J.M.C. and Y.D. commented on the manuscript. All authors have read and agreed to the published version of the manuscript.

Funding: This research was funded by the Education, Audiovisual and Culture Executive Agency (EACEA) ERASMUS+ Sport Program, grant number 2018-3291/001-001.

Acknowledgments: We thank Pia Wullinger (P.W.), Selina Moser (S.M.) and Lisa Dobner (L.D.), Bachelor students at the Technical University of Munich, who helped to prepare the surveys and to collect, analyze, and interpret data. Furthermore, we thank Jakob Buchmann, Bachelor student at the Technical University of Munich, who helped to collect and handle data. Thanks also to Anne Kelso, research assistant at the Technical University of Munich, who translated the warm-up and main question from English to German. The authors are thankful for the support of the ACTS-Consortium, too.

Conflicts of Interest: The funders had no role in the design of the study; in the collection, analyses, or interpretation of data; in the writing of the manuscript; or in the decision to publish the results.

Appendix A

Table A1. Overview of sections, questions, and response options of the first concept mapping session with students.

Section	Questions	Response Option(s)
Personal characteristics	age (years)	open-end
	gender	(a) female (b) male (c) diverse
	school's region	(a) urban (b) suburban
	school's zip-code	open-end
	educational level	(a) high school (b) junior high school
	class level	(a) 7 (b) 8
	bicycle ownership	(a) yes (b) no
	ability to cycle	(a) yes (b) no
	cycling to school	(a) yes (b) no
	cycling to school (days/week)	0–5
	shortest cycling distance home/school (km [1])	open-end
Warm-up question	Why do or don't you cycle to school?	open-end
Main question	What do you need to cycle to and from school on a daily basis?	open-end

[1] km = kilometer.

Table A2. Personal characteristics of participating students by gender.

Personal Characteristics	Female (n = 51)	Male (n = 83)	p-Value [3]	Diverse (n = 2)	Response Rate (N = 136)
Age (years in M ± SD [1])	13.1 ± 0.9	13.1 ± 0.9	0.778	13.0 ± 0.000	123
Educational level (school's region)					
(a) high school (urban)	13 (25.5%)	31 (37.3%)	0.156	0 (0%)	136
(b) junior high school (suburban)	38 (74.5%)	52 (62.7%)		2 (100%)	
Class level					
(a) 7th grade	22 (43.1%)	44 (53.0%)	0.267	0 (0%)	136
(b) 8th grade	29 (56.9%)	39 (47.0%)		2 (100%)	
Bicycle ownership					
(a) yes	43 (87.8%)	72 (100%)	0.004 **	2 (100%)	123
(b) no	6 (12.2%)	0 (0%)		0 (0%)	
Ability to cycle					
(a) yes	49 (100%)	72 (100%)	n.a. [4]	2 (100%)	123
(b) no	0 (0%)	0 (0%)		0 (0%)	
Cycling to school					
(a) yes	20 (44.4%)	51 (72.9%)	0.002 **	1 (50.0%)	117
(b) no	25 (55.6%)	19 (27.1%)		1 (50.0%)	
Cycling to school (days/week in M ± SD [1])	1.6 ± 2.0	2.7 ± 2.0	0.003 **	1.5 ± 2.1	116
Shortest cycling distance home/school (km [2] in M ± SD [1])	3.3 ± 2.6	4.0 ± 3.1	0.307	8.0 ± 9.9	122

[1] means ± standard deviation, [2] km = kilometer, [3] p-values were calculated for gender differences (female vs. male) using U-test or Chi-squared tests, [4] n.a. = not applicable, ** = 0.01 ≥ p > 0.001.

Table A3. Overview of sections, questions, and response options of the first concept mapping session with parents.

Section	Question(s)	Response Option(s)
Personal characteristics	age (years)	open-end
	gender	(a) female (b) male (c) diverse
	age of child (years)	(a) 12 (b) 13 (c) 14 (d) other
	gender of child	(a) daughter (b) son
	child's school region	(a) urban (b) suburban
	child's school zip-code of child	open-end
	educational level of child	(a) high school (b) junior high school
	class level of child	(a) 7 (b) 8
	bicycle ownership of child	(a) yes (b) no
	child's ability to cycle	(a) yes (b) no
	cycling to school of child	(a) yes (b) no
	cycling to school of child (days/week)	0–5
	shortest cycling distance home/school of child (km [1])	open-end
	bicycle ownership	(a) yes (b) no
	ability to cycle	(a) yes (b) no
	work (days/week)	0–5
	cycling to work	(a) yes (b) no
	cycling to work (days/week)	0–5
	shortest cycling distance home/work (km [1])	open-end
Warm-up question	Why does or doesn't your child cycle to school?	open-end
Main question	What does your child need to cycle to and from school daily?	open-end

[1] km = kilometer.

Table A4. Overview of sections, questions, and response options of the first concept mapping session with teachers.

Section	Question(s)	Response Option(s)
Personal characteristics	age (years)	open-end
	gender	(a) female (b) male (c) diverse
	work experience (years)	open-end
	school's region	(a) urban (b) suburban
	school's zip-code	open-end
	educational level	(a) high school (b) junior high school
	class level of target group	open-end
	cycling to school of target group (%)	open-end
	cycling to school of target group (days/week)	0–5
	bicycle ownership	(a) yes (b) no
	ability to cycle	(a) yes (b) no
	work (days/week)	0–5
	cycling to work	(a) yes (b) no
	cycling to work (days/week)	0–5
	shortest cycling distance home/work (km [1])	open-end
Warm-up question	Why do or don't your students cycle to school?	open-end
Main question	What do your students need to cycle to and from school daily?	open-end

[1] km = kilometer.

Table A5. Personal characteristics of participating parents by gender.

Personal Characteristics	Female (n = 35)	Male (n = 8)	p-Value [3]	Response Rate (N = 43)
Age (years in M ± SD [1])	46.8 ± 5.1	52.1 ± 5.2	0.034 *	42
Age of child (years in M ± SD [1])	12.6 ± 0.7	13.0 ± 0.8	0.145	42
Gender of child				
(a) daughter	(a) 12 (34.3%)	(a) 3 (37.5%)	1	43
(b) son	(b) 23 (65.7%)	(b) 5 (62.5%)		
Educational level (school's region) of child				
(a) high school (urban)	(a) 15 (42.9%)	(a) 4 (50.0%)	1	43
(b) junior high school (suburban)	(b) 20 (57.1%)	(b) 4 (50.0%)		

Table A5. Cont.

Personal Characteristics	Female (n = 35)	Male (n = 8)	p-Value [3]	Response Rate (N = 43)
Class level of child			1	43
(a) 7th grade	(a) 23 (65.7%)	(a) 6 (75.0%)		
(b) 8th grade	(b) 12 (34.3%)	(b) 2 (25.0%)		
Bicycle ownership of child			n.a. [4]	42
(a) yes	(a) 34 (100%)	(a) 8 (100%)		
(b) no	(b) 0 (0%)	(b) 0 (0%)		
Child's ability to cycle			n.a. [4]	42
(a) yes	(a) 34 (100%)	(a) 8 (100%)		
(b) no	(b) 0 (0%)	(b) 0 (0%)		
Cycling to school of child			1	40
(a) yes	(a) 22 (66.7%)	(a) 5 (71.4%)		
(b) no	(b) 11 (33.3%)	(b) 2 (28.6%)		
Cycling to school of child (days/week in M ± SD [1])	2.6 ± 2.3	3.1 ± 2.2	0.985	40
Shortest cycling distance home/school of child (km [2] in M ± SD [1])	4.3 ± 3.2	5.2 ± 3.2	0.432	42
Bicycle ownership			1	42
(a) yes	(a) 33 (97.1%)	(a) 8 (100%)		
(b) no	(b) 1 (2.9%)	(b) 0 (0%)		
Ability to cycle			n.a. [4]	42
(a) yes	(a) 34 (100%)	(a) 8 (100%)		
(b) no	(b) 0 (0%)	(b) 0 (0%)		
Work (days/week in M ± SD [1])	3.7 ± 1.5	4.9 ± 0.4	0.004 **	42
Cycling to work			0.698	38
(a) yes	(a) 12 (40.0%)	(a) 4 (50.0%)		
(b) no	(b) 18 (60.0%)	(b) 4 (50.0%)		
Cycling to work (days/week in M ± SD [1])	1.3 ± 1.9	1.8 ± 2.2	0.549	38
Shortest cycling distance home/work (km [2] in M ± SD [1])	13.0 ± 14.4	7.9 ± 5.5	0.676	39

[1] means ± standard deviation, [2] km = kilometer, [3] p-values were calculated for gender differences (female vs. male) using U-test or Chi-squared tests, [4] n.a. = not applicable, * = $0.05 \geq p > 0.01$, ** = $0.01 \geq p > 0.001$.

Table A6. Personal characteristics of participating teachers by gender.

Personal Characteristics	Female (n = 14)	Male (n = 13)	p-Value [4]	Response Rate (N = 27)
Age (years in M ± SD [1])	43.3 ± 11.5	35.3 ± 8.9	0.068	27
Work experience (years in M ± SD [1])	15.2 ± 12.0	7.2 ± 5.6	0.068	27
Educational level (school's region)			0.12	27
(a) high school (urban)	(a) 3 (21.4%)	(a) 7 (53.8%)		
(b) junior high school (suburban)	(b) 11 (78.6%)	(b) 6 (46.2%)		
Class level of target group (min/max [2])	6–9	6–9	n.a. [5]	27
Cycling to school of target group (% in M ± SD [1])	40.0%	20.0% ± 15.8%	0.277	5
Cycling to school of target group (days/week in M ± SD [1])	5.0	4.0 ± 0.8	0.264	5
Bicycle ownership			1	27
(a) yes	(a) 13 (92.9%)	(a) 13 (100%)		
(b) no	(b) 1 (7.1%)	(b) 0 (0%)		
Ability to cycle			n.a. [5]	27
(a) yes	(a) 14 (100%)	(a) 13 (100%)		
(b) no	(b) 0 (0%)	(b) 0 (0%)		
Work (days/week in M ± SD [1])	4.1 ± 0.8	4.9 ± 0.4	0.008 **	27
Cycling to work			0.107	26
(a) yes	(a) 6 (46.2%)	(a) 10 (76.9%)		
(b) no	(b) 7 (53.8%)	(b) 3 (23.1%)		
Cycling to work (days/week in M ± SD [1])	1.6 ± 2.1	2.8 ± 2.2	0.127	26
Shortest cycling distance home/work (km [3] in M ± SD [1])	8.9 ± 7.8	13.0 ± 12.9	0.382	27

[1] means ± standard deviation, [2] min/max = minimum/maximum, [3] km = kilometer, [4] p-values were calculated for gender differences (female vs. male) using U-test or Chi-squared tests, [5] n.a. = not applicable, ** = $0.01 \geq p > 0.001$.

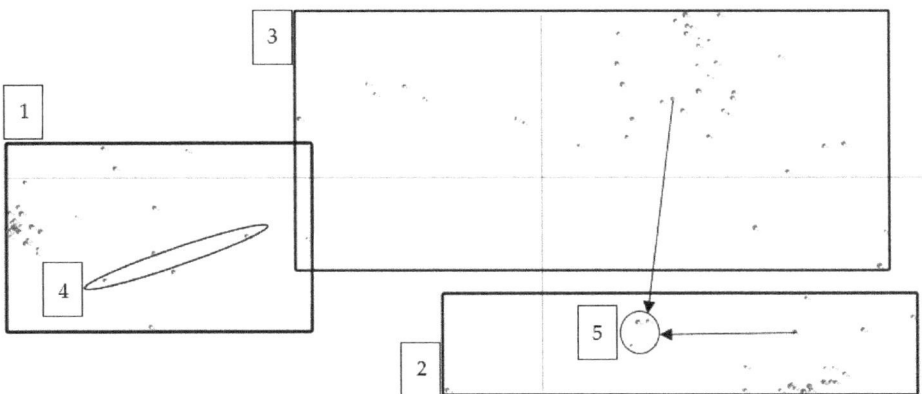

Figure A1. Concept map of girls (n = 30). Cluster 1: "bicycle and related equipment." Cluster 2: "way to school." Cluster 3: "requirements." Cluster 4: "cycle training." Cluster 5: "social behavior in road traffic." A square indicates an original cluster, and a circle indicates a newly created cluster. An arrow indicates reallocation of an answer (illustrated as a dot) into another cluster.

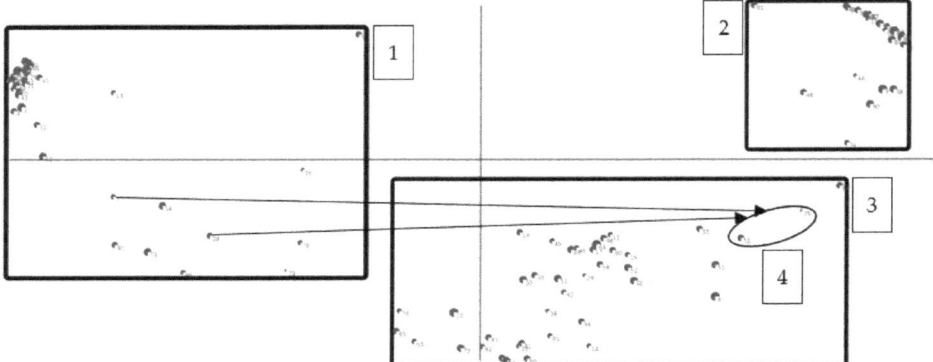

Figure A2. Concept map of boys (n = 53). Cluster 1: "bicycle and related equipment." Cluster 2: "way to school." Cluster 3: "requirements." Cluster 4: "cycle training." A square indicates an original cluster, and a circle indicates a newly created cluster. An arrow indicates reallocation of an answer (illustrated as a dot) into another cluster.

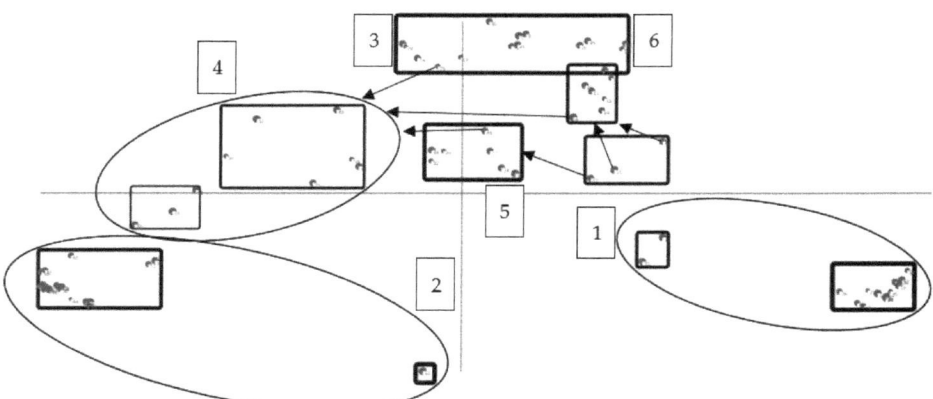

Figure A3. Concept map of mothers (n = 9). Cluster 1: "bicycle and related equipment." Cluster 2: "way to school." Cluster 3: "requirements." Cluster 4: "motivation and social aspects." Cluster 5: "role of the school." Cluster 6: "role of parents." A square indicates an original cluster, and a circle indicates a newly created cluster. An arrow indicates reallocation of an answer (illustrated as a dot) into another cluster.

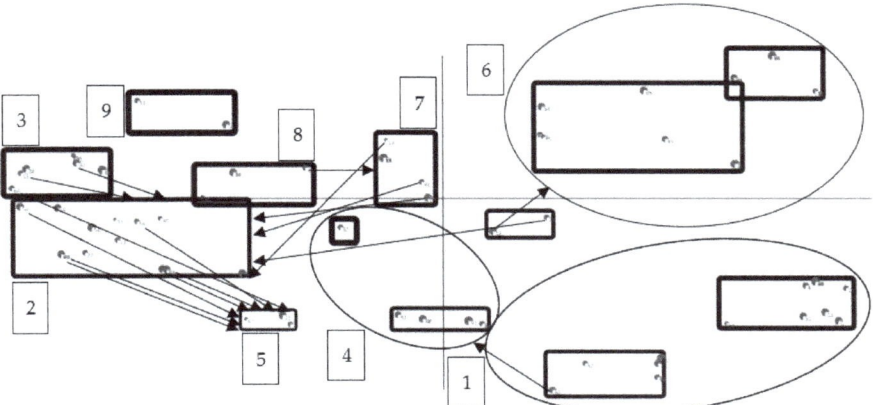

Figure A4. Concept map of female teachers ($n = 5$). Cluster 1: "bicycle and related equipment." Cluster 2: "motivation and social aspects." Cluster 3: "awareness." Cluster 4 "financial aspects." Cluster 5: "information and services." Cluster 6: "way to school." Cluster 7: "storage and changing room." Cluster 8: "role of parents." Cluster 9: "sense of safety." A square indicates an original cluster, and a circle indicates a newly created cluster. An arrow indicates reallocation of an answer (illustrated as a dot) into another cluster.

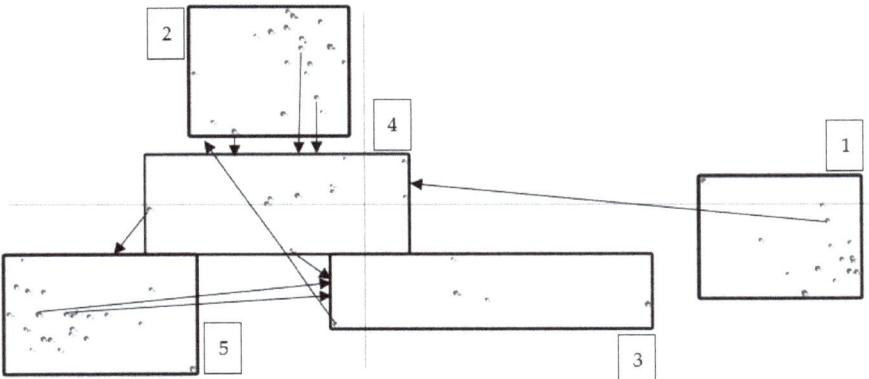

Figure A5. Concept map of male teachers ($n = 5$). Cluster 1: "bicycle and related equipment." Cluster 2: "motivation, social aspects and awareness." Cluster 3: "financial aspects." Cluster 4: "information and services." Cluster 5: "infrastructure." A square indicates an original cluster. An arrow indicates reallocation of an answer (illustrated as a dot) into another cluster.

References

1. Finger, J.D.; Varnaccia, G.; Borrmann, A.; Lange, C.; Mensink, G.B.M. Physical activity among children and adolescents in Germany. Results of the cross-sectional KiGGS Wave 2 study and trends. *J. Health Monit.* **2018**, *3*, 23–30.
2. Institute of Medicine. *Educating the Student Body: Taking Physical Activity and Physical Education to School*; The National Academies Press: Washington, DC, USA, 2013; p. 7.
3. Roth, M.A.; Millet, C.J.; Mindell, J.S. The contribution of active travel (walking and cycling) in children to overall physical activity levels: A national cross sectional study. *Prev. Med.* **2012**, *54*, 134–139. [CrossRef]

4. Larouche, R.; Saunders, T.J.; Faulkner, G.E.J.; Colley, R.; Tremblay, M. Associations Between Active School Transport and Physical Activity, Body Composition, and Cardiovascular Fitness: A Systematic Review of 68 Studies. *J. Phys. Act. Health* **2014**, *11*, 206–227. [CrossRef]
5. D'Haese, S.; De Meester, F.; De Bourdeaudhuij, I.; Deforche, B.; Cardon, G. Criterion distances and environmental correlates of active commuting to school in children. *Int. J. Behav. Nutr. Phys. Act.* **2011**, *8*, 1–10. [CrossRef]
6. Nelson, N.M.; Foley, E.; O'Gorman, D.J.; Moyna, N.M.; Woods, C.B. Active commuting to school: How far is too far? *Int. J. Behav. Nutr. Phys. Act.* **2008**, *5*, 1–9. [CrossRef]
7. EnercitEE. Available online: http://enercitee.eu/files/dokumente/Subprojects/SUSTRAMM/SustraMM_Costs_and_benefits_of_cycling.pdf (accessed on 21 March 2020).
8. Yang, X.; Telama, R.; Hirvensalo, M.; Tammelin, T.; Viikari, J.S.A.; Raitakari, O.T. Active commuting from youth to adulthood and as a predictor of physical activity in early midlife: The Young Finns Study. *Prev. Med.* **2014**, *59*, 5–11. [CrossRef] [PubMed]
9. Federal Ministry of Transport and Digital Infrastructure. Available online: https://www.bmvi.de/SharedDocs/DE/Publikationen/K/radverkehr-in-zahlen.pdf?__blob=publicationFile (accessed on 21 March 2020).
10. Schöb, A. Fahrradnutzung bei Stuttgarter Schülern. Erste Ergebnisse einer Schülerinnen- und Schülerbefragung an Stuttgarter Schulen 2005. *Stat. Inf.* **2006**, *11*, 294–317.
11. Reimers, A.K.; Jekauc, D.; Peterhans, E.; Wagner, M.O.; Woll, A. Prevalence and socio-demographic correlates of active commuting to school in a nationwide representative sample of German adolescents. *Prev. Med.* **2013**, *56*, 64–69. [CrossRef] [PubMed]
12. Schönbach, D.M.I.; Altenburg, T.M.; Marques, A.; Chinapaw, M.J.M.; Demetriou, Y. Strategies and effects of school-based interventions to promote active school transportation by bicycle among children and adolescents: A systematic review. *Int. J. Behav. Nutr. Phys. Act.*. (under review).
13. Villa-González, E.; Ruiz, J.R.; Mendoza, J.A.; Chillón, P. Effects of a school-based intervention on active commuting to school and health related fitness. *BMC Public Health* **2017**, *17*, 1–11. [CrossRef]
14. Pont, K.; Ziviani, J.; Wadley, D.; Abbott, R. The Model of Children's Active Travel (M-CAT): A conceptual framework for examining factors influencing children's active travel. *Aust. Occup. Ther. J.* **2011**, *58*, 138–144. [CrossRef] [PubMed]
15. Wilson, K.; Clark, A.F.; Gilliland, J.A. Understanding child and parent perceptions of barriers influencing children's active school travel. *BMC Public Health* **2018**, *18*, 1–14. [CrossRef] [PubMed]
16. Rodrigues, D.; Padez, C.; Machado-Rodrigues, A.M. Environmental and Socio-demographic Factors Associated with 6-10-Year-Old Children's School Travel in Urban and Non-urban Settings. *J. Urban Health* **2018**, *95*, 1–10. [CrossRef] [PubMed]
17. Aibar Solana, A.; Mandic, S.; Generelo Lanaspa, E.; Gallardo, L.O.; Zaragoza Casterad, J. Parental barriers to active commuting to school in children: Does parental gender matter? *J. Transp. Health* **2018**, *9*, 141–149. [CrossRef]
18. Hidding, L.M.; Chinapaw, M.J.M.; Altenburg, T.M. An activity-friendly environment from the adolescent perspective: A concept mapping study. *Int. J. Behav. Nutr. Phys. Act* **2018**, *15*, 1–8. [CrossRef]
19. Morton, K.L.; Atkin, A.J.; Corder, K.; Suhrcke, M.; van Sluijs, E.M.F. The school environment and adolescent physical activity and sedentary behaviour: A mixed-studies systematic review. *Obes. Rev.* **2016**, *17*, 142–158. [CrossRef]
20. Rother, T. Problemsicht. In *Schwierige Elterngespräche Erfolgreich Meistern—Das Praxisbuch. Profi-Tipps und Materialien aus der Lehrerfortbildung*; Roggenkamp, A., Rother, T., Schneider, J., Eds.; Auer: Donauwörth, Germany, 2014; pp. 6–10.
21. Hurrelmann, K. Jugendliche als produktive Realitätsverarbeiter: Zur Neuausgabe des Buches "Lebensphase Jugend". *Diskurs Kindh. Jugendforsch.* **2012**, *7*, 89–100.
22. Burke, J.G.; O'Campo, P.; Peak, G.L.; Gielen, A.C.; McDonnell, K.A.; Trochim, W.M.K. An Introduction to Concept Mapping as a Participatory Public Health Research Method. *Qual. Health Res.* **2005**, *15*, 1392–1410. [CrossRef]
23. Trochim, W.; Kane, M. Concept mapping: An introduction to structured conceptualization in health care. *Int. J. Qual. Health Care* **2005**, *17*, 187–191. [CrossRef]
24. Trochim, W.M.K. An introduction to concept mapping for planning and evaluation. *Eval. Program Plann.* **1989**, *12*, 1–16. [CrossRef]

25. Murtagh, E.M.; Dempster, M.; Murphy, M.H. Determinants of uptake and maintenance of active commuting to school. *Health Place* **2016**, *40*, 9–14. [CrossRef] [PubMed]
26. Ramírez-Vélez, R.; Beltrán, C.A.; Correa-Bautista, J.E.; Vivas, A.; Prieto-Benavidez, D.H.; Martínez-Torres, J.; Triana-Reina, H.R.; Villa-González, E.; Garcia-Hermoso, A. Factors associated with active commuting to school by bicycle from Bogotá, Colombia: The FUPRECOL study. *Ital. J. Pediatr.* **2016**, *42*, 1–9. [CrossRef] [PubMed]
27. Survalyzer. Available online: https://www.survalyzer.com/de (accessed on 20 April 2020).
28. Ariadne. Available online: http://www.minds21.org/ (accessed on 28 February 2020).
29. IBM Corp. *IBM SPSS Statistics for Windows*; Version 25.0; IBM Corp.: Armonk, NY, USA, 2017.
30. Geiser, C. *Datenanalyse mit Mplus. Eine anwendungsorientierte Einführung*, 2nd ed.; VS: Wiesbaden, Germany, 2011; p. 204.
31. Hoffmann, U.; Orthmann, P. *Schnellkurs Statistik mit Hinweisen zur SPSS-Benutzung*, 6th ed.; Sportverlag Strauß: Cologne, Germany, 2009.
32. Snijders, T.A.B.; Bosker, R.J. *Multilevel Analysis. An Introduction to Basic and Advanced Multilevel Modeling*, 2nd ed.; SAGE: Los Angeles, CA, USA, 2012; p. 18.
33. Ducheyne, F.; De Bourdeaudhuij, I.; Lenoir, M.; Cardon, G. Test-Retest Reliability and Validity of a Child and Parental Questionnaire on Specific Determinants of Cycling to School. *Pediatr. Exerc. Sci.* **2012**, *24*, 289–311. [CrossRef] [PubMed]
34. Huang, C.; Dannenberg, A.L.; Haaland, W.; Mendoza, J.A. Changes in Self-Efficacy and Outcome Expectations from Child Participation in Bicycle Trains for Commuting to and from School. *Health Educ. Behav.* **2018**, *45*, 748–755. [CrossRef] [PubMed]
35. Mendoza, J.A.; Haaland, W.; Jacobs, M.; Abbey-Lambertz, M.; Miller, J.; Salls, D.; Todd, W.; Madding, R.; Ellis, K.; Kerr, J. Bicycle Trains, Cycling, and Physical Activity: A Pilot Cluster RCT. *Am. J. Prev. Med.* **2017**, *53*, 481–489. [CrossRef]
36. Allgemeiner Deutscher Fahrrad-Club e. V. Available online: https://www.adfc.de/artikel/das-verkehrssichere-fahrrad/ (accessed on 6 July 2020).
37. Ghekiere, A.; Deforche, B.; Mertens, L.; De Bourdeaudhuij, I.; Clarys, P.; de Geus, B.; Cardon, G.; Nasar, J.; Salmon, J.; Van Cauwenberg, J. Creating Cycling-Friendly Environments for Children: Which Micro-Scale Factors Are Most Important? An Experimental Study Using Manipulated Photographs. *PLoS ONE* **2015**, *10*, 1–18. [CrossRef]
38. Ghekiere, A.; Carver, A.; Veitch, J.; Salmon, J.; Deforche, B.; Timperio, A. Does parental accompaniment when walking or cycling moderate the association between physical neighbourhood environment and active transport among 10–12 years old? *J. Sci. Med. Sport* **2015**, *19*, 149–153. [CrossRef]
39. Ahlport, K.N.; Linnan, L.; Vaughn, A.; Evenson, K.R.; Ward, D.S. Barriers to and Facilitators of Walking and Bicycling to School: Formative Results from the Non-Motorized Travel Study. *Health Educ. Behav.* **2008**, *35*, 221–244. [CrossRef]
40. Ryan, R.M.; Deci, E.L. *Self-Determination Theory. Basic Psychological Needs in Motivation, Development, and Wellness*; Guilford Press: New York, NY, USA, 2017.
41. Waka Kotahi NZ Transport Agency. Available online: http://www.feetfirst.govt.nz/assets/resources/research/reports/380/docs/380.pdf (accessed on 20 April 2020).
42. Ducheyne, F.; De Bourdeaudhuij, I.; Lenoir, M.; Cardon, G. Effects of a cycle training course on children's cycling skills and levels of cycling to school. *Accid. Anal. Prev.* **2014**, *67*, 49–60. [CrossRef]
43. Standing Conference of the Ministers of Education and Cultural Affairs. Available online: https://www.kmk.org/fileadmin/Dateien/veroeffentlichungen_beschluesse/1972/1972_07_07-Mobilitaets-Verkehrserziehung.pdf (accessed on 20 April 2020).
44. Bundesanstalt für Straßenverkehr. Geschlechtsspezifische Intervention in der Unfallprävention. *Mensch Sicherh.* **2006**, *179*, 1–108.
45. Larouche, R.; Ghekiere, A. An Ecological Model of Active Transportation. In *Children's Active Transportation*; Larouche, R., Ed.; Elsevier: Amsterdam, The Netherlands, 2018; pp. 93–103.
46. Lorenz, C. Diagnostische Kompetenz von Grundschullehrkräften. Strukturelle Aspekte und Bedingungen. Ph.D. Thesis, Otto-Friedrich-Universität Bamberg, Bamberg, Germany, 2011.
47. Hogrefe. Available online: https://dorsch.hogrefe.com/stichwort/tendenz-zur-mitte (accessed on 6 July 2020).
48. Mangione, T.W. *Mail Surveys. Improving the Quality*; SAGE: Thousand Oaks, CA, USA, 1995; p. 34.

49. Smith, W.G. *Does Gender Influence Online Survey Participation? A Record-linkage Analysis of University Faculty Online Survey Response Behavior*; San José State University: San José, CA, USA, 2008.
50. Kornet-van der Aa, D.A.; van Randeraad-van der Zee, C.H.; Mayer, J.; Borys, J.M.; Chinapaw, M.J.M. Recommendations for obesity prevention among adolescents from disadvantaged backgrounds: A concept mapping study among scientific and professional experts. *Pediatr. Obes.* **2018**, *13*, 389–392. [CrossRef] [PubMed]
51. Ariadne. Available online: http://www.minds21.org/images_public/manual%20%20ARIADNE%203.0%20%20april%202015.pdf (accessed on 22 March 2020).
52. Børrestad, L.A.B.; Andersen, L.B.; Bere, E. Seasonal and socio-demographic determinants of school commuting. *Prev. Med.* **2011**, *52*, 133–135. [CrossRef] [PubMed]
53. Fyhri, A.; Hjorthol, R. Children's independent mobility to school, friends and leisure activities. *J. Transp. Georg.* **2009**, *17*, 377–384. [CrossRef]

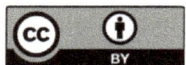

© 2020 by the authors. Licensee MDPI, Basel, Switzerland. This article is an open access article distributed under the terms and conditions of the Creative Commons Attribution (CC BY) license (http://creativecommons.org/licenses/by/4.0/).

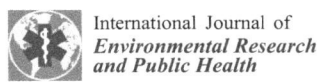

Article

Active Transportation and Obesity Indicators in Adults from Latin America: ELANS Multi-Country Study

Juan Guzmán Habinger [1], Javiera Lobos Chávez [2], Sandra Mahecha Matsudo [3,4], Irina Kovalskys [5], Georgina Gómez [6], Attilio Rigotti [7], Lilia Yadira Cortés Sanabria [8], Martha Cecilia Yépez García [9], Rossina G. Pareja [10], Marianella Herrera-Cuenca [11], Ioná Zalcman Zimberg [12], Viviana Guajardo [13], Michael Pratt [14], Cristian Cofre Bolados [15,16], Claudio Farías Valenzuela [15], Adilson Marques [17,18], Miguel Peralta [17,18], Ana Carolina B. Leme [19], Mauro Fisberg [20,21], André Oliveira Werneck [22], Danilo Rodrigues da Silva [23], Gerson Ferrari [15,*] and on behalf of the ELANS Study Group [†]

[1] Sports Medicine and Physical Activity Specialty, Science Faculty, Universidad Mayor, Santiago 8580745, Chile; juan.guzmanh@mayor.cl
[2] Datrics, Santiago 7500000, Chile; javiera@datrics.cl
[3] Science Faculty, Universidad Mayor, Santiago 8580745, Chile; sandra.mahecha@umayor.cl
[4] Academic Unit, MEDS Clinic, Santiago 7550000, Chile
[5] Nutrition Career, Faculty of Medical Sciences, Pontificia Universidad Católica Argentina, AAZ Buenos Aires C1107, Argentina; ikovalskys@gmail.com
[6] Department of Biochemistry, School of Medicine, Universidad de Costa Rica, San José 11501-2060, Costa Rica; georgina.gomez@ucr.ac.cr
[7] Department of Nutrition, Diabetes and Metabolism, School of Medicine, Pontificia Universidad Católica, Santiago 8330024, Chile; arigotti@med.puc.cl
[8] Department of Nutrition and Biochemistry, Pontificia Universidad Javeriana, Bogotá 110231, Colombia; ycortes@javeriana.edu.co
[9] College of Health Sciences, Universidad San Francisco de Quito, Quito 17-1200-841, Ecuador; myepez@usfq.edu.ec
[10] Nutrition Research Institute, Lima 15026, Peru; rpareja@iin.sld.pe
[11] Centro de Estudios del Desarrollo, Universidad Central de Venezuela (CENDES-UCV)/Fundación Bengoa, Caracas 1053, Venezuela; manyma@gmail.com
[12] Department of Psychobiology, Universidade Federal de São Paulo, São Paulo 04023-062, Brazil; iona.zimberg@gmail.com
[13] Nutrition, Health and Wellbeing Area, International Life Science Institute (ILSI) Argentina, Santa Fe Av. 1145, CABA C1059ABF, Argentina; viviana.guajardo@comunidad.ub.edu.ar
[14] Institute for Public Health, University of California San Diego, La Jolla, CA 92093-0021, USA; mipratt@health.ucsd.edu
[15] Laboratory of Sciences of Physical Activity, Sports and Health, Faculty of Medical Sciences, Universidad de Santiago de Chile, USACH, Santiago 7500618, Chile; cristian.cofre@usach.cl (C.C.B.); claudio.farias.v@usach.cl (C.F.V.)
[16] Institute of Sports Sciences, School of Sports Sciences and Physical Activity, Universidad Santo Tomas Santiago de Chile, Santiago 8370003, Chile
[17] CIPER, Faculty of Human Motricity, Universidade de Lisboa, 1499-002 Lisbon, Portugal; amarques@fmh.ulisboa.pt (A.M.); mperalta@fmh.ulisboa.pt (M.P.)
[18] ISAMB, Faculty of Medicine, Universidade de Lisboa, 1649-028 Lisbon, Portugal
[19] Department of Nutrition, School of Public Health, University of São Paulo, São Paulo 01246-904, Brazil; acarol.leme@gmail.com
[20] Department of Pediatrics, Universidade Federal de São Paulo, São Paulo 04023-061, Brazil; mauro.fisberg@gmail.com
[21] Instituto Pensi, Fundação José Luiz Egydio Setubal, Hospital Infantil Sabará, São Paulo 01227-200, Brazil
[22] Department of Nutrition, School of Public Health, Universidade de São Paulo (USP), São Paulo 01246-904, Brazil; andreowerneck@gmail.com

²³ Department of Physical Education, Federal University of Sergipe—UFS, São Cristóvão 49100-000, Brazil; danilorpsilva@gmail.com
* Correspondence: gerson.demoraes@usach.cl; Tel.: +56-9-5398-0556
† Membership of the ELANS Study Group is provided in the Acknowledgments section of the manuscript.

Received: 2 September 2020; Accepted: 21 September 2020; Published: 24 September 2020

Abstract: Purpose: The aim of this study was to determine the association between active transportation and obesity indicators in adults from eight Latin American countries. Methods: Data from the ELANS study, an observational multi-country study (n: 8336; 18–65 years), were used. Active transportation (walking and cycling) and leisure time physical activity was assessed using the International Physical Activity Questionnaire (long version). The obesity indicators considered were: body mass index, and waist and neck circumference. Results: In the total sample, the average time dedicated to active transportation was 24.3 min/day, with the highest amount of active transportation being Costa Rica (33.5 min/day), and the lowest being Venezuela (15.7 min/day). The countries with the highest proportion of active transportation were Ecuador (71.9%), and the lowest was Venezuela (40.5%). Results from linear regression analyses suggest that active transportation was significantly and independently associated with a lower body mass index (β: −0.033; 95% CI: −0.064; −0.002), but not with waist circumference (β: −0.037; 95% CI: −1.126; 0.390 and neck circumference (β: −0.007; 95% CI: −0.269; 0.130). Conclusions: Active transportation is significantly associated with a lower body mass index. Governments should incentivize this type of transportation as it could help to reduce the obesity pandemic in Latin America.

Keywords: physical activity; active transportation; Latin America; obesity; body mass index; waist circumference

1. Introduction

Approximately 39% of the world's adults are overweight or obese [1]. In Latin America, a prevalence of up to 60% of overweight and obesity has been reported [2], which is a considerable burden for public health. There has been a consistent association between overweight and obesity and cardiovascular diseases, diabetes, and some types of cancer [3]. Overweight and obesity and related comorbidities are a global epidemic that may be mitigated by the adoption of healthier lifestyles, including being physically active [4–6].

Many studies have shown that physical activity has extensive health benefits such as reducing body weight, premature mortality, and cardiovascular disease risk [5,7]. The benefits of physical activity has been extensively represented by leisure time, such as physical exercise, but evidence shows that these benefits can also be obtained through walking or cycling, as "active travel" or "active transportation" [8,9]. Active transportation has been demonstrated to be an excellent strategy for increasing physical activity level, because it is a daily behavior, an opportunity to create a healthy habit and relatively cheap alternative [10,11]. Besides, it can be integrated into everyday life particularly for those not involved or interested in engaging in leisure time physical activity [12]. Strong evidence demonstrates that physical activity related to active transportation is a crucial population-based approach, which aims to reverse the health outcomes [8,9].

Over the past two decades, the Latin American region has experienced substantial economic development due to high levels of urbanization (80%) and a unique structural, cultural and social environment, and is actually by far the most unequal region in the world [13,14]. Latin American countries are characterized by high population density patterns, the unregulated expansion of urban environments, air pollution, high crime rates, high income inequality, high levels of poverty, and population aging, which might inhibit physical activity [14–16]. Governments and nongovernmental organizations have been adopting several policies such as building public park facilities, cycling infrastructure and intervention strategies for improving active transportation (e.g., bike-sharing programs) to promote active transportation in Latin America [17–19].

Studies from Europe and the United States show that countries in which active transportation increases show decreasing obesity rates. In fact, many studies provided a contribution to the literature and filled several gaps of the association between active transportation and lower obesity indicators (body mass index) in high-income [20–22]. However, there is limited evidence on the association of active transportation and obesity indicators from Latin America representative samples [23]. In addition, Latin America has a high prevalence of physical inactivity and overweight/obesity [2,24]. Therefore, there is an urgent need to look for different strategies aiming to increase the active transportation levels and decrease obesity in the Latin American region. The aim of this study was to investigate the extent of the association between active transportation and obesity indicators in adults from eight Latin American countries.

2. Materials and Methods

2.1. Study Design and Sample

The Latin American Study of Nutrition and Health (Estudio Latinoamericano de Nutrición y Salud—ELANS) is a household-based cross-sectional survey that includes data collected from eight Latin American countries: Argentina, Brazil, Chile, Colombia, Costa Rica, Ecuador, Peru, and Venezuela. The study was based on a complex, multistage sample design, stratified by conglomerates, with all regions of each country represented, and random selection of main cities within each region according to the probability proportional to size method [25,26].

The sampling size required for necessary precision was calculated with a 95% confidence level and a maximum error of 3.5% and a survey design effect of 1.75. The sample was stratified by age, sex, and socioeconomic level. Socioeconomic levels were balanced based on national indexes used in each country [26]. Households within each secondary sampling unit were selected through systematic randomization. Considering quotas for age, sex and socioeconomic level, the selection of the participant belonging to the domicile was made using 50% of the sample's next birthday, and 50% of the sample's last birthday. Of the total sample of 9218 participants aged between 15 and 65 years, we included 8336 participants aged between 18 and 65 in this study. We excluded adolescents (15 to 17 years old) from the analyses because the ELANS study did not consider the age range of adolescents (10–19 years old) [27]. Additionally, adolescents may have restricted independent mobility that may yield different environment–physical activity associations than those observed in adults [28]. In addition, physical activity guidelines for adolescents differ from adults [29]. The rationale and design of the study is reported in more detail elsewhere [25].

All the study sites are academic-based (universities and other research institutions) and each site adhered to a common study protocol for fieldwork implementation, interviewer training, data collection and management, and the quality of control procedures. Data collection for ELANS took place from September 2014 to February 2015. The ELANS protocol was approved by the Western Institutional Review Board (#20140605) and registered at ClinicalTrials.gov (#NCT02226627). All participants of the ELANS study provided written consent.

2.2. Exclusion Criteria

During enrolment for the study, participants were excluded if they had a major physical/mental impairment that impacted on food intake and physical activity levels, were pregnant/lactating, and were ≤15 years old or ≥65 years old. For this study, we excluded participants <18 years of age from the total sample, and subjects without at least one anthropometric variable.

2.3. Active Transportation, Leisure Time and Total Physical Activity

The ELANS study employed the self-reported International Physical Activity Questionnaire-Long Form (IPAQ-LF), which was a validated measure design for Latin America [30]. IPAQ was developed to assess the physical activity levels of inhabitants from dissimilar countries [30,31]. We used a Spanish version [32] and it was adapted for all eight participating ELANS countries [14].

The ELANS study only summarized scores for active transportation and leisure time physical activity. The IPAQ-LF collected data on the reported frequency and duration (bouts at least 10 min continuously) of active transportation (walking and cycling) and leisure time physical activity (walking, moderate and vigorous physical activity) over the last seven days. Three outcomes for each domain were calculated: (1) engaging at least 10 min in active transportation and leisure time physical activity (yes, no); (2) how many days of physical activity in active transportation and leisure time physical activity; (3) how much time spent completing physical activity in active transportation and leisure time physical activity. Questions were asked separately for active transportation (walking and cycling), and leisure time physical activity (walking, moderate-intensity, and vigorous-intensity activities). Time spent in each domain was expressed as min/day.

2.4. Obesity Indicators

In each country, the obesity indicators (body weight, height, waist and neck circumferences) were evaluated in light clothing and without shoes using standard procedures and equipment. Data were collected by trained ELANS data collectors during a visit. Body weight (kg) and height (cm) were measured using a calibrated electronic scale Seca 213® (Hamburg, Germany). The measurements were taken during the end inhalation with the participant's head in the Frankfort plane [33]. The body mass index was calculated as the body weight divided by the square of body height (kg/m^2). Participants were classified as underweight: <18.5; normal weight: 18.5–24.9; overweight: 25–29.9; or obese: $\geq$30 kg/m^2 [34].

A nonstretchable tape with an accuracy of 0.1 cm was used to evaluate circumferences. Waist circumference was measured according to World Health Organization recommendations, i.e., with the participants standing, after regular expiration, to the nearest cm, midway between the lowest rib and the iliac crest on the horizontal plane with the subject in a standing position [34]. We used the "substantially increased risk of metabolic complications" cutoff defined by World Health Organization, >102 cm for men and >88 cm for women [34]. Neck circumference was measured in a plane as horizontal as possible, immediately below the laryngeal prominence, while standing erect with eyes facing forward [35] and was categorized as abnormal if the circumference was >39 cm for men and >35 cm for women [36]. All measurements were performed under strictly standardized conditions. Two measurements of the obesity indicators were performed, and the mean used for the analyses.

2.5. Sociodemographic Variables

Sociodemographics items collected by all countries included age, sex and socioeconomic level. Socioeconomic data were categorized into "low", "medium", and "high" based on the country specific indices [26]. Age was dichotomized into "18–34", "35–49", and "50–65" years. Ethnicity was classified as white, mixed (parents with dissimilar ethnicities) and other (Black, Asian, Indigenous, and Gypsy).

2.6. Statistical Analyses

Data were weighted considering sociodemographic variables, sex, age and socioeconomic level of the Latin American population to enable comparability for totals across countries. This was completed to have a representative sample of the adult population of each country. Descriptive statistics of mean, percentage and the associated 95% confidence interval (95% CI) were used to describe the sociodemographic obesity indicators (Table 1) and active transportation (Table 2). A Chi-square test was carried out to evaluate if there was a significant association between active transportation with the control variables mentioned before. For descriptive and categorical analysis, the self-reported time spent on active transportation was stratified into the following two categories: nonactive transportation (including those who reported nonwalking or cycling as part of their transportation) and active transportation (including those who reported ≥10 min of walking and/or cycling for transportation). A Pearson correlation was used to assess the association of active transportation with obesity indicators.

Table 1. Sociodemographic and obesity indicators of the population according to active transportation categories.

Variable and Category	Nonactive Transportation (%) (<10 min of Walking and/or Cycling)	Active Transportation (%) (≥10 min of Walking and/or Cycling)
n (%)	3733 (44.8)	4603 (55.2)
Country		
Argentina	565 (48.8) ***	592 (51.2) ***
Brazil	889 (48.6) ***	941 (51.4) ***
Chile	353 (44.3) ***	443 (55.7) ***
Colombia	482 (42.7) ***	646 (57.3) ***
Costa Rica	255 (35.7) ***	460 (64.3) ***
Ecuador	195 (28.1) ***	500 (71.9) ***
Peru	390 (39.0) ***	609 (61.0) ***
Venezuela	604 (59.5) ***	412 (40.5) ***
Sex		
Men	1744 (44.5)	2176 (55.5)
Women	1989 (45.0)	2427 (55.0)
Age (years)		
18–34	1733 (44.0)	2203 (56.0)
35–49	1179 (45.9)	1388 (54.1)
50–65	821 (44.8)	1012 (55.2)
Socioeconomic level		
Low	1953 (45.1)	2375 (54.9)
Medium	1428 (44.5)	1782 (55.5)
High	352 (44.1)	446 (55.9)
Ethnicity		
White	1442 (49.5) ***	1470 (50.5) ***
Mixed	1764 (42.1) ***	2429 (57.9) ***
Other	341 (41.9) ***	472 (58.1) ***
Body mass index (Kg/m^2)		
<18.5	99 (45.8) ***	117 (54.2) ***
18.5–24.9	1249 (42.7) ***	1679 (57.3) ***
25–29.9	1305 (43.9) ***	1665 (56.1) ***
≥30	1079 (48.6) ***	1143 (51.4) ***
Waist circumference (cm)		
≤102 (M) or 88 (W)	2408 (43.5) ***	3132 (56.5) ***
>102 (M) or 88 (W)	1324 (47.4) ***	1472 (52.6) ***
Neck circumference (cm)		
≤39 (M) or 35 (W)	2430 (43.7) **	3132 (56.3) **
>39 (M) or 35 (W)	1303 (47.0) **	1471 (53.0) **

Figures as percentages if not stated otherwise. Chi-square tests were used for distributions. ** $p \leq 0.01$; *** $p \leq 0.001$. M: men; W: women.

Table 2. Correlation between active transportation and obesity indicators per country.

Country	Body Mass Index (Kg/m^2)		Waist Circumference (cm)		Neck Circumference (cm)	
	r	p-Value	r	p-Value	r	p-Value
Full sample	−0.196	<0.001	−0.199	<0.001	−0.121	0.048
Argentina	−0.235	<0.001	−0.194	<0.001	−0.104	0.901
Brazil	−0.155	0.015	−0.182	<0.001	0.113	0.555
Chile	−0.184	0.015	−0.200	0.004	0.128	0.413
Colombia	−0.227	<0.001	−0.195	<0.001	−0.129	0.328
Costa Rica	−0.221	<0.001	−0.251	<0.001	−0.159	0.099
Ecuador	−0.138	0.302	−0.158	0.118	−0.114	0.702
Peru	−0.217	<0.001	−0.202	<0.001	−0.168	0.027
Venezuela	−0.231	<0.001	−0.244	<0.001	−0.184	0.006

For the calculation of the CI, an asymptotic method (wald) was used based on a normal distribution. In addition, linear regression models (β; 95% CI) per country were used to verify the relationship of active transportation (10 min/day of active transportation as the independent variable) with body mass index, waist circumference and neck circumference (dependent variables). Our first model (model 1) was adjusted for sex, age, socioeconomic level, and ethnicity. The second model was additionally adjusted for sex, age, socioeconomic level, ethnicity, and leisure time physical activity. We also adjusted for leisure time physical activity (min/day) to examine whether the associations with time spent in active transportation were independent of time spent leisure time physical activity. All analyses were made using R-studio version 1.2.5033 [37,38]. The significance level was set at $p < 0.05$.

3. Results

The average response of the surveys was 99.4%, with a range between 98.5% and 99.8%, corresponding to Peru and Ecuador, respectively. The average time dedicated to active transportation was 24.3 min/day in the total sample (those who reported nonwalking or cycling as part of their transportation). Considering the full sample, the country with the highest amount of active transportation was Costa Rica (33.5 min/day), and the lowest was Venezuela (15.7 min/day). When the nonactive transportation group (those who reported nonwalking or cycling as part of their transportation) was excluded, the average was 41.6 min/day. Costa Rica still had the highest amount of active transportation (50.3 min/day), while Venezuela had the shortest time (35.6 min/day). The average time spent on leisure time physical activity was 16.6 min/day (95% CI: 15.3; 17.9) for the group that did not engage in active transportation. Meanwhile, for the group that does at least 10 min of active transportation, it was 35.2 min/day (95% CI: 33.3; 37.1) ($p < 0.001$).

Table 1 shows a descriptive analysis of the sample, dividing the sample into those who did not complete active transportation from those who did. There was a significant association between country and active transportation ($p < 0.001$). The country with the highest proportion of active transportation was Ecuador (71.9%), and the lowest was Venezuela (40.6%). There were no statistically significant differences in the proportion of active transportation between men and women, age groups, or socioeconomic level. On the other hand, the white ethnic group had a lower proportion of active transportation than the other groups ($p < 0.001$). When comparing the proportion of active transportation by body mass index, it was observed that the prevalence of active transportation was lower among overweight and obese participants than those with normal body mass index (56.1% and 51.4% vs. 57.3%) ($p < 0.001$). The same difference is observed for waist and neck circumference, where a lower proportion of active transportation was observed among those with increased indicators compared to those with a normal waist and neck circumference (56.5% vs. 52.6% and 56.3% vs. 53.0%, respectively) ($p < 0.001$).

The correlation between the active transportation and obesity indicator (body mass index, waist and neck circumference) by country is shown in Table 2. Body mass index and waist circumference were weakly and negatively associated with all countries (except Ecuador); however, the highest correlation value was Argentina and Venezuela. Furthermore, there was a weak and negative association between active transportation and neck circumference in the full sample—Peru and Venezuela ($p < 0.05$). The highest correlation value was Venezuela. Active transportation was not associated with neck circumference in Argentina, Brazil, Chile, Colombia, Costa Rica, and Ecuador.

We also conducted two different specifications for every regression model to investigate the association between active transportation and obesity indicators as continuous variables (Table 3). The first model, adjusted for sex, age, socioeconomic level, and ethnicity, showed that active transportation was significantly associated with a lower body mass index and waist circumference, but not with neck circumference. In the second model, including leisure time physical activity, active transportation was significantly associated only with a lower body mass index. An increase of 10 min regarding active transportation per day resulted in a −0.033 Kg/m^2 change in the body mass index. No statistical association was found between active transportation with waist and neck circumference.

Table 3. Linear regression models for association of active transportation with obesity indicators.

Country	Model 1						Model 2					
	Body Mass Index (Kg/m²)		Waist Circumference (cm)		Neck Circumference (cm)		Body Mass Index (Kg/m²)		Waist Circumference (cm)		Neck Circumference (cm)	
	β (95% CI)	p-Value	β (95% CI)	p-Value	β (95% CI)	p-Value	β (95% CI)	p-Value	β (95% CI)	p-Value	β (95% CI)	p-Value
Full sample	−0.044 (−0.074; −0.014)	0.004	−0.077 (−0.150; −0.003)	0.041	−0.013 (−0.032; 0.007)	0.206	−0.033 (−0.064; −0.002)	0.036	−0.037 (−1.126; 0.390)	0.341	−0.007 (−0.269; 0.130)	0.496
Argentina	−0.074 (−0.148; 0.006)	0.059	−0.036 (−0.232; 0.160)	0.717	0.054 (0.006; 0.098)	0.023	−0.046 (−1.254; 0.333)	0.255	−0.101 (−1.538; 2.518)	0.468	0.060 (−0.123; 1.082)	0.064
Brazil	−0.030 (−0.101; 0.041)	0.407	−0.059 (−0.236; 0.119)	0.515	0.001 (−0.050; 0.053)	0.969	−0.038 (−1.116; 0.357)	0.313	−0.034 (−2.172; 1.496)	0.718	−0.006 (−0.600; 0.474)	0.818
Chile	−0.012 (−0.111; 0.088)	0.821	−0.058 (−0.306; 0.190)	0.646	0.009 (−0.049; 0.068)	0.752	−0.006 (−1.085; 0.964)	0.908	−0.058 (−3.151; 1.986)	0.656	0.014 (−0.469; 0.740)	0.661
Colombia	−0.071 (−0.137; −0.003)	0.038	−0.162 (−0.323; 0.007)	0.053	−0.025 (−0.065; 0.016)	0.230	−0.06 (−1.302; 0.096)	0.091	−0.138 (−3.093; 0.327)	0.113	−0.012 (−0.536; 0.304)	0.588
Costa Rica	−0.081 (−0.172; 0.012)	0.083	−0.129 (−0.352; 0.099)	0.262	−0.056 (−0.106; −0.007)	0.027	−0.072 (−1.658; 0.216)	0.131	−0.097 (−3.271; 1.326)	0.407	−0.054 (−1.043; −0.032)	0.037
Ecuador	0.043 (−0.054; 0.139)	0.381	−0.018 (−0.229; 0.192)	0.868	−0.025 (−0.085; 0.034)	0.407	0.055 (−0.450; 1.553)	0.006	0.021 (−1.961; 2.380)	0.850	−0.020 (−0.82; 0.415)	0.520
Peru	−0.025 (−0.111; 0.061)	0.563	−0.088 (−0.292; 0.117)	0.403	−0.070 (−0.123; −0.017)	0.009	−0.017 (−1.066; 0.718)	0.702	−0.051 (−2.636; 1.612)	0.636	−0.067 (−1.221; −0.128)	0.016
Venezuela	−0.043 (−0.161; 0.068)	0.463	−0.141 (−0.430; 0.113)	0.308	−0.058 (−0.134; 0.010)	0.114	−0.029 (−1.445; 0.859)	0.618	−0.101 (−3.737; 1.720)	0.468	−0.049 (−1.215; 0.240)	0.189

Model 1: adjusted for sex, age, socioeconomic level, and ethnicity. Model 2: Model 1 + leisure time physical activity.

4. Discussion

This is the first multi-country study with a representative sample of Latin Americans to determine the extent of association between active transportation and obesity indicators in adults. In general, we demonstrated that a greater amount of time on active transportation was associated with a lower body mass index. This association was independent of age, sex, socioeconomic level, ethnicity and leisure time physical activity. These are novel results that reflect what has been reported in some countries and multinational studies [21,39].

Our findings are compatible with other studies that reported a lower body mass index associated with active transportation [40,41]. Flint et al. [42] studied the association of active commuting and body mass index in a cross-sectional study of more than 15,000 people in the United Kingdom. Active commuting was associated with a lower body mass index—0.97 Kg/m^2 and 0.87 Kg/m^2 in men and women, respectively. Later, the same author [21] showed similar results in a cross-sectional study of more than 264,000 middle-aged adults. They found a lower body mass index—1.0 Kg/m^2 and 0.67 Kg/m^2 in men and women, respectively. Laverty et al. [39] carried out a multinational study of six middle-income countries, with more than 40,000 participants. They found that ≥150 min/week of active transportation was associated with a lower body mass index of 0.54 Kg/m^2. Wojan et al. [43] searched for this association in the United States in a study of 12,405 adults. They found that active commuting produced an average treatment effect of −1.83 Kg/m^2.

Different from previous studies [39,41], we did not find an association between active transportation and waist circumference. This was observed when the analysis was adjusted for leisure time physical activity (model 2), indicating a potential co-existence of physical activity in these different contexts and reinforcing a stronger association of leisure time physical activity with waist circumference compared to transport physical activity. Concerning neck circumference, although studies have found associations with moderate to vigorous physical activity [44], their relationship with active transportation in adults has not been describe before. Here, we observed that active transportation was associated with a lower neck circumference in Costa Rica and Peru only, which can be related to the higher prevalence of active transportation in these countries. However, further studies are needed in order to explore specific amounts and intensities of transport physical activity associated with obesity indicators.

We found that the mean time spent in active transportation was 24.3 min/day. Latin America has low levels of active transportation compared to European countries, such as Germany or Sweden [45–47]. Only about one-fifth of the time for transportation is spent in active transportation in Latin America [13]. This is especially important considering that 27% to 47% of people in Latin America do not achieve the physical activity recommendations for health [47]. In a previous study, we showed that the prevalence of physical inactivity (<150 min/week) was 40.6% (95% CI: 38.8, 42.5); ranging from 26.9% (Chile) to 47% (Costa Rica and Venezuela). Physical inactivity was greater in Argentina (43.7%; 95% CI: 38.1, 49.5), Brazil (43.5%; 95% CI: 39.4, 47.7), Costa Rica (48.0%; 95% CI: 42.1, 53.9) and Venezuela (47.1%; 95% CI: 42.1, 52.3) [47]. In this context, promoting public policies aimed to encourage this type of transport, as it can help more people achieve the physical activity recommendation for health [43]. This could help to significantly decrease the disease burden associated with physical inactivity [5,48]. Other countries have estimated that moderate increases in active transportation lead to savings in national public health services. For example, in the United Kingdom, it was found that an increase of 1 km in walking and 3 km in cycling per day would save £17 billion for the national health system in 20 years [49].

Moreover, those who change their mode of commuting gain weight if they shift from cycling or walking to car travel, but lose weight when shifting from cars to active commuting [50]. Martin et al. [40] showed that changing from private transport to active commuting decreased body mass index by 0.32 Kg/m^2. Conversely, shifting from active commuting to private transport increased body mass index by 0.34 Kg/m^2. As established before, urban factors impact on the choice of transport modality [13,23]. One of the strategies to increase active transportation in the population is to invest in creating neighborhoods and cities that favor this type of transport [18,23]. This could be a key to reducing the obesity pandemic that exists in Latin America and the world. Several countries in this region have invested in infrastructure to encourage the use of active transportation—as is the case of some cities, such as Bogotá in Colombia, which invested in creating exclusive bike paths [18]. Our results are consistent with the findings reported in high-income countries. Therefore, they are generalizable to some extent for other middle-income countries.

The strengths of this study include the large sample from eight Latin American countries and standardized objective anthropometric indicators (body mass index, waist circumference and neck circumference). Given that a representative sample of these countries was studied, these results can be extrapolated to the rest of the adult population of these eight Latin American countries. Waist circumference is a well-established indicator of central obesity, a key factor in cardiovascular disease risk and metabolic syndrome [51]. While neck circumference is an indicator, which is still under study [36,52,53], its relationship with active transportation had not been previously reported in adults.

Within the limitations, we found that part of the sample (418 participants, 5.01%) was not classified by ethnicity. When using a subjective active transport measurement (IPAQ), there may be reporting bias [54]. From the four domains of physical activity, only the active transportation and leisure time physical activity sections were included. This decision was made for two reasons: (i) due to the greater relevance of these domains for targeted physical activity programming and policy efforts [30] and (ii) the weak validity of occupational and home-based physical activity questions [55]. The cross-sectional design of this study limits generalizability and limits conclusions regarding of causality. There is a possibility of reverse causality and residual confusion; it could be that obese people less actively travel.

5. Conclusions

This study supports that active transportation is significantly associated with a lower body mass index. Incentive active transportation could help to reduce the obesity pandemic and help more people to meet physical activity recommendations in Latin America. These findings are consistent with existing evidence from other regions of the world. For these reasons, the generation of public policies aiming to promote active transportation in Latin America should be prioritized.

Author Contributions: Conceptualization, J.G.H., J.L.C. and G.F.; Formal analysis, J.G.H., and J.L.C.; Investigation I.K., G.G., A.R., L.Y.C.S., M.C.Y.G., R.G.P., M.H.-C., I.Z.Z., V.G., M.P. (Michael Pratt) and M.F.; Funding acquisition, M.F. and I.K.; Writing—original draft: J.G.H.; Writing—review and editing: C.C.B., C.F.V., A.M., M.P. (Miguel Peralta), S.M.M., A.C.B.L., A.O.W., D.R.d.S. and G.F.; Statistical analysis, J.L.C. All authors have read and agreed to the published version of the manuscript.

Funding: Fieldwork and data analysis compromised in ELANS protocol was supported by a scientific grant from the Coca Cola Company, and by a grant and/or support from Instituto Pensi/Hospital Infantil Sabara, International Life Science Institute of Argentina, Universidad de Costa Rica, Pontificia Universidad Católica de Chile, Pontificia Universidad Javeriana, Universidad Central de Venezuela (CENDES-UCV)/Fundación Bengoa, Universidad San Francisco de Quito, and Instituto de Investigación Nutricional de Peru. André Werneck is supported by the São Paulo Research Foundation (FAPESP) with a PhD scholarship (FAPESP process: 2019/24124-7). This paper presents independent research. The views expressed in this publication are those of the authors and not necessarily those of the acknowledged institutions. The funding sponsors had no role in study design; the collection, analyses, or interpretation of data; writing of the manuscript; or in the decision to publish the results.

Acknowledgments: The authors would like to thank the staff and participants from each of the participating sites who made substantial contributions to ELANS. The following are members of ELANS Study Group: Chairs: Mauro Fisberg and Irina Kovalskys; Co-chair: Georgina Gómez Salas; Core Group Members: Attilio Rigotti, Lilia Yadira Cortés Sanabria, Georgina Gómez Salas, Martha Cecilia Yépez García, Rossina Gabriella Pareja Torres and Marianella Herrera-Cuenca; Steering committee: Berthold Koletzko, Luis A. Moreno and Michael Pratt; Accelerometry analysis: Priscila Bezerra Gonçalves, and Claudia Alberico; Physical activity advisor: Gerson Ferrari. Nutrition Advisors: Regina Mara Fisberg and Agatha Nogueira Previdelli. Project Managers: Viviana Guajardo, and Ioná Zalcman Zimberg.

Conflicts of Interest: M.F. has received fees and consultancy payments from biotechnology, pharmaceutical and food and beverage companies. He has also received fees, payments for consulting and financing research studies without any restrictions, from government sources and nonprofit entities. The rest of the authors also have no conflict of interest to declare. None of the entities mentioned had or have any role in the design or preparation of this manuscript.

References

1. World Health Organisation (WHO) Obesity and Overweight. Available online: https://www.who.int/en/news-room/fact-sheets/detail/obesity-and-overweight (accessed on 12 August 2020).
2. Kovalskys, I.; Fisberg, M.; Gomez, G.; Pareja, R.G.; Yepez Garcia, M.C.; Cortes Sanabria, L.Y.; Herrera-Cuenca, M.; Rigotti, A.; Guajardo, V.; Zalcman Zimberg, I.; et al. Energy intake and food sources of eight Latin American countries: Results from the Latin American Study of Nutrition and Health (ELANS). *Public Health Nutr.* **2018**, *21*, 2535–2547. [CrossRef]
3. Abdelaal, M.; le Roux, C.W.; Docherty, N.G. Morbidity and mortality associated with obesity. *Ann. Transl. Med.* **2017**, *5*, 161. [CrossRef] [PubMed]
4. Mytton, O.T.; Ogilvie, D.; Griffin, S.; Brage, S.; Wareham, N.; Panter, J. Associations of active commuting with body fat and visceral adipose tissue: A cross-sectional population based study in the UK. *Prev. Med.* **2018**, *106*, 86–93. [CrossRef] [PubMed]
5. Piercy, K.L.; Troiano, R.P.; Ballard, R.M.; Carlson, S.A.; Fulton, J.E.; Galuska, D.A.; George, S.M.; Olson, R.D. The Physical Activity Guidelines for Americans. *JAMA* **2018**, *320*, 2020–2028. [CrossRef] [PubMed]
6. Jakicic, J.M.; Davis, K.K. Obesity and physical activity. *Psychiatr. Clin. N. Am.* **2011**, *34*, 829–840. [CrossRef]
7. Kokkinos, P. Physical activity, health benefits, and mortality risk. *ISRN Cardiol.* **2012**, *2012*, 718789. [CrossRef]
8. Celis-Morales, C.A.; Lyall, D.M.; Welsh, P.; Anderson, J.; Steell, L.; Guo, Y.; Maldonado, R.; Mackay, D.F.; Pell, J.P.; Sattar, N.; et al. Association between active commuting and incident cardiovascular disease, cancer, and mortality: Prospective cohort study. *BMJ* **2017**, *357*, j1456. [CrossRef]
9. Schafer, C.; Mayr, B.; Fernandez La Puente de Battre, M.D.; Reich, B.; Schmied, C.; Loidl, M.; Niederseer, D.; Niebauer, J. Health effects of active commuting to work: The available evidence before GISMO. *Scand. J. Med. Sci. Sports* **2020**. [CrossRef]
10. Andersen, L.B. Active commuting: An easy and effective way to improve health. *Lancet Diabetes Endocrinol.* **2016**, *4*, 381–382. [CrossRef]
11. Menai, M.; Charreire, H.; Feuillet, T.; Salze, P.; Weber, C.; Enaux, C.; Andreeva, V.A.; Hercberg, S.; Nazare, J.A.; Perchoux, C.; et al. Walking and cycling for commuting, leisure and errands: Relations with individual characteristics and leisure-time physical activity in a cross-sectional survey (the ACTI-Cites project). *Int. J. Behav. Nutr. Phys. Act.* **2015**, *12*, 150. [CrossRef]
12. Vaara, J.P.; Vasankari, T.; Fogelholm, M.; Koski, H.; Kyrolainen, H. Cycling but not walking to work or study is associated with physical fitness, body composition and clustered cardiometabolic risk in young men. *BMJ Open Sport Exerc. Med.* **2020**, *6*, e000668. [CrossRef] [PubMed]
13. Ferrari, G.L.M.; Kovalskys, I.; Fisberg, M.; Gomez, G.; Rigotti, A.; Sanabria, L.Y.C.; García, M.C.Y.; Torres, R.G.P.; Herrera-Cuenca, M.; Zimberg, I.Z.; et al. Socio-demographic patterns of public, private and active travel in Latin America: Cross-sectional findings from the ELANS study. *J. Transp. Health* **2020**, *16*, 100788. [CrossRef]
14. Salvo, D.; Reis, R.S.; Sarmiento, O.L.; Pratt, M. Overcoming the challenges of conducting physical activity and built environment research in Latin America: IPEN Latin America. *Prev. Med.* **2014**, *69* (Suppl. S1), S86–S92. [CrossRef] [PubMed]
15. Lund, C.; De Silva, M.; Plagerson, S.; Cooper, S.; Chisholm, D.; Das, J.; Knapp, M.; Patel, V. Poverty and mental disorders: Breaking the cycle in low-income and middle-income countries. *Lancet* **2011**, *378*, 1502–1514. [CrossRef]
16. United Nations. *World Urbanization Prospects: The 2011 Revision: Data Tables and Highlights 2011 Rev.*; United Nations publication: New York, NY, USA, 2012.
17. Montes, F.; Sarmiento, O.L.; Zarama, R.; Pratt, M.; Wang, G.; Jacoby, E.; Schmid, T.L.; Ramos, M.; Ruiz, O.; Vargas, O.; et al. Do health benefits outweigh the costs of mass recreational programs? An economic analysis of four Ciclovia programs. *J. Urban Health* **2012**, *89*, 153–170. [CrossRef]
18. Gomez, L.F.; Sarmiento, R.; Ordonez, M.F.; Pardo, C.F.; de Sa, T.H.; Mallarino, C.H.; Miranda, J.J.; Mosquera, J.; Parra, D.C.; Reis, R.; et al. Urban environment interventions linked to the promotion of physical activity: A mixed methods study applied to the urban context of Latin America. *Soc. Sci. Med.* **2015**, *131*, 18–30. [CrossRef]

19. Hoehner, C.M.; Ribeiro, I.C.; Parra, D.C.; Reis, R.S.; Azevedo, M.R.; Hino, A.A.; Soares, J.; Hallal, P.C.; Simoes, E.J.; Brownson, R.C. Physical activity interventions in Latin America: Expanding and classifying the evidence. *Am. J. Prev. Med.* **2013**, *44*, e31–e40. [CrossRef]
20. Berglund, E.; Lytsy, P.; Westerling, R. Active Traveling and Its Associations with Self-Rated Health, BMI and Physical Activity: A Comparative Study in the Adult Swedish Population. *Int. J. Environ. Res. Public Health* **2016**, *13*, 455. [CrossRef]
21. Flint, E.; Cummins, S. Active commuting and obesity in mid-life: Cross-sectional, observational evidence from UK Biobank. *Lancet Diabetes Endocrinol.* **2016**, *4*, 420–435. [CrossRef]
22. Larouche, R.; Faulkner, G.; Tremblay, M.S. Active travel and adults' health: The 2007-to-2011 Canadian Health Measures Surveys. *Health Rep.* **2016**, *27*, 10–18.
23. Sallis, J.F.; Cerin, E.; Kerr, J.; Adams, M.A.; Sugiyama, T.; Christiansen, L.B.; Schipperijn, J.; Davey, R.; Salvo, D.; Frank, L.D.; et al. Built Environment, Physical Activity, and Obesity: Findings from the International Physical Activity and Environment Network (IPEN) Adult Study. *Annu. Rev. Public Health* **2020**, *41*, 119–139. [CrossRef] [PubMed]
24. Guthold, R.; Stevens, G.A.; Riley, L.M.; Bull, F.C. Worldwide trends in insufficient physical activity from 2001 to 2016: A pooled analysis of 358 population-based surveys with 1.9 million participants. *Lancet Glob. Health* **2018**, *6*, e1077–e1086. [CrossRef]
25. Ferrari, G.L.M.; Kovalskys, I.; Fisberg, M.; Gomez, G.; Rigotti, A.; Sanabria, L.Y.C.; Garcia, M.C.Y.; Torres, R.G.P.; Herrera-Cuenca, M.; Zimberg, I.Z.; et al. Methodological design for the assessment of physical activity and sedentary time in eight Latin American countries—The ELANS study. *MethodsX* **2020**, *7*, 100843. [CrossRef]
26. Fisberg, M.; Kovalskys, I.; Gomez, G.; Rigotti, A.; Cortes, L.Y.; Herrera-Cuenca, M.; Yepez, M.C.; Pareja, R.G.; Guajardo, V.; Zimberg, I.Z.; et al. Latin American Study of Nutrition and Health (ELANS): Rationale and study design. *BMC Public Health* **2016**, *16*, 93. [CrossRef] [PubMed]
27. World Health Organisation (WHO). Adolescent Health. Available online: https://www.who.int/southeastasia/activities/adolescent-health (accessed on 1 September 2020).
28. Guthold, R.; Stevens, G.A.; Riley, L.M.; Bull, F.C. Global trends in insufficient physical activity among adolescents: A pooled analysis of 298 population-based surveys with 1.6 million participants. *Lancet Child Adolesc. Health* **2020**, *4*, 23–35. [CrossRef]
29. Hallal, P.C.; Andersen, L.B.; Bull, F.C.; Guthold, R.; Haskell, W.; Ekelund, U.; Lancet Physical Activity Series Working Group. Global physical activity levels: Surveillance progress, pitfalls, and prospects. *Lancet* **2012**, *380*, 247–257. [CrossRef]
30. Hallal, P.C.; Gomez, L.F.; Parra, D.C.; Lobelo, F.; Mosquera, J.; Florindo, A.A.; Reis, R.S.; Pratt, M.; Sarmiento, O.L. Lessons learned after 10 years of IPAQ use in Brazil and Colombia. *J. Phys. Act. Health* **2010**, *7* (Suppl. 2), S259–S264. [CrossRef]
31. Craig, C.L.; Marshall, A.L.; Sjostrom, M.; Bauman, A.E.; Booth, M.L.; Ainsworth, B.E.; Pratt, M.; Ekelund, U.; Yngve, A.; Sallis, J.F.; et al. International physical activity questionnaire: 12-country reliability and validity. *Med. Sci. Sports Exerc.* **2003**, *35*, 1381–1395. [CrossRef]
32. Medina, C.; Barquera, S.; Janssen, I. Validity and reliability of the International Physical Activity Questionnaire among adults in Mexico. *Rev. Panam. Salud Publica/Pan Am. J. Public Health* **2013**, *34*, 21–28.
33. Lohman, T.G.; Roche, A.F.; Martorell, R. *Anthropometric Standardization Reference Manual*, 3rd ed.; Human Kinetics Press: Champaign, IL, USA, 1988; Volume 24.
34. World Health Organisation (WHO). *WHO Waist Circumference and Waist–Hip Ratio: Report of a WHO Expert Consultation*; WHO: Geneva, Switzerland, 2008.
35. Cornier, M.A.; Despres, J.P.; Davis, N.; Grossniklaus, D.A.; Klein, S.; Lamarche, B.; Lopez-Jimenez, F.; Rao, G.; St-Onge, M.P.; Towfighi, A.; et al. Assessing adiposity: A scientific statement from the American Heart Association. *Circulation* **2011**, *124*, 1996–2019. [CrossRef]
36. Onat, A.; Hergenc, G.; Yuksel, H.; Can, G.; Ayhan, E.; Kaya, Z.; Dursunoglu, D. Neck circumference as a measure of central obesity: Associations with metabolic syndrome and obstructive sleep apnea syndrome beyond waist circumference. *Clin. Nutr.* **2009**, *28*, 46–51. [CrossRef] [PubMed]
37. R Core Team. R: A Language and Environment for Statistical Computing. 2019. Available online: http://www.R-project.org/ (accessed on 10 June 2020).

38. RStudio Team Studio: Integrated Development for R. 2019. Available online: http://www.rstudio.com/ (accessed on 10 June 2020).
39. Laverty, A.A.; Palladino, R.; Lee, J.T.; Millett, C. Associations between active travel and weight, blood pressure and diabetes in six middle income countries: A cross-sectional study in older adults. *Int. J. Behav. Nutr. Phys. Act.* **2015**, *12*, 65. [CrossRef] [PubMed]
40. Martin, A.; Panter, J.; Suhrcke, M.; Ogilvie, D. Impact of changes in mode of travel to work on changes in body mass index: Evidence from the British Household Panel Survey. *J. Epidemiol. Community Health* **2015**, *69*, 753–761. [CrossRef] [PubMed]
41. Steell, L.; Garrido-Mendez, A.; Petermann, F.; Diaz-Martinez, X.; Martinez, M.A.; Leiva, A.M.; Salas-Bravo, C.; Alvarez, C.; Ramirez-Campillo, R.; Cristi-Montero, C.; et al. Active commuting is associated with a lower risk of obesity, diabetes and metabolic syndrome in Chilean adults. *J. Public Health (Oxf.)* **2018**, *40*, 508–516. [CrossRef]
42. Flint, E.; Cummins, S.; Sacker, A. Associations between active commuting, body fat, and body mass index: Population based, cross sectional study in the United Kingdom. *BMJ* **2014**, *349*, g4887. [CrossRef]
43. Wojan, T.R.; Hamrick, K.S. Can Walking or Biking to Work Really Make a Difference? Compact Development, Observed Commuter Choice and Body Mass Index. *PLoS ONE* **2015**, *10*, e0130903. [CrossRef]
44. Luis de Moraes Ferrari, G.; Kovalskys, I.; Fisberg, M.; Gomez, G.; Rigotti, A.; Sanabria, L.Y.C.; Garcia, M.C.Y.; Torres, R.G.P.; Herrera-Cuenca, M.; Zimberg, I.Z.; et al. Association of moderate-to-vigorous physical activity with neck circumference in eight Latin American countries. *BMC Public Health* **2019**, *19*, 809. [CrossRef]
45. Buehler, R.; Pucher, J.; Merom, D.; Bauman, A. Active travel in Germany and the U.S. Contributions of daily walking and cycling to physical activity. *Am. J. Prev. Med.* **2011**, *41*, 241–250. [CrossRef]
46. Eriksson, J.S.; Ekblom, B.; Kallings, L.V.; Hemmingsson, E.; Andersson, G.; Wallin, P.; Ekblom, O.; Ekblom-Bak, E. Active commuting in Swedish workers between 1998 and 2015-Trends, characteristics, and cardiovascular disease risk. *Scand. J. Med. Sci. Sports* **2020**, *30*, 370–379. [CrossRef]
47. Ferrari, G.L.M.; Kovalskys, I.; Fisberg, M.; Gomez, G.; Rigotti, A.; Sanabria, L.Y.C.; Garcia, M.C.Y.; Torres, R.G.P.; Herrera-Cuenca, M.; Zimberg, I.Z.; et al. Socio-demographic patterning of objectively measured physical activity and sedentary behaviours in eight Latin American countries: Findings from the ELANS study. *Eur. J. Sport Sci.* **2019**, 1–12. [CrossRef]
48. Schauder, S.A.; Foley, M.C. The relationship between active transportation and health. *J. Transp. Health* **2015**, *2*, 343–349. [CrossRef]
49. Jarrett, J.; Woodcock, J.; Griffiths, U.K.; Chalabi, Z.; Edwards, P.; Roberts, I.; Haines, A. Effect of increasing active travel in urban England and Wales on costs to the National Health Service. *Lancet* **2012**, *379*, 2198–2205. [CrossRef]
50. Flint, E.; Webb, E.; Cummins, S. Change in commute mode and body-mass index: Prospective, longitudinal evidence from UK Biobank. *Lancet Public Health* **2016**, *1*, e46–e55. [CrossRef]
51. Ashwell, M.; Gunn, P.; Gibson, S. Waist-to-height ratio is a better screening tool than waist circumference and BMI for adult cardiometabolic risk factors: Systematic review and meta-analysis. *Obes. Rev.* **2012**, *13*, 275–286. [CrossRef] [PubMed]
52. Ben-Noun, L.L.; Sohar, E.; Laor, A. Neck circumference as a simple screening measure for identifying overweight and obese patients. *Obes. Res.* **2001**, *9*, 470–477. [CrossRef]
53. Alzeidan, R.; Fayed, A.; Hersi, A.S.; Elmorshedy, H. Performance of neck circumference to predict obesity and metabolic syndrome among adult Saudis: A cross-sectional study. *BMC Obes.* **2019**, *6*, 1–8. [CrossRef] [PubMed]
54. Ferrari, G.L.M.; Kovalskys, I.; Fisberg, M.; Gomez, G.; Rigotti, A.; Sanabria, L.Y.C.; Garcia, M.C.Y.; Torres, R.G.P.; Herrera-Cuenca, M.; Zimberg, I.Z.; et al. Comparison of self-report versus accelerometer—Measured physical activity and sedentary behaviors and their association with body composition in Latin American countries. *PLoS ONE* **2020**, *15*, e0232420. [CrossRef]
55. Luis de Moraes Ferrari, G.; Kovalskys, I.; Fisberg, M.; Gomez, G.; Rigotti, A.; Sanabria, L.Y.C.; Garcia, M.C.Y.; Torres, R.G.P.; Herrera-Cuenca, M.; Zimberg, I.Z.; et al. Original research Socio-demographic patterning of self-reported physical activity and sitting time in Latin American countries: Findings from ELANS. *BMC Public Health* **2019**, *19*, 1723. [CrossRef]

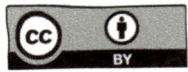

© 2020 by the authors. Licensee MDPI, Basel, Switzerland. This article is an open access article distributed under the terms and conditions of the Creative Commons Attribution (CC BY) license (http://creativecommons.org/licenses/by/4.0/).

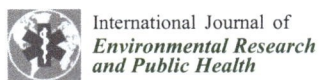 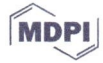

Article

The Profile of Bicycle Users, Their Perceived Difficulty to Cycle, and the Most Frequent Trip Origins and Destinations in Aracaju, Brazil

Mabliny Thuany [1], João Carlos N. Melo [1], João Pedro B. Tavares [1], Filipe M. J. Santos [1], Ellen C. M. Silva [1], André O. Werneck [2], Sayuri Dantas [3], Gerson Ferrari [4,*], Thiago H. Sá [2] and Danilo R. Silva [1]

1. Department of Physical Education, Federal University of Sergipe (UFS), São Cristóvão 49100-000, Brazil; mablinysantos@gmail.com (M.T.); joaofghc@gmail.com (J.C.N.M.); jp.edf1@gmail.com (J.P.B.T.); filipe.matheusef@gmail.com (F.M.J.S.); ellencmendesilva@gmail.com (E.C.M.S.); danilorpsilva@gmail.com (D.R.S.)
2. Center for Epidemiological Research in Nutrition and Health (NUPENS), University of São Paulo (USP), São Paulo 01246-904, Brazil; andreowerneck@gmail.com (A.O.W.); thiagoherickdesa@gmail.com (T.H.S.)
3. Non-Governmental Organization Associação Ciclo Urbano, Aracaju 49070-376, Brazil; sayuriods@gmail.com
4. Physical Activity, Sport and Health Sciences Laboratory, Faculty of Medical Sciences, University of Santiago, Chile (USACH), Santiago 7500618, Chile
* Correspondence: gerson.demoraes@usach.cl; Tel.: +56-95398-0556

Received: 29 June 2020; Accepted: 3 September 2020; Published: 30 October 2020

Abstract: The objective of this study was to describe the profile of bicycle users, their perceived difficulty to cycle, and the most frequent trip origins and destinations in Aracaju, Northeast Brazil. Our cross-sectional study sampled 1001 participants and we collected information through structured interviews. Aged ≥15 years, participants were residents of all Aracaju's neighborhoods and used a bicycle for commuting to work or for leisure. We observed that bicycle users in Aracaju are predominantly employed male subjects, aged between 18 and 40 years, and were the heads of their households. Most of the them reported "work" as the main reason for their bicycle trips and, "health" and "practicality" aspects as their main motivations for using bicycles. In general, the neighborhoods in the north and center of the city were identified as the most difficult for cycling, and the easiest trips occurred in places with cycle paths. As a conclusion of this study, we reaffirm the need for intersectoral actions that create favorable environments for active commuting and more sustainable cities.

Keywords: transportation; exercise; sedentary behavior; urbanization; city planning

1. Introduction

Increased physical inactivity is currently a major challenge in several countries [1], mainly due to its association with an increased risk of chronic noncommunicable diseases, such as cardiovascular diseases, different types of cancer, and mental disorders [2,3]. Most people do not comply with the minimum recommended levels of physical activity to prevent diseases and to protect health, i.e., according to the World Health Organization's physical activity guidelines [4]. In this sense, the adoption of different strategies to provide an active lifestyle emerges as the most viable alternative for the promotion of physical activity [1,5], such as changes in the urbanized environment of cities to enable active commuting [6].

Given that commuting is seen as a daily practice among adult populations and that at least 30 min a day are spent on this activity [7], active alternatives, such as the use of bicycles, can be applied as a strategy to increase total physical activity. Commuting by bicycle provides additional benefits, such as contributing to air and noise pollution reduction, increasing social engagement, and reducing road traffic injuries [8–12]. Active commuting by bicycle can be considered as an accessible and relatively "easy" way to promote physical activity among different age groups (children, adults, and older adults) [13–16] and cultures/countries [17,18]. However, despite the relevance of this approach, there is limited information about the effectiveness of these strategies or even the adherence of the population to them, particularly in low- and middle-income settings [19–21].

Previous studies report the influence of individual and environmental variables on the use of bicycles for transport, including sex, age, economic status, and education, in addition to proximity between the point of origin and the destination [19,22–24]. In the Brazilian context, the accessibility of bicycle use as a means of transport is a topic of discrepancy. Reis, et al. [25] compared the prevalence of bicycle use for transportation among three cities in different states and regions of Brazil, observing differences between Recife (Pernambuco, Northeast, 16.0%), Curitiba (Paraná, South, 9.6%), and Vitória (Espírito Santo, Southeast, 8.8%). In another study conducted in Rio Claro (São Paulo, Southeast), Teixeira, et al. [26] found a much greater prevalence of bicycle use for transportation (28.3%). Although it seems clear that men, younger adults, and lower education/economic status were associated with greater use of bicycles for transportation [8,25–27] in both studies, some specificities should be considered in the low- and middle-income contexts. For example, Reis, et al. [25] observed a higher prevalence of bicycle use in the city with the highest crime rate (Recife), which was not expected. However, this was also the city with the lowest human development index, highest unemployment rate, and social inequalities, suggesting that bicycle use could not be an option in low-income regions. Thus, understanding the profile of bicycle users and their relations with specific characteristics of the cities is justified in order to provide better conditions for those who already use the bicycle, and to create opportunities for other population subgroups to use bicycles for transport.

Aracaju city (Sergipe, Northeast) is known as of the first Brazilian capitals to implement the proposal for mobility on bicycles in 2005 (implementing networks of cycle paths and on flat land). However, only 11.9% of the population reported active commuting (walking and cycling) in 2018 [28], and there is no available information on the use of the bicycle for transport. Given that Aracaju's street design favors the use of bicycles for commuting, studies on bicycle flow within available structures would contribute to the development of strategies for urban planning, acting as an important way to increase health, environment, and sustainability indicators in that context. However, information about bicycle users, their perceptions about the city, and the most frequent trip origins and destinations could foster public policies in urban planning. Thus, we researched the profile of bicycle users, their perceived difficulty to cycle, and the most frequent origins and destinations of bicycle travel in Aracaju, Brazil.

2. Methods

2.1. Design

We used a cross-sectional method, carried out in Aracaju, Brazil. Aracaju is the state capital of Sergipe, with about 657 thousand inhabitants (2019), and a Human Development Index of 0.770 (2010). The population's average income in 2010 was 3.1 times the minimum wage (approximately USD 200) and 56.6% of public spaces were forested [29].

2.2. Sample and Data Procedures

The information in this study was obtained from the "Origin and Destination of Biking Trips in the City of Aracaju, Survey," over a one-year period (June 2014 to June 2015). The survey was conducted with bicycle users that were approached personally in all 40 neighborhoods of the city, respecting the proportionality of the population of each neighborhood [29]. The structured interviews were conducted by 17 trained advisors on weekdays, from 2:00 PM to 7:00 PM. This convenience sample consisted of 1001 bicycle users. The city neighborhoods were organized into bordering zones (north, south, central, and expansion). It is important to note that the set of neighborhoods, communities, and villages that make up the Expansion Zone have been incorporated to Aracaju by legal decision. All participants were provide with information about the objectives of the study, which was conducted in accordance with the ethical standards of the institutional and/or national research committee, respecting the 1964 Helsinki Declaration and its further amendments, or comparable ethical standards. The study was approved by the Ethics Committee of the Federal University of Sergipe (CAAE: 16418619.7.0000.5546).

2.3. Instrument

The questionnaire used was prepared by the nongovernmental organization "Associação Ciclo Urbano—Aracaju," consisting of 23 items and divided into (a) cyclist profile: sex (male and female), age (categorized into five age groups: up to 18 years, 18 to 30 years, 30 to 40 years, 40 to 50 years, and over 50 years), and family role (head of family, spouse, child, or relative); (b) socioeconomic information: work status (employed and not employed), educational level (below upper secondary,, secondary, and above secondary), activity sector (commerce, industry, construction, education, and health), monthly income (up to one minimum wage and above one minimum wage), and automotive vehicle ownership (yes or no); (c) characteristics of the origin and destination of trips made by bicycles: reason for the trip (work, school, leisure, shopping, and others), location of origin and destination (Aracaju neighborhood), region's access conditions (easy, difficult), bicycle parking conditions (public, paid parking, and free parking), motivation to ride a bicycle (health, practicality, leisure, economic, and two options), departure and arrival period of the day (morning, afternoon, and night), time spent commuting (0 to 15 min, 15 to 30 min, 30 to 45 min, 45 to 60 min, and over 60 min), whether the destination is a different neighborhood (yes or no), and the type of trip origin and destination (nonrecreational or recreational).

2.4. Statistical Analysis

Descriptive information was presented using absolute and relative frequencies. To compare the profile of bicycle users with Aracaju's population, we restricted the analysis to adult participants and used the information provided by the Brazilian 2013 National Health Survey, which is the closest survey to the reference year with representative information of the adult population of Aracaju [30] (% and 95% confidence intervals). The perception analysis of cycling difficulty in neighborhoods was determined by the relative frequency of citations used (easy or difficult). Absolute frequencies of commuting between neighborhoods were used to verify the main trip origin and destination, and the main neighborhoods cited as the origin or destination. Main trip origins and destinations were defined as those representing at least 0.9% of the total mentioned. The Aracaju Mobility Master Plan (2016) was used to identify bike lanes that were implemented until 2015. Finally, the information was presented in the form of a map with an origin and destination analysis. It was carried out using a cross-reference table to check the main neighborhoods in which there was a greater flow of bicycle users entering and leaving, in addition to identifying the main trip origin and destination of the interviewees. The maps were built using the CorelDRAW Graphics Suite 2019 software (Corel Corporation, Ottawa, ON, Canada). All analyses were performed using SPSS 22.0 software (IBM, Armonk, NY, USA).

3. Results

Table 1 shows information on bicycle user profiles. It shows that the sample was predominantly composed of men, aged 18 to 40 years, who were heads of their households and were employed. Most reported schooling at primary and secondary levels, and work in civil construction and health sectors; 66.7% reported "work" as the main reason for their travel. Most individuals reported not having their own automotive vehicle and having income of up to one minimum wage. Most participants reported "healthy" and "practicality" as their main motivation to ride a bicycle.

Table 1. Characteristics of Bicycle Users and Aracaju's Population.

Variable	Bicycle Users % (n)	Population * % (CI 95%)
Sex		
Female	11.5 (102)	55.1 (50.0 to 60.1)
Male	88.5 (782)	44.9 (39.9 to 50.0)
Age		
18–30	34.5 (305)	26.1 (21.8 to 30.8)
30–40	30.8 (272)	24.1 (19.9 to 28.7)
40–50	20.5 (181)	19.2 (15.6 to 23.4)
>50	14.3 (126)	30.7 (26.3 to 35.4)
Family Role		
Head of Family	60.9 (538)	-
Spouse	14.0 (124)	-
Child	19.5 (172)	-
Relative	5.7 (50)	-
Work status		
Employed	88.9 (786)	54.2 (49.3 to 59.2)
Not employed	11.1 (98)	45.7 (40.8 to 50.7)
Education		
Below Secondary	54.3 (480)	38.9 (34.1 to 43.8)
Secondary	32.0 (285)	39.3 (34.5 to 44.2)
Beyond Secondary	13.7 (121)	21.9 (17.9 to 26.5)
Activity Sector		
Commerce	20.7 (179)	-
Industry	10.0 (79)	-
Construction	33.9 (268)	-
Education	2.8 (22)	-
Health	30.6 (242)	-
Monthly Income		
Up to one minimum wage	78.7 (695)	-
Above one minimum wage	21.3 (189)	-
Automotive Vehicle Ownership		
No	78.4 (693)	49.0 (44.0 to 54.1)
Yes	21.6 (191)	51.0 (45.9 to 56.0)
Reason for Trip		
Work	66.7 (590)	-
School	2.9 (26)	-
Leisure	12.7 (112)	-
Shopping	6.4 (57)	-
Others	11.2 (99)	-
Motivation to Ride a Bicycle		
Health	26.4 (229)	-
Practicality	25.3 (219)	-
Leisure	7.5 (65)	-
Economic	19.3 (167)	-
Two options	21.5 (186)	-

Table 1. *Cont.*

Variable	Bicycle Users % (n)	Population * % (CI 95%)
Time Spent Commuting		
0 to 15 min	22.7 (200)	-
15 to 30 min	36.4 (321)	-
30 to 45 min	18.1 (160)	-
45 to 60 min	13.9 (123)	-
>60 min	8.8 (78)	-
Is your destination a different neighborhood?		
Yes	82.6 (730)	-
No	17.4 (154)	-
Type of Trip Origin and Destination		
Nonrecreational	96.6 (854)	-
Recreational	3.4 (30)	-

Note: Time spent commuting refers to the total time spent commuting from the place of departure to destination. CI = confidence interval. * Based on the Brazilian 2013 National Health Survey.

Figure 1 presents the perceived degree of difficulty for cycling in city neighborhoods. In general, Center (23%) and Porto Dantas (13%) were pointed out as neighborhoods in which cycling was the most difficult for cycling, while 13 de Julho (14%), Atalaia (13%), Siqueira Campos (13%), and Jabotiana (12%) were cited as the ones in which cycling was the easiest.

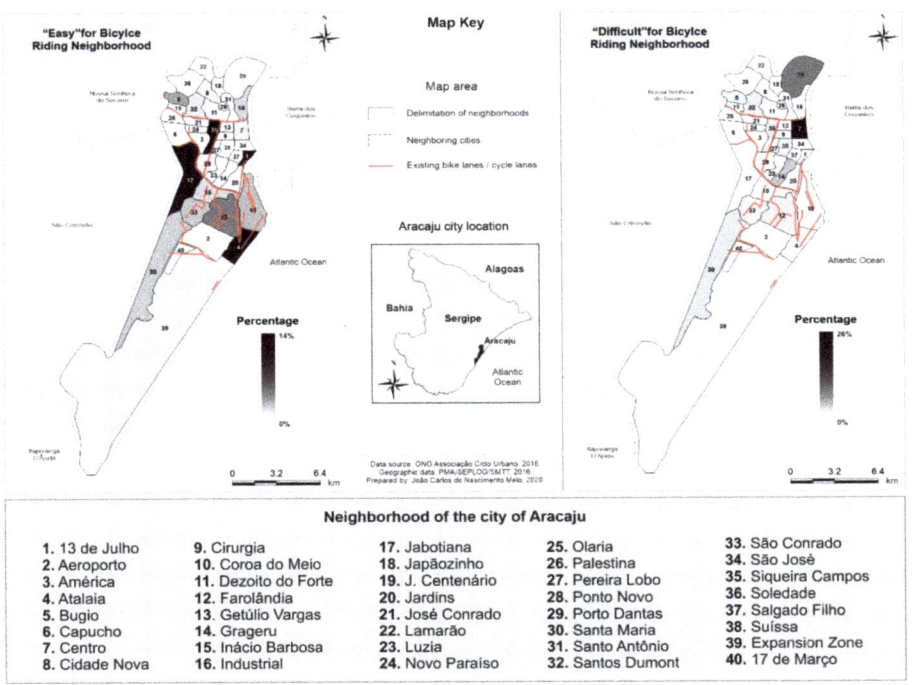

Figure 1. Perception of the difficulty of cycling in Aracaju/Sergipe.

Figure 2 shows the most frequent trip origins and destinations among the participants. The main destination was Santa Maria neighborhood (10.9%), followed by Atalaia (5.3%), Farolândia (5.7%), and Santos Dumont (6%). Regarding the trip origin and destination, Center (6.6%), Farolândia (5.9%), and Siqueira Campos (5.6%) were the most reported. In addition, there is a greater tendency to move toward neighborhoods close to the point of departure, with 23% of the total trips occurring within the neighborhood of origin (especially the José Conrado (50%) and the Expansion Zone (77%) neighborhoods).

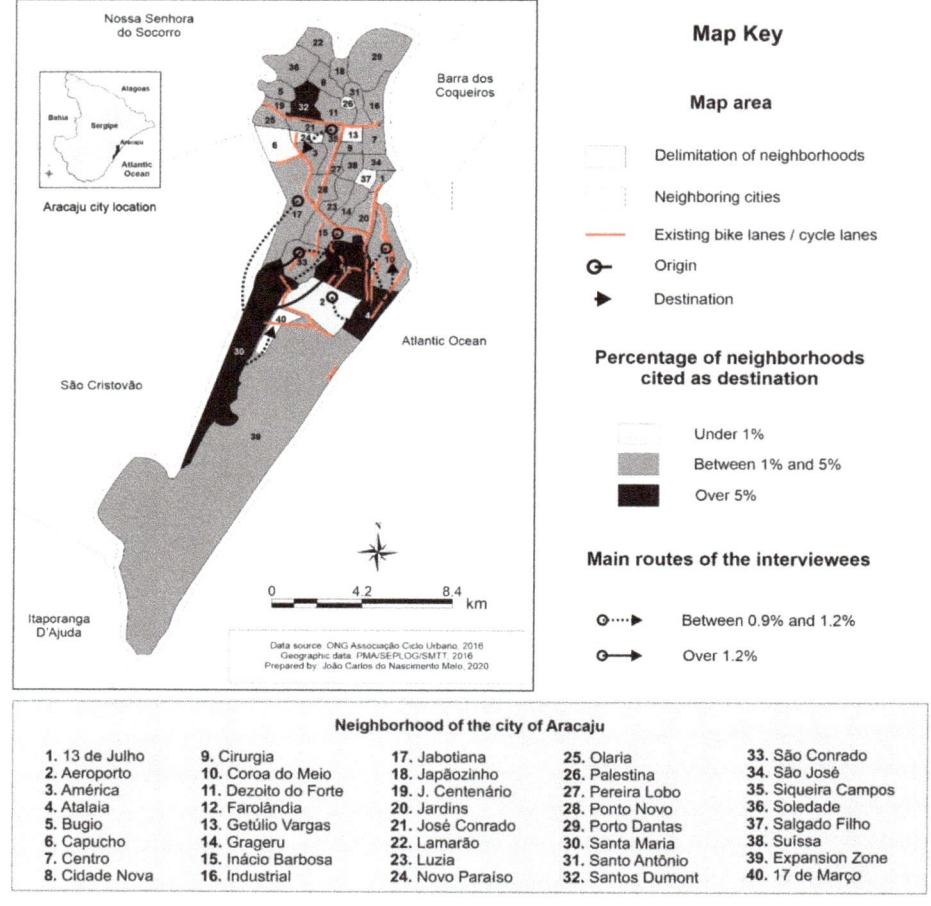

Figure 2. Main Trajectories of Bike Riders in Aracaju/Sergipe.

4. Discussion

This study aimed to describe the profile of bicycle users, their perceived difficulty to cycle, and the most frequent trip origins and destinations in the city of Aracaju. The results indicated that (1) the 60-km cycle paths distributed in the city of Aracaju serve mostly men, younger adults, and people with lower educational levels, as compared with the population of Aracaju; (2) the use of active commuting is associated with going to work, especially in the lowest income group; (3) most bicycle users move from central to peripheral areas; and (4) the majority of the participants spent an average of 15 to 30 min (per cycling trip). This information is vital to develop strategies to improve current bicycle user conditions and to create new opportunities for less represented population groups, especially in developing countries.

Bicycle user profiles differed greatly from those of Aracaju's population in general, which reinforces the fact that some population subgroups are more inclined to use bicycles for transportation. The initial results confirm data from previous studies in Brazilian cities showing a similar bicycle user profile, including a higher proportion of adult young men [8,25–27]. This behavior in men is associated with a duality in terms of stimuli directed at boys and girls in childhood, with a tendency to maintain these habits in adulthood [31], culminating in less use of bicycles by women in particular and less engagement in physical activities in general. Another factor is the perception of safety, which tends to be different between sexes, making factors related to "lack of lighting during commuting," "driver-cyclist behavior in traffic," and "public insecurity" great obstacles, especially among women [16,32]. Some studies [8,26] also showed greater use of bicycles among workers in areas with a higher representation of men (e.g., construction and industry).

Considering that most participants who traveled by bicycle did not own automotive vehicles—a proportion higher than that observed in the population of Aracaju (78.4% vs. 49.0%)—the socioeconomic structure of the population may be a factor that explains these results. In previous studies, this factor has already been negatively associated with levels of active transport [33] and were observed more frequently in low-income regions. Bicycles tend to be a "cheaper" mode of transport due to inaccessibility of a private vehicle, high fares, and lack of quality in public transport.

Safety issues in public transport and the lack of adequate infrastructure for bicycle use tend to "disable" environments that favor walking or cycling as means to travel to work [34]. Our results indicated that, in general, the districts of the North and Central Zones were identified as the most difficult to cycle in, which may be associated with the fact that most of the Aracaju cycle system is concentrated in the South Zone [35]. In previous studies, not having bike paths, conservation of streets and avenues, car traffic, and rough surfaces were examples of variables that could impact bicycle users' perception of neighborhoods [36,37].

The origin and destination of the trips indicated greater commuting from central areas to peripheral areas of the city. One of the possible explanations may be associated with the growth in investments in civil construction, industry, and commerce in the South Zone of the city, leading people to move to the peripheral regions of the city for work. In addition, a large part of the participants reported working in these sectors (33.9%, 20.7%, and 10.0%, for construction, commerce, and industry, respectively). Another explanation for these results could be the data collection times, which were concentrated in the afternoon and may represent the commute home from work. It was noted that the most frequently cited trip origins and destinations by respondents (Figure 2) involved commuting between adjacent or nearby neighborhoods. Previous studies identified that distances under 10 kilometers were more feasible to retain the use of the bicycle as a means of daily commuting [38–40]. In the present study, the most participants spent an average of 15 to 30 min (per trip) on daily commuting. This behavior shows a viability threshold for this mode of transport and can offer health benefits [41]. Other actions could improve and facilitate the use of cycle paths. The equitable distribution of schools, jobs, and sectors necessary for day-to-day activities can help people from places with longest trip origins and destinations [42,43].

The practical application of the study is to use this data as an aid in producing public policies to improve the infrastructure of cycle paths and expand cycle routes. Understanding the behavior and profile of bicycle users may also inform political decisions regarding active transport and urban planning. Although this was a nonrepresentative sample and interviews are likely to provide report bias, this study analyzes the profile and characteristics of trip origins and destinations and the perception of bicycle users in a specific social, economic, and climate context regarding active commuting.

5. Conclusions

Bicycle users are predominantly represented by men, aged between 18 and 40 years, from low income families in Aracaju, Brazil. In general, the use of active commuting is associated with going to work, mainly because this form of transport is more practical and healthier than public and private transport. The study reported a tendency of travel from central to peripheral areas, which may be associated with the workplaces. Considering that some bicycle users report the economic factor as a motivation to use bicycles and that women and adolescents are underrepresented in this scenario, the present study reaffirms the need for intersectoral actions to enable the construction of a safer city through expansion of bicycle networks with safe dimensions and accessibility.

Author Contributions: All authors contributed to the study conception and design. Material preparation and data analysis were performed by M.T., J.C.N.M., J.P.B.T., F.M.J.S., and D.R.S. The first draft of the manuscript was written by M.T. Substantial writing-review and editing were performed by E.C.M.S., A.O.W., S.D., G.F., T.H.S., and D.R.S. All authors have read and agreed to the published version of the manuscript.

Funding: This research received no specific grant from any funding agency in the public, commercial, or not-for-profit sectors. Mabliny Thuany is supported by the Foundation for Support to Research and Technological Innovation of the State of Sergipe (FAPITEC). André Werneck is supported by the São Paulo Research Foundation (FAPESP) with a PhD scholarship (FAPESP process: 2019/24124-7). This paper presents an independent research. The views expressed in this publication are those of the authors and not necessarily those of the acknowledged institutions.

Conflicts of Interest: Authors declare no conflicts of interest.

References

1. World Health Organization. Physical Inactivity: A Global Public Health Problem. Available online: https://www.who.int/dietphysicalactivity/factsheet_inactivity/en/ (accessed on 25 April 2020).
2. Firth, J.; Siddiqi, N.; Koyanagi, A.; Siskind, D.; Rosenbaum, S.; Galletly, C.; Allan, S.; Caneo, C.; Carney, R.; Carvalho, A.F.; et al. The Lancet Psychiatry Commission: A blueprint for protecting physical health in people with mental illness. *Lancet Psychiatry* **2019**, *6*, 675–712. [CrossRef]
3. Lee, I.M.; Shiroma, E.J.; Lobelo, F.; Puska, P.; Blair, S.N.; Katzmarzyk, P.T. Effect of physical inactivity on major non-communicable diseases worldwide: An analysis of burden of disease and life expectancy. *Lancet* **2012**, *380*, 219–229. [CrossRef]
4. World Health Organization. *Global Recommendations on Physical Activity for Health*; WHO Guidelines Review Committee: Geneva, Switzerland, 2010.
5. Gomes, G.A.; Kokubun, E.; Mieke, G.I.; Ramos, L.R.; Pratt, M.; Parra, D.C.; Simoes, E.; Florindo, A.A.; Bracco, M.; Cruz, D.; et al. Characteristics of physical activity programs in the Brazilian primary health care system. *Cad. Saude Publica* **2014**, *30*, 2155–2168. [CrossRef] [PubMed]
6. Stevenson, M.; Thompson, J.; de Sá, T.H.; Ewing, R.; Mohan, D.; McClure, R.; Roberts, I.; Tiwari, G.; Giles-Corti, B.; Sun, X.; et al. Land use, transport, and population health: Estimating the health benefits of compact cities. *Lancet* **2016**, *388*, 2925–2935. [CrossRef]
7. Schantz, P. Distance, duration, and velocity in cycle commuting: Analyses of relations and determinants of velocity. *Int. J. Environ. Res. Public Health* **2017**, *14*, 1166. [CrossRef]
8. Sa, T.H.; Duran, A.C.; Tainio, M.; Monteiro, C.A.; Woodcock, J. Cycling in Sao Paulo, Brazil (1997-2012): Correlates, time trends and health consequences. *Prev. Med. Rep.* **2016**, *4*, 540–545. [CrossRef]
9. Saunders, L.E.; Green, J.M.; Petticrew, M.P.; Steinbach, R.; Roberts, H. What are the health benefits of active travel? A systematic review of trials and cohort studies. *PLoS ONE* **2013**, *8*, e69912. [CrossRef]
10. Götschi, T.; Garrard, J.; Giles-Corti, B. Cycling as a part of daily life: A review of health perspectives. *Transp. Rev.* **2015**, *36*, 45–71. [CrossRef]
11. Johansson, C.; Lovenheim, B.; Schantz, P.; Wahlgren, L.; Almstrom, P.; Markstedt, A.; Stromgren, M.; Forsberg, B.; Sommar, J.N. Impacts on air pollution and health by changing commuting from car to bicycle. *Sci. Total Environ.* **2017**, *584–585*, 55–63. [CrossRef]
12. Savan, B.; Cohlmeyer, E.; Ledsham, T. Integrated strategies to accelerate the adoption of cycling for transportation. *Transp. Res. Part. F Traffic Psychol. Behav.* **2017**, *46*, 236–249. [CrossRef]
13. Trapp, G.S.; Giles-Corti, B.; Christian, H.E.; Bulsara, M.; Timperio, A.F.; McCormack, G.R.; Villaneuva, K.P. On your bike! A cross-sectional study of the individual, social and environmental correlates of cycling to school. *Int. J. Behav. Nutr. Phys. Act.* **2011**, *8*, 123. [CrossRef] [PubMed]
14. Gatersleben, B.; Appleton, K.M. Contemplating cycling to work: Attitudes and perceptions in different stages of change. *Transp. Res. Part A Policy Pract.* **2007**, *41*, 302–312. [CrossRef]

15. Kohl, H.W.; Craig, C.L.; Lambert, E.V.; Inoue, S.; Alkandari, J.R.; Leetongin, G.; Kahlmeier, S. The pandemic of physical inactivity: Global action for public health. *Lancet* **2012**, *380*, 294–305. [CrossRef]
16. Heesch, K.C.; Sahlqvist, S.; Garrard, J. Gender differences in recreational and transport cycling: A cross-sectional mixed-methods comparison of cycling patterns, motivators, and constraints. *Int J. Behav. Nutr. Phys. Act.* **2012**, *9*, 106. [CrossRef]
17. Te Velde, S.J.; Haraldsen, E.; Vik, F.N.; De Bourdeaudhuij, I.; Jan, N.; Kovacs, E.; Moreno, L.A.; Dossegger, A.; Manios, Y.; Brug, J.; et al. Associations of commuting to school and work with demographic variables and with weight status in eight European countries: The ENERGY-cross sectional study. *Prev. Med.* **2017**, *99*, 305–312. [CrossRef] [PubMed]
18. Aparicio-Ugarriza, R.; Mielgo-Ayuso, J.; Ruiz, E.; Avila, J.M.; Aranceta-Bartrina, J.; Gil, A.; Ortega, R.M.; Serra-Majem, L.; Varela-Moreiras, G.; Gonzalez-Gross, M. Active commuting, physical activity, and sedentary behaviors in children and adolescents from Spain: Findings from the ANIBES Study. *Int. J. Environ. Res. Public Health* **2020**, *17*, 668. [CrossRef] [PubMed]
19. Bauman, A.E.; Reis, R.S.; Sallis, J.F.; Wells, J.C.; Loos, R.J.F.; Martin, B.W. Correlates of physical activity: Why are some people physically active and others not? *Lancet* **2012**, *380*, 258–271. [CrossRef]
20. Pollack Porter, K.M.; Prochnow, T.; Mahoney, P.; Delgado, H.; Bridges Hamilton, C.N.; Wilkins, E.; Umstattd Meyer, M.R. Transforming city streets to promote physical activity and health equity. *Health Aff.* **2019**, *38*, 1475–1483. [CrossRef]
21. Sallis, J.F.; Cerin, E.; Conway, T.L.; Adams, M.A.; Frank, L.D.; Pratt, M.; Salvo, D.; Schipperijn, J.; Smith, G.; Cain, K.L.; et al. Physical activity in relation to urban environments in 14 cities worldwide: A cross-sectional study. *Lancet* **2016**, *387*, 2207–2217. [CrossRef]
22. Pinjari, A.R.; Pendyala, R.M.; Bhat, C.R.; Waddell, P.A. Modeling the choice continuum: An integrated model of residential location, auto ownership, bicycle ownership, and commute tour mode choice decisions. *Transportation* **2011**, *38*, 933–958. [CrossRef]
23. Werneck, A.O.; Baldew, S.S.; Miranda, J.J.; Díaz Arnesto, O.; Stubbs, B.; Silva, D.R. Physical activity and sedentary behavior patterns and sociodemographic correlates in 116,982 adults from six South American countries: The South American physical activity and sedentary behavior network (SAPASEN). *Int. J. Behav. Nutr. Phys. Act.* **2019**, *16*, 68. [CrossRef]
24. Mitáš, J.; Cerin, E.; Reis, R.S.; Conway, T.L.; Cain, K.L.; Adams, M.A.; Schofield, G.; Sarmiento, O.L.; Christiansen, L.B.; Davey, R.; et al. Do associations of sex, age and education with transport and leisure-time physical activity differ across 17 cities in 12 countries? *Int. J. Behav. Nutr. Phys. Act.* **2019**, *16*, 121. [CrossRef] [PubMed]
25. Reis, R.S.; Hino, A.A.; Parra, D.C.; Hallal, P.C.; Brownson, R.C. Bicycling and walking for transportation in three Brazilian cities. *Am. J. Prev. Med.* **2013**, *44*, e9–e17. [CrossRef] [PubMed]
26. Teixeira, I.; Nakamura, P.; Smirmaul, B.; Fernandes, R.; Kokubun, E. Fatores associados ao uso de bicicleta como meio de transporte em uma cidade de médio porte. *Rev. Bras. Ativ. Fis. Saúde* **2013**, *18*, 698. [CrossRef]
27. Kienteka, M.; Reis, R.S.; Rech, C.R. Personal and behavioral factors associated with bicycling in adults from Curitiba, Paraná State, Brazil. *Cad. Saude Publica* **2014**, *30*, 79–87. [CrossRef] [PubMed]
28. Ministério da Saúde do Brasil. *Vigilância de fatores de risco e proteção para doenças crônicas por inquérito telefônico—VIGITEL*; Ministério da Saúde: Brasília, Brasil, 2019, 2018.
29. Instituto Brasileiro de Geografia e Estatística (IBGE). Sergipe. Available online: https://cidades.ibge.gov.br/brasil/se/aracaju/panorama (accessed on 25 April 2020).
30. Instituto Brasileiro de Geografia e Estatística (IBGE). Pesquisa nacional de saúde 2013: Ciclos de vida. Available online: https://biblioteca.ibge.gov.br/visualizacao/livros/liv94522.pdf (accessed on 9 August 2020).
31. Telama, R.; Yang, X.; Leskinen, E.; Kankaanpaa, A.; Hirvensalo, M.; Tammelin, T.; Viikari, J.S.; Raitakari, O.T. Tracking of physical activity from early childhood through youth into adulthood. *Med. Sci. Sports Exerc.* **2014**, *46*, 955–962. [CrossRef] [PubMed]
32. Heim LaFrombois, M.E. (Re)Producing and challenging gender in and through urban space: Women bicyclists' experiences in Chicago. *Gend. Place Cult.* **2019**, *26*, 659–679. [CrossRef]
33. Sa, T.H.; Salvador, E.P.; Florindo, A.A. Factors associated with physical inactivity in transportation in Brazilian adults living in a low socioeconomic area. *J. Phys. Act. Health* **2013**, *10*, 856–862. [CrossRef]
34. Providelo, J.K.; Sanches, S.P. Percepções de indivíduos acerca do uso da bicicleta como modo de transporte. *Transportes* **2010**, *18*, 53–61. [CrossRef]

35. Superintendência Municipal de Transporte e Trânsito (SMTT). Plano diretor de mobilidade de Aracaju. Available online: http://smttaju.com.br/mobilidade-urbana/PLANO-DIRETOR-DE-MOBILIDADE.pdf (accessed on 25 April 2020).
36. Sivasankaran, S.K.; Balasubramanian, V. Exploring the severity of bicycle-vehicle crashes using latent class clustering approach in India. *J. Saf. Res.* **2020**, *72*, 127–138. [CrossRef]
37. Yan, X.; Ma, M.; Huang, H.; Abdel-Aty, M.; Wu, C. Motor vehicle-bicycle crashes in Beijing: Irregular maneuvers, crash patterns, and injury severity. *Accid. Anal. Prev.* **2011**, *43*, 1751–1758. [CrossRef] [PubMed]
38. Cervero, R.; Duncan, M. Walking, bicycling, and urban landscapes: Evidence from the San Francisco Bay Area. *Am. J. Public Health.* **2003**, *93*, 1478–1483. [CrossRef]
39. Xing, Y.; Handy, S.L.; Mokhtarian, P.L. Factors associated with proportions and miles of bicycling for transportation and recreation in six small US cities. *Transp. Res. D Transp. Environ.* **2010**, *15*, 73–81. [CrossRef]
40. Zahran, S.; Brody, S.D.; Maghelal, P.; Prelog, A.; Lacy, M. Cycling and walking: Explaining the spatial distribution of healthy modes of transportation in the United States. *Transp. Res. D Transp. Environ.* **2008**, *13*, 462–470. [CrossRef]
41. Mueller, N.; Rojas-Rueda, D.; Salmon, M.; Martinez, D.; Ambros, A.; Brand, C.; de Nazelle, A.; Dons, E.; Gaupp-Berghausen, M.; Gerike, R.; et al. Health impact assessment of cycling network expansions in European cities. *Prev. Med.* **2018**, *109*, 62–70. [CrossRef] [PubMed]
42. Goenka, S.; Andersen, L.B. Urban design and transport to promote healthy lives. *Lancet* **2016**, *388*, 2851–2853. [CrossRef]
43. Krizek, K.J.; Stonebraker, E.W. Assessing options to enhance bicycle and transit integration. *Transp. Res. Rec.* **2011**, *2217*, 162–167. [CrossRef]

Publisher's Note: MDPI stays neutral with regard to jurisdictional claims in published maps and institutional affiliations.

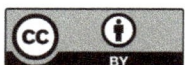

© 2020 by the authors. Licensee MDPI, Basel, Switzerland. This article is an open access article distributed under the terms and conditions of the Creative Commons Attribution (CC BY) license (http://creativecommons.org/licenses/by/4.0/).

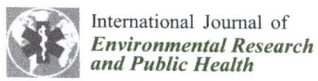

Article

Active Transport to School May Reduce Psychosomatic Symptoms in School-Aged Children: Data from Nine Countries

Dorota Kleszczewska [1,*], Joanna Mazur [2,3], Jens Bucksch [4], Anna Dzielska [3], Catherina Brindley [4] and Agnieszka Michalska [5]

1. Institute of Mother and Child Foundation, 01-211 Warsaw, Poland
2. Collegium Medicum, University of Zielona Góra, 65-046 Zielona Góra, Poland; joanna.mazur@hbsc.org
3. Department of Child and Adolescent Health, Institute of Mother and Child, 01-211 Warsaw, Poland; anna.dzielska@imid.med.pl
4. Department of Natural and Sociological Sciences, Heidelberg University of Education, 69120 Heidelberg, Germany; bucksch@ph-heidelberg.de (J.B.); brindley@ph-heidelberg.de (C.B.)
5. Department of Biomedical Foundations of Development and Sexology, Faculty of Education, University of Warsaw, 01-211 Warsaw, Poland; michalska.agg@gmail.com
* Correspondence: dorota.kleszczewska@imid.med.pl; Tel.: +48-606-371-850

Received: 15 October 2020; Accepted: 21 November 2020; Published: 24 November 2020

Abstract: It is widely proven that being physically active and avoiding sedentary behaviour help to improve adolescents' well-being and keep them in better health in general. We aimed to investigate the relationship between modes of transport to school and subjective complaints among schoolchildren. Analyses were based on the HBSC (Health Behaviour in School-aged Children) surveys conducted in 2017/18 in nine countries (N = 55,607; mean age 13.43 ± 1.64 yrs.). The main outcome showed that health complaints consisted of somatic and psychological complaints. Transport to school was characterized by mode of getting there (walking, biking, or another passive mode). A total of 46.1% of students walked and 7.3% cycled to school; 46.6% commuted by passive means. Biking to school was more frequent in Denmark (37.9%), Norway (26.5%), and Germany (26.6%). The multivariate generalized linear model adjusted for age, gender, country, and school proximity showed that biking to school is protective against reports of health complaints. The beta parameters were equal to −0.498 ($p < 0.001$) for the general HBSC-SCL index, −0.208 ($p < 0.001$) for the somatic complaint index, and −0.285 ($p < 0.001$) for the psychological complaints index. Young people who actively commute to school are less likely to report health complaints, especially psychological symptoms.

Keywords: physical activity; wellbeing; active transport; youth; school; mental health; psychosomatic complaints

1. Introduction

Improving the health of young people is currently one of the priority areas of public health activities. For this reason, it is worth paying attention to non-specific health complaints, which are lately more often communicated by young people [1]. They are described in the literature as "psychosomatic complaints" and include physical symptoms such as backache, headache, and abdominal pain, as well as mental symptoms including fatigue, irritability, or difficulty falling asleep [2]. Non-specific health complaints may also occur due to unhealthy everyday habits, i.e., sleep deficits [3,4], cigarette smoking, or sitting for too long in front of a TV or computer screen [5].

A physically active life and avoiding long episodes of sedentary behaviour help prevent non-specific health complaints and improve well-being among adolescents [6–8]. A study involving over 171,000 teenagers from 37 countries revealed that young people who lead physically active, healthy lifestyles experience psychosomatic symptoms less frequently [9]. In particular, the protective functions of physical activity are well established in the context of mental health [10]. Physical activity goes far beyond sports. According to WHO recommendations, moderate to intense physical activity is important, including daily activities that require energy expenditure, such as cleaning, walking upstairs, or active transport to school (ATS) [11]. A key to changing to a more active lifestyle is to implement more physical activity into daily life, including active travel, which does not require financial costs or making huge changes in one's course of everyday life. [12]. Over the last two decades, studies have shown that ATS plays a significant role in improving adolescent health in many countries [13–15]. Existing studies have focused mainly on walking and cycling as two forms of active transport [16]. Cycling to school enables young people to meet the WHO recommendations for daily physical activity to a greater extent [17], reduces the risk of obesity [18], improves overall body fitness, and ensures proper blood circulation [19]. ATS also strengthens positive effects on mental health, helping students perform better in school. This positive effect on mental well-being is significant, as is the joy that physical activity generates and the contact with nature while walking or cycling. It is assumed that ATS can help one build a sense of independence and self-confidence as well as concern for the environment [20].

However, ATS has changed throughout the last decades. Several decades ago, walking to school was the norm in most societies [21], while in more economically developed countries today, children are usually "chauffeured" or driven to school in their parents' cars [22]. A British study showed a 9% drop in walking to school in 1975–1994 among children aged 5–10 [23]. A similar tendency was recorded in Switzerland, indicated by a 7% decrease in ATS rates among children aged 6–14 between 1994 and 2005 [24]. A 20% decrease in ATS rates was recently recorded in Czechia among adolescents aged 11–15 years [25]. However, a gender difference is well established in active travel, showing that boys are more likely to walk or cycle to school than girls [26]. Moreover, there is a clear link between age and the declining prevalence of ATS [27]. Furthermore, ATS seems to vary by socio-ecological determinants, as patterns of ATS differ between countries according to geographical and cultural backgrounds [26]. Finally, when analysing ATS, the distance to school is one of the strongest predictors for the likelihood of undertaking ATS [28].

When analysing the international literature, we were not aware of any study on the relationship between modes of transport to school and psychosomatic complaints of adolescents in international samples. This contribution refers to data from the international HBSC (Health Behaviour in School-aged Children) study. The HBSC Symptom Check List (HBSC-SCL) has been part of the HBSC questionnaire since the beginning. Gender and age-related demographic determinants and selected psychosocial and behavioural correlates, including those related to physical activity, have been extensively discussed [4,5,7,10]. To our knowledge, no research on the protective effect of active transport to school has been conducted so far based on HBSC data. The authors of this paper assume that this could be a valuable contribution in this matter. We examine the relationship between non-specific somatic complaints among adolescents and ATS for nine European countries of various geographical backgrounds. We hypothesize that ATS is significantly associated with psychosomatic complaints in adolescents and that the protective effect of cycling is greater than that of other forms of ATS, including walking. The aim of the study was to investigate the relationship between modes of transport to school and subjective complaints among schoolchildren. We have set the following research questions:

1. Are there cross-country differences in terms of active transport to and from school?
2. Do young people who use active forms of transport to school report psychosomatic complaints less frequently?
3. Does cycling reduce the incidence of psychosomatic complaints in adolescents more than other forms of active transport to school?
4. Do difficulties in getting to school by active transport moderate the above relationships (duration of travel)?

2. Materials and Methods

The HBSC network provides data on health behaviour and outcomes for children and adolescents from 49 countries over a four-year study period. Our data are derived from the last survey cycle of the international HBSC research carried out in the 2017/18 school year. HBSC has developed as a unique mandatory tool for psychosomatic complaints in children and adolescents. For the 2018 study wave, nine member states optionally collected data on ATS. The international sample of the countries covering the topic of ATS and psychosomatic complaints includes 56,834 individuals from nine countries and regions: Azerbaijan (N = 4582), Czechia (N = 11,553), Denmark (N = 2837), Germany (N = 4147), Ireland (N = 3806), Norway (N = 2759), Poland (N = 5191), Scotland (N = 4892), and Wales (N = 15,840). Surveys were conducted in schools according to a standardized procedure described in the international research protocol [29]. The response rate on the student level varied by country, from 53.7% in Germany to 99.3% in Azerbaijan.

The international sample consisted of 49.3% boys and 50.7% girls. The percentage of boys ranged from 47.3% (Germany) to 50.6% (Ireland). Students were categorized into three age groups: 11-year-olds (35.4%), 13-year-olds (34.6%), and 15-year-olds (30.0%). The mean age was 13.43 years (SD = 1.64) and ranged from 13.05 in Norway to 13.59 in Poland.

2.1. Variables

2.1.1. Psychosomatic Complaints

Psychosomatic complaints were self-reported. The HBSC Symptom Checklist (HBSC-SCL) includes eight symptoms and is a validated scale that has been used for all HBSC study waves throughout the HBSC process [30]. The adolescents reported how often they had experienced particular complaints in the last 6 months according to a 5-category response scale (from rarely or never to almost daily), coded from 0 to 4. The total (HBSC-SCL) scale range is 0–32 points. We also created two independent indexes: (1) somatic complaints (HBSC-SCL_S) including headache, abdominal pain, back pain, and dizziness, and (2) psychological complaints (HBSC-SCL_P) including depression, nervousness, irritability or bad mood, and difficulty sleeping. These both had index ranges of 0–16 points. Higher scores on individual scales represent greater psychosomatic complaints. In the combined international sample, the HBSC-SCL index has a single-factor structure with reliability of $\alpha = -0.804$. The HBSC-SCL_S and HBSC-SCL_P indexes are also homogeneous and have a reliability of 0.673 and 0.744, respectively. The percentage of missing data was 3.8% for the entire HBSC-SCL scale and for subscales was 2.8% (HBSC-SCL_S) and 3.4% (HBSC-SCL_P).

2.1.2. Active Transport to School

Students self-reported how they usually get to and from school. There were five mutually exclusive categories of answers: (1) on foot; (2) by bicycle; (3) by bus, train, tram, or metro; (4) by car, motorbike, or scooter; and (5) other means. For this study, three groups of students were identified, creating a single variable based on their answers about getting to school and back home. In the absence of data on a one-way route, students were categorized based on the second type of available information. Individual categories of this variable are:

- walking–if the bicycle was not used and the student usually walked at least one way;
- riding a bicycle–if the bicycle was used at least one way;
- not using active transport–other cases, assumed to be passive ones.

Moreover, the travel to school difficulty index (TSDI), ranging from 1 to 10 points, was defined as an important covariate to control for this effect as the impact of difficulties in active commuting to school which may translate into increased school stress. This index is a measure of the interaction between a typical mode of transport and how long it takes to get to school (estimated only one way). This type of index was assumed to be an approximate measure of the location of the school in relation to home. It illustrates the difficulties with commuting, which may translate into increased school stress. The index ranges from 1 to 10, with "1" indicating a short duration (<5 min) by car and "10" indicating a trip more than 30 min by car. Three experts independently scored the TSDI taking into account the duration of the travel to school and the means of transport. A common version was then discussed and accepted. The TSDI index was created especially for this study. The description of coding rules and definition of the Travel to School Difficulty Index (TSDI) index are given in Table S1 in Supplementary Materials.

2.2. Statistical Analysis

To characterize the description of the sample, we used a chi-square test to compare the categories of ATS in groups according to gender, age, and country. The correlation between the symptom indexes and the TSDI variable was examined with the Spearman coefficient.

Kolmogorov–Smirnov test for normality (with Lilliefors correction) indicated that all applied scales were not normally distributed: SCL_T: KS = 0.11, $p < 0.001$; SCL_S: KS = 0.18, $p < 0.001$; SCL_P: KS = 0.13, $p < 0.001$; TSDI: KS = 0.16, $p < 0.001$). So, non-parametric analyses were conducded.

The mean values of the SCL_T, SCP_S, and SCL_P indexes were compared in groups of active and passive commutes to school using a nonparametric Kruskal–Wallis test. Similar calculations for each of the nine countries are provided as supplementals.

We used a generalized linear model (the GENLIN procedure of the SPSS software, IBM SPSS Statistics for Windows, Version 25.0, IBM Corp: Armonk, NY, USA) in the multivariate analysis and included gender, age group, country, or region and the predominant way of reaching school according to the three predefined categories as predictors of successive complaint indexes. The reference categories were as follows: 15-year-olds, girls, students from Azerbaijan, and young people not using active forms of transport from or to school. We also estimated models specific to the nine countries, presenting the values of beta parameters at levels related to active transport (walking, biking).

3. Results

3.1. Prevalence of Psychosomatic Complaints

The burden of non-specific psychosomatic complaints is presented in Table 1. In the total sample of students from three grades, the average overall symptom index (HBSC-SCL) was 8.28 ± 6.52 (median 7.00) and ranged from 5.64 in Azerbaijan to 9.15 in Poland. Similarly, the two sub-indexes (HBSC-SCL_S and HBSC-SCL_P) had the lowest values in Azerbaijan and the highest in Germany and Poland. Girls reported psychosomatic complaints significantly more often than boys. This applies to the general index and its two domains. In the international sample, the mean HBSC-SCL indexes were 7.12 ± 5.88 for boys and 9.39 ± 6.90 for girls ($p < 0.001$). Significant differences among girls were noted in all countries except Azerbaijan. The lack of gender-related differences in that country mainly concerned the HBSC-SCL_S subscale ($p = 0.270$), because in the case of the HBSC-SCL_P sub-scale, the results were already significant, although at the border of statistical significance ($p = 0.044$).

There was also a clearly increasing burden of psychosomatic symptoms in subsequent age groups. The mean overall HBSC-SCL_T index was as follows: 11-year-olds, 7.00 ± 5.97; 13-year-olds, 8.40 ± 6.54; and 15-year-olds, 9.56 ± 6.80 ($p < 0.001$). Age-related differences were statistically significant in all nine countries. This was confirmed for the overall HBSC-SCL_T index as well as the HBSC-SCL-S and HBSC-SCL-P sub-indexes (data not shown).

Table 1. Mean indices of psychosomatic complaints reported by students from nine countries.

Country /WHO Region	HBSC-SCL [1] (n-53491)		HBSC-SCL_S [2] (n-54052)		HBSC-SCL_P [3] (n-53741)	
	Mean	SD	Mean	SD	Mean	SD
Azerbaijan	5.64	6.87	2.40	3.44	3.22	4.06
Czechia	8.33	5.82	2.66	2.73	5.63	3.89
Denmark	7.80	5.96	2.91	3.05	4.86	3.71
Germany	8.16	5.89	3.58	3.18	4.56	3.52
Ireland	8.32	6.57	3.07	3.22	5.18	4.05
Norway	7.48	5.98	2.72	2.96	4.72	3.69
Poland	9.15	6.48	3.08	3.09	6.02	4.29
Scotland	8.50	6.87	3.15	3.37	5.31	4.26
Wales	8.89	6.91	3.36	3.37	5.49	4.34
Total	8.28	6.52	3.04	3.19	5.20	4.14

[1] HBSC-SCL–total index of psychosomatic symptoms; [2] HBSC-SCL_S–index of somatic symptoms; [3] HBSC-SCL_P–index of psychological symptoms.

3.2. Active Transport to School

In total, almost half of the respondents (46.6%) reported using passive forms of commuting to school. The results of the chi-sq test indicate that there is a statistically significant association between countries and active transport to school (chi-sq (1, N = 55,607) = 14,942.61, $p < 0.001$). The proportion ranged from 16.5% in Azerbaijan to 68.4% in Ireland. Almost the same number of students reported walking to school, as the proportion was 46.1%, ranging from 25.4% in Denmark to 81.2% in Azerbaijan; 7.3% of students reported using a bicycle as a means of transport. Students in Denmark (37.9%), Norway (26.5%), and Germany (26.6%) were more likely to cycle to school than young people from other countries (Table 2). The difference between countries is significant at $p < 0.001$ (chi-sq = 14,942.6; df = 16).

Table 2. Characteristics of commuting to school in nine countries.

Country /WHO Region	Means of Transport (%) (N-55607)			Level of TSDI [1] (N-55409)	
	Passive	Walking	Biking	Mean	SD
Azerbaijan	16.5	81.2	2.3	4.37	1.94
Czechia	35.0	62.1	2.9	4.29	1.88
Denmark	36.7	25.4	37.9	4.34	1.81
Germany	54.6	18.9	26.6	4.97	1.94
Ireland	68.4	27.9	3.7	3.78	2.05
Norway	33.8	39.8	26.5	4.52	1.82
Poland	41.1	52.8	6.1	4.32	2.00
Scotland	46.8	51.8	1.4	4.10	1.98
Wales	62.3	36.5	1.2	4.64	2.11
Total	46.7	46.1	7.3	4.41	2.00

[1] TSDI–transport to school difficulty index.

The total sample showed an association between the gender and age of respondents and the use of active transport on the way to school. Girls use active forms less often, and boys ride bicycles more frequently (chi-sq (2, N = 55,607) = 325,12, $p < 0.001$). Moreover, 11-year-old students are also more active on their way to school than the two older age groups. The frequency of using a bicycle as a means of transport decreases with age (chi-sq (4, N = 55,256) = 223.90, $p < 0.001$).

On the TSDI, ranging from 1 to 10, the surveyed young people assessed the level of complexity of reaching their schools at 4.41 points on average (SD = 2.00). As presented in Table 2, the TSDI values ranged from 3.78 in Ireland to 4.97 in Germany (F(8,55400) = 139.12; $p < 0.001$)). Mean results were similar for boys and girls (4.42 vs. 4.4; t(55407) = 0.999; $p = 0.318$). However, their values were higher in the two older age groups (13- and 15-year-olds) as compared to the 11-year-olds (13-year-olds: 4.07 ± 1.94, 4.55 ± 2.00, and 4.66 ± 2.02, respectively; F(2,55066) = 456.40; $p < 0.001$).

3.3. Psychosomatic Complaints in Relation to Mode of Transport to School

In total, the highest values of the general index HBSC-SCL and two partial indexes were reported by adolescents who did not use any forms of active transport (Table 3, Table S2). The values of all three indexes were lower in the group of people walking to school and were the lowest in the case of cycling. For the general index (SCL_T) and that of psychological complaints (SCL_P), differences were found depending on the modes of AST in eight countries (except Scotland), while for SCL_S, differences were significant in six countries (Azerbaijan, Czechia, Denmark, Ireland, Germany, and Norway).

Table 3. Psychosomatic complaints according to mode of transport to school in the combined sample from nine countries.

Transport to School	SCL_T [1]		SCL_S [2]		SCL_P [3]	
	Mean	SD	Mean	SD	Mean	SD
Passive mode	8.57	6.57	3.18	3.24	5.34	4.15
Walking	8.15	6.57	2.94	3.16	5.17	4.20
Biking	7.27	5.72	2.76	2.97	4.48	3.58
Kruskal–Wallis test	-		-		-	
Chi-sq	141.22		133.28		125.52	
df	2		2		2	
p	<0.001		<0.001		<0.001	

[1] SCL_T–total index of psychosomatic symptoms; [2] SCL_S–index of somatic symptoms; [3] SCL_P–index of psychological symptoms.

The level of difficulty in getting to school measured by the TSDI correlated significantly with the indexes of complaints, but the values of respective Spearman's correlation coefficients were low (for HBSC-SCL, rho = 0.070; for HBSC-SCL_S, rho = 0.066, and for HBSC-SCL_P, rho = 0.061). The only country showing no statistically significant correlation between HBSC-SCL_T and TSDI was Denmark. The highest correlation coefficients of TSDI with HBSC-SCL_T were recorded in Ireland (rho = 0.151), Scotland (rho = 0.107), and Poland (rho = 0.076). Relatively higher values of Spearman's correlation coefficients were also observed in Ireland in relation to the sub-indexes HBSC-SCL_S (rho = 0.134) and HBSC-SCL_P (rho = 0.137).

Table 4 presents a comparison of groups differing in the mode of AST, taking into account age, gender, country, and the TSDI. The results of the generalized linear model indicate that gender and age are significant predictors of psychosomatic complaints. Using Azerbaijan as the reference category (i.e., the country where young people report subjective complaints the least frequently), HBSC-SCL values increased in the remaining eight countries and were the highest in Poland and Wales. Cycling to school remains a factor in reducing HBSC-SCL values. Walking to school did not significantly affect the variability of HBSC-SCL after adjusting for other factors ($p = 0.086$). An increase in TSDI values by one unit increased the HBSC-SCL value by 0.210.

In analogous generalized linear models estimated for partial indexes (unpublished data), the protective effect of cycling to school was maintained. When the dependent variable was the somatic complaint index, the value of parameter B for the variable relating to cycling was −0.208 (SE = 0.0580) –$p < 0.001$. In the model for mental complaints, the value of parameter B with the variable relating to cycling was −0.285 (SE = 0.0749)–$p < 0.001$. In the first case, walking to school was not found to significantly influence the variability of HBSC-SCL_S (beta = 0.020; $p = 0.499$). In the second case, complaints of a psychological nature (HBSC-SCL_P) increased slightly in the group who reported usually walking (beta = 0.080; $p = 0.035$).

It is also worth mentioning that the protective effect of ATS varies by country. Table 5 shows the beta linear regression coefficients estimated in specific models for nine countries. It includes results adjusted for gender, age, and TSDI modification. The protective effect of cycling to school was significant in four countries (Czechia, Denmark, Germany, and Norway), while the protective effect of walking was only evident in Azerbaijan.

Table 4. Generalized linear regression model for total index of psychosomatic symptoms (HBSC-SCL) estimated on the combined sample from nine countries (N-53016).

Parameter	B	SE(B)	Wald Statistics	df	p
(Constant)	6.940	0.1342	2675.525	1	0.000
Age category					
11 yrs	−2.402	0.0682	1238.425	1	0.000
13 yrs	−1.165	0.0674	298.659	1	0.000
15 yrs (ref.)					
Gender					
Boys	−2.252	0.0546	1704.425	1	0.000
Girls (ref.)					
Mode of transport to school					
Walking	0.102	0.0596	2.941	1	0.086
Biking	−0.498	0.1181	17.790	1	0.000
Passive mode (ref.)					
TSDI [1]	0.210	0.0139	228.058	1	0.000
Country/WHO region					
Czechia	2.702	0.1130	571.464	1	0.000
Denmark	2.542	0.1595	253.785	1	0.000
Germany	2.486	0.1429	302.617	1	0.000
Ireland	2.925	0.1445	409.642	1	0.000
Norway	2.270	0.1579	206.752	1	0.000
Poland	3.534	0.1307	731.153	1	0.000
Scotland	3.027	0.1333	516.126	1	0.000
Wales	3.304	0.1113	882.060	1	0.000
Azerbaijan (ref.)					
(Scale)	39.075	0.2400			

[1] TSDI—transport to school difficulty index.

Table 5. Beta parameters related to the effect of active transport to school estimated by country-specific generalized linear regression models for total index of psychosomatic symptoms (HBSC-SCL).

Country /WHO Region	Effect of Biking			Effect of Walking		
	Beta	SE	p	Beta	SE	p
Azerbaijan	0.190	0.7377	0797	−1.426	0.2783	<0.001
Czechia	−0.669	0.3368	0.047	−0.112	0.1164	0.337
Denmark	−0.593	0.2589	0.022	0.619	0.2864	0.031
Germany	−0.707	0.2109	0.001	0.309	0.2416	0.202
Ireland	−0.142	0.5667	0.802	0.934	0.2346	<0.001
Norway	−0.867	0.3005	0.004	−0.207	0.2664	0.436
Poland	−0.323	0.3839	0.400	0.169	0.1826	0.357
Scotland	0.085	0.8315	0.919	0.234	0.1945	0.230
Wales	1.303	0.5152	0.011	0.327	0.1132	0.004

4. Discussion

The aim of the study was to examine whether ATS reduces the prevalence of non-specific psychosomatic complaints in adolescents from nine countries or regions of the WHO European region. We analyzed a sample of 56,834 students aged 11–15 surveyed in the HBSC round 2017/18. Adjusted for other factors, cycling showed a protective effect against psychosomatic complaints in Czechia, Denmark, Germany, and Norway, and walking showed a protective association for children and adolescents in Azerbaijan. The analyses of the protective function of active transport highlighted several issues. Above all, it is clear that ATS enhances adolescent health. This supports the main hypothesis of the paper—that ATS is significantly associated with psychosomatic complaints, depending on cross-country differences. Thus, this contribution is part of a wide range of international research on active transport as an important element of describing the current situation regarding the health and activity levels of adolescents [29]. According to our knowledge and the international literature, there have been no studies verifying to what extent active transport is associated with non-specific psychosomatic complaints in adolescents, though many studies have shown a positive association with cardiovascular, weight-, and fitness-related outcomes in adolescents. There are also some studies of adult populations showing protective effects in terms of depression and the relationship between ATS and adolescents' mental health, defined as well-being [31,32].

ATS, as well as engaging in any physical activity, depends largely on culture, family education, and the promotion of a healthy lifestyle at school and in the community. It is also influenced by the level of socio-economic development of a given country [33]. In countries of higher economic status, such as Germany or Denmark, young people are more likely to use bicycles thanks to better infrastructure. In these countries, young people can use bicycle paths, and schools have designated storage spaces for bicycles [34], enhancing the sense of security. According to our analyses, cycling (not walking to school) has the greatest impact on non-specific somatic complaints in these countries. We might also argue that adolescents in countries with less developed economies walk more often, and therefore, walking to school is not an additional part of overall physical activity and does not show health benefits. A small percentage of teenagers use bicycles, which makes it difficult to estimate health effects of cycling to school among this age group. Walking may be the result of an informed decision or the absence of a public transport network. Azerbaijan turned out to be the only country where walking to school protected against psychosomatic complaints.

In analysing the differences between countries adolescent ATS frequency, it is worth bearing legislation in mind. For example, age limits apply to children going to school or riding bicycles independently. In Poland, a 9-year-old child with parental consent may return home on foot, but by bicycle only if they have a bicycle card, starting at the age of 13. Public transport and school buses provided by municipalities can provide attractive alternatives or leave young people from the countryside with no choice.

An interesting finding of our analyses is the negative relationship between age and the frequency of cycling to school. The decline in this mode of AST in older years may result from the general age-related decline in physical activity, but also from school changes. After moving to a secondary school, students often need to travel to another town or cover a longer distance within a particular city [35]; this finding is in accordance with other studies [18] in terms of the TSDI, which is our measure of interaction between the time needed to get to school and the means of transport. Adding this factor significantly improved the quality of the fit of the models. It was assumed that a difficult, prolonged commute to school intensifies perceived stress, influencing the occurrence of non-specific psychosomatic complaints in adolescents. In many studies based on HBSC data, school stress and general stress are mentioned as the main predictors of SCL values [36]. In the international literature, the distance to school is mentioned mainly as a barrier to physical activity [37,38]. In our models, the SCL burden increases as the correction index increases, therefore showing the opposite association for ATS indicators.

In terms of analysing country differences, it is also worth taking physical conditions into accounts, such as geography, topography, and weather. In some countries, during winter, young people choose only passive modes of commuting [39]. In countries such as Scotland, Wales, and Ireland, cycling does not show a protective association with psychosomatic complaints, even though bicycle use is relatively popular. In Wales, bicycle commuters report more frequent symptoms. Similarly, the association with walking from school in Ireland and Denmark was negative, whereas cycling had a positive effect. One explanation could be the distance to school. However, the shorter the distance to school, the less the commute would affect health.

The mode of active or passive transport to school varies by gender. Girls use active forms of transport less frequently, which may be due in part to their general reluctance to engage in physical activity. In the case of active travel, safety issues also play a role in explaining this difference, since boys are allowed more independent mobility. All the more worrying is the fact that with age, the burden of psychosomatic complaints increases in girls, along with the decrease in physical activity. Potrebny et al. confirmed this in an extensive longitudinal study conducted in 1994–2014 on a sample of teenagers from Norway [40]. They showed that health complaints affect teenage boys to a lesser extent than girls, and that the difference is more pronounced in terms of mental health issues. Teenage girls' lack of ATS may also be a manifestation of reverse dependency. Adolescent girls are more likely to experience non-specific complaints, which discourage them from engaging in physical activity, including ATS [41]. It can also be assumed that parents more often declare their willingness to drive their daughters to school, being concerned with their safety and bearing in mind their reported worse well-being [42]. Further research should address this gender issue specifically to understand and promote active travel in girls.

One of our most important findings is the greater protective effect of ATS in relation to psychological rather than somatic complaints. This is in line with studies that describe the positive effects of physical activity on the mental health of adolescents [8]. It seems that both cycling and walking to school can build self-esteem based on greater independence. Often, ATS is carried out in a peer group and improves relations with schoolmates, creating opportunities for discussions and joint planning of extracurricular activities [34]. It also should be highlighted that young people who are in better health and in better mood engage in physical activity more often and probably are also more willing to actively commute to school. In these cases, lack of subjective health complaints could be a cause of ATS not an effect [43].

When analysing the issue of ATS, it is important to consider the differences in methodological assumptions of the conducted research. This article uses three simple ATS-related questions available as an optional package in the HBSC protocol. We defined secondary indicators on this basis, affecting the results obtained. The main limitations of the conducted research stemmed from the design of the research tool and not considering other factors. Among the limitations, we highlight the cross-sectional character of the study and the fact that data were self-reported by adolescents. We treated modes of transport as mutually exclusive categories according to the HBSC protocol. In planning the analyses, we adopted a number of simplifications, leaving two forms of active transport: walking and cycling. This approach is used in other studies [44]. The use of other equipment/modes and all mixed forms of movement are summarized in one category. The international literature draws attention to the growing popularity of scooters or skateboards and the emergence of electric devices, which are attractive but result in lower energy expenditure [45]. In some studies, public transport is also treated as a form of physical activity if young people have to cover some part of the way on foot [46]. We added a covariate to our methods, the index of difficulty in getting to school (TSDI). This is our measure of the interaction between the time needed to get to school and the means of transport. It seems that its inclusion is a strength of the paper, counterbalancing the above-mentioned limitations. It should be also mentioned that the response rate in some countries was relatively low, e.g., 53.7% in Germany. This could be considered as a limitation of the present study.

When examining adolescents' ATS in the context of the reduction of non-specific psychosomatic complaints, one should also bear potential negative effects in mind. Walking or cycling in a city with poor air quality can generate a number of complaints, such as headaches and nausea. Deterioration of well-being can also be aggravated by noise and crowds [47]. Nevertheless, a recent systematic review analysing the health impact of active transportation showed that the positive health effects of active transport outweigh the negative influences of air pollution. In our paper, these negative effects are partially illustrated by the TSDI modification factor.

5. Conclusions

Considering the significant burden for students with various somatic or psychological symptoms, demonstrating the beneficial effects of ATS may help to set new directions for carrying out interventions. It would be valuable to take cross-country determinants of active travel to school into consideration while planning such interventions. Young people who cycle to school are less likely to report health complaints, especially psychological symptoms. Research on this subject should take into account the cross-country differences. Promoting cycling seems to be particularly beneficial to psychological health but is not common among the studied countries.

Supplementary Materials: The following are available online at http://www.mdpi.com/1660-4601/17/23/8709/s1, Figure S1: Mode of transport to school by age and gender., Table S1. Level of subjective complaints by mode of transport to school.

Author Contributions: Conceptualization, D.K. and J.M., J.B.; methodology, D.K., J.M.; software, J.B., A.D., C.B.; validation, D.K., J.M., J.B., A.D., C.B., and Z.Z.; formal analysis, D.K., A.D., C.B., A.M.; investigation, D.K., J.M., J.B., A.D.; resources, A.D., C.B., A.M.; data curation, J.M., J.B.; writing—original draft preparation, D.K., J.M., J.B.; writing—review and editing, A.D., C.B., A.M.; visualization, D.K., A.M.; supervision, D.K., J.M.; project administration, D.K., A.M.; funding acquisition, D.K., A.M. All authors have read and agreed to the published version of the manuscript.

Funding: Erasmus+ project number EAC-A05-2017.

Conflicts of Interest: The authors declare no conflict of interest.

References

1. Van Geelen, S.M.; Hagquist, C. Are the time trends in adolescent psychosomatic problems related to functional impairment in daily life? A 23-year study among 20,000 15–16 year olds in Sweden. *J. Psychosom. Res.* **2016**, *87*, 50–56. [CrossRef]
2. Eriksen, H.R.; Ursin, H. Sensitization and subjective health complaints. *Scand. J. Psychol.* **2002**, *43*, 189–196. [CrossRef]
3. Segura-Jiménez, V.; Carbonell-Baeza, A.; Keating, X.D.; Ruiz, J.R.; Castro-Piñero, J. Association of sleep patterns with psychological positive health and health complaints in children and adolescents. *Qual. Life Res.* **2015**, *24*, 885–895. [CrossRef]
4. Paiva, T.; Gaspar, T.; Matos, M.G. Sleep deprivation in adolescents: Correlations with health complaints and health-related quality of life. *Sleep Med.* **2015**, *16*, 521–527. [CrossRef]
5. Kleszczewska, D.; Małkowska -Szkutnik, A.; Nałęcz, H.; Mazur, J. Sedentary behavior and non-specific psychosomatic health complaints of school-aged children. *Pediatr. Pol. Pol. J. Paediatr.* **2017**, *92*, 553–560. [CrossRef]
6. Ng, K.W.; Sudeck, G.; Marques, A.; Borraccino, A.; Boberova, Z.; Vasickova, J.; Tesler, R.; Kokko, S.; Samdal, O. Associations Between Physical Activity and Perceived School Performance of Young Adolescents in Health Behavior in School-Aged Children Countries. *J. Phys. Act. Health* **2020**, *17*, 698–708. [CrossRef]
7. Husárová, D.; Veselská, Z.D.; Sigmundová, D.; Gecková, A.M. Age and Gender Differences in Prevalence of Screen Based Behaviour, Physical Activity and Health Complaints among Slovak School-aged Children. *Cent. Eur. J. Public Health* **2015**, *23*, S30–S36. [CrossRef]
8. Verhoeven, H.; Simons, D.; Van Dyck, D.; Van Cauwenberg, J.; Clarys, P.; De Bourdeaudhuij, I.; de Geus, B.; Vandelanotte, C.; Deforche, B. Psychosocial and Environmental Correlates of Walking, Cycling, Public Transport and Passive Transport to Various Destinations in Flemish Older Adolescents. *PLoS ONE* **2016**, *11*, e0147128. [CrossRef]
9. Marques, A.; Demetriou, Y.; Tesler, R.; Gouveia, É.R.; Peralta, M.; Matos, M.G. Healthy Lifestyle in Children and Adolescents and Its Association with Subjective Health Complaints: Findings from 37 Countries and Regions from the HBSC Study. *Int. J. Environ. Res. Public Health* **2019**, *16*, 3292. [CrossRef]
10. Kleszczewska, D.; Szkutnik, A.M.; Siedlecka, J.; Mazur, J. Physical Activity, Sedentary Behaviours and Duration of Sleep as Factors Affecting the Well-Being of Young People against the Background of Environmental Moderators. *Int. J. Environ. Res. Public Health* **2019**, *16*, 915. [CrossRef]

11. WHO Global Recommendations on Physical Activity for Health. Available online: https://apps.who.int/iris/bitstream/handle/10665/44399/9789241599979_eng.pdf;sequence=1 (accessed on 10 October 2020).
12. Gardner, B.; de Bruijn, G.J.; Lally, P. A systematic review and meta-analysis of applications of the Self-Report Habit Index to nutrition and physical activity behaviours. *Ann. Behav. Med.* **2011**, *42*, 174–187. [CrossRef] [PubMed]
13. Faulkner, G.E.; Buliung, R.N.; Flora, P.K.; Fusco, C. Active school transport, physical activity levels and body weight of children and youth: A systematic review. *Prev. Med.* **2009**, *48*, 3–8. [CrossRef] [PubMed]
14. Saunders, L.E.; Green, J.M.; Petticrew, M.P.; Steinbach, R.; Roberts, H. What are the health benefits of active travel? A systematic review of trials and cohort studies. *PLoS ONE* **2013**, *8*, e69912. [CrossRef] [PubMed]
15. Tudor-Locke, C.; Ainsworth, B.E.; Popkin, B.M. Active commuting to school: An overlooked source of childrens' physical activity? *Sports Med.* **2001**, *31*, 309–313. [CrossRef]
16. Carver, A.; Timperio, A.F.; Hesketh, K.D.; Ridgers, N.D.; Salmon, J.L.; Crawford, D.A. How is active transport associated with children's and adolescents' physical activity over time? *Int. J. Behav. Nutr. Phys. Act.* **2014**, *8*, 126. [CrossRef]
17. Schönbach, D.M.I.; Altenburg, T.M.; Chinapaw, M.J.M.; Marques, A.; Demetriou, Y. Strategies and effects of promising school-based interventions to promote active school transportation by bicycle among children and adolescents: Protocol for a systematic review. *Syst. Rev.* **2019**, *8*, 4–9. [CrossRef]
18. Mendoza, J.A.; Watson, K.; Nguyen, N.; Cerin, E.; Baranowski, T.; Nicklas, T.A. Active commuting to school and association with physical activity and adiposity among US youth. *J. Phys. Act. Health* **2011**, *8*, 488–495. [CrossRef]
19. Cooper, A.R.; Wedderkopp, N.; Jago, R.; Kristensen, P.L.; Moller, N.C.; Froberg, K.; Page, A.S.; Andersen, L.B. Longitudinal associations of cycling to school with adolescent fitness. *Prev. Med.* **2008**, *47*, 324–328. [CrossRef]
20. Biddle, S.J.; Ciaccioni, S.; Thomas, G.; Vergeer, I. Physical activity and mental health in children and adolescents: An updated review of reviews and an analysis of causality. *Psychol. Sport Exerc.* **2019**, *42*, 146–155. [CrossRef]
21. Aubert, S.; Barnes, J.D.; Abdeta, C.; Abi Nader, P.; Adeniyi, A.F.; Aguilar-Farias, N.; Andrade Tenesaca, D.S.; Bhawra, J.; Brazo-Sayavera, J.; Cardon, G.; et al. Global Matrix 3.0 Physical Activity Report Card Grades for Children and Youth: Results and Analysis From 49 Countries. *J. Phys. Act. Health* **2018**, *15*, S251–S273. [CrossRef]
22. Larouche, R.; Saunders, T.J.; Faulkner, G.; Colley, R.; Tremblay, M. Associations between active school transport and physical activity, body composition, and cardiovascular fitness: A systematic review of 68 studies. *J. Phys. Act. Health* **2014**, *11*, 206–227. [CrossRef] [PubMed]
23. Black, C.; Collins, A.; Snell, M. Encouraging walking: The case of journey-to-school trips in compacturban areas. *Urban Stud.* **2001**, *38*, 1121–1141. [CrossRef]
24. Grize, L.; Bringolf-Isler, B.; Martin, E.; Braun-Fahrlander, C. Trend in active transportation to school among Swiss school children and its associated factors: Three cross-sectional surveys 1994, 2000 and 2005. *Int. J. Behav. Nutr. Phys. Act.* **2010**, *7*, 1–8. [CrossRef] [PubMed]
25. Pavelka, J.; Sigmundová, D.; Hamřík, Z.; Kalman, M.; Sigmund, E.; Mathisen, F. Trends in Active Commuting to School among Czech Schoolchildren from 2006 to 2014. *Cent. Eur. J. Public Health* **2017**, *25* (Suppl. 1), S21–S25. [CrossRef] [PubMed]
26. Rothman, L.; Macpherson, A.K.; Ross, T.; Buliung, R.N. The decline in active school transportation (AST): A systematic review of the factors related to AST and changes in school transport over time in North America. *Prev. Med.* **2018**, *111*, 314–322. [CrossRef] [PubMed]
27. Ikeda, E.; Stewart, T.; Garrett, N.; Egli, V.; Mandic, S.; Hosking, J.; Witten, K.; Hawley, G.; Tautolo, E.S.; Rodda, J.; et al. Built environment associates of active school travel in New Zealand children and youth: A systematic meta-analysis using individual participant data. *J. Transp. Health* **2018**, *9*, 117–131. [CrossRef]
28. Chillón, P.; Evenson, K.R.; Vaughn, A.; Ward, D.S. A systematic review of interventions for promoting active transportation to school. *Int. J. Behav. Nutr. Phys. Act.* **2011**, *8*, 10. [CrossRef]
29. Inchley, J.; Currie, D.; Budisavljevic, S.; Torsheim, T.; Jåstad, A.; Cosma, A.; Colette, K.; Arnarsson, A.M. *Spotlight on Adolescent Health and Well-Being. Findings from the 2017/2018 Health Behaviour in School-Aged Children (HBSC) Survey in Europe and Canada. International Report*; World Health Organization Regional Office for Europe: Copenhagen, Denmark, 2020; ISBN 978-92-890-5500-0.

30. Bójko, M.; Dzielska, A.; Kleszczewska, D.; Kowalewska, A.; Korzycka, M.; Malinowka-Cieślik, M.; Małkowska-Szkutnik, A.; Mazur, A.; Oblacińska, A.; Ostręga, W.; et al. *Zdrowie Uczniów w 2018 Roku Na Tle Nowego Modelu Badań HBSC*; Instytut Matki i Dziecka: Warsaw, Poland, 2018; ISBN 978-83-951033-3-9.
31. Sun, Y.; Liu, Y.; Tao, F.B. Associations between Active Commuting to School, Body Fat, and Mental Well-being: Population-Based, Cross-Sectional Study in China. *J. Adolesc. Health* **2015**, *57*, 679–685. [CrossRef]
32. Waygood, E.O.D.; Friman, M.; Olsson, L.E.; Taniguchi, A. Transport and child well-being: An integrative review. *Travel Behav. Soc.* **2017**, *9*, 32–49. [CrossRef]
33. Roth, M.A.; Millett, C.J.; Mindell, J.S. The contribution of active travel (walking and cycling) in children to overall physical activity levels: A national cross sectional study. *Prev. Med.* **2012**, *54*, 134–139. [CrossRef]
34. Mandic, S.; Hopkins, D.; Bengoechea, E.; Moore, A.; Sandretto, S.; Coppell, K.; Ergler, C.; Keall, M.; Rolleston, A.; Kidd, G.; et al. Built environment changes and active transport to school among adolescents: BEATS Natural Experiment Study protocol. *BMJ Open* **2020**, *10*, e034899. [CrossRef]
35. Vanwolleghem, G.; Van Dyck, D.; De Meester, F.; De Bourdeaudhuij, I.; Cardon, G.; Gheysen, F. Which Socio-Ecological Factors Associate with a Switch to or Maintenance of Active and Passive Transport during the Transition from Primary to Secondary School? *PLoS ONE* **2016**, 11. [CrossRef]
36. Tabak, I.; Mazur, J. Social support and family communication as factors protecting adolescents against multiple recurrent health complaints related to school stress. *Dev. Period Med.* **2016**, *20*, 27–39.
37. Yang, Y.; Xue, H.; Liu, S.; Wang, Y. Is the decline of active travel to school unavoidable by-products of economic growth and urbanization in developing countries? *Sustain. Cities Soc.* **2019**, *47*, 101446. [CrossRef]
38. Salmon, J.; Timperio, A. Prevalence, trends and environmental influences on child and youth physical activity. *Med. Sport Sci.* **2007**, *50*, 183–199. [CrossRef]
39. Aibar, A.; Bois, J.E.; Generelo, E.; Bengoechea, E.G.; Paillard, T.; Zaragoza, J. Effect of Weather, School Transport, and Perceived Neighborhood Characteristics on Moderate to Vigorous Physical Activity Levels of Adolescents From Two European Cities. *Environ. Behav.* **2015**, *47*, 395–417. [CrossRef]
40. Potrebny, T.; Wiium, N.; Haugstvedt, A.; Sollesnes, R.; Torsheim, T.; Wold, B.; Thuen, F. Health complaints among adolescents in Norway: A twenty-year perspective on trends. *PLoS ONE* **2019**, *14*, e0210509. [CrossRef]
41. Haugland, S.; Wold, B. Subjective health complaints in adolescence–reliability and validity of survey methods. *J. Adolesc.* **2001**, *24*, 611–624. [CrossRef]
42. Leslie, E.; Kremer, P.; Toumbourou, J.W.; Williams, J.W. Gender differences in personal, social and environmental influences on active travel to and from school for Australian adolescents. *J. Sci. Med. Sport* **2010**, *13*, 597–601. [CrossRef]
43. Patnode, C.; Lytle, L.; Ericsson, D.; Sirard, J.; Barr-Anderso, D.; Story, M. The relative influence of demographic, individual, social, and environmental factors on physical activity among boys and girls. *Int. J. Behav. Nutr.* **2010**, *7*, 79. [CrossRef]
44. Larsen, K.; Buliung, R.N.; Faulkner, G. School travel route measurement and built environment effects in models of children's school travel behavior. *J. Transp. Land Use* **2015**, *9*, 5–23. [CrossRef]
45. Fang, K.; Handy, S. Skateboarding for transportation: Exploring the factors behind an unconventional mode choice among university skateboard commuters. *Transportation* **2019**, *46*, 263–283. [CrossRef]
46. Frazer, A.; Voss, C.; Winters, M.; Naylor, P.J.; Higgins, J.W.; McKay, H. Differences in adolescents' physical activity from school-travel between urban and suburban neighbourhoods in Metro Vancouver, Canada. *Prev. Med. Rep.* **2015**, *2*, 170–173. [CrossRef]
47. Mueller, N.; Rojas-Rueda, D.; Cole-Hunter, T.; de Nazelle, A.; Dons, E.; Gerike, R.; Götschi, T.; Int Panis, L.; Kahlmeier, S.; Nieuwenhuijsen, M. Health impact assessment of active transportation: A systematic review. *Prev. Med.* **2015**, *76*, 103–114. [CrossRef]

Publisher's Note: MDPI stays neutral with regard to jurisdictional claims in published maps and institutional affiliations.

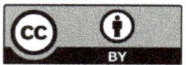

© 2020 by the authors. Licensee MDPI, Basel, Switzerland. This article is an open access article distributed under the terms and conditions of the Creative Commons Attribution (CC BY) license (http://creativecommons.org/licenses/by/4.0/).

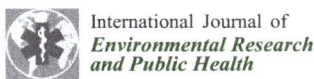 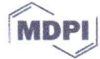

Article

The Association between the Regular Use of ICT Based Mobility Services and the Bicycle Mode Choice in Tehran and Cairo

Hamid Mostofi [1,*], Houshmand Masoumi [2,3] and Hans-Liudger Dienel [1]

[1] Mobility Research Cluster, Department of Work, Technology and Participation, Technische Universität Berlin, 10587 Berlin, Germany; hans-liudger.dienel@tu-berlin.de
[2] Center for Technology and Society, Technische Universität Berlin, 10623 Berlin, Germany; masoumi@ztg.tu-berlin.de
[3] Department of Transport and Supply Chain Management, College of Business and Economics, University of Johannesburg, Johannesburg 2006, South Africa
* Correspondence: mostofidarbani@tu-berlin.de

Received: 8 October 2020; Accepted: 23 November 2020; Published: 25 November 2020

Abstract: Regarding the sharp growth rate of ICT (information and communication technology)—based mobility services like ridesourcing, it is essential to investigate the impact of these new mobility services on the transport mode choices, particularly on active mobility modes like cycling. This impact is more important in the MENA context (the Middle East and North Africa), where cycling does not constitute the main mobility mode in the modal split of most MENA cities. This paper studies the relationship between the regular use of ICT-based mobility services like ridesourcing and the tendency to cycle to near destinations. This paper contains the analysis of 4431 interviews in two large cities of the MENA region (Cairo and Tehran). This research uses logistic regression to analyze and compare the odds of cycling among regular and non-regular users of ridesourcing by considering the socio-economic, land use, and perception variables. The findings indicate that the odds of cycling among the regular users of ridesourcing are 2.30 and 1.94 times greater than these odds among non-regular ridesourcing users in Tehran and Cairo, respectively. Therefore, the regular users of ridesourcing are more likely to cycle to their near destinations than non-regular ridesourcing users in these cities.

Keywords: ICT-based mobility services; cycling; the active mobility mode; nonmotorized mode choices; ridesourcing; ride hailing; MENA region

1. Introduction

Nonmotorized transport modes such as biking are sustainable modes in urban transportation systems, and are reliable and effective in terms of energy use and healthiness without environmental pollution [1–7]. In comparison to motorized modes, such as a private car, a bicycle is a cheaper door-to-door mobility mode. Moreover, compared to walking, urban biking is 3.6 times faster [8,9] and requires less energy (35% of the walking calories) for the same travel [10,11]. At this time, traffic congestion and environmental pollution are common in many cities worldwide due to high car dependency [12–14]. Therefore, cycling is a practical solution to reduce CO_2 emissions and help cities' sustainability in economic and social aspects [15–17]. Therefore, the international advice is to develop the bicycle's share in the cities' modal splits [18–21]. However, biking is not a substantial mode for daily travel purposes in some MENA cities, such as Cairo and Tehran, which is entirely different from the cycling mode share in European cities. For example, the share of biking is less than 1 percent in the modal split in Iranian cities [22]. However, cycling constitutes around 40 percent of daily trips in bicycle-friendly cities in Europe, such as Copenhagen and Amsterdam [23]. Some studies indicate different reasons for the low cycling rate in Tehran and Cairo, such as car-oriented urban forms, topographic conditions, sociocultural attitudes (women rarely use bikes), and the lack of suitable infrastructure [24–28]. Moreover, ICT (information and communication technology) has considerably affected the urban mobility system, as it offers real-time trip information, sourcing, and communication instruments between service providers and users. Moreover, the ICT-based mobility services have been developed very fast, such as online ridesharing and sourcing modes, in which services information technologies are the major component. The ICTs have also changed the concepts of distance, accessibility, and individual lifestyles, which consequently have a potential influence on mobility behaviors, particularly nonmotorized mode choice [29–32]. This influence is gaining more importance in the cities where the share of nonmotorized modes is low.

This study investigates the association between the regular usage of ICT-based mobility services such as ridesourcing and the cycling mode choice in Tehran and Cairo. The primary assumption of this research is related to the principle that the frequent usage of one mobility mode affects other mode choices [33]. We conducted 4431 face-to-face interviews in Cairo and Tehran in 2017. Among ICT-based mobility services, such as online car-sharing and bike-sharing, this study focuses only on the online ridesourcing platforms because there was no considerable online bike and car-sharing in these two cities in 2017. Ridesourcing is a door-to-door mobility service in which commuters and drivers interact through ICT and GPS platforms, such as Uber and Lyft in many western countries, "Careem" in Cairo, and "Snapp" in Tehran [34]. As commuters are able to "source" a ride from a pool of drivers by ICT-based platforms, this mobility service is named ridesourcing [35]. Passengers use their smartphone apps to book, pay, and rate the quality of the services. In the MENA countries, ridesourcing has seen a sharp growth rate among other mobility modes.

Regarding the Uber report, Egypt is the biggest market of this company in the MENA region, with 157,000 drivers and 4 million users in 2017 [36]. The first ridesourcing company in Iran was Snapp, established in 2014 with a growth rate of 70% per month, with a big network of 120,000 active drivers to give services to 0.5 million users in 2016 [37,38]. These figures show the rapid growth of these new emerging travel modes in Tehran and Cairo, and indicate a potential impact on these cities' mode choice behaviors.

Ridesourcing Adaptation and Biking Mode Choice

It is necessary to study whether ICT-based mobility services support or compete with sustainable modes like cycling, in order to evaluate their role in the sustainability of urban transport systems [39–41]. There is a debate around ridesourcing that it encourages commuters to shift from sustainable mobility modes, like nonmotorized modes, to car travels. Regarding the findings in the global north, the adoption rate of ridesourcing is remarkably higher among young people with higher incomes and educational degrees [42,43]. Moreover, Alemi et al. (2017) mentioned a positive correlation between ridesourcing usage and the regular use of smartphones for daily activities such as shopping, entertainment, and travel [42]. Feigon and Murphy (2018) reported that ridesourcing was used for an average travel distance of between three and six kilometers in five American cities [44], indicating its possible impact on the cycling mode choice. Alemi et al. (2018) showed that due to the ridesourcing adaptation, the younger generation decreased their nonmotorized mobility choices, such as walking and biking, more so than the older people [42]. Gehrke et al. (2019) indicated the high probability of a modal shift from walking and cycling to near destinations or under poor weather conditions to ridesourcing in Boston [45]. Becker et al. (2017) mentioned that although ridesourcing can fill gaps in the public transport network, in many situations, it decreases public transport usage and nonmotorized modes, which indicates a substitution impact in favor of car dependency [46]. Circella et al. (2018) mentioned that around 40% of ridesourcing users have decreased their walking and biking, while 10% of users have increased these nonmotorized modes in California [47]. On the other hand, ridesourcing services in some countries provide more motorized mobility options for disabled people with health issues, by employing trained drivers to help passengers with walkers, wheelchairs, and other equipment [39,48].

2. Materials and Methods

This research includes 3 main research questions: (1) Are the socio-economic variables of the respondents who use bicycles significantly different from those who do not use this mode? (2) Is there a significant association between regular ridesourcing use and the odds of cycling? (3) what are the main subjective barriers and reasons for not cycling among regular ridesourcing users?

We conducted a large sample size of face-to-face interviews in Cairo and Tehran in different neighborhoods to answer these three questions. Regarding the literature review about the urban forms in Cairo and Tehran, the compactness, population density, urban forms, and road network forms in these two cities have correlations with the periods of urban construction and development [49]. The newly developed neighborhoods are centerless and have less population density and compactness than older neighborhoods in Tehran and Cairo. As such, we chose six neighborhoods in each city in three different urban forms (two neighborhoods in each urban form) to gather adequate samples. These three different urban forms are traditional parts (historical), transitional parts (in between), and newly developed parts. The traditional (historical) neighborhoods in both cities are discernible center with high density and compact urban forms. Transitional neighborhoods were constructed from 1930 till 1980 with lower density and compactness than the old parts. The new parts, which were developed after 1980, are centerless neighborhoods and are located in the peripheral parts of Tehran and Cairo. The interviewers conducted face-to-face interviews with the residents of these neighborhoods who were selected randomly in 2017. The total observations are 4431 interviews for these two cities, including 2369 interviews in Tehran and 2062 interviews in Cairo.

Many studies reported that the cycling mode choice has an association with age [49–51], socio-economic parameters, road network and land use parameters [52,53], the safety of cycling paths with physical separation from the motorized network [54], efficient facilities [55,56], and the gently graded topography of cities [57]. Therefore, we designed three main sections in the questionnaire, which are (1) socio-economic variables, (2) mobility behavior variables, and (3) the land use parameters of the neighborhood. The socio-economic factors included gender, age, monthly household expenditure and income, car ownership, and having a driving license. The variable of car ownership is a binary variable, which indicates whether the household has at least one car or not. The variable of possession of a driving license is also a binary variable, indicating whether the respondent has a driving license or not. The economic factors of income and monthly expenses were assessed in Egyptian pound (the Egyptian currency) and Iranian rial (Iranian currency).

2.1. The Mobility Behavior Variables

The mobility behavior section includes questions in two main subsections, which are the main modes for common daily travel purposes and the tendency towards cycling to near destinations. The regular trip purposes include study or work trips and non-work/study trips within and out of the respondents' neighborhoods. We defined a binary variable, "ridesourcing use", to study the impact of ridesourcing adaptation as the main mode on the tendency to cycle. This variable categorizes the interviewees into 2 groups: (1) regular users; (2) non-regular users. The regular users of ridesourcing are defined as the commuters who frequently use ridesourcing as the major mobility mode for a minimum of one of their daily trip purposes. The non-regular users are the commuters who do not use and adopt ridesourcing as their major mobility mode for their everyday trip purposes. Therefore, "ridesourcing use" is a dichotomized variable that is collectively exhaustive and mutually exclusive. Therefore, this variable classified all observations of the Tehran and Cairo samples into 2 classes, and these two classes do not have the same observation.

In the second subsection, the respondents answered whether they cycle to a near destination inside their neighborhood. This question aims to capture the tendency of respondents to cycle inside their neighborhoods to a destination that is near based on their subjective perception of distance. Therefore, in this question, we did not mention the distance in meters or kilometers. We mentioned the term of "near destination" to understand whether the respondent tends to cycle even to a destination that he/she perceives as a near destination. The dichotomized variable is defined as "bicycle use for a near destination," coded 1 and 0 for the yes and no responses, respectively. Additionally, the respondents were asked about their main reason for not cycling to near destinations. The respondents could only choose one major reason for the multiple-choice question. These options were designed in the present form to collect subjective reasons for not cycling. This question asks for the interviewees' perceptions about cycling to a near destination. We designed the answers to this multiple-choice question following the review of research and reports about cycling barriers in the MENA cities [58–63]. The options include four factors, which are (1) cultural and social problems, (2) lack of biking facilities, (3) disabled/too old, (4) takes too much time/it is slow.

2.2. The Land Use Parameters of the Neighborhood

Regarding the role of the land use and road network factors in the tendency to cycle, two parameters were measured, indicating the neighborhoods' connectivity. These parameters are "link–node ratio (%)" and "intersection density". Link–node ratio (%) is the number of links (street segments) divided by nodes (street intersections) within the 600 m catchment of every interviewee's house. A bigger link–node ratio indicates the greater connectivity of the road network in the interviewee's neighborhood. This parameter illustrates how many possible routes there are in the neighborhood per each node for cycling. However, the link–node ratio is unrelated to the size of the intersections or blocks [64]. Intersection density (nodes/ha is the sum of intersections per unit area in a 600 m catchment area of the interviewee's house) is related to the size of blocks in a neighborhood [65]. The bigger intersection density suggests more connectivity in a neighborhood because of the smaller blocks and the shorter cycling distances inside this neighborhood. The full details of the neighborhood characteristics in this survey were published [66].

2.3. Analysis Methods

2.3.1. Comparison of the Demographic Variables

We compared the socio-economic parameters of two groups of respondents who use bicycles and who do not use this mode for a near destination in the samples of Cairo and Tehran. First, the Kolmogorov–Smirnov test was applied to check whether the distribution of the continuous socio-economic variables is normal. The result indicates a p-value less than 0.001 for the variables of age, monthly household income, and monthly household living costs, indicating their distributions are not normal. Therefore, we applied nonparametric tests, such as the Mann–Whitney U test and the median test, to evaluate whether the differences in the distribution and median of the mentioned continuous variables are significant across the binary variable (bicycle use) at the confidence level of 95%. The H_0 of the Mann–Whitney U test indicates that the distribution of each socio-economic variable is the same between two values of the binary variable "bike use". The H_0 of the median test assumes that the continuous variable has a similar median between two groups of respondents who ride a bicycle and do not ride it for a near destination. Regarding gender and household car ownership variables, the hypotheses are defined for each variable about the significant correlation between bicycle use and gender variables. We applied the Chi-square test to test this hypothesis at a confidence level of 95%.

2.3.2. Association between Frequent Ridesourcing Use and Odds of Cycling

We used binary logit models (logistic regression) to compare the probability of cycling between regular and non-regular users of ridesourcing in each sample of these MENA cities at significance levels of 0.05. The odds of bicycle use for a near destination are the probability of cycling over the probability of not cycling, which are response variables in the logit models. The transformation from probability to odds is monotonous, indicating the odds increase (decrease) as the probability increases (decrease). The binary logit model is structured by the equations below, where P is the probability of cycling to

a near destination, $1 - P$ is the probability of not cycling, β_0 is the constant, and β_i is the coefficient related to each explanatory variable.

$$ln\left(\frac{P}{1 - P}\right) = \beta_0 + \beta_1 x_1 + \beta_2 x_2 + \beta_3 x_3 + \ldots + \beta_n \tag{1}$$

$$P = \frac{e^{(\beta_0 + \beta_1 x_1 + \ldots + \beta_n x_n)}}{1 + e^{(\beta_0 + \beta_1 x_1 + \ldots + \beta_n x_n)}} \tag{2}$$

The logistic model reveals the effects of the independent variables on the odds of bike use (probability of bike use/probability of no bike use). The exponentiated coefficient changes the cycling odds to a unit increase in the independent variable by holding other regressors constant. Suppose the odds ratio of an independent variable is greater than 1. In that case, it is suggested that by keeping other regressors constant, the odds of bike use increase (decrease) by increasing (decreasing) this independent variable. If the odds ratio is 1 for an estimator, it suggests that this estimator's change does not change the cycling odds. When the odds ratio of one estimator is less than 1, it indicates a decrease in biking odds caused by an increase in this estimator if other independent variables are constant. Some transport studies estimate the odds ratio to show the impacts of the explanatory variables on the odds of mode choices. However, the estimation of average marginal effects is an intuitive technique and a useful way to directly explain the probability changes and interpret the results of the estimations more understandably. The logistic regression is nonlinear; therefore, the effect of one unit change in an explanatory variable is averaged over all observations to estimate the average marginal effects. The average marginal effects of an independent variable are the average change in probability of the dependent variable when the given independent variable changes by one unit and the other is constant. We used the add-on package "margins" in R to calculate the average marginal effects. Therefore, in addition to the odds ratio, we also report the average marginal effects of each explanatory variable.

We checked the risk of multicollinearity among the independent variables of one pair or more of explanatory variables being highly correlated together and causing unreliable estimations. The regressors were selected to avoid high multicollinearity among variables and to control confounding effects. Therefore, the regressors (independent variables) in the logistic regression are regular ridesourcing, household car ownership, gender, age, monthly household income, intersection density, and link–node ratio. Checking the correlation matrix might be useful in order to detect multicollinearity, but it is not enough. The sufficient diagnostics are performed by linear regression between the variables to check the variance inflation factor (VIF), tolerance, and the condition index. If the correlation coefficient among two independent variables is greater than 0.90, it indicates a high multicollinearity risk in the logit model [67,68]. We checked the correlation matrix, and we did not find a correlation greater than 0.8 for both samples of Cairo and Tehran. Furthermore, we performed the linear regression among the different combinations of explanatory variables and then checked the VIF, tolerance, and condition index. The VIF for an estimator in the regression model is the ratio of the variance of the overall model to the variance of a model that includes only the given estimator. Hair et al. (2010) indicated that if the VIF is greater than 5, there is a concern for multicollinearity among independent variables [68]. As we checked the VIFs for different combinations of the estimators, the VIFs of all estimators in the combination of regular ridesourcing, household car ownership, gender, age, income, intersection density and link–node ratio are less than 4.0 in both the Cairo and Tehran models. Then, we checked the tolerances of the mentioned variables, which is the amount of variability in one estimator that is not explained by the other estimators. Tolerance values less than 0.2 indicate the risk of multicollinearity among estimators. Having checked the tolerance values for the mentioned independent variables, all of them were bigger than 0.3, indicating the low risk of multicollinearity. Moreover, we checked the condition indices. Condition indices above 15 indicate a risk of multicollinearity. The estimated condition indices were below 15 in the linear regressions among the aforementioned estimators. Moreover, we checked the interactions between the variables, such as monthly household income–age, monthly household income–gender and gender–age, in the two logit models of Cairo and Teheran, and estimated their coefficients. The coefficients of the interaction terms between these variables were not significant at the 95% confidence level in the models of both cities. For example, the coefficient of the interaction age–monthly household income has a Wald chi-square = 2.610, and a p-value = 0.106 in the Tehran model, and a Wald chi-square = 0.364 and p-value = 0.547 in the Cairo model. Therefore, we did not consider the interaction terms between the variables in either model. We applied the Omnibus test to check if the regression model with estimators is an improvement of the baseline model without estimators. Moreover, the Hosmer and Lemeshow test was applied to check if the regression result was correctly specified, and the results were appropriately fitted to the observed data. If the p-value of the Hosmer and Lemeshow test is less than 0.05, it suggests a significant difference between the observed values and the model's estimated values [69].

3. Results

3.1. Demographic Profile

Among the 2062 interviews in Cairo, 224 respondents mentioned that they use a bicycle for a near destination, and this result for Tehran is 254 out of 2369 interviews. Table 1 shows the socio-economic parameters, including age, gender, household income, household living cost and household car ownership, for the two groups of respondents who use and do not use a bike for a near destination in Tehran and Cairo.

The Chi-square test suggests significant associations ($p < 0.001$) between the variables of "bicycle use for a near destination" and household car ownership and gender in the Cairo sample. This means that men are substantially more likely to cycle to a near destination than women in Cairo. Moreover, 58.5% of bike users and 70.5% of non-bike users have at least one household car, which indicates a different rate in car ownership among users and non-users of bikes in Cairo. Furthermore, the Mann–Whitney U test indicates a significant association between bike use and age at the 99% confidence level. Furthermore, the median test suggests that the medians of age are different across bike users and non-users for a near destination at the 0.05 level ($p < 0.05$). The mean and median of bike riders' age are 25.6 and 24.0, respectively, which indicates they are significantly younger than non-bike riders in the Cairo sample.

The medians and the Mann–Whitney U tests do not reject the H_0 (null hypotheses) for the variables of monthly household income and living costs across variables of bike use in the Cairo sample. This means that there are no significantly different distributions and medians in monthly household living expenses and income between bike users and non-users.

In the Tehran sample, the Chi-square test indicates a significant association at the 0.001 level among the variables of gender and bike use. This suggests that men cycle considerably more than women in Tehran. The Mann–Whitney U test rejects the null hypothesis for age at the 99% confidence level, which is similar to the result of this test in the Cairo sample. Furthermore, the median test reveals that the median age is significantly different across users and non-users of bikes. Therefore, the respondents who tend to use bikes to travel to a near destination are significantly younger than those who do not have this tendency. Moreover, these tests do not reject the H_0 for the variables of monthly household income and living expenses across users and non-users of bikes at the 0.05 level in the Tehran sample. Therefore, like the Cairo sample, these two tests indicate that the monthly household living costs and income are not significantly different between the users and non-users of bikes.

Table 1. The socio-economic parameters in the Tehran and Cairo samples.

Do You Use Bicycle for a Near Destination?		Tehran						Cairo					
		No		Yes				No		Yes			
		N	%	N	%			N	%	N	%		
Gender	Female	1242	52.4%	38	15.0%			887	42.9%	29	12.9%		
	Male	1128	47.6%	216	85.0%			1181	57.1%	195	87.1%		
Age group	<25	348	14.7%	91	35.8%			502	24.3%	111	49.6%		
	25 ≤ age < 45	1246	52.6%	121	47.6%			1008	48.7%	98	43.8%		
	45 ≤ age < 60	550	23.2%	34	13.4%			416	20.1%	13	5.8%		
	60≤	226	9.5%	8	3.1%			142	6.9%	2	0.9%		
Having driving license	No	569	24.0%	81	31.9%			1095	53.0%	131	58.4%		
	Yes	1801	76.0%	173	68.1%			973	47.00%	93	41.6%		
Having household car	Yes	2118	89.4%	209	82.3%			1457	70.5%	131	58.5%		
	No	252	10.6%	45	17.7%			611	29.5%	93	41.5%		
		Mean	Median	Mean	Median			Mean	Median	Mean	Median		
Age		38.76	37.00	31.35	28.00			35.96	33.00	26.56	25.00		
Household income (Euros) [1]		1315.99	1169.00	1435.61	1169.00			7143.68	6000.00	6918.42	5000.00		
Household income (country currency)		55,271,580 [3]	49,098,000 [3]	60,295,620 [3]	49,098,000 [3]			150,017.28 [2]	126,000 [2]	145,286.82 [2]	105,000 [2]		
Monthly living cost (Euros) [1]		1048.36	935.00	1302.18	935.00			6401.05	5500.00	6192.66	5000.00		
Monthly living cost (country currency)		44,031,120 [3]	39,270,000 [3]	54,691,560 [3]	39,270,000 [3]			134,422.05 [2]	1,155,000 [2]	130,045.86 [2]	105,000 [2]		

[1] The amount is converted into EUR based on the central bank's exchange rates in 2017 in Egypt and Iran, [2] Egyptian pound (Egyptian currency), [3] Iranian rial (Iranian Currency).

3.2. The Logit Models for Cycling to a Near Destination

The logistic regression model is used to compare the odds of bike use between regular ridesourcing users and the non-regular users for each sample of Cairo and Tehran. For the categorical variable of ridesourcing use, we defined the non-regular ridesourcing user as the reference mode in the logistic regression. The Omnibus test shows a significant difference at the 0.001 level between the log-likelihoods of the model with estimators and the baseline model (without estimators), with Chi-square values of 233.955 and 274.906 for the samples of Cairo and Tehran, respectively.

The Hosmer and Lemeshow test indicates that the goodness of fit for both the Cairo and Tehran models is appropriate. The *p*-value of this test is 0.773 for the Cairo sample and 0.092 for the Tehran sample. Table 2 shows the Omnibus test results, the Hosmer and Lemeshow test, and the Nagelkerke R squared for the logistic regressions. The coefficients of estimators are shown in Tables 3 and 4 for Tehran and Cairo samples, respectively.

Table 2. The results of the Omnibus test and the Hosmer and Lemeshow test for biking.

Tests	Cairo	Tehran
Omnibus Tests of Model Coefficients		
Chi-square	233.955	274.906
p-value	<0.001	<0.001
−2 Log likelihood	1121.058	1281.290
Nagelkerke R Square	0.221	0.224
Hosmer and Lemeshow Test		
Chi-square	4.850	13.645
p-value	0.773	0.092

Table 3. Binary logit regression for cycling to near destination in Tehran.

Tehran		B	S.E.	Wald	AME	S.E.	Sig.	Exp(B)
Ridesourcing use	Regular users = 1 Non-regulars = 0	0.833	0.373	4.892	0.0605	0.0276	0.026	2.301
Gender	Female = 1. Male = 0	−2.057	0.196	110.183	−0.1494	0.0171	<0.001	0.128
Monthly household Income	Iranian rial	0.000	0.000	2.8614	0.000	0.000	0.091	1.000
Having a household car	No = 1. Yes = 0	0.324	0.217	2.227	0.0236	0.0155	0.136	1.383
Age	Year	−0.058	0.006	84.497	−0.0042	0.0005	<0.001	0.944
Link–node ratio	%	0.025	0.005	24.597	0.0018	0.0004	<0.001	1.025
Intersection density	Node/hectare	0.130	0.044	8.495	0.0094	0.0032	0.004	1.138
Constant		−4.123	0.927	19.801			<0.001	0.016

AME: Average Marginal Effects, S.E.: Standard Error.

Tehran's model suggests three significant variables with a *p*-value < 0.001 level—gender, age, and link–node ratio. The model also indicates that the ridesourcing use and intersection density variables are significant at levels 0.05 and 0.01, respectively. As "ridesourcing use" is a binary variable, its exponentiated coefficient shows the odds ratio of cycling for regular users relative to the non-regular ridesourcing users. The odds of cycling for the regular ridesourcing users are 2.30 times more than these odds for non-regular users, when fixing all other regressors as constant. The average marginal effects of ridesourcing use indicate that being regular users of ridesourcing services increases the probability of cycling to a near destination by 6.0%. Therefore, the results reveal that regular ridesourcing users are more likely to cycle to a near destination than non-regular users. The marginal effects of gender indicate that the cycling probability of women is 14.9% less than men. Moreover, the model suggests that the odds of biking for women are 87% less than for men with the same other independent variables. Each unit increase of link–node ratio (percent) raises the odds of cycling by 2.5% and the cycling probability by 0.2%. Each unit increase in intersection density (node/hectare) increases biking odds by 13.8% and biking probability by around 1%. Therefore, Tehranians living in a neighborhood with better intersection density and node–link ratio are more likely to cycle to a near destination. The model of

Tehran indicates that the odds ratio and average marginal effects of age are 0.94 and −0.004, respectively. Therefore, a one-year increase in age decreases the biking odds by 6% and the biking probability by 0.4%. This means younger citizens are more likely to bike than older citizens in Tehran.

Table 4. Binary logit regression for cycling to near destination in Cairo.

Cairo		B	S.E.	Wald	AME	S.E.	Sig.	Exp(B)
Ridesourcing use	Regular users = 1 Non-regulars = 0	0.663	0.302	4.815	0.0531	0.0234	0.028	1.940
Gender	Female = 1, Male = 0	−1.991	0.221	81.261	−0.1542	0.0172	<0.001	0.137
Monthly household Income	Egyptian pound	0.000	0.000	0.003	0.000	0.000	0.953	1.000
Having a household car	No = 1, Yes = 0	0.894	0.181	24.431	0.0692	0.0139	<0.001	2.445
Age	Year	−0.08	0.009	81.777	−0.0062	0.0007	<0.001	0.924
Link–node ratio	%	0.010	0.008	1.721	0.0008	0.0006	0.190	1.010
Intersection density	Node/hectare	−0.026	0.061	0.188	−0.0020	0.0047	0.665	0.974
Constant		−1.130	1.402	0.633			0.426	0.323

AME: Average Marginal Effects, S.E.: Standard Error.

Table 4 illustrates the binary logit regression for Cairo with three statistically significant variables at the significant level of 0.001: household car ownership, gender, and age. Furthermore, the variable ridesourcing is significant at the 0.05 level. The model shows that the cycling odds for the regular ridesourcing users are 1.94 times greater than non-regular users by controlling for other independent variables. Moreover, the average marginal effects of regular ridesourcing are 5.3%. This result suggests that regular users are more likely to cycle to a near destination than non-regular users of ridesourcing. This result is similar to the Tehran sample, whereby regular users of ridesourcing are also more likely to use bikes than non-regular users. Like the Tehran model, the average marginal effects of gender are −15.4%, and the odds of biking for women are 86% less than these odds for men, with the same values for the other regressors. Moreover, the people who do not have a household car have biking odds 2.44 times and a biking probability 7.0% greater than those who have at least one household car. The model indicates that the odds ratio of biking and the average marginal effects of age are 0.92 and −0.006, respectively. The increase of one year in age decreases the cycling odds by 8%, and its probability by 0.6%. Therefore, older citizens are less likely to cycle than younger ones. Moreover, the model suggests that the coefficients of the variables income, intersection density, and link–node ratio are not significant at the 95% confidence level. Therefore, the binary logistic regression results reveal that these variables do not contribute to the estimation of the odds and probability of cycling to a near destination, and the other variables have a more significant influence on the tendency to cycle in the Cairo sample.

3.3. Reasons for Not Cycling

We asked about subjective barriers to and reasons for not cycling to a near destination in the interviews in Cario and Tehran. The form of this question is multiple-choice, but the respondents should choose only one reason out of the four reasons, which are (1) cultural and social problems, (2) lack of biking facilities, (3) being disabled or too old, and (4) it is slow or takes too much time. We asked this question in the present form to collect subjective reasons correlated with the way citizens decide about not cycling to near destinations in their neighborhoods. The subjective reasons are usually highly correlated together and constitute a package of factors for mode choice. However, we asked respondents to choose one reason in order to find the dominant and major subjective obstacle to cycling. This question type might be useful for urban planners to understand which problems are more influential on the tendency of citizens toward cycling. For example, suppose the cycling facilities in a neighborhood are improved. In that case, the person who mentioned "lack of biking facilities" as the main reason for not cycling is more likely to cycle than the person who replied "being disable or too old" as the main reason for not biking. Social and cultural problems address social barriers to cycling for women in public spaces, inconvenience during cycling in public areas, and fear of harassment. The answer "lack of biking facilities" indicates the lack of bicycle infrastructures like bike lanes, excluding motorized modes in the road network and public shared bikes. The findings are presented in Figures 1 and 2 for regular and non-regular users of ridesourcing in both cities. Figures 3 and 4 illustrate the reasons for not cycling among female and male respondents in Tehran and Cairo.

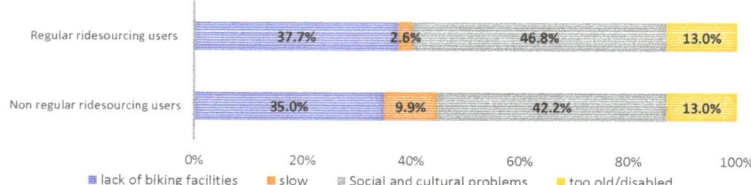

Figure 1. Reasons for not cycling among regular and non-regular ridesourcing users in the Tehran sample.

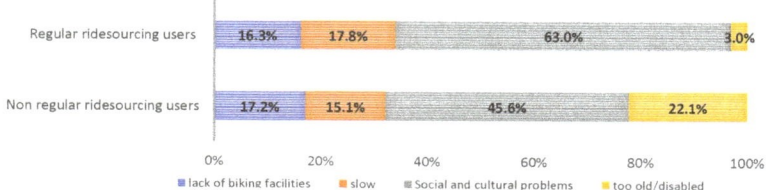

Figure 2. Reasons for not cycling among regular and non-regular ridesourcing users in the Cairo sample.

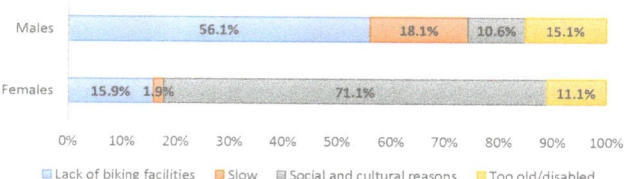

Figure 3. Reasons for not cycling among female and male respondents in the Tehran sample.

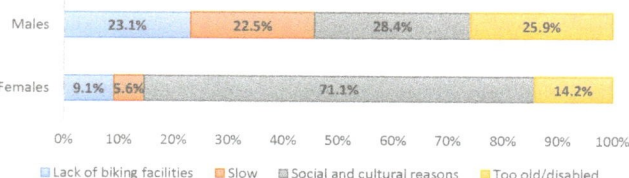

Figure 4. Reasons for not cycling among female and male respondents in the Cairo sample.

The results of this question in the Tehran sample indicate that the major reasons for regular ridesourcing users not cycling are "social and cultural problems" and "lack of cycling facilities", which 46.8% and 37.7% of regular users mentioned, respectively. These two reasons were also selected more than the other reasons by the non-regular users in this sample. This finding indicates that the perceptions of social and cultural problems and the lack of cycling facilities are the main reasons for regular and non-regular ridesourcing users not cycling to a nearby destination in Tehran. Moreover, Figure 3 shows that 71.1% of female respondents who do not cycle indicate the social and cultural problem as their main reason for not cycling in Tehran. However, 10.6% of male respondents mentioned the social and cultural problems as their major reason for not cycling. Therefore, Figure 3 shows that the social and cultural problems are substantial barriers for women wishing to cycle in Tehran.

In Cairo, the major reasons of regular ridesourcing users for not cycling are "social and cultural problems" (63%), "It is slow/takes too much time" (17.8%), and "the lack of biking facilities" (16.3%). The non-regular users reasoned "social and cultural problems", "too old or disabled", and "the lack of biking facilities", with 45.6%, 22.1%, and 17.2%, respectively.

Figure 4 indicates that 71% of female respondents in the Cairo sample mentioned the social and cultural problems as their main reason for not cycling, while 28.4% of males cited this option as their major reason. Therefore, as in the Tehran sample, social and cultural problems are significant barriers against women cycling. Moreover, the reason "the lack of biking facilities" was mentioned by the regular users in Tehran almost two times more than these users in Cairo. Furthermore, 13% of regular users in Tehran stated the reason "too old/disabled," which is noticeably more than Cairene regular users (3%), and is the lowest observed reason in the Cairo sample.

4. Discussion

We used large samples in Cairo (2062 interviews) and Tehran (2369 interviews) to study the effect of the frequent use of ICT-based mobility services on the tendency toward bike use. The findings show that a low percentage of the respondents use bikes for a near destination, which is 10.9% in Tehran and 10.7% in Cairo. This result confirms the other research's conclusion that bicycles are not a substantial mobility mode in Tehran and Cairo [22,25,26,28,70,71]. Therefore, our findings show that bicycles' share in the modal split of these cities is lower than in most western countries, such as in Europe [23,24,72]. As such, our findings emphasize the necessity of raising public awareness about the social and health benefits of cycling, as well as the improvement of the bike facilities to encourage citizens to use this mobility mode more.

4.1. The Relationship between the Tendency toward Biking and Frequent Ridesourcing Use

Regarding the growing share of ICT-based mobility modes, such as ridesourcing, it is necessary to investigate the impact of these new emerging transport services on mobility behaviors. This effect on the bike mode choice is particularly important in the MENA region, which has a low share in the cities' modal mobility split. However, the studies in this field often come from western countries, while there is little research in developing countries like the MENA region. Moreover, with the emergence and rapid rise of ridesourcing in the modal split of MENA cities, it is essential to analyze the impacts of this new mobility mode on people's mode choice behaviors in this region. Cairo and Tehran are the two largest cities in this region, with similarities in urban development in recent years. The development of urban forms in both cities is more car-oriented rather than sustainable mobility modes-oriented. Moreover, transportation network companies launched their services in a similar period with the same growth rate. Therefore, we studied the impacts of ridesourcing on citizens' bike mode choices in these two cities as a case study in the MENA region. Among ICT-based mobility services, such as ridesourcing, online car and bike sharing, we focused on ridesourcing to study the correlation between the regular use of this mobility mode and bike use for near destinations in Tehran and Cairo. Other ICT-based mobility modes have not been developed enough to be considered in these two cities' modal splits. Some western studies investigated the modal shift from active mobility modes like cycling to ridesourcing by counterfactual questions in their interviews and questionnaires [35,42–44,73,74]. These counterfactual questions ask, "what would you have done if ridesourcing services had not been available?". The interviewees should think about a manipulated memory to answer this kind of question. However, this study categorized the respondents into the two groups of regular ridesourcing users who adopt ridesourcing for their everyday trip purposes and non-regular ridesourcing users. Then, we studied their current tendency toward cycling to a near destination via the question framed in the present tense, intended as the think-forward question, "Do you use a bike for a near destination?".

Thus, we analyzed the association between the frequent use of ridesourcing and present tendency towards cycling, instead of the past modal shift among these mobility modes.

We applied binary logistic regressions to analyze the association between frequent ridesourcing use and the odds of biking to near destinations. The results revealed that the odds of cycling for the frequent ridersourcing users are 2.30 (in Tehran) and 1.94 times (in Cairo) more than these odds for non-regular users. Furthermore, the average marginal effects of being a regular ridesourcing user are 6.0 and 5.3% in the models of Tehran and Cairo, respectively. This means that in these cities, people who have adopted ICT mobility modes, such as ridesourcing, as their major mobility mode are more likely to cycle to a near destination than the non-regular users of ridesourcing. This result is in contrast to some western studies that suggest frequent ridesourcing use has a negative association with biking. For example, 40% of regular ridesourcing users in Californian reported that they decreased cycling [47].

Moreover, the studies in American cities reported a substitution of active modes, such as biking, in the range of 9% and 13% of total ridesourcing trips in San Francisco, Boston, and Denver [35,45,73]. Moreover, a similar study in Chinese cities reported that 6.5% of ridesourcing users reduced walking and biking in the Chinese cities [75]. The finding of this paper, that in Tehran and Cairo, where cycling does not constitute a considerable travel mode, the adaptation of ridesourcing has a positive association with the likelihood of cycling, is important. It shows that the regular users of ridesourcing who adopt information technologies in their mobility modes tend toward cycling more than non-regular ridesourcing. Therefore, this finding indicates the potential for online-based bike-sharing services in Tehran and Cairo because the people who regularly use online-based ridesourcing also might use more online bike-sharing for their near destinations in these two cities.

4.2. Socio-Economic Variables

The associations between the socio-economic parameters and bike use for a near destination were studied in Tehran and Cairo. The findings indicate that women are significantly less likely to cycle to a near destination than men in both cities. Other transport studies also confirm this result in the MENA region, finding that women do not use bicycles because of cultural and social problems [71,76–78]. However, in the high cycling countries, such as Belgium and the Netherlands, women within the 20–65 age group use bicycles more than men [79,80]. Moreover, the findings indicate that younger people tend to use bikes more than older citizens in both cities, which is similar to the findings of studies in western countries such as the UK [81,82] and the MENA region [78]. Although many studies indicate the important role of cycling and its health benefits for the older ages [65], our findings showed that older people have a significantly lower tendency to cycle. Although the association between biking and aging might be negative in higher cycling countries, the share of cycle traveling in the older age groups is high. For example, cycling decreases with aging in Denmark, but still, among people who are 70–74 years old, cycling constitutes 12% of all their travels, which is similar among Germans who are 65 and older. Moreover, Dutch people over 65 years old make 24% of all their trips by bike [65].

Additionally, the logistic regression results indicate that Cairenes who have at least one household car are significantly less likely to use a bike for a near destination than those who do not have household cars. This finding is similar to studies in some American cities [83]. However, the Tehran model does not suggest a significant association between the probability of biking and car ownership, which is similar to the findings of Fishman et al. (2013) and Carse et al. (2013) [84,85]. In addition, the logit models of the Tehran and Cairo samples do not indicate a significant coefficient for the variable of income at the 95% confidence level. Moreover, the Mann–Whitney U and median test results do not show significant differences in the distributions and medians of monthly household incomes and living expenses among users and non-users of bikes. Therefore, these findings indicate that a tendency towards cycling does not have a significant association with the incomes of citizens in Cairo and Tehran.

4.3. Impact of Land Use Parameters

We used two land use parameters to analyze the correlation between the connectivity of neighborhoods and the tendency towards cycling among regular and non-regular users of ridesourcing. Tehran's binary logit model reveals that the connectivity variables have significant odds ratios bigger than 1, which are 1.138 and 1.025 for intersection density and link–node ratio, respectively. In other words, by improving the connectivity of the neighborhoods, Tehranians are more likely to cycle to close destinations inside their neighborhoods. This result is the same in the related studies in both the western context [86–89] and the MENA context [56,90], which indicated that increasing the connectivity of neighborhoods increases the nonmotorized mode choices, such as bicycles, which promote physical activity. However, these land use variables do not have significant odds ratios in the Cairo logit regression. As such, the Cairo model shows that the probability of biking to a near destination is more associated with the other parameters, such as gender, age, and household car ownership. In other words, because of the impacts of the other factors, the probability of cycling in neighborhoods with good connectivity is not significantly different from the neighborhoods with low link–node ratio and intersection density. This finding is similar to some studies in the western context [60] and the MENA cities [91,92], indicating that other parameters such as social and cultural factors have more substantial effects than land use factors (i.e., connectivity) on nonmotorized mode choices such as cycling.

Moreover, some studies indicate the important role of terrain slope and the elevation profile of cities in their citizens' cycling behaviors and mode choices [93–95]. The average terrain slope, which is calculated in percentage, has a negative correlation with the tendency to cycle [96]. If the slope of a road is more 3%, it is not convenient to cycle and control bikes, and consequently, the citizens are less likely to cycle in this condition. [97]. In Tehran, the slope direction decreases from the north to the south, which means the ground height reduces gradually from the north to the south of Tehran. Regarding the topographic studies in Tehran, most areas have a slope between 0 and 3%, and some small residential districts in the north of this city have a slope of more than 3% [97]. Therefore, for most parts of Tehran (except some districts in the north part), the steep slopes of roads are not major barriers for cycling. Two high plateaus surround Cairo in the east and the west. According to the topographic studies in Egypt, Cairo's average terrain slope is below that of the most bicycle-friendly cities in the world [98]. Therefore, the average terrain slope of the neighborhoods does not make a problem for cycling in Cairo.

4.4. Reasons for Not Cycling

The most observed reasons for Tehranian regular ridesourcing users not cycling are "social and cultural problems" and "lack of biking facilities". In the Cairo sample, the main excuses of regular ridesourcing users for not cycling include "social and cultural problems", "It is slow/takes too much time", and "the lack of biking facilities". The social problems are the most observed reason in both cities, which refer to social barriers to women cycling in public spaces in the MENA countries, inconvenience in public areas, and fear of harassment. Davies et al. (2001) also reported social and cultural problems as the main barrier against cycling in some British cities in 2001 [99]. However, the problems women face when cycling are the dominant social barrier in Tehran and Cairo. Regarding this barrier in the MENA region, it is necessary to raise public awareness about the health benefits and positive environmental impacts of cycling, and encourage women to use bikes through cultural programs.

4.5. The Necessity for Improvement in Biking Infrastructure

The lack of cycling infrastructures is the second and third most observed reason for not cycling among regular ridesourcing users in Tehran and Cairo, respectively. Some studies indicate the important role of appropriate biking infrastructure in raising the tendency toward biking. Dill and Carr (2003) indicated that improving biking infrastructure is associated with increasing bike use [100]. Moreover, developing special bicycle facilities, such as bike lanes and adding traffic lights for cycling, decreases the risk of crashes and injuries and significantly improves cycling safety in cities, which consequently encourages citizens to bicycle to their destinations more often. Therefore, these cities need to improve the cycling infrastructure by increasing the special bike lanes, city bikes, and bike-sharing services. The findings of this section confirm the suggestion of other similar studies, that increasing cycling among citizens needs to be addressed by infrastructural improvements and changes in social and individual perspectives on cycling [101–104].

4.6. Limitation and Further Research

In this paper, we studied the subjective reasons for not cycling in Tehran and Cairo. The findings indicate the social and cultural problems as the major barriers to cycling in both cities. Therefore, we suggest further qualitative and quantitative research into the impacts of social and cultural problems on cycling in more detail, in order to distinguish the different social aspects in this field. Moreover, in this study, we did not access the precise data of slope roads around the houses of each of the respondents. Therefore, further research is proposed to study the impact of different road slopes among the neighborhoods on citizens' tendencies to cycle in Tehran and Cairo. Moreover, we propose further research to gather more detailed data of the physiological conditions related to respondents' age, so as to develop the models of bicycle mode choice in these two cities, with more explanatory variables and their interactions.

5. Conclusions

This research studied the relationship between the regular use of ICT-based mobility services such as ridesourcing and the biking mode choice in the MENA region (Tehran and Cairo). Its findings suggest that although cycling does not have a considerable share in Tehran and Cairo's modal split, the frequent ridesourcing users are more likely to use bicycles than non-frequent users. This finding shows the potential for online bike-sharing in both cities where this online mobility mode has not been developed considerably in recent years. Following this, the people who regularly use online-based ridesourcing also might use online bike-sharing more often for their near destinations in these two cities. Moreover, the findings indicate that women and elderly citizens are significantly less likely to cycle to a near destination than men in both cities.

Furthermore, the built environment parameters of the neighborhood, such as intersection density and link–node ratio, have a significant positive correlation with the probability of biking in Tehran. The reasons for not cycling are studied among regular ridesourcing users, and the results show that social and cultural problems are the main barriers to the use of bicycles in both cities. Therefore, our findings suggest developing a new shape of online bike-sharing, raising awareness of the health and environmental benefits of cycling, particularly among women and older people, as well as improving bike facilities to promote the share of cycling in Tehran and Cairo.

Author Contributions: Conceptualization, H.M. (Hamid Mostofi); methodology, H.M. (Hamid Mostofi); resources and data, H.M. (Houshmand Masoumi); formal analysis, H.M. (Hamid Mostofi); writing—original draft preparation, H.M. (Hamid Mostofi); writing—review and editing, H.M. (Hamid Mostofi), H.M. (Houshmand Masoumi) and H.-L.D. All authors have read and agreed to the published version of the manuscript.

Funding: This study was undertaken by the support of the German Research Foundation (DGF) as the research project Urban Travel Behavior in Large Cities of MENA Region (UTB-MENA) with the project number MA6412/3-1.

Acknowledgments: We acknowledge support by the German Research Foundation and the Open Access Publication Fund of Technical University of Berlin.

Conflicts of Interest: The authors declare no conflict of interest. The funders had no role in the design of the study; in the collection, analyses, or interpretation of data; in the writing of the manuscript, or in the decision to publish the results.

References

1. Rietveld, P. *Biking and Walking: The Position of Nonmotorized Transport Modes in Transport Systems*; Tinbergen Institute Discussion Papers 01-111/3; Tinbergen Institute: Amsterdam, The Netherlands, 2001.
2. Litman, T. Burwell Issues in sustainable transportation international. *J. Glob. Environ. Issues* **2006**, *6*, 331–347. [CrossRef]
3. Frank, L.; Schmid, T.; Sallis, J.; Chapman, J.; Selens, B. Linking objectively measured physical activity with objectively measured urban form. *Am. J. Prev. Med.* **2005**, *28*, 117–125. [CrossRef] [PubMed]
4. Frank, L.; Engelke, P. The Built Environment and Human Activity Patterns: Exploring the Impacts of Urban Form on Public Health. *J. Plan. Literat.* **2001**, *16*, 202–218. [CrossRef]
5. Doorley, R.; Pakrashi, V.; Ghosh, B. Quantifying the health impacts of active travel: Assessment of methodologies. *Transp. Rev.* **2015**, *35*, 559–582. [CrossRef]
6. Jarrett, J.; Woodcock, J.; Griffiths, U.K.; Chalabi, Z.; Edwards, P.; Roberts, I.; Haines, P. Effect of increasing active travel in urban England and Wales on costs to the National Health Service. *Lancet* **2012**, *379*, 2198. [CrossRef]
7. Mueller, N.; Rojas-Rueda, D.; Cole-Hunter, T.; Nazelle, A.; Dons, E.; Gerike, R.; Goetschi, T.; Panis, L.; Kahlmeier, S.; Nieuwenhuijsen, M. Health impact assessment of active transportation: A systematic review. *Prev. Med.* **2015**, *76*, 103–114. [CrossRef]
8. David, K.S.; Sullivan, M. Expectations for walking speeds: Standards for students in elementary schools. *Pediatr. Phys. Ther.* **2005**, *17*, 120–127. [CrossRef]
9. Bernardi, S.; Rupi, F. An analysis of bicycle travel speed and disturbances on off-street and on-street facilities. *Transp. Res. Procedia* **2015**, *5*, 82–94. [CrossRef]
10. Suzuki, D.; Hanington, I. *Everything Under the Sun: Toward a Brighter Future on a Small Blue Planet*; Greystone: Vancouver, BC, Canada, 2012.
11. Lowe, M.D. *The Bicycle: Vehicle for a Small Planet*; Worldwatch Institute: Washington, DC, USA, 1989.
12. Kenworthy, J.; Laube, F. *The Millennium Cities Database for Sustainable Transport*; International Union of Public Transport, Brussels, and Institute for Sustainability and Technology Policy: Perth, Australia, 2001.
13. Litman, T. *The Costs of Automobile Dependency and the Benefits of Balanced Transportation*; Victoria Transport Policy Institute: Victoria, BC, Canada, 2002.
14. American Public Transportation Association, Transit Ridership APTA Report, Third Quarter 2017. Available online: http://www.apta.com/resources/statistics/Documents/Ridership/2017-q3-ridership-APTA.pdf (accessed on 30 August 2020).
15. Macmillan, A.; Connor, J.; Witten, K.; Kearns, R.; Rees, D.; Woodward, A. The societal costs and benefits of commuter bicycling: Simulating the effects of specific policies using system dynamics modeling. *Environ. Health Perspect.* **2014**, *122*, 335–344. [CrossRef]
16. Sun, Y.; Mobasheri, A.; Hu, X.; Wang, W. Investigating Impacts of Environmental Factors on the Cycling Behavior of Bicycle-Sharing Users. *Sustainability* **2017**, *9*, 1060. [CrossRef]
17. Scotini, R.; Skinner, I.; Racioppi, F.; Fusé, V.; Bertucci, J.D.O.; Tsutsumi, R. Supporting Active Mobility and Green Jobs through the Promotion of Cycling. *Int. J. Environ. Res. Public Health* **2017**, *14*, 1603. [CrossRef] [PubMed]
18. Eryig~it, S.; Ter, Ü. The effects of cultural values and habits on bicycle use—Konya sample. *Procedia Soc. Behav. Sci.* **2014**, *140*, 178–185. [CrossRef]
19. Lanzendorf, M.; Busch-Geertsema, A. The cycling boom in large German cities—Empirical evidence for successful cycling campaigns. *Transp. Policy* **2014**, *36*, 26–33. [CrossRef]
20. Heinen, E.; Maat, K.; Wee, B. The role of attitudes toward characteristics of bicycle commuting on the choice to cycle to work over various distances. *Transp. Res. D Transp. Environ.* **2011**, *16*, 102–109. [CrossRef]
21. Rietveld, P.; Daniel, V. Determinants of bicycle use: Do municipal policies matter? *Transp. Res. A Policy Pract.* **2004**, *38*, 531–550. [CrossRef]
22. Tehran Times. Cycling Holds Less than 1% Share of Urban Transport in Iran. 24 September 2019. Available online: https://www.tehrantimes.com/news/440456/Cycling-holds-less-than-1-share-of-urban-transport-in-Iran (accessed on 22 July 2020).
23. Fishman, E.; Böcker, L.; Helbich, M. Adult active transport in the Netherlands: An analysis of its contribution to physical activity requirements. *PLoS ONE* **2015**, *10*, e0121871. [CrossRef]

24. Elharoun, M.; Shahdah, U.E.; El-Badawy, S.M. Developing a Mode Choice Model for Mansoura city in Egypt. *Int. J. Traffic Transp. Eng.* **2018**, *8*, 528–542. [CrossRef]
25. Elserafi, T. Challenges for Cycling and Walking in New Cities in Egypt Experience of ElsheikhL Zayad City. *J. Eng. Appl. Sci.* **2019**, *66*, 703–725.
26. Aladdini, P.; Fayezi, E. Promoting urban sustainability through alternative measures of transportation: Bike-sharing pilot project to measure achievements and challenges in Tehran. *J. Sociol. Stud. Urban* **2011**, *1*, 77–90.
27. Alireza, E.; Amir, S. Promoting active transportation modes in school trips. *Transp. Policy* **2015**, *37*, 203–211. [CrossRef]
28. Shirzadi Babakan, A.; Alimohammadi, A.; Taleai, M. An agent-based evaluation of impacts of transport developments on the modal shift in Tehran, Iran. *J. Dev. Eff.* **2015**, *7*, 230–251. [CrossRef]
29. Gössling, S. ICT and transport behaviour: A conceptual review. *Int. J. Sustain. Transp.* **2017**. [CrossRef]
30. Line, T.; Jain, J.; Lyons, G. The role of ICTs in everyday mobile lives. *J. Transp. Geogr.* **2011**, *19*, 1490–1499. [CrossRef]
31. Shaheen, S.; Adam, C.; Ismail, Z.; Beaudry, K. *Smartphone Applications to Influence Travel Choices: Practices and Policies*; Report No. FHWA-HOP-16-023; Federal Highway Administration: Washington, DC, USA, 2016. Available online: https://ops.fhwa.dot.gov/publications/fhwahop16023/fhwahop16023.pdf (accessed on 26 May 2020).
32. Samaha, A.; Mostofi, H. Predicting the Likelihood of Using Car-Sharing in the Greater Cairo Metropolitan Area. *Urban Sci.* **2020**, *4*, 61. [CrossRef]
33. Bamberg, S.; Ajzen, I.; Schmidt, P. Choice of travel mode in the theory of planned behavior: The roles of past behavior, habit, and reasoned action. *Basic Appl. Soc. Psychol.* **2003**, *25*, 175–187. [CrossRef]
34. SAE International. *Taxonomy and Definitions for Terms Related to Shared Mobility and Enabling Technologies*; Special Report: J3163_201809; SAE International: Washington, DC, USA, 2018. [CrossRef]
35. Rayle, L.; Dai, D.; Chan, N.; Cervero, R.; Shaheen, S. Just a better taxi? A survey-based comparison of taxis, transit, and ridesourcing services in San Francisco. *Transp. Policy* **2016**, *45*, 168–178. [CrossRef]
36. Hamdi, N.; Mourad, M.; Knecht, E.; Potter, M. Egypt Passes Law Regulating Uber, Careem Ride-Sharing Services. Available online: https://www.reuters.com/article/us-egypt-uber/egypt-passes-law-regulating-uber-careem-ride-sharing-services-idUSKBN1I81VG (accessed on 7 September 2018).
37. Alkhalisi, Z.; Daftari, A. The Ride-Hailing App that Rules Tehran's Busy Streets. Available online: https://money.cnn.com/2017/07/30/technology/iran-snapp-ride-hailing/ (accessed on 24 May 2020).
38. The Guardian. Snapp: How Tehran's Answer to Uber is Changing How People Travel, and Live. Available online: https://www.theguardian.com/cities/2017/jul/31/snapp-how-tehran-answer-to-uber-is-changing-how-people-travel-and-live (accessed on 30 August 2020).
39. Tirachini, A. Ride-hailing, travel behaviour and sustainable mobility: An international review. *Transportation* **2019**, *47*, 2011–2047. [CrossRef]
40. Mostofi, H.; Masoumi, H.; Dienel, H.-L. The Association between Regular Use of Ridesourcing and Walking Mode Choice in Cairo and Tehran. *Sustainability* **2020**, *12*, 5623. [CrossRef]
41. Mostofi, H.; Masoumi, H.; Dienel, H.-L. The Relationship between Regular Use of Ridesourcing and Frequency of Public Transport Use in the MENA Region (Tehran and Cairo). *Sustainability* **2020**, *12*, 8134. [CrossRef]
42. Alemi, F.; Circella, G.; Handy, S.; Mokhtarian, P. What influences travelers to use Uber? Exploring the factors affecting the adoption of on-demand ride services in California. *Travel Behav. Soc.* **2018**, *13*, 88–104. [CrossRef]
43. Clewlow, R.; Mishra, G. *Disruptive Transportation: The Adoption, Utilization, and Impacts of Ride-Hailing in the United States*; Research Report UCD-ITS-RR-17-07; Institute of Transportation Studies, University of California: Davis, CA, USA, 2017; Available online: https://itspubs.ucdavis.edu/wp-content/themes/ucdavis/pubs/download_pdf.php?id=2752 (accessed on 24 August 2020).
44. Feigon, S.; Colin, M. *Shared Mobility and the Transformation of Public Transit*; TCRP Research Report; 188 Transportation Research Board: Washington, DC, USA, 2016. [CrossRef]
45. Gehrke, S.R.; Felix, A.; Reardon, T.G. Substitution of Ride-Hailing Services for More Sustainable Travel Options in the Greater Boston Region. *Transp. Res. Rec.* **2019**, *2673*, 438–446. [CrossRef]

46. Becker, H.; Ciari, F.; Axhausen, K.W. Comparing car-sharing schemes in Switzerland: User groups and usage patterns. *Transp. Res. Part A Policy Pract.* **2017**, *97*, 17–29. [CrossRef]
47. Circella, G.; Alemi, F. Transport Policy in the Era of Ride Hailing and Other Disruptive Transportation Technologies. *Adv. Transp. Policy Plan.* **2018**, 119–144. Available online: http://transp-or.epfl.ch/heart/2018/abstracts/5400.pdf (accessed on 28 August 2020).
48. Rodier, C. *The Effects of Ride Hailing Services on Travel and Associated Greenhouse Gas Emissions*; White Paper; National Center for Sustainable Transportation: Davis, CA, USA, 2018.
49. Dill, J.; Voros, K. Factors affecting bicycling demand: Initial survey findings from the Portland, Oregon, region. *Transp. Res. Rec.* **2007**, *2031*, 9–17. [CrossRef]
50. Woodcock, J.; Tainio, M.; Cheshire, J.; O'Brien, O.; Goodman, A. Health effects of the London bicycle sharing system: Health impact modelling study. *BMJ* **2014**, *348*, g425. [CrossRef]
51. Pucher, J.; Buehler, R. Making cycling irresistible: Lessons from the Netherlands, Denmark and Germany. *Trans. Rev. A Transnatl. Transdiscipl. J.* **2008**, *28*, 495–528. [CrossRef]
52. Masoumi, H.; Gouda, A.A.; Layritz, L.; Stendera, P.; Matta, C.; Tabbakh, H.; Fruth, E. Urban Travel Behavior in Large Cities of MENA Region: Survey Results of Cairo, Istanbul, and Tehran. 2018. Available online: https://www.researchgate.net/publication/326175506_Urban_Travel_Behavior_in_Large_Cities_of_MENA_Region_Survey_Results_of_Cairo_Istanbul_and_Tehran (accessed on 9 November 2020).
53. Krizek, K.; Handy, S.; Forsyth, A. Explaining changes in walking and bicycling behavior: Challenges for transportation research. *Environ. Plan. B* **2009**, *36*, 725–740. [CrossRef]
54. Li, Z.; Wang, W.; Liu, P.; Ragland, R.D. Physical environments influencing bicyclists' perception of comfort on separated and on-street bicycle facilities. *Transp. Res. Part D* **2012**, *17*, 256–261. [CrossRef]
55. Schoner, J.E.; Cao, J.; Levinson, D.M. Catalysts and magnets: Built environment and bicycle commuting. *J. Transp. Geogr.* **2015**, *47*, 100–108. [CrossRef]
56. Basu, S.; Vasudevan, V. Effect of Bicycle Friendly Roadway Infrastructure on Bicycling Activities in Urban India. *Procedia Soc. Behav. Sci.* **2013**, *104*, 1139–1148. [CrossRef]
57. Majumdar, B.B.; Mitra, S. Investigating the Relative Influence of Various Factors in Bicycle Mode Choice. *Procedia Soc. Behav. Sci.* **2013**, *104*, 1120–1129. [CrossRef]
58. Etminani-Ghasrodashti, R.; Ardeshiri, M. Modeling travel behavior by the structural relationships between lifestyle, built environment and non-working trips. *Transport. Res. Pol. Pract.* **2015**, *78*, 506–518. [CrossRef]
59. Etminani-Ghasrodashti, R.; Ardeshiri, M. The impacts of built environment on home-based work and non-work trips: An empirical study from Iran. *Transport. Res. Pol. Pract.* **2016**, *85*, 196–207. [CrossRef]
60. Shahangian, R.; Kermanshah, M.; Mokhtarian, P.L. Gender differences in response to policies targeting commute to automobile-restricted central business district. *J. Transp Res. Board* **2012**, *2320*, 80–89. [CrossRef]
61. Al-Atawi, A.; Saleh, W. Travel behavior in Saudi Arabia and the role of social factors. *Transport* **2014**, *29*, 269–277. [CrossRef]
62. Danaf, M.; Abou-Zeid, M.; Kaysi, I. Modeling travel choices of students at a private, urban university: Insights and policy implications. *Case Stud. Transp. Pol.* **2014**, *2*, 142–152. [CrossRef]
63. Handy, S.; Cao, X.; Mokhtarian, P. Correlation or Causality between the Built Environment and Travel Behavior? Evidence from Northern California. *Transp. Res. Part D* **2005**, *10*, 427–444. [CrossRef]
64. Kuzmyak, J.R.; Kockelman, K.; Bowman, J.; Bradle, M.; Lawton, K.; Pratt, R.H. *Estimating Bicycling and Walking for Planning and Project Development*; Task 3 Interim Report- NCHRP Project, Transportation Research Board; The National Academies Press: Washington, DC, USA, 2011; Volume 3, pp. 8–78.
65. Bartholomew, K.; Ewing, R. Land Use–Transportation Scenarios and Future Vehicle Travel and Land Consumption: A Meta-Analysis. *J. Am. Plan. Assoc.* **2008**, *75*, 13–27. [CrossRef]
66. Masoumi, H. A discrete choice analysis of transport mode choice causality and perceived barriers of sustainable mobility in the MENA region. *Transp. Policy* **2019**, *79*, 37–53. [CrossRef]
67. Pallant, J. *SPSS Survival Manual: A Step by Step Guide to Data Analysis Using SPSS*, 4th ed.; Allen & Unwin Book Publishers: Crows Nest, QLD, Australia, 2010.
68. Hair, J.F.; Black, W.C.; Babin, B.J.; Anderson, R.E.; Tatham, R.L. *Multivariate Data Analysis*, 7th ed.; Pearson: New York, NY, USA, 2010.
69. Hosmer, D.W.; Lemeshow, S. A goodness-of-fit test for the multiple logistic regression model. *Commun. Stat.* **1980**, *9*, 1043–1069. [CrossRef]

70. El-Geneidy, A.; Diab, E.; Jacques, C.; Mathez, A. 2014 Sustainable Urban Mobility in the Middle East and North Africa, Global Report on Human Settlements. 2013. Available online: https://www.researchgate.net/publication/260087548_Sustainable_Urban_Mobility_in_the_Middle_East_and_North_Africa_Thematic_study_prepared_for_Global_Report_on_Human_Settlements_2013 (accessed on 1 September 2019).
71. Malek Husseini, A.; Dargahi, M.M.; Haji Sharifi, A.; Karami Nejad, T.; Ramezandadeh Lasbooyi, M. Investigating the factors in the use of bike sharing system in urban development: A case-study of Haft Hoz and Madaen area. *J. Geogr. Urban Plan. Perspect. Zagros* **2012**, *11*, 159–179.
72. Salarvandian, F.; Dijst, M.; Helbich, M. Impact of Traffic Zones on Mobility Behavior in Tehran, Iran. *J. Transp. Land Use* **2017**, *10*, 965–982. [CrossRef]
73. Henao o, A.; Marshall, W.E. The Impact of Ride-Hailing on Vehicle Miles Traveled. *Transportation* **2019**, *46*, 2173–2194. [CrossRef]
74. Hampshire, R.; Simek, C.; Fabusuyi, T.; Di, X.; Chen, X. Measuring the Impact of an Unanticipated Suspension of Ride-Sourcing in Austin, Texas. *SSRN Electron. J.* **2017**. [CrossRef]
75. Tang, B.-J.; Li, X.-Y.; Yu, B.; Wei, Y.-M. How app-based ride-hailing services influence travel behavior: An empirical study from China. *Int. J. Sustain. Transp.* **2019**, *14*, 554–568. [CrossRef]
76. Ramdani, N. Saudi Women Are Allowed to Cycle-But Only Around in Circles. The Women's Blog. The Guardian. 2013. Available online: https://www.theguardian.com/lifeandstyle/the-womens-blog-with-jane-martinson/2013/apr/03/saudi-women-allowed-to-cycle (accessed on 2 September 2020).
77. Noury, A.; Speciale, B. Constraints and women's education: Evidence from Afghanistan under radical religious rule. *J. Comp. Econ.* **2016**, *44*, 821–841. [CrossRef]
78. Elfiky, U. *Cycling around Delta Cities in Egypt: Applicable Cycling Program within Kafr Elshiekh City, Second International Conference on Sustainable Architecture and Urban Development*; University of Jordan: Amman, Jordan, 2010; pp. 377–393. Available online: https://www.irbnet.de/daten/iconda/CIB22652.pdf (accessed on 2 September 2020).
79. Witlox, F.; Tindemans, H. Evaluating bicycle-car transport mode competitiveness in an urban environment: An activity-based approach. *World Transp. Policy Pract.* **2004**, *10*, 32–42.
80. Harms, L.; Bertolini, L.; Brömmelstroet, M.T. Spatial and social variations in cycling patterns in a mature cycling country: Exploring differences and trends. *J. Transp. Health* **2014**, *1*, 232–242. [CrossRef]
81. Office for National Statistics. 2011 Census Analysis-Cycling to Work. London: Author. Parliamentary Office for Science and Technology. Peak Car Use in Britain, a Briefing for the Commons Transport Select Committee. 2013. Available online: http://www.parliament.uk/documents/commons-committees/transport/POST-briefing-on-peak-car.pdf (accessed on 2 September 2020).
82. Aldred, R.; Woodcock, J.; Goodman, A. Does More Cycling Mean More Diversity in Cycling? *Transp. Rev.* **2016**, *36*, 28–44. [CrossRef]
83. Handy, S.L.; Xing, Y.; Buehler, T.J. Factors associated with bicycle ownership and use: A study of six small U.S. cities. *Transportation* **2010**, *37*, 967–985. [CrossRef]
84. Fishman, E.; Washington, S.; Haworth, N. Bike Share: A Synthesis of the Literature. *Transp. Rev. A Transnatl. Transdiscipl. J.* **2013**, *33*, 148–165. [CrossRef]
85. Carse, A.; Goodman, A.; Mackett, R.L.; Panter, J.; Ogilvie, D. The factors influencing car use in a cycle-friendly city: The case of Cambridge. *J. Transp. Geogr.* **2013**, *28*, 67–74. [CrossRef] [PubMed]
86. Ewing, R.; Cervero, R. Travel and the Built Environment: A Meta-Analysis. *J. Am. Plan. Assoc.* **2010**, *76*, 265–294. [CrossRef]
87. Reilly, M.K.; Landis, J. Influence of Urban form and Land Use on Mode Choice: Evidence from the 1996 Bay Area Travel Survey. In Proceedings of the 81st Annual Meeting of the TRB, Washington, DC, USA, 1 September 2003.
88. Cervero, R.; Radisch, C. Travel choices in pedestrian versus automobile oriented neighborhoods. *Transp. Policy* **1995**, *3*, 127–141. [CrossRef]
89. Langlois, M.; Wasfi, R.A.; Ross, N.A.; El-Geneidy, A.M. Can transit-oriented developments help achieve the recommended weekly level of physical activity? *J. Transp. Health* **2016**, *3*, 181–190. [CrossRef]
90. Soltani, A.; Shams, A. Analyzing the influence of neighborhood development pattern on modal choice. *J. Adv. Transp.* **2017**, *2017*, 4060348. [CrossRef]

91. Arabani, M.; Amani, B. Evaluating the Parameters Affecting Urban Trip-Generation. *Iran. J. Sci. Technol. Trans. B Eng.* **2007**, *31*, 547–560.
92. Soltani, A.; Esmaeili-Ivaki, Y. The Influence of Urban Physical Form on Trip Generation, Evidence from Metropolitan Shiraz, Iran. *Indian J. Sci. Technol.* **2011**, *4*, 1168–1174. [CrossRef]
93. Kerr, J.; Emond, J.A.; Badland, H.; Reis, R.; Sarmiento, O.; Carlson, J.; Natarajan, L. Perceived neighborhood environmental attributes associated with walking and cycling for transport among adult residents of 17 cities in 12 countries: The IPEN study. *Environ. Health Perspect.* **2016**, *124*, 290–298. [CrossRef]
94. Winters, M.; Brauer, M.; Setton, E.M.; Teschke, K. Built environment influences on healthy transportation choices: Bicycling versus driving. *J. Urban Health* **2010**, *87*, 969–993. [CrossRef]
95. Yang, Y.; Wu, X.; Zhou, P.; Gou, Z.; Lu, Y. Towards a Cycling-Friendly City: An Updated Review of the Associations between built Environment and Cycling Behaviors (2007–2017). *J. Transp. Health* **2019**, *14*, 100613. [CrossRef]
96. Saelens, B.E.; Handy, S.L. Built environment correlates of walking: A review. *Med. Sci. Sport. Exerc.* **2008**, *40* (Suppl. S7), S550–S566. [CrossRef] [PubMed]
97. Azadeh del, Y.; Anari, M.; Khorami Sarif, M.; Varasteh, M. A Model to Estimate the Slope of the Combined System of Passageways and a Bicycle Network Proposal for Continuity and Facilitating Cycling (A Case Study of Tehran, Iran). In Proceedings of the 16th International Conference of Traffic and Transportation in Iran, Tehran, Iran, 28–29 February 2016; Available online: https://civilica.com/doc/717439/ (accessed on 1 October 2020).
98. Anwer Zayed, M. Towards an index of city readiness for cycling. *Int. J. Transp. Sci. Technol.* **2016**, *5*, 210–225. [CrossRef]
99. Davies, D.; Gray, S.; Gardner, G.; Harland, G. *A Quantitative Study of the Attitudes of Individuals to Cycling*; TRL Report 481; Transport Research Laboratory: Crowthorne, UK, 2001.
100. Dill, J.; Carr, T. Bicycle Commuting and Facilities in Major, U.S. Cities: If You Build Them, Commuters Will Use Them. *Transp. Res. Rec.* **2003**, *1828*, 116–123. [CrossRef]
101. Gatersleben, B.; Appleton, K.M. Contemplating cycling to work: Attitudes and perceptions in different stages of change. *Transp. Res. Part A Policy Pract.* **2007**, *41*, 302–312. [CrossRef]
102. Newby, L. On the right tracks: Cycle planning best practice and its potential in Leicester. In *Research Report No 3. Best Practice Research Unit*; Leicester Environment City Trust Leicester: Leicester, UK, 1993.
103. Akar, G.; Clifton, K.J. Influence of Individual Perceptions and Bicycle Infrastructure on Decision to Bike. *Transp. Res. Rec.* **2009**, *2140*, 165–172. [CrossRef]
104. Wardman, M.; Hatfield, R.; Page, M. The UK national cycling strategy: Can improved facilities meet the targets? *Transp. Policy* **1997**, *4*, 123–133. [CrossRef]

Publisher's Note: MDPI stays neutral with regard to jurisdictional claims in published maps and institutional affiliations.

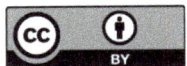

© 2020 by the authors. Licensee MDPI, Basel, Switzerland. This article is an open access article distributed under the terms and conditions of the Creative Commons Attribution (CC BY) license (http://creativecommons.org/licenses/by/4.0/).

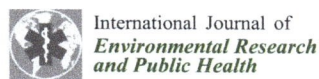 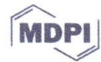

Article

Traffic Safety Perception, Attitude, and Feeder Mode Choice of Metro Commute: Evidence from Shenzhen

Yuanyuan Guo [1], Linchuan Yang [2,*], Wenke Huang [3] and Yi Guo [4]

1. Department of Geography and Resource Management, The Chinese University of Hong Kong, Hong Kong 999077, China; guoyuanyuan@link.cuhk.edu.hk
2. Department of Urban and Rural Planning, School of Architecture and Design, Southwest Jiaotong University, Chengdu 611756, China
3. The Research Center for Artificial Intelligence, Peng Cheng Laboratory, Shenzhen 518000, China; hwk727@163.com
4. Department of Geography, Hong Kong Baptist University, Hong Kong 999077, China; 18481744@life.hkbu.edu.hk
* Correspondence: yanglc0125@swjtu.edu.cn; Tel.: +86-028-6636-6683

Received: 15 November 2020; Accepted: 11 December 2020; Published: 15 December 2020

Abstract: Like many other transit modes, the metro provides stop-to-stop services rather than door-to-door services, so its use undeniably involves first- and last-mile issues. Understanding the determinants of the first- and last-mile mode choice is essential. Existing literature, however, mostly overlooks the mode choice effects of traffic safety perception and attitudes toward the mode. To this end, based on a face-to-face questionnaire survey in Shenzhen, China, this study uses the two-sample t-test to confirm the systematic differences in traffic safety perception and attitudes between different subgroups and develops a series of multinomial logistic (MNL) models to identify the determinants of first- and last-mile mode choice for metro commuters. The results of this study show that: (1) Walking is the most frequently used travel mode, followed by dockless bike-sharing (DBS) and buses; (2) Variances in traffic safety perception and attitude exist across gender and location; (3) Vehicle-related crash risks discourage metro commuters from walking to/from the metro station but encourage them to use DBS and buses as feeder modes; (4) DBS–metro integration is encouraged by the attitude that DBS is quicker than buses and walking, and positive attitudes toward the bus and DBS availability are decisive for the bus–metro and DBS–metro integration, respectively; and (5) Substantial differences exist in the mode choice effects of traffic safety perception and attitudes for access and egress trips. This study provides a valuable reference for metro commuters' first- and last-mile travel mode choice, contributing to developing a sustainable urban transport system.

Keywords: traffic safety; attitude; perception; objective factor; subjective factor; dockless bike-sharing; vehicle-related crash; last mile; multinomial logistic; Shenzhen; China

1. Introduction

Cities are now encountering a large number of transport-related problems (mainly attributed to the extensive use of private cars or car dependency), including traffic congestion, deteriorated traffic safety situation, air pollution, increased vehicle emissions, environmental degradation, and excessive consumption of natural sources. "Reclaiming the city from cars" has constantly been advocated. Some of these vexing problems (e.g., air pollution) even adversely affect the population's health [1–3]. Additionally, as a sustainable travel mode, transit (e.g., high-speed rail, metro, commuter rail, light rail, tram, bus rapid transit, and conventional bus transit) provides a high-capacity, medium-/long-distance, and low-emission transport service for residents. It contributes to overcoming car dependence and redressing a wide variety of contemporary cumbersome urban problems [4]. Hence, transit has received immense popularity and gained substantial interest in recent years and has also been promoted in a host of cities worldwide to facilitate people's sustainable travel [5–7]. However, in general, it offers stop-to-stop services (rather than door-to-door services) and thus cannot cover every location of a city [8]. Poor transit accessibility, particularly in periphery areas, makes it hard, if not impossible, to reach a goal of offering convenient transport services, thereby generating first- and last-mile challenges for commuters [9,10].

The metro is a popular transit mode implemented in a multitude of cities, particularly large cities. Many motorized (e.g., private car, bus, and taxi) and non-motorized (e.g., walk, bicycle, and scooter) modes have been encouraged to serve as the feeder modes of the metro (or first-/last-mile modes before/after riding the metro), thereby attracting more commuters to use the metro. In a great many car-oriented U.S. metropolitan areas, park-and-ride is preferable, due in part to high car ownership and poor transit service [11]. In European cities where cycling is pervasive and even viewed as a cultural norm, bike-and-ride has gained enormous popularity [12]. By contrast, East Asian cities such as Shanghai and Hong Kong tend to encourage the bus (e.g., feeder bus and public bus) as a way of connecting the metro [13,14]. In addition to these traditional feeder modes, new types of shared mobility services, such as bike-sharing and ride-sourcing, have recently been introduced to promote metro use. For example, Ma et al. [15] suggest that for a 10% increase in bike-sharing ridership, Metrorail ridership increases by 2.8% in Washington. The majority of dockless bike-sharing (DBS) bikes are distributed around metro stations in Chinese cities [16]. These newly shared mobility services contribute to solving the first- and last-mile problem [17].

However, the decision-making process of the feeder mode choice is complicated and is determined by various factors. Previous studies offer insights into why individuals use specific transfer modes to connect transit [18]. They mainly focus on "hard" factors such as socio-economic and demographic characteristics, mandatory policies or requirements (e.g., wearing a helmet), and the physical environment such as topography, weather conditions, and the built environment at the origin and destination and around metro stations [7,19–23]. For instance, if parking space is available, people with cars and young adults with bicycles will be likely to drive or ride, respectively, to transit stations, [7,19]; transfer distance is fundamental to mode choice because different transfer modes usually correspond to different distance ranges (e.g., if the walking distance to a transit station goes beyond a certain threshold, residents will not choose to walk to transit) [23]; cycling-related facilities, such as sheltered parking spaces and bicycle lanes, contribute to a bike-friendly environment, thereby attracting bike-sharing–metro integration [24]. Besides, "soft" factors on the psychological aspect, such as attitude and perception, are postulated to determine travel behaviors, which has prominently been discussed in socio-psychological theories such as the theory of planned behavior (TPB) [25]. Traditional travel behavior literature also recurrently suggests that traffic safety and individual attitudes are crucial in shaping travel mode choice (e.g., [18,19]). The perceived traffic safety/risk affects the choice of self-controlled travel modes, such as driving and cycling [26–28]. The role of attitudes in mode choices could be as important as or even more important than the physical environment and socio-economic characteristics [29–31], but this is still inconclusive. For example, individuals with favorable attitudes toward a specific travel mode may likely use that mode [18,32]. Even though the effects of traffic safety perception and attitudes on mode choice are widely acknowledged, to the knowledge of the authors, limited studies have investigated (1) the impacts of the two psychological factors on the feeder mode choice of the metro; and (2) how the impacts vary across metro commuters' first- and last-mile trips.

To this end, based on a case study of Shenzhen, China, this study explores how the perceived traffic safety and the attitude toward transfer modes correlate to the feeder mode choice of metro commuters. A field questionnaire survey was conducted at many metro stations in Shenzhen, in which the metro commuter's transfer mode for the access/egress trip has been examined. The two-sample t-test is used to confirm the systematic differences in traffic safety perception and attitudes between different subgroups, and a series of multinomial logistic (MNL) models is developed to identify the determinants of first- and last-mile mode choice for metro commuters. The study aims to address the following four research questions: (1) What is the mode share of access/egress trips in today's Chinese mega cities? (2) Do traffic safety perceptions and attitudes vary by gender and location? (3) Are perceived traffic safety and attitudes toward transfer modes important in determining the transfer mode choice? (4) Are the effects of perceived traffic safety and attitudes toward the mode different between access and egress trips? We believe that this study contributes to the promotion of green and healthy urban mobility and serves as a valuable reference for Chinese mega cities and other settings with similar traffic conditions.

The remainder of the paper is organized as follows. Section 2 introduces existing feed modes. Section 3 reviews the literature on the effects of perceived traffic safety and attitudes on feeder mode choice. Section 4 presents the study context, questionnaire survey, and methodologies. Section 5 offers the analyses of feeder mode share, the individual variance in perceived traffic safety and attitude, and the modeling results. Section 6 provides policy implications, research limitations, and avenues for future research. The final section (Section 7) concludes the paper.

2. Summary of Existing Feed Modes

Walking, a travel mode with economic, environmental, social, and health impacts [10,33], is often used to reach a transit station (walk-and-ride). However, it requires the use of the human body as a travel machine. Therefore, it is significantly restricted by travel distance [21]. Generally, the willingness to walk can be well described by distance decay curves: after 800–1000 m, the mode share of walking declines sharply.

The bicycle's integration with transit (bike-and-ride) is also common for commuters. The synergy of the bicycle and transit for access/egress trips can be summarized into three patterns: bicycle-and-transit, transit-and-bicycle, and bicycle-on-transit (taking a bicycle on transit) [34,35]. There are many preconditions for the bicycle-and-transit and transit-and-bicycle patterns, such as the ownership of bicycles, available secure parking spaces, and parking facilities (e.g., shelter and parking dock) around transit stations [36]. However, the bicycle-on-transit pattern is usually constrained by the parking space or capacity on transit, which may bring conflicts between regular transit passengers and bicycle–transit users [35]. Recently, bike-sharing services, including docked and dockless programs, have been introduced to various cities (e.g., Paris, Singapore, and Shanghai). This makes the bike–metro integration smarter, greener, and more economical because there is no need to bring bikes on transit and worry about the issues of theft and maintenance [16,37].

As for motorized feeder modes, the motorcycle (two-/three-wheeled motor vehicle), which usually carries 1–2 passengers, has a similar function with the taxi in many developing countries, such as China, Thailand, Vietnam, and India [38,39]. Motorcycle drivers always wait at large-scale residential areas and the exits of transit stations and solicit passengers. They often ride through narrow spaces during traffic jams. Thus, as for passengers, the motorcycle is fast (or time-saving) and easy to access. Moreover, in larger metropolitan areas, feeder buses, which are commonly operated in two forms—demand-responsive transit and fixed-route transit [40]—have been introduced by transit agencies to residents, especially those with poor transit accessibility. They perform well when the to-transit distance is long [22].

The private car is an option to access transit stations, and it involves two manners: park & ride and kiss & ride (i.e., passenger drop-off) [21]. The availability of park & ride facilities is a key factor for commuters with cars [20]. However, using the private car as the feeder mode of transit, particularly for the park & ride pattern, is more common in remote locations than downtown [41].

Other modes such as traditional and electric scooters, e-bike, taxi, and ride-hailing can serve as the feeder modes of transit. However, few empirical studies have discussed their integration with transit [42].

3. Related Studies

3.1. Perceived Traffic Safety and Last-Mile Mode Choice

Traffic safety is usually measured by how unlikely accidents occur. It is reported that traffic accidents kill about 1.2 million people all over the world each year [43]. Traffic safety is determined by many factors, such as road characteristics, climate and weather, and—perhaps most importantly—vehicle speeds [44]. Previous research confirmed that the higher the speed, the greater the possibility of traffic accidents [28,45].

Perceived traffic safety refers to individuals' perceived likelihood of an accident-free traffic outcome (i.e., avoiding traffic accident and crash) [43,46]. It varies from person to person based on their background (information and experience) and how they deal with risks [47,48]. For example, Salonen indicated that men have a higher level of traffic safety awareness, in-vehicle security, and emergency management than women [43]. Bordagaray et al. confirmed that young adults (aged 34 years or below) perceive traffic safety as less important than older people do [1]. Moreover, the built environment is associated with people's safety perceptions. Intersection density and the presence of major road crossings en-route were found to insensibly affect the individual's perception of safety, such as the fear of collision [28]. Safety concerns also come from heavy traffic, such as high volume/speed of vehicles on streets [49,50].

Furthermore, the perception of traffic safety may significantly affect mode choice decision [51]. According to the TPB model, perceived behavior control, which means the perceived difficulty in or ease of performing a behavior, is one of the socio-cognitive factors determining the individual's behavioral intention [25]. Moreover, a model for passenger transport developed by Van Wee [52] summarizes elements shaping travel behavior, including activity locations, transport resistances, needs, opportunities, and abilities. Typically, travel resistance consists of time, money, and other non-monetary costs, such as the perceived risk of traffic. Specifically, the perception that a certain type of transport mode is unsafe can be a psychological barrier to its use [53]. According to some empirical studies, the number of occurred crashes can directly affect the safety perception of pedestrians and bicyclists [54], thereby influencing active transport behaviors. Aziz et al. [55] also indicated that decreasing traffic crashes on pedestrians and bicyclists led to an increase in the likelihood of walking and cycling behavior. A recent study focusing on new safety challenges that autonomous vehicles (AVs) introduce indicates that, among road users, cyclists have the lowest level of perceived safety, followed by pedestrians and drivers, when their activities are near an AV [56].

3.2. Attitude and Last-Mile Mode Choice

Attitude can be defined as "global and relatively stable evaluations that people do about persons, things or ideas" [57]. Thus, attitudes involve positive or negative views that people have in terms of any aspect of reality [32,58]. According to existing literature [50,52,53], travel-related attitudes are usually connected to preferences for destinations, routes, activities, and modes of transport. A more general understanding of travel-related attitudes may also correlate with the individual's beliefs (e.g., environmentalism) [59].

Some behavior theories, such as the theory of reasoned action (TRA) and its extension, namely the TPB, emphasized that the individual's travel behavior is significantly influenced by attitudes. In TRA and TPB models, attitude is a predictor of the individual's behavioral intention, which is a predictor of behaviors [25,60,61]. Travel behavior literature has well recognized the role of attitude in shaping travel behavior [32,62,63]. In particular, the individual's attitude toward travel modes is evidenced to affect mode choice. For example, positive attitudes toward walking and cycling are related to frequent physical activities (through active travel), discouraging the motorized mode usage (e.g., car and bus) [32]. Thøgersen [64] found that a good attitude toward transit can predict transit use among Danish residents based on a panel survey during 1998–2000. Tran et al. [59] investigated the specific attitudes toward cars and buses and how such attitudes affect mode choice. They concluded that attitudes toward car use significantly affect the bus utility. Through a qualitative study in Porto (Portugal), Beirão and Sarsfield Cabral [65] also demonstrated the significant role of attitude in influencing the mode switch (from the car and public transit) for commuters. They suggested that improving the levels or images of public transit services could be effective to attract occasional public transport users and car users. Additionally, the relative attitudes among transport modes play a crucial role in affecting mode choice. He and Thøgersen [66] revealed that people's favorable attitudes toward transit (relative to cars) make transit more attractive. In a similar vein, people who prefer cars to public transport tend to travel by car.

In addition to the specific attitude toward the travel mode, the travel behavior effects of general attitudes with a broad concept have been studied. For example, a positive attitude toward physical activity promotes bicycling and walking behaviors [67]. Based on samples of Swedish commuters, Johansson et al. [27] found that attitudes toward flexibility and comfort influence mode choice. Additionally, some studies incorporated attitudes to analyze the influences of environmental awareness and sustainability concerns about mode choice and demonstrated the role of these attitudes [32,68].

However, studies on the effect of traffic safety and attitude toward mode choice are still scarce in terms of the specific condition of feeder trips. Previous studies have mostly investigated mode choice for general trips but paid limited attention to the first- and last-mile trips. Therefore, more sophisticated analyses are indispensable to explore the associations between traffic safety, attitude, and feeder mode choice.

4. Data and Methodology

4.1. Study Area: Shenzhen

Shenzhen, a famous international metropolis located on the southern coast of China and adjacent to Hong Kong, is selected as our study area. In 2019, Shenzhen had a population of 13.44 million and covered an area of 1997 km^2, indicating a high population density (6730 people/km^2). Shenzhen had a vast amount of GDP in 2019 (390.34 billion dollars), ranking third in China. Over the last ten years, Shenzhen has widely been known as one of the Tier 1 cities in China (the other three cities are Beijing, Shanghai, and Guangzhou) [69]. Compared to other Asian modern cities, the GDP of Shenzhen is only smaller than Tokyo but larger than Singapore, Hong Kong, and Seoul. Additionally, Shenzhen has a large-scale metro system, which has opened since 28 December 2004. As of October 2020, Shenzhen has 11 metro lines, 237 metro stations, and a total mileage of 411 km (Figure 1). The daily ridership in 2018 was 5.14 million [37], ranking fourth in Mainland China. It is comparable to Hong Kong and Seoul but falls behind Tokyo. Therefore, Shenzhen is a representative modern city in China and also in East Asia.

The metro is an important travel mode for commuters, accounting for over 40% of trips taken by residents [37]. According to an online report issued by the Shenzhen Rail Transit Construction Headquarters Office, the average daily metro ridership and the per-km passenger volume in 2019 were 5.57 million and 19.2 thousand, respectively (Top Five in Mainland China) [70]. After the city has officially been designated as a "Transit Metropolis (*gongjiao dushi*)" by the Ministry of Transport of China, the local government has implemented a series of policy measures, such as establishing bus stops and allocating shared bikes (i.e., public bicycle and DBS) around metro stations, to promote the seamless connection between the metro and its feeder modes.

Although Shenzhen witnessed an accomplished development of public transit, it experienced a sharp growth of private cars over the last decade. As of 2018, the number of motor vehicles in Shenzhen was approximately 3.37 million, and the total length of the road was 6443 km. This means that the density of motor vehicles (522.58 vehicles/km) is very high, which may result in an increased risk of traffic safety issues such as pedestrian/bicycle/vehicle-related crashes. Obviously, traffic safety issues are more acute in metro catchment areas with concentrated populations and vehicles than in other areas.

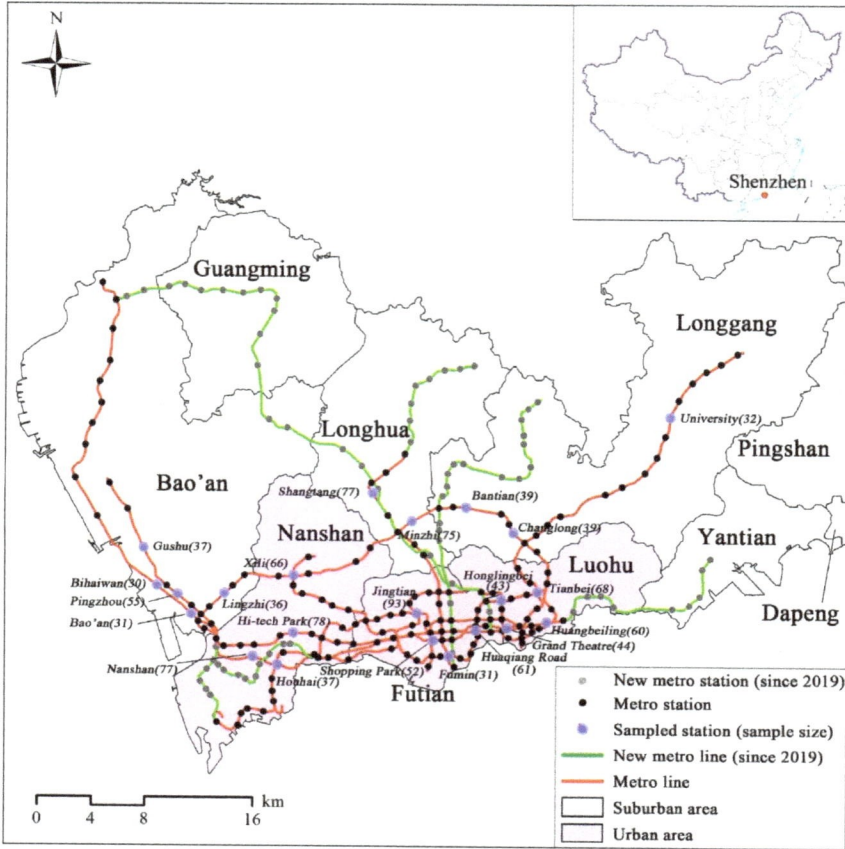

Figure 1. Study context of Shenzhen. Note: Since 2019, 70 new metro stations and 114.3 km metro lines have been built [37].

4.2. Data and Variables

4.2.1. Data

As formerly mentioned, this study aims to identify factors influencing the feeder mode of the metro, paying special attention to perceived traffic safety and attitude; and feeder mode includes walking, DBS, private bicycles, buses, taxi/Didi, cars, scooters, and other modes. We, therefore, collected the data by conducting a field questionnaire survey at 22 randomly selected metro stations in Shenzhen, China, between October and November in 2019 (Figure 1). During the survey, rainy days were excluded. Metro users who entered or left from the metro station during 7:30 a.m. and 9:00 a.m. were randomly selected as the survey samples. Given that metro commuters are usually in a hurry during the morning peak time, the respondents were requested to keep a leaflet with a quick response (QR) code. Thus, metro passengers can complete the questionnaire in their leisure time by scanning the QR code.

The questionnaire was composed of several parts, including transfer mode choice, the individual's perceptions of and attitudes toward specific transport modes, and socio-demographic characteristics. In this study, traffic safety concerns were measured in a subjective way by considering two safety issues: pedestrian–bicycle crash and pedestrian/bicycle–vehicle crash. Metro users' attitudes toward typical first-/last- mile travel modes were investigated. Additionally, relative attitudes of metro users, such as DBS versus walking and DBS versus bus, were recorded. Furthermore, questions on the attitude toward metro users' ability to access DBS and buses and the attitude toward daily physical activities were asked.

Questions related to traffic safety perception were designed by referring to the "Neighborhood Environment Walkability Scale (NEWS)" questionnaire, which includes questions on individuals' perceptions of the environment [71]. Based on the NEWS, a four-point Likert scale (i.e., "strongly disagree" = 1, "somewhat disagree" = 2, "somewhat agree" = 3, and "strongly agree" = 4) was adopted to assess the perceived traffic safety. Similarly, individual's attitudes were evaluated by the four-point Likert scale, thereby making the results comparable to those of perceived traffic safety.

We received 1702 questionnaires, 1167 of which were valid (valid rate = 68.57%). The number of valid questionnaires for each metro station ranged from 30 to 93 (Figure 1). Among valid samples, 1086 respondents chose walking, DBS, or buses in access trips, while 1108 adopted one of these three modes to finish their egress trips. These three popular feeder modes account for 93.06% and 94.94% of the total trips in the access and egress scenarios, respectively, while other modes (e.g., private bicycle, taxi, Didi, and scooter) constitute less than 7%.

4.2.2. Variables

Table 1 shows the measurements and descriptive statistics of perceived traffic safety variables, attitude variables, and socio-demographic characteristics.

The average score of bicycle crash is approximately 3 ("somewhat agree"), which is modestly larger than vehicle crash. This observation indicates that the bicycle-related crash could be a major safety concern for metro users in first-/last-mile trips and may significantly affect metro commuters' first-/last-mile mode choice. Similarly, metro commuters may face a risk of crashes with vehicles along their feeder routes. As for the transport mode, metro riders usually have a positive attitude or fondness toward non-motorized modes (including walking and cycling) but a negative attitude toward the bus (the average score is only 2.3).

As for the access trip connecting home and the metro station, DBS/bus availability involves how easy to find DBS bikes/bus stops around their home. In terms of the egress trip connecting the metro station and the workplace, DBS/bus availability means that how easy to find DBS bikes/bus stops around metro exits. However, we observe that many metro users agree that it is not easy to find a DBS bike for both access and egress trips. By contrast, metro users hold an attitude that the bus stop is relatively easy to access. Moreover, respondents usually want to have some daily physical activities.

Table 1 indicates that more male passengers (59%) participated in the survey than female passengers (41%); most respondents were young (84% aged 35 years or below), well-educated (88% hold a bachelor degree or above), and middle-income earners (68% earn between 5000 and 14,999 RMB monthly); the respondents usually did not own a bicycle; and minimal differences in socio-demographic characteristics existed between the two scenarios. However, most access trips occurred in suburban areas (56.54%), while egress trips were largely concentrated in urban areas (79.69%). This observation indicates the jobs-housing imbalance in Shenzhen: Many metro commuters live in suburban areas because of low housing rent but work in urban areas with more job opportunities.

The feeder trip distance is calculated via a geographic information system by connecting the geo-coded home/workplace addresses and the metro station reported by the respondents. The result shows that metro users have a longer transfer distance of home–metro feeder trips (access trip, 766 m) than that of the workplace–metro feeder trips (egress trip, 565 m).

Table 1. Measurements and statistics of variables of safety, attitude, and socio-demographic characteristics (N (access trips) = 1086; N (egress trips) = 1108).

Variable	Description	Category and/or Code	Mean/Percentage Access Trip	Mean/Percentage Egress Trip
Explanatory variables: safety and attitude				
Bicycle crash	I have safety concerns about crashes with a bicycle along the feeder trip.		3.04	3.15
Vehicle crash	I have safety concerns about crashes with a vehicle along the feeder trip.		2.45	2.43
Cycling	I like to ride a bicycle.		3.09	3.09
Walking	I like to walk.		3.15	3.14
Bus	I like to take a bus.	Strongly disagree = 1;	2.34	2.33
DBS	I like DBS.	Somewhat disagree = 2;	2.97	2.97
DBS vs. walking	I think DBS is quicker than walking to connect the metro.	Somewhat agree = 3; and	2.80	2.81
DBS vs. bus	I think DBS is quicker than buses to connect the metro.	Strongly agree = 4	2.76	2.77
Easy to take a bus	I think it is easy to take a bus to connect the metro.		2.95	2.88
Easy to find DBS	I think it is easy to search for a DBS bike to connect the metro.		2.29	2.60
Physical activity	I would like to have daily physical activities.		3.14	3.14
Control variables: socio-demographic characteristics				
Gender	Male or female	Female	41.16%	41.34%
		Male	58.84%	58.66%
Age	/	<25 years	32.23%	32.13%
		26 to 35 years	51.66%	52.08%
		36 to 45 years	12.80%	12.73%
		>46 years	3.31%	3.07%
Education	Education status	Middle school or below	1.93%	1.99%
		High school	9.85%	10.11%
		University/College	75.32%	75.00%
		Graduate institute	12.89%	12.91%
Income	Monthly personal income	<4999 RMB	11.97%	11.82%
		5000 to 9999 RMB	44.94%	44.68%
		10,000 to 14,999 RMB	23.39%	23.29%
		>15,000 RMB	19.71%	20.22%
Bicycle ownership		No	89.32%	88.36%
		Yes	10.68%	11.64%
Location	Location of the feeder trip	Urban area	43.46%	79.69%
		Suburban area	56.54%	20.31%
Transfer distance	The Euclidean distance of the trip (km)		0.766	0.565

4.3. Methodology

This study applies two analysis approaches, namely the two-sample (two-tailed) t-test and the multinomial logistic (MNL) model.

First, the two-tailed t-test is widely used to determine the statistical significance of difference between the means of two groups. In this study, it was performed to identify the variance in traffic safety perception and attitude among groups segmented by gender and location (male vs. female groups, and passenger groups working/living in urban areas vs. those working/living in suburban areas).

Second, the MNL model is a popular method to relate a nominal (or categorical) outcome variable to its predictors [72]. One of its assumptions is that the random components of the utilities of different choices (error terms) are independent and identically distributed according to a Gumbel distribution (extreme value distribution). Moreover, the MNL model has the property of proportional substitution across alternatives (e.g., independent from irrelevant alternatives, or IIA) (recall the red bus-blue bus problem). In this study, feeder mode choices are typically nominal outcomes (with no natural ordering) and composed of three categories (i.e., walking, DBS, and bus). Thus, the MNL model fits well with our research and thus was used to identify how the factors of perceived traffic safety and attitudes are associated with first-/last-mile mode choice under two scenarios of access and egress feeder trips. More information on the MNL model can be found in [73].

Two kinds of transfer trips, namely access trips and egress trips, were considered. Thus, two MNL models (*Access* MNL model and *Egress* MNL model) are developed. As the name explicitly states, the *Access* MNL model scrutinizes the determinants of feeder mode choice for access trips, while the *Egress* MNL model does so for egress trips. Additionally, collinearity was assessed by calculating the variance inflation factor (VIF), and the result shows that the VIF values of all variables were less than 5.

5. Results

5.1. Feeder Mode Choice of the Metro

Figure 2 presents the share of the three feeder modes. It suggests that walking is the most frequently used mode by metro commuters for first- and last-mile trips, which is in line with many previous studies [22,23,34]. For either access or egress trips, the mode share of walking (more than 70%) is far larger than DBS (approximately 15%), closely followed by buses (about 10%). The relatively high share of DBS as the feeder mode of the metro demonstrates the popularity of DBS–metro integration in the study context. Compared with the share of the traditional docked bike-sharing (public bicycles) (4.4% in Nanjing [22] and 7.04% in Beijing) [23], DBS accounts for a larger market share, which reveals that it outperforms public bicycles in serving as the feeder mode of the metro. Furthermore, walking is more commonly adopted in egress trips than in access trips (difference in mode share = 5%). Few differences are observed between the two scenarios for DBS–metro integration, while metro users have a higher willingness to transfer by buses for home-metro connection than workplace-metro connection.

Table 2 reveals the feeder mode choice of men and women. It indicates that feeder mode choices substantially differ across genders. The male group has a similar share of walking with the female group but a higher share of DBS and a lower share of buses for access trips. As for egress trips, the differences in the share of three feeder modes between the two groups are subtle.

Table 3 shows the feeder mode choice in urban and suburban areas. Walking is preferable for metro users who live/work in urban areas than those living/working in suburban areas. A possible explanation for this observation is that the metro transit system is less developed in suburban areas, thereby generating a longer transfer distance unsuitable for walking but suitable for riding buses.

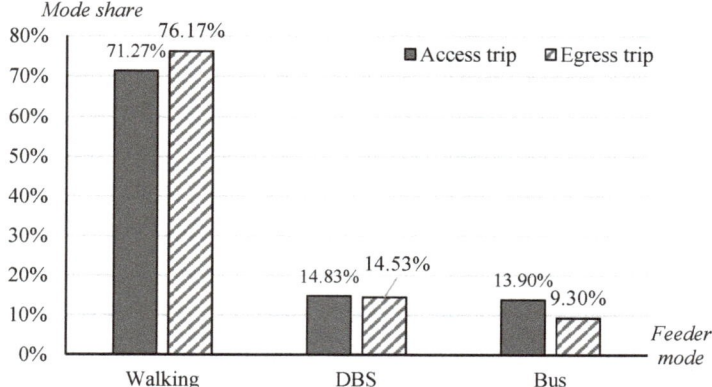

Figure 2. Share of the three feeder modes.

Table 2. Feeder mode choice of men and women.

Mode	Access Trip		Egress Trip	
	Female	Male	Female	Male
Walking	72.71%	70.27%	76.64%	75.85%
DBS	11.41%	17.21%	13.54%	15.23%
Bus	15.88%	12.52%	9.83%	8.92%

Table 3. Feeder mode choice in urban and suburban areas.

Mode	Access Trip		Egress Trip	
	Urban Area	Suburban Area	Urban Area	Suburban Area
Walking	75.85%	67.75%	80.29%	60.00%
DBS	16.31%	13.68%	12.68%	21.78%
Bus	7.84%	18.57%	7.02%	18.22%

5.2. Variance in Perceived Traffic Safety and Attitude

Ample evidence shows that traffic safety perception is associated with gender [56,74] and location [75]. We, therefore, considered the variance in perceived traffic safety across genders and home/workplace locations. However, the variance in attitudes is usually correlated with socio-demographic characteristics, such as gender [43], so we made a comparison between male and female groups. We calculated the mean difference along two dimensions (gender (female versus male) and location (urban versus suburban areas)) and conducted two-sample t-tests. The mean differences were obtained as follows: male metro users minus female metro users, and metro users with a home/workplace located in urban areas minus those with a home/workplace situated in suburban areas.

Table 4 shows the result of the two-sample t-test. The perceived traffic safety significantly varies across gender and location. Compared with male metro users, female counterparts perceive a higher risk of vehicle-related crashes but a statistically equivalent risk of bicycle-related crashes. Moreover, the perceived risk of bicycle and vehicle crashes could be more obvious in suburban areas than in urban areas for access trips (connecting the home and the metro), but the reverse is true for egress trips (connecting the workplace and the metro).

Table 4. Two-sample t-test results of individual variance in perceived traffic safety and attitude.

Variable	Male vs. Female Passengers			Urban vs. Suburban Location		
	Difference of Mean	F	Sig.	Difference of Mean	F	Sig.
Access feeder trip (home-side, N = 1086)						
Bicycle crash	0.049	1.120	0.290	0.210 ***	21.074	0.000
Vehicle crash	−0.071 *	2.003	0.097	0.152 ***	9.311	0.002
Cycling	0.051	1.193	0.275			
Walking	0.038	0.613	0.434			
Bus	−0.004	0.008	0.929			
DBS	0.028	0.457	0.499			
DBS vs. walking	0.162 ***	10.068	0.002			
DBS vs. bus	0.030	0.339	0.561			
Easy to take a bus	−0.111 **	4.371	0.037			
Easy to find DBS	0.113 **	4.299	0.038			
Physical activity	0.119 ***	11.400	0.001			
Egress feeder trip (workplace-side, N = 1108)						
Bicycle crash	0.040	0.813	0.367	−0.124 **	5.169	0.023
Vehicle crash	−0.103 **	4.031	0.045	−0.187 ***	8.960	0.003
Cycling	0.044	0.875	0.350			
Walking	0.038	0.630	0.427			
Bus	−0.003	0.004	0.947			
DBS	0.034	0.665	0.415			
DBS vs. walking	0.146 ***	8.147	0.004			
DBS vs. bus	0.045	0.754	0.385			
Easy to take a bus	0.007	0.017	0.897			
Easy to find DBS	0.049	0.785	0.376			
Physical activity	0.123 ***	12.462	0.000			

Note: *** $p < 0.01$; ** $p < 0.05$; * $p < 0.1$.

Table 4 reveals no significant difference in attitudes toward feeder modes (i.e., cycling, walking, bus, and DBS) between male and female metro users. However, compared with female metro users, male counterparts are more likely to hold an attitude that DBS is quicker than walking to connect the metro. Moreover, male metro users also have a higher willingness to carry out some daily physical activities than their female counterparts. Such a result is consistent with the work of Lee [76], which reveals that the female is less likely to be active than the male. Additionally, it is observed that the attitudes toward searching buses and DBS differ between male and female groups for their access trips connecting home and the metro. We found that female metro users think it is easier to take a bus but more difficult to search for DBS bikes around their home than male metro users. It is possible that compared with the female, the male is more likely to overestimate the bus waiting time, which is measured by a ratio of perceived waiting time to actual waiting time [77].

5.3. MNL Modeling Results

Tables 5 and 6 present the MNL modeling results for access and egress trips, respectively, using walking as the reference group. The Pseudo R^2 of *Access* and *Egress* MNL models (0.237 and 0.206) indicate that the MNL models have acceptable goodness of fit. Obviously, the MNL models can explain more variances in the access integrated use than the egress integrated use.

5.3.1. The Role of Perceived Traffic Safety

The vehicle-related safety concern has significant effects on the feeder mode choice, while bicycle-related safety risk does not play such a significant role. The perception of bicycle-related crashes only affects mode choice between DBS and walking for access trips. A one-unit increase in the score of the perceived bicycle-related crash decreases the odds for choosing DBS relative to walking by 23.6% (= 1−0.764), holding all the other variables constant.

A higher perceived risk of the vehicle-related crash encourages the choices of DBS and buses rather than walking to/from the metro station. For instance, high-speed vehicles crossing the intersections may make pedestrians feel dangerous. Thus, the exposures to vehicle-related crashes are deterrents for walk–metro users. Bikeway can provide cyclists with safety protection from the vehicle crash, and the bus is a sheltered mode protecting commuters from slight collisions with vehicles. For access trips, we see a 35.4% and 46.4% increase in the odds for opting for DBS and buses, respectively, relative to walking for a one-unit increase in the perceived risk of the vehicle-related crash, while the values for egress trips are 30.2% and 31.6%, respectively. This finding indicates that metro passengers are more affected by vehicle-related safety risks for access trips than for egress trips.

5.3.2. The Role of Attitude

Specific attitudes toward transport modes are observed to have an essential role in determining mode choice. As many previous studies concluded, bike-sharing mostly replaces walking for travel [78,79]. Our results reveal that a positive attitude toward DBS and cycling behavior but a negative attitude toward walking can significantly promote the likelihood of adopting DBS rather than walking as the feeder mode. More specifically, every one-unit higher in the score of cycling attitude can increase the odds for choosing DBS relative to walking by 87.8% (= 1.878–1) for access trips and 27.6% (= 1.276–1) for egress trips; a one-unit increase in the DBS attitude score increased the odds for opting for DBS relative to walking by 127.9% (= 2.279–1) and 60.9% (= 1.609–1) for access and egress trips, respectively. However, the odds for adopting DBS relative to walking will decrease by more than 30% for each unit in an increase in the walking–attitude score (OR = 0.700 in the *Access* model and OR = 0.647 in the *Egress* model). Similarly, by comparing the coefficients of the same variable, we find that favorable attitudes toward DBS and cycling behavior also promote the substitution effect of DBS to buses as the feeder mode. Moreover, it is found that the attitude toward buses does not significantly affect mode choice. We only observe that a negative attitude toward walking increases the possibility of choosing buses for an access trip, particularly when the bus service is easily perceived to be offered around the home. This observation is reasonable.

Relative attitudes between travel modes are also crucial to metro passengers' feeder mode choice. If metro users think that DBS is faster than walking to connect the metro station, they will have a higher possibility of adopting DBS as the feeder mode (OR = 1.631 in the *Access* model and OR = 1.921 in the *Egress* model). Moreover, a relative attitude that DBS is quicker than buses can increase the odds of choosing DBS as an egress mode. Our results are consistent with the study by Heinen and Bohte [18].

Tables 5 and 6 also show significant effects of the attitude toward DBS/bus availability on the feeder mode choice, mostly applicable for the access trip scenario. It shows that, for access trips, an attitude of easy access to the bus stop can add the willingness to take buses rather than walk for connecting the metro. Moreover, a positive attitude of searching for DBS bike around the home significantly increases the odds of DBS–metro integration. This outcome indicates a self-reinforcing effect in terms of the attitudes toward the DBS/bus availability. Furthermore, the perception of ease of searching for DBS bikes is crucial for replacing walking with DBS for both access and egress trips. However, the attitude toward physical activity is insignificant in affecting the feeder mode choice.

5.3.3. The Role of Socio-Demographic Characteristics

The socio-demographic characteristics are strongly related to the feeder mode choice. This outcome is in line with existing literature [22,23,80]. More specifically, our results show that DBS is preferable for males than females to finish their access trips, while no significant difference exists between genders for egress trips. Age and income significantly affect the feeder mode choice of egress trips, but not that of access trips. Compared to those under 25 years, young adults (26 to 35 years) have a higher willingness to opt for DBS relative to walking (OR = 1.745) in egress trips. However, older adults prefer using buses (relative to walking) for egress trips. Interestingly, we found that middle- and high-incomers (monthly income > 5000 RMB) are more likely to walk than taking buses as their major mode for access trips. Buses are usually crowded during peak hours and lack privacy, which is what high earners care about.

Table 5 shows that, compared with urban peers, suburban respondents are more likely to transfer by buses than walking for the access trip (home-to-metro); and that compared with suburban residents, urban peers are more likely to use DBS than walking for the access trip. The two findings are reasonable. On the one hand, metro accessibility is lower in suburban areas, and access distance to the metro station is longer. Suburban commuters cannot reach the metro by walking as their urban peers do, so buses are preferable for them (relative to walking). On the other hand, cycling infrastructures are more developed in urban areas than in suburban areas, leading to a higher willingness to transfer by DBS. Thus, DBS is more prevalent in cities than in suburban areas.

Table 6 indicates that for egress trips (metro-to-workplace), walking is more likely adopted in urban areas, while DBS and buses are more prevalent in suburban areas. Three possible reasons could be proposed. First, in urban areas, the dense distribution of the metro system in urban areas makes it unnecessary to transfer by DBS and buses because of the short transfer distance. Second, the heavy traffic condition in urban areas (e.g., traffic congestion) may be perceived to be unsafe by cyclists, whereas riding buses is time-consuming and unnecessary in most cases in urban areas of Shenzhen, a quintessential transit-dependent city. Third, the high quality of pedestrian infrastructures in urban areas means high walkability, which is friendly to pedestrians.

Moreover, transfer distance is significantly associated with the feeder mode choice, which is in agreement with previous studies [16,23]. Our results also show that DBS and buses are attractive for long-distance trips in the two scenarios. Additionally, the coefficient of the variable *Transfer distance* in the *Bus* model is larger than that in the *DBS* model, indicating that the substitution effect between bus and walking is more significant than that between DBS and walking when the transfer distance is reasonably long.

Table 5. Results of the access MNL model (reference group: walking, $N = 1086$).

Variable	DBS				Bus			
	Coef.	Odds Ratio	Std.	z	Coef.	Odds Ratio	Std.	z
Safety and attitude variables								
Bicycle crash	−0.269 **	0.764	0.146	−1.99	0.028	1.028	0.135	0.19
Vehicle crash	0.303 **	1.354	0.135	2.39	0.381 ***	1.464	0.127	2.82
Cycling	0.630 ***	1.878	0.164	3.84	0.069	1.071	0.164	0.42
Walking	−0.357 ***	0.700	0.148	−2.60	−0.285 *	0.752	0.138	−1.92
Bus	−0.018	0.982	0.282	−0.07	0.318	1.374	0.258	1.13
DBS	0.824 ***	2.279	0.180	4.14	−0.213	0.809	0.199	−1.18
DBS vs. walking	0.489 ***	1.631	0.158	3.13	0.277 *	1.319	0.156	1.75
DBS vs. bus	−0.028	0.972	0.183	−0.16	−0.260	0.771	0.171	−1.42
Easy to take a bus	−0.396 **	0.673	0.201	−2.36	0.599 ***	1.821	0.168	2.98
Easy to find DBS	0.605 ***	1.832	0.129	5.05	−0.098	0.906	0.120	−0.76
Physical activity	−0.263	0.768	0.192	−1.38	−0.153	0.858	0.191	−0.80
Control variables								
Gender (reference: female)								
Male	0.342 *	1.407	0.222	1.59	−0.181	0.835	0.215	−0.81
Age (reference: under 25 years)								
26–35 years	0.187	1.206	0.263	0.78	0.138	1.148	0.241	0.53
36–45 years	−0.468	0.626	0.358	−1.28	0.366	1.442	0.367	1.02
Over 46 years	−0.387	0.679	0.644	−0.63	−0.015	0.985	0.613	−0.02
Education (reference: middle school or below)								
High school	−0.137	0.872	0.758	−0.19	−0.379	0.684	0.728	−0.50
College/University	−0.276	0.759	0.718	−0.40	−0.573	0.564	0.694	−0.80
Graduate institute	−0.523	0.593	0.786	−0.69	−0.419	0.658	0.753	−0.53

Table 5. Cont.

Variable	DBS				Bus			
	Coef.	Odds Ratio	Std.	z	Coef.	Odds Ratio	Std.	z
Income (reference: <4999 RMB)								
5000 to 9999 RMB	0.132	1.141	0.323	0.39	−0.608 *	0.544	0.336	−1.89
10,000 to 14,999 RMB	0.206	1.229	0.401	0.54	−1.134 ***	0.322	0.379	−2.83
>15,000 RMB	−0.239	0.788	0.413	−0.56	−0.781 *	0.458	0.423	−1.89
Bicycle ownership (reference: no)								
Yes	0.203	1.225	0.322	0.65	0.600 *	1.822	0.314	1.86
Home location (reference: urban area)								
Suburban area	−0.351 *	0.704	0.236	−1.69	0.397 *	1.487	0.208	1.68
Transfer distance	0.972 ***	1.001	0.158	5.98	1.298 ***	1.001	0.163	8.21
Intercept	−6.378 ***	0.002	1.249	−5.16	−3.678 ***	0.025	1.237	−2.95
Pseudo R^2				0.237				
Log-likelihood				−661.507				

Note: *** $p < 0.01$; ** $p < 0.05$; * $p < 0.1$.

Table 6. Results of the egress MNL model (reference group: walking, $N = 1108$).

Variable	DBS				Bus			
	Coef.	Odds Ratio	Std.	z	Coef.	Odds Ratio	Std.	z
Safety and attitude variables								
Bicycle crash	−0.186	0.830	0.163	−1.38	−0.089	0.915	0.135	−0.55
Vehicle crash	0.264 **	1.302	0.144	2.13	0.275 *	1.316	0.124	1.91
Cycling	0.244 *	1.276	0.181	1.65	−0.015	0.985	0.147	−0.08
Walking	−0.435 ***	0.647	0.163	−3.23	−0.255	0.775	0.135	−1.56
Bus	0.029	1.029	0.322	0.11	0.140	1.150	0.259	0.43
DBS	0.475 ***	1.609	0.200	2.60	0.068	1.070	0.183	0.34
DBS vs. walking	0.653 ***	1.921	0.170	4.02	0.079	1.082	0.162	0.47
DBS vs. bus	0.428 **	1.535	0.201	2.42	−0.127	0.881	0.177	−0.63
Easy to take a bus	−0.202	0.817	0.204	−1.27	0.066	1.069	0.160	0.33
Easy to find DBS	0.261 **	1.298	0.135	2.35	0.053	1.055	0.111	0.40
Physical activity	0.236	1.266	0.213	1.26	0.047	1.048	0.187	0.22
Control variables								
Gender (reference: female)								
Male	0.141	1.152	0.246	0.68	−0.034	0.967	0.208	−0.14
Age (reference: under 25 years)								
26–35 years	0.557 **	1.745	0.296	2.32	−0.015	0.986	0.240	−0.05
36–45 years	0.387	1.473	0.385	1.14	0.791 **	2.207	0.340	2.06
Over 46 years	0.302	1.353	0.570	0.51	1.026 *	2.789	0.594	1.80
Education (reference: middle school or below)								
High school	−0.321	0.725	0.697	−0.48	−1.021	0.360	0.671	−1.46
College/University	−0.996	0.369	0.647	−1.56	−1.381 **	0.251	0.638	−2.13
Graduate institute	−1.419 *	0.242	0.754	−1.94	−1.299 *	0.273	0.730	−1.72
Income (reference: <4999 RMB)								
5000 to 9999 RMB	0.028	1.029	0.367	0.09	−0.219	0.803	0.313	−0.60
10,000 to 14,999 RMB	−0.502	0.605	0.444	−1.36	−0.589	0.555	0.368	−1.33
>15,000 RMB	−1.180 ***	0.307	0.476	−2.78	−0.706	0.493	0.425	−1.48
Bicycle ownership (reference: no)								
Yes	0.215	1.240	0.341	0.72	0.406	1.500	0.298	1.19
Workplace location (reference: urban area)								
Suburban area	0.445 *	1.560	0.272	1.91	0.489 *	1.630	0.233	1.80
Transfer distance	1.143 ***	1.001	0.194	5.96	1.605 ***	1.002	0.192	8.29
Intercept	−6.796 ***	0.001	1.275	−5.42	−2.282 *	0.102	1.255	−1.79
Pseudo R^2				0.206				
Log-likelihood				−622.990				

Note: *** $p < 0.01$; ** $p < 0.05$; * $p < 0.1$.

6. Discussion

Like many other transit modes, the metro offers commuters stop-to-stop services instead of door-to-door services. First- and last-mile issues are, therefore, inevitable for metro trips [10]. A synergy between the metro and other travel modes, either motorized (e.g., bus and car) or non-motorized (e.g., walking and cycling), brings potentials to promote urban mobility through addressing the first- and last-mile problem [11,21]. Identifying the determinants of the feeder mode choice is, therefore, dispensable for understanding the first-/last-mile behavior of metro commuters.

This study contributes to the literature in three aspects. First, we explored the feeder mode choices of metro commuters in the Chinese mega-city context featured with unique characteristics of feeder behaviors, thereby generating diverse targeted implications for improving the seamless connection of metro transit. Second, the discussion of DBS, the newly emerged transport mode that has profoundly reshaped feeder mode choices, enriches the traditional transport research on multimodal behavior. Third, we compared the effects of traffic safety perception and attitudes on the feeder mode choices between access and egress feeder trip scenarios, which have been scarcely discussed in the literature.

This study provides a useful reference to guide metro users to choose reasonable feeder modes for connecting the metro transit with optimal utilities. Its findings also provide DBS/bus operators and the local government with a valuable reference for the management and improvement of the first- and last-mile. For instance, setting sideways and exclusive bikeways may improve safety perception, thereby encouraging active travel modes (e.g., walking and cycling) for connecting the metro transit [24]. Appropriate distributions of DBS bikes and bus stops near origins/destinations in metro catchment areas and close to metro entrances/exits are indispensable for fostering a good attitude toward DBS/bus usage [16]. During peak hours at metro entrances/exits, DBS bikes are excessively allocated and parked disorderly, whereas the queue for the bus is usually long, clogging the road. Thus, effective management for metro connection around metro entrances/exits is necessarily provided by local transport departments or bureaus. Moreover, available feeder services (e.g., bus lines, fare discount scheme, smart card, and real-time information system) and people-friendly facilities (e.g., bicycle parking space, protected shelters, benches, sidewalks, and exclusive bikeways) in metro catchment areas are suggested to be offered by local transport departments or bureaus [24,38]. More attention and efforts should be paid to suburban areas where feeder services and facilities are less equipped. These measures aiming at a seamless metro transit connection contribute to promoting metro usage or facilitating the modal shift from the car to the metro transit, thereby benefiting sustainable development urban transport. Furthermore, in today's era with diversified last-mile travel choices, we hope that our topic can ignite a tremendous fascination from local and international researchers.

However, there are some limitations that deserved future research. First, limited by the questionnaire design, we only include two traffic safety variables (bicycle crash and vehicle crash) in the MNL models. As such, more perceived safety factors such as in-vehicle safety in buses and cars should be considered in future studies [43]. Second, attitude factors are insufficiently considered. For example, the attitudes toward economic cost and environmental awareness, which this study fails to capture, may affect the decision-making process of feeder trip mode choice. Third, attitudes may be shaped by objective, physical factors. For example, the attitude towards bus/PBS availability is likely related to the objective level of service. In a similar vein, perceived traffic safety is possibly associated with the actual number of accidents. As such, exploring the interplay between objective factors and (subjective) attitudes (e.g., objectively measured and perceived service quality) is worthy of examination. Fourth, future studies can be devoted to exploring the relationships between traffic safety, attitude, socio-demographic characteristics, and feeder mode choice by revealing the underlying mediation or moderation effects. Last but not least, as travel behavior is jointly shaped by socio-economic variables, the physical environment (built environment + natural environment), and perceptions or attitudes, examining the relative importance of all the independent variables and determining which category plays a larger role in shaping travel behavior is worthy of investigation. Machine learning techniques (e.g., support vector machine, decision tree, random forest, gradient boosting decision tree, and extreme gradient boosting model) are recommended to be adopted in future studies.

7. Conclusions

In a departure from existing literature, this study explores how perceived traffic safety and attitude factors are associated with metro commuters' feeder mode choice during the morning peak time. Our analysis results basically answer our four research questions (see Section 1) and can be listed as follows. (1) Walking is the most frequently used mode for connecting the metro (accounting for over 70%), followed by DBS and buses. The high feeder mode share of walking and DBS is unique in the context of Mainland Chinese mega cities, which differs from European and North American cities; (2) Variances in traffic safety perception and attitude exist across gender and space; (3) The variance in the attitude toward the feeder mode between genders is minimal (or subtle), but men's attitude toward the DBS/bus availability remarkably differs from women's; (4) The vehicle-related crash risk usually discourages walking but supports the DBS and buses as transfer modes, whereas the bicycle-related crash is a barrier of transfer by DBS for access trips; (5) Positive attitudes toward cycling and DBS make DBS competitive as a feeder mode. A good attitude toward walking promotes walk–metro integration, but the attitude toward buses does not matter in the feeder mode choice; and (6) Perceived traffic safety and attitudes toward the mode play different roles in shaping first- and last-mile mode choices.

Author Contributions: Conceptualization, Y.G. (Yuanyuan Guo) and L.Y.; Methodology, Y.G. (Yuanyuan Guo) and L.Y.; Software, Y.G. (Yuanyuan Guo) and L.Y.; Validation, W.H. and Y.G. (Yi Guo); Formal analysis, Y.G. (Yuanyuan Guo); Writing—original draft preparation, Y.G. (Yuanyuan Guo) and L.Y.; Writing—review and editing, W.H. and Y.G. (Yi Guo); Supervision, L.Y.; Project administration, Y.G. (Yuanyuan Guo) and L.Y. All authors have read and agreed to the published version of the manuscript.

Funding: This study is sponsored by the National Natural Science Foundation of China (No. 51778530).

Acknowledgments: The authors are grateful to the three reviewers for their helpful comments.

Conflicts of Interest: The authors declare no conflict of interest.

References

1. Huang, W.; Guo, Y.; Xu, X. Evaluation of real-time vehicle energy consumption and related emissions in China: A case study of the Guangdong–Hong Kong–Macao greater Bay Area. *J. Clean. Prod.* **2020**, *263*, 121583. [CrossRef]
2. Sommar, J.N.; Johansson, C.; Lövenheim, B.; Markstedt, A.; Strömgren, M.; Forsberg, B. Potential effects on travelers' air pollution exposure and associated mortality estimated for a mode shift from car to bicycle commuting. *Int. J. Environ. Res. Public Health* **2020**, *17*, 7635. [CrossRef]
3. Wang, K.; Wang, X. Providing sports venues on mainland China: Implications for promoting leisure-time physical activity and national fitness policies. *Int. J. Environ. Res. Public Health* **2020**, *17*, 5136. [CrossRef]
4. Cheng, Y.H.; Liu, K.C. Evaluating bicycle-transit users' perceptions of intermodal inconvenience. *Transp. Res. Part A Policy Pract.* **2012**, *46*, 1690–1706. [CrossRef]
5. Yang, L.; Chu, X.; Gou, Z.; Yang, H.; Lu, Y.; Huang, W. Accessibility and proximity effects of bus rapid transit on housing prices: Heterogeneity across price quantiles and space. *J. Transp. Geogr.* **2020**, *88*, 102850. [CrossRef]
6. Yang, L.; Chau, K.W.; Szeto, W.Y.; Cui, X.; Wang, X. Accessibility to transit, by transit, and property prices: Spatially varying relationships. *Transp. Res. Part D Transp. Environ.* **2020**, *85*, 102387. [CrossRef]
7. Qin, H.; Guan, H.; Wu, Y. Analysis of park-and-ride decision behavior based on Decision Field Theory. *Transp. Res. Part F Psychol. Behav.* **2013**, *18*, 199–212. [CrossRef]
8. Wang, R.; Chen, L. Bicycle-transit integration in the United States, 2001–2009. *J. Public Transp.* **2013**, *16*, 95–119. [CrossRef]

9. Park, K.; Choi, D.A.; Tian, G.; Ewing, R. Not parking lots but parks: A joint association of parks and transit stations with travel behavior. *Int. J. Environ. Res. Public Health* **2019**, *16*, 547. [CrossRef]
10. Zhao, R.; Yang, L.; Liang, X.; Guo, Y.; Lu, Y.; Zhang, Y.; Ren, X. Last-mile travel mode choice: Data-mining hybrid with multiple attribute decision making. *Sustainability* **2019**, *11*, 6733. [CrossRef]
11. Duncan, M.; Cook, D. Is the provision of park-and-ride facilities at light rail stations an effective approach to reducing vehicle kilometers traveled in a US context? *Transp. Res. Part A Policy Pract.* **2014**, *66*, 65–74. [CrossRef]
12. Pucher, J.; Buehler, R. Integrating bicycling and public transport in North America. *J. Public Transp.* **2009**, *12*, 79–104. [CrossRef]
13. Wu, S.S.; Zhuang, Y.; Chen, J.; Wang, W.; Bai, Y.; Lo, S.M. Rethinking bus-to-metro accessibility in new town development: Case studies in Shanghai. *Cities* **2019**, *94*, 211–224. [CrossRef]
14. Wang, J.J.; Po, K. Bus routing strategies in a transit market: A case study of Hong Kong. *J. Adv. Transp.* **2001**, *35*, 259–288. [CrossRef]
15. Ma, T.; Liu, C.; Erdoğan, S. Bicycle sharing and transit: Does Capital Bikeshare affect Metrorail ridership in Washington, D.C.? *Transp. Res. Rec. J. Transp. Res. Board* **2015**, *2534*, 1–9. [CrossRef]
16. Guo, Y.; He, S.Y. Built environment effects on the integration of dockless bike-sharing and the metro. *Transp. Res. Part D Transp. Environ.* **2020**, *83*, 102335. [CrossRef]
17. Hern, S.O.; Estgfaeller, N. A scientometric review of powered micromobility. *Sustainability* **2020**, *12*, 9505.
18. Heinen, E.; Bohte, W. Multimodal commuting to work by public transport and bicycle: Attitudes toward mode choice. *Transp. Res. Rec. J. Transp. Res. Board* **2014**, *2015*, 111–122. [CrossRef]
19. Bachand-Marleau, J.; Larsen, J.; El-Geneidy, A. Much-anticipated marriage of cycling and transit. *Transp. Res. Rec. J. Transp. Res. Board* **2011**, *2247*, 109–117. [CrossRef]
20. Chalermpong, S.; Wibowo, S.S. Transit station access trips and factors affecting propensity to walk to transit stations in Bangkok, Thailand. *J. East. Asia Soc. Transp. Stud.* **2007**, *7*, 1806–1819.
21. Cervero, R. Walk-and-ride: Factors influencing pedestrian access to transit. *J. Public Transp.* **2001**, *3*, 1–23. [CrossRef]
22. Ji, Y.; Fan, Y.; Ermagun, A.; Cao, X.; Wang, W.; Das, K. Public bicycle as a feeder mode to rail transit in China: The role of gender, age, income, trip purpose, and bicycle theft experience. *Int. J. Sustain. Transp.* **2017**, *11*, 1–23. [CrossRef]
23. Zhao, P.; Li, S. Bicycle-metro integration in a growing city: The determinants of cycling as a transfer mode in metro station areas in Beijing. *Transp. Res. Part A Policy Pract.* **2017**, *99*, 46–60. [CrossRef]
24. Griffin, G.P.; Sener, I.N. Planning for bike share connectivity to rail transit. *J. Public Transp.* **2016**, *19*, 1–22. [CrossRef]
25. Ajzen, I. The theory of planned behavior. *Organ. Behav. Hum. Decis. Process.* **1991**, *50*, 179–211. [CrossRef]
26. Elias, W.; Shiftan, Y. The influence of individual's risk perception and attitudes on travel behavior. *Transp. Res. Part A Policy Pract.* **2012**, *46*, 1241–1251. [CrossRef]
27. Johansson, M.V.; Heldt, T.; Johansson, P. The effects of attitudes and personality traits on mode choice. *Transp. Res. Part A Policy Pract.* **2006**, *40*, 507–525. [CrossRef]
28. Guliani, A.; Mitra, R.; Buliung, R.N.; Larsen, K.; Faulkner, G.E.J. Gender-based differences in school travel mode choice behaviour: Examining the relationship between the neighbourhood environment and perceived traffic safety. *J. Transp. Heal.* **2015**, *2*, 502–511. [CrossRef]
29. Bagley, M.N.; Mokhtarian, P.L. The impact of residential neighborhood type on travel behavior: A structural equations modeling approach. *Ann. Reg. Sci.* **2002**, *36*, 279–297. [CrossRef]
30. Schwanen, T.; Mokhtarian, P.L. What affects commute mode choice: Neighborhood physical structure or preferences toward neighborhoods? *J. Transp. Geogr.* **2005**, *13*, 83–99. [CrossRef]
31. McMillan, T.E. The relative influence of urban form on a child's travel mode to school. *Transp. Res. Part A Policy Pract.* **2007**, *41*, 69–79. [CrossRef]
32. Arroyo, R.; Ruiz, T.; Mars, L.; Rasouli, S.; Timmermans, H. Influence of values, attitudes towards transport modes and companions on travel behavior. *Transp. Res. Part F Traffic Psychol. Behav.* **2020**, *71*, 8–22. [CrossRef]
33. Lee, J.M. Exploring Walking behavior in the streets of New York City using hourly pedestrian count data. *Sustainability* **2020**, *12*, 7863. [CrossRef]

34. Krizek, K.; Stonebraker, E. Bicycling and transit a marriage unrealized. *Transp. Res. Rec. J. Transp. Res. Board* **2010**, *2144*, 161–167. [CrossRef]
35. Singleton, P.; Clifton, K. Exploring synergy in bicycle and transit use. *Transp. Res. Rec. J. Transp. Res. Board* **2014**, *2417*, 92–102. [CrossRef]
36. Martens, K. Promoting bike-and-ride: The Dutch experience. *Transp. Res. Part A Policy Pract.* **2007**, *41*, 326–338. [CrossRef]
37. Guo, Y.; Yang, L.; Lu, Y.; Zhao, R. Dockless bike-sharing as a feeder mode of metro commute? The role of the feeder-related built environment: Analytical framework and empirical evidence. *Sustain. Cities Soc.* **2020**, 104947.
38. Rastogi, R.; Krishna Rao, K.V. Travel characteristics of commuters accessing transit: Case study. *J. Transp. Eng.* **2003**, *129*, 684–694. [CrossRef]
39. Pongprasert, P.; Kubota, H. Switching from motorcycle taxi to walking: A case study of transit station access in Bangkok, Thailand. *IATSS Res.* **2017**, *41*, 182–190. [CrossRef]
40. Chandra, S.; Bari, M.E.; Devarasetty, P.C.; Vadali, S. Accessibility evaluations of feeder transit services. *Transp. Res. Part A Policy Pract.* **2013**, *52*, 47–63. [CrossRef]
41. Schiller, P.L.; Kenworthy, J. *An Introduction to Sustainable Transportation: Policy, Planning and Implementation*, 2nd ed.; Routledge: London, UK, 2010.
42. Campbell, A.A.; Cherry, C.R.; Ryerson, M.S.; Yang, X. Factors influencing the choice of shared bicycles and shared electric bikes in Beijing. *Transp. Res. Part C Emerg. Technol.* **2016**, *67*, 399–414. [CrossRef]
43. Salonen, A.O. Passenger's subjective traffic safety, in-vehicle security and emergency management in the driverless shuttle bus in Finland. *Transp. Policy* **2018**, *61*, 106–110. [CrossRef]
44. Gargoum, S.A.; El-basyouny, K. Exploring the association between speed and safety: A path analysis approach. *Accid. Anal. Prev.* **2016**, *93*, 32–40. [CrossRef]
45. Giles-Corti, B.; Wood, G.; Pikora, T.; Learnihan, V.; Bulsara, M.; Van Niel, K.; Timperio, A.; McCormack, G.; Villanueva, K. School site and the potential to walk to school: The impact of street connectivity and traffic exposure in school neighborhoods. *Heal. Place* **2011**, *17*, 545–550. [CrossRef]
46. Hamed, M.M.; Al Rousan, T.M. Impact of perceived risk on urban commuters' route choices. *Road Transp. Res.* **1998**, *7*, 46–62.
47. Syafriharti, R.; Kombaitan, B.; Kusumantoro, I.P.; Syabri, I. Relationship between train users' perceptions of walkability with access and egress mode choice. In *MATEC Web of Conferences*; EDP Sciences: Les Ulis, France, 2018; Volume 147, pp. 1–9.
48. Adams, J.G.U. Evaluating the effectiveness of road safety measures. *Traffic Eng. Control* **1988**, *29*, 344–352.
49. Cho, G.; Rodríguez, D.A.; Khattak, A.J. The role of the built environment in explaining relationships between perceived and actual pedestrian and bicyclist safety. *Accid. Anal. Prev.* **2009**, *41*, 692–702. [CrossRef]
50. Kerr, J.; Emond, J.A.; Badland, H.; Reis, R.; Sarmiento, O.; Carlson, J.; Sallis, J.F.; Cerin, E.; Cain, K.; Conway, T.; et al. Perceived neighborhood environmental attributes associated with walking and cycling for transport among adult residents of 17 cities in 12 countries: The IPEN study. *Environ. Health Perspect.* **2016**, *124*, 290–298. [CrossRef]
51. Zhang, C.Q.; Zhang, R.; Gan, Y.; Li, D.; Rhodes, R.E. Predicting transport-related cycling in Chinese employees using an integration of perceived physical environment and social cognitive factors. *Transp. Res. Part F Traffic Psychol. Behav.* **2019**, *64*, 424–439. [CrossRef]
52. Van Wee, B. Verkeer en transport. In *Verkeer en Vervoer in hoofdlijnen (Outlining Traffic and Transport)*; Van Wee, B., Anne Annema, J., Eds.; Coutinho: Bussum, The Netherlands, 2009.
53. Schepers, P.; Hagenzieker, M.; Methorst, R.; Van Wee, B.; Wegman, F. A conceptual framework for road safety and mobility applied to cycling safety. *Accid. Anal. Prev.* **2014**, *62*, 331–340. [CrossRef]
54. Dill, J.; Carr, T. Bicycle commuting and facilities in major U.S. cities: If you build them, commuters will use them. *Transp. Res. Rec. J. Transp. Res. Rec.* **2003**, 116–123. [CrossRef]
55. Aziz, H.M.A.; Nagle, N.N.; Morton, A.M.; Hilliard, M.R.; White, D.A.; Stewart, R.N. Exploring the impact of walk–bike infrastructure, safety perception, and built-environment on active transportation mode choice: A random parameter model using New York City commuter data. *Transportation* **2018**, *45*, 1207–1229. [CrossRef]

56. Pyrialakou, V.D.; Gkartzonikas, C.; Gatlin, J.D.; Gkritza, K. Perceptions of safety on a shared road: Driving, cycling, or walking near an autonomous vehicle. *J. Safety Res.* **2020**, *72*, 249–258. [CrossRef]
57. Morales, J.F.; Moya, M.; Gaviria, E.; Cuadrado, I. *Psicología Social*; McGraw-Hill: Madrid, Spain, 2007.
58. Eagly, A.H.; Chaiken, S. *The Psychology of Attitudes*; Harcourt Brace Jovanovich College Publishers: Fort Worth, TX, USA, 1993; ISBN 0155000977.
59. Tran, Y.; Yamamoto, T.; Sato, H.; Miwa, T.; Morikawa, T. The analysis of influences of attitudes on mode choice under highly unbalanced mode share patterns. *J. Choice Model.* **2020**, *36*, 100227. [CrossRef]
60. Fishbein, M.; Ajzen, I. *Belief, Attitude, Intention, and Behavior: An Introduction to Theory and Research*; Addison-Wesley: Reading, MA, USA, 1975.
61. Gärling, T.; Gillholm, R.; Gärling, A. Reintroducing attitude theory in travel behavior research: The validity of an interactive interview procedure to predict car use. *Transportation* **1998**, *25*, 129–146. [CrossRef]
62. Hunecke, M.; Haustein, S.; Böhler, S.; Grischkat, S. Attitude-based target groups to reduce the ecological impact of daily mobility behavior. *Environ. Behav.* **2010**, *42*, 3–43. [CrossRef]
63. Ye, R.; Titheridge, H. Satisfaction with the commute: The role of travel mode choice, built environment and attitudes. *Transp. Res. Part D Transp. Environ.* **2017**, *52*, 535–547. [CrossRef]
64. Thøgersen, J. Understanding repetitive travel mode choices in a stable context: A panel study approach. *Transp. Res. Part A Policy Pract.* **2006**, *40*, 621–638. [CrossRef]
65. Beirão, G.; Sarsfield Cabral, J.A. Understanding attitudes towards public transport and private car: A qualitative study. *Transp. Policy* **2007**, *14*, 478–489. [CrossRef]
66. He, S.Y.; Thøgersen, J. The impact of attitudes and perceptions on travel mode choice and car ownership in a Chinese megacity: The case of Guangzhou. *Res. Transp. Econ.* **2017**, *62*, 57–67. [CrossRef]
67. Tran, Y.; Yamamoto, T.; Sato, H. The influences of environmentalism and attitude towards physical activity on mode choice: The new evidences. *Transp. Res. Part A Policy Pract.* **2020**, *134*, 211–226. [CrossRef]
68. Liu, D.; Du, H.; Southworth, F.; Ma, S. The influence of social-psychological factors on the intention to choose low-carbon travel modes in Tianjin, China. *Transp. Res. Part A Policy Pract.* **2017**, *105*, 42–53. [CrossRef]
69. Bao, Z.; Lu, W. Developing efficient circularity for construction and demolition waste management in fast emerging economies: Lessons learned from Shenzhen, China. *Sci. Total Environ.* **2020**, *724*, 138264. [CrossRef]
70. Xie, M. Shenzhen Ranks First in Urban Rail Transit Network Density in China with the Average Daily Passenger Flow of the Whole Network of 5.568 Million in 2019. Available online: http://k.sina.com.cn/article_1677991972_6404202402000n77w.html?from=news&subch=onews (accessed on 1 May 2020).
71. Cerin, E.; Saelens, B.E.; Sallis, J.F.; Frank, L.D. Neighborhood Environment Walkability Scale: Validity and development of a short form. *Med. Sci. Sports Exerc.* **2006**, *38*, 1682. [CrossRef]
72. Nickkar, A.; Banerjee, S.; Chavis, C.; Bhuyan, I.A.; Barnes, P. A spatial-temporal gender and land use analysis of bikeshare ridership: The case study of Baltimore City. *City, Cult. Soc.* **2019**, *18*, 100291. [CrossRef]
73. Washington, S.P.; Karlaftis, M.G.; Mannering, F.L. *Statistical and Econometric Methods for Transportation Data Analysis*, 2nd ed.; Chapman and Hall/CRC: Boca Raton, FL, USA, 2011.
74. Ham, N.; Field, J.; Kirkwood, B. Gender differences and areas of common concern in the driving behaviors and attitudes of adolescents. *J. Safety Res.* **1996**, *27*, 163–173.
75. Najaf, P.; Thill, J.C.; Zhang, W.; Fields, M.G. City-level urban form and traffic safety: A structural equation modeling analysis of direct and indirect effects. *J. Transp. Geogr.* **2018**, *69*, 257–270. [CrossRef]
76. Lee, Y.S. Gender differences in physical activity and walking among older adults. *J. Women Aging* **2005**, *17*, 55–70. [CrossRef] [PubMed]
77. Psarros, I.; Kepaptsoglou, K.; Karlaftis, M.G. An empirical investigation of passenger wait time perceptions using hazard-based duration models. *J. Public Transp.* **2011**, *14*, 109–122. [CrossRef]
78. Shaheen, S.; Zhang, H.; Martin, E.; Guzman, S. China's Hangzhou public bicycle understanding: Early adoption and behavioral response to bikesharing. *Transp. Res. Rec. J. Transp. Res. Board* **2011**, *2247*, 33–41. [CrossRef]

79. Fishman, E.; Washington, S.; Haworth, N. Bikeshare's impact on active travel: Evidence from the United States, Great Britain, and Australia. *J. Transp. Heal.* **2014**, *2*, 135–142. [CrossRef]
80. Lin, J.; Zhao, P.; Takada, K.; Li, S.; Yai, T.; Chen, C. Built environment and public bike usage for metro access: A comparison of neighborhoods in Beijing, Taipei, and Tokyo. *Transp. Res. Part D Transp. Environ.* **2018**, *63*, 209–221. [CrossRef]

Publisher's Note: MDPI stays neutral with regard to jurisdictional claims in published maps and institutional affiliations.

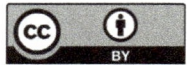

© 2020 by the authors. Licensee MDPI, Basel, Switzerland. This article is an open access article distributed under the terms and conditions of the Creative Commons Attribution (CC BY) license (http://creativecommons.org/licenses/by/4.0/).

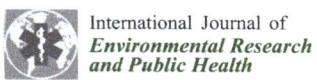

Article

Why Do Students Walk or Cycle for Transportation? Perceived Study Environment and Psychological Determinants as Predictors of Active Transportation by University Students

Monika Teuber * and Gorden Sudeck

Institute of Sports Science, University of Tübingen, 72074 Tübingen, Germany; gorden.sudeck@uni-tuebingen.de
* Correspondence: monika.teuber@uni-tuebingen.de

Abstract: University students are particularly at risk to suffer from physical and psychological complaints and for not fulfilling health-oriented physical activity (PA) recommendations. Since PA is linked with various benefits for health and educational outcomes, the group of students is of particular interest for PA promotion. Although active commuting has been identified as a relevant domain of PA in order to gain the various benefits of PA, little knowledge is available with respect to university students. This study tested conditions in the study environment, as well as personal motivators and barriers, as determinants for the active transportation of university students. Using a cross-sectional convenience sample of a university in the southwest of Germany (n = 997), we applied factor analyses to bundle relevant information on environmental and psychological determinants (adapted NEWS-G; adapted transport-related items from an Australian university survey) and blockwise hierarchical regressions. The objective was to analyze associations between the bundled determinants and self-reports on PA for transport-related walking and cycling (measured by the EHIS-PAQ). Results revealed associations between transport-related cycling and the perceived study environment (e.g., high automobile traffic) as well as certain personal motivators and barriers (e.g., time effort or weather conditions). The study contributes to the knowledge about determinants that are important for the development and improvement of public health interventions for students in a university setting.

Keywords: active transportation; physical activity; perceived study environment; psychological determinants; motivators; barriers; university students; socio-ecological approaches

Citation: Teuber, M.; Sudeck, G. Why Do Students Walk or Cycle for Transportation? Perceived Study Environment and Psychological Determinants as Predictors of Active Transportation by University Students. *IJERPH* **2021**, *18*, 1390. https://doi.org/10.3390/ijerph18041390

Academic Editor: Paul B. Tchounwou
Received: 21 December 2020
Accepted: 28 January 2021
Published: 3 February 2021

Publisher's Note: MDPI stays neutral with regard to jurisdictional claims in published maps and institutional affiliations.

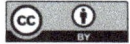

Copyright: © 2021 by the authors. Licensee MDPI, Basel, Switzerland. This article is an open access article distributed under the terms and conditions of the Creative Commons Attribution (CC BY) license (https://creativecommons.org/licenses/by/4.0/).

1. Introduction

Academic studies often impose high demands on university students, which can be associated with negative effects on health. Students suffer more often from perceived stress [1] and from physical and psychological complaints than their peers [1–4]. As health is positively related with physical activity (PA) and less sedentary behavior, these behaviors can provide starting points for improving the students' health: because students who are more physically active through sports or everyday activities have fewer complaints and a greater sense of well-being than inactive students [2,4–6]. For the same reason, active transportation is associated with less obesity, less cardiovascular risk factors, and higher physical fitness for students [7,8].

Since the transition from school to university often marks a particular risk for becoming physically inactive [9], the group of students is of particular interest for PA promotion in order to gain health benefits. According to current guidelines for health-enhancing PA, about half of the students in the United States, Canada, and China, 40% in Australia, and 67% in Europe are not sufficiently physically active [10]. Reasons for students' physical inactivity are increasing self-employment, increasing academic workload with resulting problems in time management regarding work and social demands [8], and an increasing distance from home to university [11].

To counteract this, the promotion of PA in university settings is necessary. Due to the increasing number of people who will study, universities have a growing potential to reach a large mass of young adults in order to promote positive PA behavior, which will last in later life. However, in contrast to school settings, the promotion of PA is not yet widespread in university settings, which leads to a gap between school-based and workplace-oriented approaches of PA promotion. Moreover, the knowledge about determinants of PA in university students is scarce, but this knowledge is necessary to guide evidence-based PA promotion in university settings [12].

Since the 2000s, PA promotion research has emphasized that the physical and social environment play an important role for PA behavior. Socio-ecological approaches increasingly have taken this into account and complement individually-focused approaches [12]. For example, Bauman and colleagues [12] as well as Bucksch and colleagues [13] differ between personal/individual and contextual/environmental factors that contribute to differences in PA behaviors. According to these basic ideas, Figure 1 schematically depicts individual and contextual factors of students' PA behavior which are important to understand in order to develop and improve interventions for active transportation, which can lead to an higher level of physical activity and in turn to a better health status [12]. Adapted to the university setting, the perspective of students' individual conditions is integrated into the perspective of the surrounding conditions of the study environment, increasing the extent of the effect radius of the PA promotion when regarded together [14–17]. Hence, this adaption follows public health and socio-ecological approaches [13,15,18].

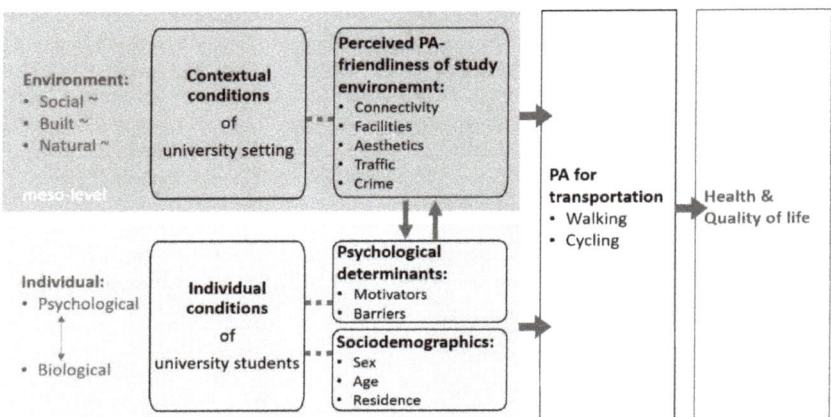

Figure 1. Schematic representation of the socio-ecological approach of PA promotion adapted to the university setting (own presentation based on Bucksch et al. (2012) [13] and Bauman et al. (2012) [12]).

Some empirical studies in the university setting already exist, which have revealed several factors important for the active transportation behavior of students [19–30]. The results show basically that encouraging students to commute to university by bicycle or by foot is linked with the learning environment as well as with the campus environment, which deliver more or less activity-friendly physical environments.

The connectivity of the street network has been identified as an important determinant for the cycling behavior of students [22,24,27,28,30]. This refers, for example, to intersection density [28], street connectivity [24], and bicycle racks installed on buses to extend the commuting distance [20]. Such improvements to the cycling infrastructure reduce effort and time demands, which in turn mitigate the negative impact of distance [21,22,26,28,29] and increase the likelihood of cycling for commuting reasons [30].

In addition, the availability and proximity of walking or cycling facilities encourage students to cycle more [19–21,23,25,27,28,30]. However, also in terms of active commuting in general, the perception of walking and cycling facilities are positively associated with active commuting to university [23].

The feeling of safety also contributes to increased active transportation of students. Traffic safety, for example, based on traffic-calming measures [22], has been shown to be important for the active commuting of students [19,22,27]. On the other hand, safety concerns can lead to avoidance of active commuting. Such is the case, for example, with high automobile traffic including sharing the roadway with automobile traffic [19]. Moreover, crime issues are related to students' active transportation behavior [21,25,27,28]; this refers to personal safety as well as to bicycle security such as secure bicycle-parking racks and lockers, and a high degree of safety against bicycle theft [22,25,27].

Finally, there are the aesthetic aspects, which are positively related to active transportation and are expressed, for example, by the "attractiveness of the surroundings" [27] (p. 72).

In addition to environmental conditions, potential personal motivators, and barriers among students' active forms of transportation are also known from empirical studies [19,20,22,23,25,26,28]. For example, motivators such as concerns for the environment increase the probability of choosing bicycles [28]. Barriers such as travel costs [26,28] or inclement weather [25] prevent students from active transportation. In addition to the barrier of time effort [26], there are other types of effort that prevent students from active transportation such as planning [23], inconvenience, time constraints [21], or physiological discomfort [27].

The current state of research leaves open questions regarding the environmental and personal determinants of active transportation behavior in university settings. So far, only a few studies have dealt with such questions by considering environmental and psychological determinants together. Especially the environmental variables have been less studied, but are thought to have widespread effects for active transportation behavior [12]. Furthermore, there is less known about the differentiation in various modes of active transportation, as most often only general PA or a specific mode of transportation is considered. In addition, there is a lack of consistent measurement methods. Since the relationship of the environment to physically active behavior has also been studied in the community neighborhood, various survey instruments have been established in the communities for assessing the neighborhood environment [17,18,31–41]. None are yet available for the study environment. Therefore, there is a lack of both a general more extensive survey procedure of the PA-friendliness of the study environment and investigations on how this relates to the two transport-related modes of PA, walking and cycling.

2. Purpose of the Study

The present study addresses the question of which conditions of the study environment as well as personal motivators and barriers are related to the active transportation behavior of university students. Relationships are considered separately for transport-related walking and cycling because different modes of transportation can have different interactions with the environment.

This question is addressed because students are particularly at risk of not fulfilling health-oriented PA recommendations and active transportation has been shown to be a relevant domain of PA that brings various health-promoting benefits of PA. As students suffer from physical and psychological complaints, promoting active transportation could counteract this. This requires specific knowledge of socio-ecological determinants. So far only a few studies have considered both personal and environmental determinants together [22,23,27].

By this study, additional specific knowledge about why students walk or cycle will be gained to support the implementation of specific interventions in the university setting to improve personal health and, beyond that, public health.

To achieve the purpose of the study, two steps are carried out. Since there is no established survey instrument available for the study environment, in a first step the questionnaire for the Neighborhood Environment Walkability Scale for Germany (NEWS-G) was adapted to the study environment. NEWS-G offers a comprehensive collection of environmental characteristics across several sub-chapters and is one of the most widespread measurement procedures of the perceived PA environment [31]. The adapted version should represent a coherent construct for friendliness of the study environment regarding transport-related PA. For the individual perspective, motivators/barriers that are interrelated will be exploratively clustered so that the relationships between them are considered. In the second step, regression analyses will be conducted to empirically identify associations between individual as well as environmental factors and the two separate outcomes of transport-related walking and cycling in terms of health-enhancing activity. We assume that, in the context of the socio-economic approach, both psychological and environmental factors are related to the active transportation behavior of university students.

3. Materials and Methods

3.1. Design, Setting, and Sample

The cross-sectional convenience sample for this study (n = 997) was formed by students at the University of Tübingen in southwestern Germany who completed the survey. The University of Tübingen represents an urban university setting integrated into an urban hilly landscape. It consists of eight faculties plus a further five interfaculty institutes. More than 200 courses of study are offered. The cross-sectional study was conducted as part of the PA promoting project "BeTa*Balance*" of the university sports organization at the Institute of Sports Science of the University of Tübingen. The study was performed online for three weeks during the end of the university time of the summer semester in 2018 and addressed all students at the university. The online questionnaire was distributed via the university's mailing list and Facebook posts, as well as outreach campaigns in cafeterias and at university meeting points (e.g., the University library and lecture halls) using flyers with a QR code leading to the link for the online questionnaire. The Ethics Commission of the Faculty of Economics and Social Sciences at the University of Tübingen gave a positive vote for the study procedures.

Of a total of 999 returned questionnaires, 997 form the sample of this study, since two cases were not usable due to incomplete answers. Among the participants were 718 female students (72%), 232 male students (23.3%), and 47 (4.7%) did not provide any gender information. The average age of the surveyed students was 23.4 years (SD = 3.45), with an age range from 18 to 42 years. A total of 224 students (22.5%) of the sample reported that they are not living in town and commute to the university town (Table 1). In total, 26,151 students were registered in the summer semester 2018 of the University of Tübingen (state 15 May 2018), resulting in a response rate of 3.8%. Of these, 58.2% were female and 42.8% were male. The sample in this study showed a shift toward more female students.

3.2. Measures

3.2.1. Physical Activity: Transport-Related Walking and Cycling

To assess PA, the instrument from the European Health Interview Survey (EHIS-PAQ) was used, which records domain-specific information on PA for transport-related walking and transport-related cycling [42]. The questionnaire enables the determination of activity volume in different activity domains. In the domain of active transportation, the participants answered the following questions, each worded in the same way, but separately for walking and cycling in relation to a typical week: (a) "In a typical week, on how many days do you walk/bicycle for at least 10 min continuously to get to and from places?" and (b) "How much time do you spend walking/bicycling in order to get to and from places on a typical day?" Activity volumes were determined in accordance with the procedure in the validation studies [42] and were subsequently indicated as duration per week (minutes or hours). Time values were transformed in metabolic equivalent (MET) values using 3.3 as a factor for computing MET-minutes for walking and 6.0 for cycling, which corresponds to the procedure in the validation studies [42]. As a guideline, 1 MET equals the energy expenditure in the state of complete rest [43].

Table 1. Overview of the sample as well as of the study variables according to physical activity (dependent variables), perceived study environment, and personal motivators for and barriers to PA.

Variables (Number of Items of the Scale)		n	f	f (%)				
Sociodemographic characteristics								
Residence: resident in university town		997	773	77.5				
Residence: not resident in university town			224	22.5				
Gender: female		950	718	24.4				
Gender: male			232	75.6				

	r/α	n	M	SD	min	max	Skewness	Kurtosis
Age		994	23.40	3.45	18	42	1.37	3.25
Physical activity								
Transportation walking (METh/week) [1]		993	9.31	9.17	0	40.15	1.55	2.11
Transportation cycling (METh/week) [2]		991	8.71	12.21	0	51.00	1.63	2.19
Perceived study environment								
Active transportation: uphill (1)		994	2.56	0.99	1	4	−0.02	−1.03
Active transportation: connectivity (1)		996	2.20	0.81	1	4	0.22	−0.47
Active transportation: walking/cycling facilities (2)	0.51	993	1.55	0.57	1	4	1.04	1.06
Aesthetics (3)	0.60	992	2.24	0.59	1	4	0.07	−0.11
High automobile traffic (3)	0.69	989	2.32	0.63	1	4	0.24	−0.26
General crime (1)		997	1.25	0.53	1	4	2.32	5.75
Bicycle-related crime (1)		990	2.19	2.00	1	4	0.47	−0.12
Psychological determinants-Motivators								
Study-related motivator (2)	0.53	971	2.78	0.84	1	4	−0.19	−0.82
Personal benefits (2)	0.42	983	3.00	0.75	1	4	−0.33	−0.65
Instrumental extrinsic (2)	0.43	888	2.55	0.93	1	4	−0.11	−0.97
Avoid air pollution (1)		983	2.69	0.07	1	4	−0.14	−1.01
Psychological determinants-Barriers								
Personal (3)	0.69	975	1.77	0.68	1	4	0.87	0.29
Discomfort with study life (3)	0.77	837	2.11	0.88	1	4	0.41	−0.87
External (2)	0.48	990	2.25	0.82	1	4	0.45	−0.55

[1] Factor 3.3 for computing MET-minutes for walking. [2] Factor 6.0 for computing MET-minutes for cycling.

3.2.2. Contextual Conditions: Perceived PA-Friendliness of the Study Environment

For the assessment of the perceived study environment, the German version of the Neighborhood Environment Walkability Scale (NEWS-G) [44] was contextualized to the university setting. Thus, it can be applied to everyday study life and it records the PA friendliness of the study environment. The following two sections were relevant for this article: (1) opportunities for walking and cycling (including land use mix–access, street connectivity, walking/cycling facilities, and environmental design) and (2) (traffic) safety (including crime) (Appendix A Table A1). Both areas consider relevant factors of leisure-related resources, appearance, and land use, and they are also congruent with the categories of the instrument "Neighborhood Active Living Potential" [45]. Both sections of the adapted version of NEWS-G consist of different statements for which the participants had to indicate their degree of agreement: 1 = totally disagree; 2 = more likely to disagree; 3 = more likely to agree; 4 = totally agree. For the purpose of the main analysis, the items of the study environment were bundled to main factors in the pre-analysis to get a dimensionally reduced yet statistically coherent measurement of the perceived PA-friendliness of the study environment (see Section 4.1.1).

3.2.3. Individual Conditions: Psychological Determinants of Active Transportation—Motivators and Barriers

The survey instrument of Shannon et al. (2006) guided the measurement of motivators and barriers. This instrument was used in a study with university students in order to analyze motivators and barriers for active commuting [26]. All items include statements, which should be rated according to the extent to which they either motivate or prevent one toward or from engaging in active transportation behavior (e.g., Mot1, "Potential to save money", or Bar1, "Inappropriate weather" with the answer choices: 1 = not at all, 2 = a little, 3 = strong, 4 = very strong). There was also an option, "I cannot judge", which was included in this study for further analysis as an item-nonresponse, since a simultaneous increase in the proportion of people who claim to have no opinion does not allow for the attribution of an actual lack of opinion [46–48].

In addition, two items were added (Mot5, and Mot8) which describe study-related motivator-items. Both were supplemented by the reasons for doing sports or PA, which were asked in the questionnaire for the study "GEDA 2014/2015-EHIS" [49] (p. 118) (Appendix A Table A2).

For barriers, three items were added which should account for the hilly conditions of the university setting (Bar2), study-related barriers (Bar5), and barriers relating to mood or desire (Bar12). Here, concerns of "GEDA 2014/2015-EHIS" [49] (p. 118) and the study by Krämer and Fuchs [50] (p. 174) were used to complement the specific areas (Appendix A Table A3).

Again, factor analyses were applied to obtain dimensionally reduced data on barriers and motivators for active transportation. This was done in the pre-analysis in order to bundle relevant information to be considered later in the main analysis (see Section 4.1.2).

3.3. Statistical Analysis

In a first step (pre-analyses), exploratory factor analyses (EFA) were conducted separately for the items measuring the study environment as well as for the psychological determinants of active transportation (in terms of motivators and barriers). Therefore, the IBM SPSS 25 software package was used. The decision regarding the number of factors extracted was based on both statistical indices (eigenvalue scree plot, commonalities h^2, factor loadings, and internal consistency of bundled items r/α) as well as content-related fit with the literature and the dimensions measured by the NEWS-G.

In a second step (main analyses), blockwise hierarchical regression analyses using IBM SPSS AMOS 25 software was applied. This was done in order to analyze associations between self-reports on PA, the perceived study environment, and psychological determinants of active transportation. Dependent variables were, separately, transport-related walking (A) and cycling (B). Firstly, in the blockwise procedure, sociodemographic factors were included as predictors (sex, age, and whether or not a resident in the university town). Secondly, determinants of the perceived study environment were included, and thirdly the psychological determinants of motivators and barriers were added as predictors in the regression model.

Missing values were estimated in the main analysis using the full information maximum likelihood (FIML) method implemented in AMOS 25. This was done in the case when at least one item of a scale measure was missing. In those cases, no mean value was calculated for the respective scale measure that could be included in the main analysis. Accordingly, the number of cases n for certain scales was reduced due to missing scale mean values.

For the evaluation of the global model fit, the root mean square error of approximation (RMSEA) [51], the comparative fit index (CFI) [52], and the minimum of discrepancy in relation to the degrees of freedom (CMIN/DF) were used [51,52]. In order to compare the different models within the hierarchical blockwise approach, information on the determination of variance (R^2) and the change of R^2 compared to the previous model were calculated.

Furthermore, the regression models were specified in a way that included significant correlations between the predictors. This led to an acceptable and good model fit, which ensures the model-based estimation of missing values. In addition to tests for statistical significance ($\alpha < 0.05$), effect sizes were determined and interpreted—according to small effects in agreement with Cohen (1988) [53]—if the standardized regression coefficient is equal to or higher than $\beta \geq 0.10$.

4. Results

4.1. Pre-Analyses: Exploratory Factor Analyses

4.1.1. Contextual Conditions: Perceived PA-Friendliness of the Study Environment

The bundling of the 14 initial items for the perceived study environment resulted in a differentiation of seven factors. A comparison of the finally derived factors and their content fit with the categories of the NEWS-G [44] and were adapted for the study environment as reported in Appendix A (Table A1). In this bundling process, we considered the subsequent categories of the NEWS-G: (C) "Land use mix–access", (D) "Street connectivity", (E) "Walking/Cycling facilities", (F) "Aesthetics", (G) "Pedestrian/automobile traffic safety", (H) "Crime safety". The EFA with 14 items initially proposed a five-factor solution, however, the results of the EFA led to the elimination of two items in order to improve the reliability of the factor regarding traffic safety. This concerns two items of category G, pedestrian/automobile traffic safety (Item G3, "The traffic speed in most surrounding streets is normally low (30 km/h or less)", and item G6, "There are crosswalks and pedestrian signals to help walkers cross busy streets in my study environment"). The item wordings, item descriptives, factor loadings, and communalities are reported in Appendix A (Table A4).

For the remaining items, statistical- and content-based criteria indicated a preference for a more differentiated seven-factor solution after keeping individual items that could not be bundled well to one factor, but which contributed to a variance explanation with reasonable communalities. They were either included as a single item in the further analyses after a content-wise comparison with the categories of the NEWS-G, or were assigned to other content-wise suitable factors after statistical verification by reliability analyses. The derived seven factors reflect the following areas of the perceived PA-friendliness of the study environment:

- The factor, "active transportation: walking/cycling facilities", contains two items (E1, and E3), both of which originally belonged to the category E "Walking/cycling facilities" of the NEWS-G. They combine aspects of available sidewalks and the proximity of bicycle or pedestrian trails. They showed a significant inter-item-correlation ($r = 0.51$).
- The factor, "aesthetics", comprises three items, which refer to the corresponding category of the NEWS-G (F1, F3, and F5). They refer to trees along the streets, interesting things to look at, and a lot of nature in the study environment. The internal consistency of the factor was rather low, but still satisfactory with respect to group-based analyses (Cronbach's $\alpha = 0.60$).
- The factor, "high automobile traffic", bundles three items that represent the difficulty, unpleasantness, or insecure feeling when walking/cycling due to much traffic and the noticeable exhaust fumes from cars or buses. This factor showed a satisfying internal consistency (Cronbach's $\alpha = 0.69$).
- "General crime" is presented by a single item, which describes the unsafe feeling during the day due to crime (New2). It was separated from another crime-related item.
- "Bicycle-related crime" is represented by a single item (New3). This item describes the unsafe feeling of leaving even a locked bicycle in the study environment.
- The factor, "active transportation: uphill", is reflected by one single item which describes the limited number of routes for getting from place to place due to a hilly landscape (C7). It was the only item that covers the category C "Land use mix–access" from the NEWS-G.
- The factor, "active transportation: connectivity", is described by one single item which stands for alternative (walking/biking) routes for getting from place to place (D5). It originally belonged to the category D "Street connectivity" from the NEWS-G.

4.1.2. Individual Conditions: Psychological Determinants of Active Transportation—Motivators and Barriers

The analyses to bundle psychological determinants of active transportation resulted in a differentiation of four factors for motivators and three factors for barriers. To arrive at these results, the following steps were taken. The EFA for motivators suggested the formation of two factors, after having previously removed item Mot6 (opportunity to socialize) due to a very low communality value ($h^2 = 0.23$). Mainly based on content-related considerations as well as on information of internal consistency statistics, and inter-item-correlations, we decided to split up two factors and preferred a four-factor solution. The item wordings, item descriptives, factor loadings, and communalities of motivators are reported in Appendix A (Table A5).

- The topic, "comfort with study life", includes two items, which describe the motivation of active transportation because of being more efficient for study and work and because of the active balance between and after courses. The items showed a high inter-item-correlation ($r = 0.53$).
- The factor, "personal benefits", comprises two items with motivators such as joy, health, and fitness. According to the results of the EFA, they belong to the same factor as the study-related items. As mentioned above, we preferred to separate the study-related items and other personal benefits in order to be able to be more specific regarding the university setting. The items showed a satisfactory inter-item-correlation ($r = 0.43$).
- The label, "instrumental extrinsic benefits", summarizes two items regarding the potential to save money and to avoid the search for a parking space. These items showed a satisfactory inter-item correlation of $r = 0.43$.
- The topic, "avoid air pollution", is reflected by one single item that was separated from the former extrinsic benefits factor. It revealed the lowest factor loading ($\lambda = 0.48$) and did not fit to the content of the other instrumental extrinsic benefits.

The EFA for barriers to PA suggested using three factors, after having previously removed two items due to overlap with items of the perceived study environment regarding the hilly landscape and the lack of secure bicycle parking facilities. Regarding the results of the EFA, two more items were excluded that could not be satisfactorily assigned to one factor due to statistical reasons (Bar3, and Bar10). Additionally, item Bar10, which refers to the lack of knowledge of the quickest and easy routes, had the lowest communality ($h^2 = 0.34$). The item wordings, item descriptives, factor loadings, and communalities are reported in Appendix A (Table A6). For the remaining items, the following three factors were considered:

- Factor, "discomfort with study life" (Cronbach's $\alpha = 0.77$), consists of three items that describe barriers related to everyday life at university such as an uncomfortable feeling participating in university courses after physical exertion, the necessity of bringing a change of clothes, or the lack of or poor changing/shower facilities (Bar5, Bar6, and Bar7).
- The factor, "personal barriers" (Cronbach's $\alpha = 0.69$), summarizes three items which describe barriers of physical effort, time effort, and bad mood (Bar4, Bar11, and Bar12).
- The factor, "external barriers" (Cronbach's $\alpha = 0.65$), comprises two items which describe barriers referring to the weather conditions and time of day (Bar1 and Bar2).

Tables A2 and A3 in Appendix A summarize the results regarding the motivators and barriers for PA. Moreover, Table 1 gives an overview for the finally considered determinants of active transportation behavior and provides descriptive information.

4.2. Main Results: Regression Models

The main analysis consisted of two separate analyses for the respective dependent variables of transport-related walking (A) and transport-related cycling (B). For each type of transportation mode, bivariate correlations and a separate regression model were calculated. In the basis model, we included the three sociodemographic indicators (sex, age, resident in university town; Model A0 and Model B0). We then added blockwise the indicators of the perceived study environment (models A1 and B1) and the indicators for personal motivators and barriers (models A2 and B2) (see Tables 2 and 3).

Table 2. Results of the blockwise multivariate regression models A1 (predictors—sociodemographics, and perceived study environment) and A2 (A1 plus motivators and barriers) for the active transportation by walking.

Walk	Model A1		Model A2 (A1 Plus Motivators and Barriers)	
Predictors	β	p	β	p
Sociodemographic				
Sex	0.03	0.33	0.02	0.56
Age	0.00	0.92	−0.01	0.88
Resident in university town	−0.06	0.07	−0.07	0.03 *
Perceived study environment				
Active transportation: uphill	−0.01	0.68	0.01	0.87
Active transportation: connectivity	0.03	0.31	0.03	0.41
Active transportation: walking/cycling facilities	0.03	0.40	0.03	0.45
Aesthetics	0.07	0.04 *	0.05	0.16
High automobile traffic	0.01	0.84	0.00	0.96
General crime	−0.02	0.59	−0.02	0.61
Bicycle-related crime	0.06	0.09	0.07	0.04 *
Psychological determinants-Motivators				
Study-related motivator			0.02	0.71
Personal benefits			0.07	0.12
Instrumental extrinsic			−0.06	0.08
Avoid air pollution			0.05	0.22
Psychological determinants-Barriers				
Personal			0.02	0.69
Discomfort with study life			−0.08	0.04 *
External			0.01	0.79
R^2	0.01		0.03	
ΔR^2	0.01		0.02	
RMSEA	0.03		0.04	
CFI	0.95		0.95	
CMIN/DF	1.772		2.396	

RMSEA: Root Mean Square Error of Approximation; CFI: Comparative Fit Index; CMIN/DF: ratio of Chi-square (minimum discrepancy) to its Degrees of Freedom; * The probability of error is less than 5%.

4.2.1. Regression Analyses for Walking

The regression models for active transportation by walking showed good global fit indices (CMIN/DF = 1.52–2.40; RMSEA = 0.023–0.037). There was also an improvement of variance clarification by the number of predictors added to the model (R^2 = 0.005–0.032). Altogether five of 17 predictors in the model showed associations with the weekly amount of walking, all of which had a standardized regression coefficient β lower than 0.10. Most associations were found among the motivator predictors (see Appendix A Table A7).

In the multivariate Model A1 including sociodemographic variables and determinants of the perceived study environment, only aesthetics showed a significant regression coefficient, which was lower than 0.10 (β = 0.07). When adding psychological determinants in Model A2, this association disappeared, but three other associations were statistically significant: not living in the university town (β = −0.07), bicycle-related crime (β = 0.07), and the barrier related to discomfort with study life (β = −0.08). All of them showed regression coefficients smaller than β < 0.10.

Table 3. Results of the blockwise multivariate regression models B1 (predictors—sociodemographics, and perceived study environment) and B2 (A1 plus motivators & barriers) for the active transportation by cycling.

Cycle	Model B1		Model B2 (B1 Plus Motivators & Barriers)	
Predictors	β	p	β	p
Sociodemographic:				
Sex	−0.06	0.07	−0.04	0.22
Age	0.02	0.52	0.01	0.80
Resident in university town	0.20	<0.01 ***	0.14	<0.01 ***
Perceived study environment:				
Active transportation: uphill	−0.08	0.02 *	0.01	0.70
Active transportation: connectivity	−0.00	0.96	−0.03	0.26
Active transportation: walking/cycling facilities	−0.04	0.22	−0.07	0.02 *
Aesthetics	0.02	0.56	−0.05	0.12
High automobile traffic	0.12	<0.01 ***	0.08	0.01 **
General crime	−0.07	0.04 *	−0.02	0.52
Bicycle-related crime	−0.14	<0.01 ***	−0.13	<0.01 ***
Psychological determinants-Motivators:				
Study-related motivator			−0.01	0.71
Personal benefits			0.13	0.00 **
Instrumental extrinsic			0.06	0.08
Avoid air pollution			0.05	0.11
Psychological determinants-Barriers:				
Personal			−0.24	<0.01 ***
Discomfort with study life			0.04	0.23
External			−0.23	<0.01 ***
R^2	0.08		0.24	
ΔR^2	0.03		0.16	
RMSEA	0.03		0.04	
CFI	0.955		0.957	
CMIN/DF	1.767		2.401	

* The probability of error is less than 5%. ** The probability of error is less than or equal to 1%. *** The probability of error is less than or equal to 0.1%.

4.2.2. Regression Analyses for Cycling

The regression models for active transportation by cycling showed adequate to good global fit indices (CMIN/DF = 1.52–2.41; RMSEA = 0.023–0.038). There was also an improvement of variance clarification reached by blockwise including the sets of different predictors to the model (R^2 = 0.05–0.24). Altogether, 12 of 17 predictors showed associations with the weekly amount of cycling, whereas all of the psychological determinants were present. For most predictors, the standardized regression coefficients were considered small to medium size (|0.06| < r < |0.38|) (see Appendix A Tables A8 and A9).

In the multivariate Model B1 including sociodemographic variables and variables of the perceived study environment, five predictors showed a significant regression coefficient, but for two of them it was lower than 0.10. The highest regression coefficient was found for the predictor of resident in the university town (β = 0.20), followed by bicycle-related crime (β = −0.14), and high automobile traffic (β = 0.118). When adding psychological determinants in Model B2, all associations became smaller or, in the case of high automobile traffic, showed a regression coefficient smaller than β < 0.10 (β = 0.08). The following associations remained with a small to medium regression coefficient: resident in the university town ($\beta = 0.14$) and bicycle-related crime ($\beta = -0.13$). While the association with "active transportation: uphill" disappeared, "walking/cycling facilities" were statistically significant but with a regression coefficient smaller than $\beta < 0.10$. Additionally, three other associations were statistically significant: personal barriers ($\beta = -0.24$), external barriers ($\beta = -0.23$), and personal benefits ($\beta = 0.13$).

5. Discussion

Using a socio-ecological approach in a university setting, the present study addresses the question of which conditions of the study environment as well as individual motivators and barriers are related to students' transport-related walking and cycling. Results show that there were no relevant predictors associated with the amount of transport-related walking: neither sex, age, and place of living nor the study environment or personal motivators and barriers were substantially linked with transport-related walking. In contrast, transport-related cycling was associated with predictors from both depicted conditions of students' PA behavior, which are important to understand for developing and improving public health interventions: resident in university town, personal benefits, personal barriers, and external barriers relying on individual conditions and high automobile traffic, and bicycle-related crime relying on contextual conditions. Bearing in mind the social-ecological approach of the study, the results reveal multivariate relationships between the level of cycling for transportation and both environmental and individual conditions.

To investigate these relationships, the present study has firstly bundled factors for the perceived study environment regarding the established survey instruments for neighborhood environment NEWS-G and statistical indices of EFA. The same was done for psychological determinants of students for active transportation regarding the study of Shannon et al., (2006) [26]. This procedure has enabled us to link the study environment based upon an adaption of the NEWS-G as well as psychological determinants with the active transport behavior of students, something that has not yet been investigated much in German-speaking countries. So far, only Molina-Gracia et al., (2010) in Spain have used parts of the NEWS besides other aspects to analyze the active commuting of students to university, namely "walking/cycling facilities" (E) [23]. A short version without adaption was used by Peachey and Baller (2015) in a mid-Atlantic undergraduate university with the NEWS-Abbreviate to distinguish environmental characteristics of the living environment between on-campus neighborhoods and off-campus neighborhoods, and to bring this into connection with general PA [54]. While the NEWS assesses the environment of the neighborhood, none of the previous studies used an adaption to access the environment of the study area. Titze et al., (2007) developed a questionnaire based on the literature and focus groups with a special relation to cycling for transportation and the environment along the transport route of students [27]. With the adaption of NEWS-G to the study environment in this study, we wanted to rely on an established survey procedure of the perceived environment and bring it together with the PA-friendliness of the study environment for transport-related PA. The conceptually and empirically derived factors covered areas of the environmental conditions in relation to the study environment: land use mix–access, connectivity, walking/cycling facilities, aesthetics, automobile traffic, and crime safety. The last two factors showed significant correlations for the convenience sample with students' cycling for transportation, but none showed associations with walking.

That "high automobile traffic" is positively associated with cycling is contrary to the expected result. This association was slightly weakened by adding psychological determinants into the regression model. It seems paradoxical that sampled students' perceived difficulties, unpleasantness, or insecure feeling when active traveling due to much traffic and noticeable exhaust fumes from cars or buses, is positively related to cycling for transportation. The same contrary effect was found in multinomial regression analysis from Titze et al., (2007) [27] for regular cyclists, who cycle more than three times a week. For irregular cyclists, the perception of traffic did not show any effect at all. One possible explanation is that cyclists are more exposed to the problem and therefore more likely to report it [27]. Further studies should investigate moderation analyses based on a representative sample, whereby psychological determinants should be integrated as moderators between the study environment and active commuting—especially cycling for transportation.

There is a negative correlation between bicycle-related crime and cycling. Students' unsafe feeling for leaving even a locked bicycle in the study environment is negatively related to cycling for transportation. This association has repeatedly been reported in the literature [22,25,27]. For example, Rybarczyk and Gallagher (2014) [25] showed that general crime was the strongest barrier for cycling among students and staff of the university, but also bicycle theft was represented under the three most highly ranked barriers. Rybarczyk and Gallagher concluded that the implementation of law enforcement and safe bicycle facility may promote cycling. This was also suggested by Shannon et al., (2006) [26].

Regarding individual conditions, personal barriers showed the strongest associations with cycling. This is in line with the conclusion of Shannon et al., (2006) that reducing barriers to using active transportation modes is likely to be more effective than promoting the benefits of active modes [26]. Further, Rybarczuk and Gallagher (2014) showed that students indicated that any bicycle barrier would cause a decrease in cycling [25]. Our study results reinforce the premise that students' personal barriers such as physical effort, time effort, and bad mood are negatively related to cycling for transportation. Such personal barriers of time constraints, inconvenience, or physiological discomfort are in accordance with previous findings [21,27]. The same applies to students' external barriers such as the weather or the time of day. These external inhibiting factors were also found in previous studies [25,26,28]. Nordfjærn et al., (2019) [55] recently showed that those who strongly prioritized convenience tended to use a car for transportation modes. However, the increased awareness of the negative consequences was related to a more use of active transportation and less car use. A positive association with cycling for transportation applies to students' personal benefits for active transportation such as joy, health, and fitness. This finding is also in line with the positive relation between emotional satisfaction and regular cycling as found by Titze et al., (2007) [27]. It is also in accordance with the association between strong priorities of PA and less public transportation mode use and more use of active transportation found by Nordfjærn et al., (2019) [55]. Overall, the inclusion of the set of psychological factors in the model improved the variance explanation for the cycling behavior of university students, indicating their important role for individual decisions related to transport-related cycling. However, Nordfjærn et al., (2019) showed that besides psychological variables, situational constraints were more important for mode use than psychological variables and are important to consider as well, for example, car ownership or longer walking time [55].

Regarding sociodemographic variables of the sampled students, the association between residence in the university town and cycling was slightly weakened by adding psychological determinants into the regression model but was still significant at medium level. Students' residence in the university town was positively associated with cycling for transportation. This is in line with the negative impact of distance found in previous studies [21,22,26,28,29] and also with the association between longer walking time from students' residence to university and the more use of public transportation for less active transportation recently showed by Nordfjærn et al., (2019) [55]. Moreover, Zannat et al., (2020) [56] revealed in terms of city planning the travel time besides the provision of infrastructure as influencing factors for active and public transportation of university students. Furthermore, the factor "personal barriers" of our study, which covers the barrier of time effort, is negatively associated with cycling on a medium level and reinforces this interpretation.

The result that there were no relevant contextual and individual predictors for students' transport-related walking has already been shown in both the university and community setting. Missing statistical significance for the probability of use of walking for students with environmental incentives was also the case in the results of Rybarczuk and

Gallagher (2014) [25]. In communal settings, walking for transportation shows a different association than walking for leisure, which is associated with recreation facilities and aesthetics and green spaces [13,17,36,37]. That the results of this study, which investigated only the domain of active transportation, did not show such correlations, suggests that students were not likely to choose walking as an active mode of transportation for contextual or individual reasons, but rather that it was purely a means of getting from point A to point B. However, in terms of active commuting by students in general, positive associations with the perception of walking and cycling facilities [23], traffic and crime safety [19,21,22,25,27,28], and aesthetic aspects such as the "attractiveness of the surroundings" [27] (p. 72) exist, which could not be shown in this study for walking.

Furthermore, active transportation cannot only be considered in the perspective of promoting PA but also in the perspective of promoting more sustainable modes of transport which in turn has effects on the environment, on the economy, and on the health of people [57]. Some recent studies have dealt with the importance of using sustainable means of transport by the university community [56,57]. The authors of these studies also showed that the mode of transportation is conditioned by particularities of university campuses such as bike share systems [58], tailored and strategically-placed point-of-choice prompts, through which students should switch to active transportation [59], or the distribution of the university scheduled classes on the days of the week [60]. However, in order to make use of the potential to increase cycling among students Grimes and Baker (2020) [58] revealed that bike share systems conditions in university settings must be tailored to the target group, Chim et al., (2020) [60] pointed out that there is only a positive association of university courses on weekdays with more time spent cycling if students cycle to classes anyway, and Irwin (2019) [61] showed that uncontrollable factors for example time, built environment, and weather affected the participation in activities. Thus, just like the results of our study, these findings show that the combination of environmental conditions and personal psychological determinants is important to consider. In addition to tailored measures offered by the university to promote sustainable and active transportation, also competing modes of transportation bring further psychological factors into play. Cruz-Rodriguez et al., (2020) [57] analyzes students' feelings and emotions provoked by alternative means of transport. In addition to various electric means of transportation, only the use of bicycles showed associations with the possibility of PA, but, for example, the feeling of freedom or getting around quickly in the city or avoiding traffic jams were also present for scooters and motorcycles [57]. Further studies should include deeper psychological backgrounds of transportation choice. To take advantage of the synergies between promoting PA and sustainability, further studies should additionally compare competing modes of transportation such as scooters and motorcycles.

Strengths and Limitations

Certain limitations must be considered when interpreting the results. Due to the cross-sectional study design, we could not identify causal associations. In addition, the study was conducted in the summertime, which could have an influence on the reported active commuting information due to better weather [19]. Furthermore, regarding the shift toward more female students in the convenience sample of the study, possible sampling bias cannot be excluded. Some studies report a gender difference in favor of male students with regard to the use of bicycles for active transportation [28,30], but other studies did not found different travel patterns between male and female students [23,62]. Agarwal and North (2012) [19] found some gender differences regarding the perception of barriers to cycling. Accordingly, generalizability of the associations would still need to be empirically verified.

The measuring instrument for the study environment was empirically used for the first time. Although the study has attempted to bundle information for both study environment and psychological determinants to better account for psychometric properties of the factors, some variables were measured as single items. For study environment the categories "land use mix–access", "connectivity," "general crime", and "bicycle-related crime" were only covered with one item each. For psychological determinants, the motivator item "avoid air pollution" was considered separately due to content and statistical indices. It is possible that the single items contributed to the absence of associations due to their lower variance. However, it has not been uncommon to include single items in this area of research to date [19,21,26]. Further development is thus needed for measurement procedures. For some areas, the present study provides indications. Our study did form a factor, which dealt with study-related psychological determinants. Furthermore, factors relying on personal benefits, on instrumental extrinsic benefits, and on avoiding air pollution were formed for motivators. Factors for barriers were discomfort with study life, personal barriers, and external barriers. Overall, further surveys in other universities are necessary to concretize and validate the adapted NEWS-G for the study environment as well as to confirm the factors formed.

In addition, the measuring instrument for the study environment captures the self-assessed perception of the students and thus does not provide an objective measure of the survey. This can lead to distortions, for example, as people who frequently walk or cycle outside might perceive traffic more strongly [40]. The importance of perception can only be filtered out and captured through a combination of objective and self-assessed measurement of physical environmental characteristics [41].

Despite the limitations, this study provides some strengths. It tried for the first time to assess not the living environment but the specific study environment with reference to an established survey instrument, so it can be used for campus as well as urban universities. This is important due to the fact that the transfer of results from campus universities is difficult to universities, which are not structured as closed geographical spaces, but the urban university is integrated into urban landscape [24,63].

In addition, referring to socio-ecological approaches could confirm the relationship between transport-related PA and both contextual as well as individual determinants. Further, it provides initial multivariate results on active transportation and its relation to contextual and individual determinants from Germany. Furthermore, since this study differentiated the PA domains into the different modes of transportation, walking and cycling, it could show that the compositional and contextual conditions are different for both modes. So for promoting PA it is important to distinguish between the needs of pedestrians and cyclists [20].

To sum up, in relation to other studies with respect of university students which considered both personal and environmental determinants together in relation with active transportation, the scientific value of the presented study lies in the insights into the contextual conditions of the study environment, the consideration of associated correlates through the factor bundling, and separate information for transport-related cycling and transport-related walking.

6. Conclusions

Current findings confirm on a regression-analytical basis the postulated socio-ecological relationships between both contextual as well as individual factors and transport-related cycling, but not with transport-related walking. In total, the students' amount of cycling a week is positively associated with the students' residence in the university town, high automobile traffic, and personal benefits such as joy and health, and negatively associated with bicycle-related crime, personal barriers such as physical or time effort, and external barriers such as weather conditions. It should be noted that there might be a partial correlation between "high automobile traffic" and psychological determinants which indicate a moderation role of psychological determinants.

Possible strategies leading to an adequate infrastructure for universities may be the implementation of safe bicycle racks, bicycle routes, or more student residences in town. Additionally, academic training programs that indicate the benefits of transport-related cycling may students help to understand the associations between cycling and health, environment, sports and recreation. This can increase motivation to use the bicycle for transportation and lead to consolidate the bicycle culture in transportation in the university community. Given the current climate change and the increasing physical inactivity of society, a cycling culture can advance alternative means of transportation and thus have positive effects on the economy, environment, and health. As PA is linked with various benefits for health and educational outcomes, the results contribute to the understanding of the correlates of active commuting. This is important especially for university students who are particularly at risk of not fulfilling health-oriented PA recommendations. Therefore, the present study supplements specific knowledge about determinants that are important for developing and improving public health interventions for students in a university setting.

Author Contributions: Conceptualization, M.T. and G.S.; methodology, M.T. and G.S.; formal analysis, M.T.; investigation, M.T. and G.S.; resources, G.S.; data curation, M.T.; writing—original draft preparation, M.T.; writing—review and editing, M.T. and G.S.; supervision, G.S.; project administration, M.T. and G.S.; funding acquisition, G.S. All authors have read and agreed to the published version of the manuscript.

Funding: This research was funded by the Allgemeiner Deutscher Hochschulsportverband (adh) (German University Sports Federation) and the Techniker Krankenkasse, health insurance fund.

Institutional Review Board Statement: Translation of the Ethics Committee Statement of the Faculty of Economics and Social Sciences of the University of Tübingen (original version: German): "From our point of view, there are no concerns for the project as you have presented it, since you inform the participating persons in detail about the purpose of the study, explicitly assure the voluntary nature of the survey, obtain a declaration of consent for the storage and analysis of the data, and the data are collected and processed anonymously." The study was conducted according to the guidelines of the Declaration of Helsinki, and approved by the Ethics Committee of the Faculty of Economics and Social Sciences of the University of Tübingen (protocol code A2.54-077_aa, 26 June 2018).

Informed Consent Statement: Informed consent was obtained from all subjects involved in the study.

Data Availability Statement: The data presented in this study are available on request from the corresponding author.

Acknowledgments: We would like to thank Ingrid Arzberger, Head of University Sports at the University of Tübingen, for providing the resources and co-applying for the funding. We would like to thank the participating students in the master course of the sports science program at the University of Tübingen and again Ingrid Arzberger for their support during the project conduction. We acknowledge support by Open Access Publishing Fund of University of Tübingen.

Conflicts of Interest: The authors declare no conflict of interest. The funders had no role in the design of the study; in the collection, analyses, or interpretation of data; in the writing of the manuscript, or in the decision to publish the results.

Appendix A

Table A1. Comparison of the finally selected items and their category bundled by the factor analysis and content fit in this article with the adapted categories of the NEWS-G [1] [44] for the study environment asked in the survey.

Original Items NEWS-G [1]	Adapted Items of the Survey [2]	Finally Selected Items and Their Factor (Bolds) [3]
	(2) Opportunities for walking and cycling:	
(C) Land use mix–access (1 of 7 adopted in the survey)	C7: There are many canyons/hillsides in my study environment that limit the number of routes for getting from place to place.	**Active transportation: uphill** C7: There are many canyons/hillsides in my study environment that limit the number of routes for getting from place to place.

Table A1. Cont.

Original Items NEWS-G [1]	Adapted Items of the Survey [2]	Finally Selected Items and Their Factor (Bolds) [3]
(D) Street connectivity (1 of 6 adopted in the survey)	D5: There are many alternatives (walking/biking) routes for getting from place to place in my study environment. You do not always have to take the same route.	**Active transportation: connectivity** D5: There are many alternatives (walking/biking) routes for getting from place to place in my study environment. You do not always have to take the same route.
(E) Walking/Cycling facilities (2 of 5 adopted in the survey)	E1: There are sidewalks on most of the streets in my study environment. E3: There are bicycle or pedestrian trails in or near my study environment that are easy to get to.	**Active transportation: walking/cycling facilities** E1: There are sidewalks on most of the streets in my study environment. E3: There are bicycle or pedestrian trails in or near my study environment that are easy to get to.
(F) Aesthetics (3 of 6 adopted in the survey)	F1: There are trees along the streets in my study environment. F3: There are many interesting things to look at while walking in my study environment. F5: There is a lot of nature in my study environment that is beautiful to look at (such as landscapes, viewpoints).	**Aesthetics** F1: There are trees along the streets in my study environment. F3: There are many interesting things to look at while walking in my study environment. F5: There is a lot of nature in my study environment that is beautiful to look at (such as landscapes, viewpoints).
(3) (Traffic) safety:		
(G) Pedestrian/Traffic safety (4 of 8 adopted in the survey; 1 own addition in the survey)	G2: There is so much traffic along nearby streets that it makes it difficult or unpleasant to walk in my study environment G3: The traffic speed in most surrounding streets is normally low (30 km/h or less). G6: There are crosswalks and pedestrian signals to help walkers cross busy streets in my study environment. G8: When walking in my study environment there are a lot of noticeable exhaust fumes (e.g., from cars and buses). New1: Because of the heavy traffic in my study environment, one feels insecure when walking/cycling [4].	**High automobile traffic** G2: There is so much traffic along nearby streets that it makes it difficult or unpleasant to walk in my study environment. G8: When walking in my study environment there are a lot of noticeable exhaust fumes (e.g., from cars and buses). New1: Because of the heavy traffic in my study environment, one feels insecure when walking/cycling.[4]
(H) Crime safety (0 of 6 adopted in the survey; 2 own additions in the survey)	New2: I feel unsafe in my study environment during the day due to crime [4]. New3: It is unsafe to leave even a locked bicycle in my study environment [5].	**General crime** New2: I feel unsafe in my study environment during the day due to crime [4]. **Bicycle-related crime** New3: It is unsafe to leave even a locked bicycle in my study environment [5].

[1] Neighborhood Environment Walkability Scale—Germany. [2] adapted categories of the NEWS-G for the study environment asked in the survey. [3] newly formed by factor analysis and content fit in this article. [4] for reasons of condensation, a summarized generalized statement of the respective category of the NEWS-G was newly formed. [5] due to previous evidence on the relationship between bicycle thefts and active camouflage transport behavior of students, a new specific item on crime was formed.

Table A2. Comparison of the final construct of motivator items newly formed by the factor analysis and content fit in this article.

Original Items	Adapted Items of the Survey	Final Factors [1]
To compensate for sedentary activities [2]	Mot5: Active balance between and after courses.	Comfort with study life
To improve my physical performance [2]	Mot8: Being more efficient for study and work.	
Improvement to health/fitness [3]	Mot3: Improvement to health/fitness	Personal benefits
Enjoyment gained from current mode [3] & Gain sense of enjoyment [2]	Mot7: Enjoyment in transportation	

Table A2. Cont.

Original Items	Adapted Items of the Survey	Final Factors [1]
Potential to save money [3]	Mot1: Potential to save money	Instrumental extrinsic benefits
Avoid the need to find parking [3] & Unable to obtain parking permit [3]	Mot2: Avoiding the search for a parking space.	
Personal contribution to reducing air pollution levels [3]	Mot4: Personal contribution to reducing air pollution levels	Avoid air pollution
Opportunity to socialize [3]	Mot6: Opportunity to socialize	Not included due to statistical reason

[1] Newly formed by factor analysis and content fit in this article. [2] Own items according to the study "GEDA 2014/2015-EHIS" [44] (p. 118). [3] Motivator items (Shannon et al., 2006) [26].

Table A3. Comparison of the final construct of barrier items newly formed by the factor analysis and content fit in this article.

Original Items	Adapted Items of the Survey	Final Factors [1]
I do not feel safe enough to be physically active outdoors alone [2] & I feel too fat to exercise	Bar5: I feel uncomfortable participating in university courses after physical exertion.	Discomfort with study life
Necessity of bringing a change of clothes [3]	Bar6: Necessity of bringing a change of clothes	
Lack of or poor changing/shower facilities at University of Western Australia (UWA) [3]	Bar7: Lack of or poor changing/shower facilities	
Physical effort involved [3]	Bar4: Physical effort involved	Personal barriers
Time involved [3]	Bar11: Time involved	
I lack motivation, I have no interest [2] & I am not in the mood [4].	Bar12: I lack motivation, I´m not in the mood.	
Weather (rain, wind, or heat) [3]	Bar1: Inappropriate weather	External barriers
Need to travel to/from UWA at night [3]	Bar2: Inappropriate time of day.	
-	Bar9: There are too many hills/climbs on the paths [5]	Not included due to redundancy with study environment
Lack of secure bicycle parking facilities at UWA [3]	Bar8: Lack of secure bicycle parking facilities	Not included due to redundancy with study environment
Lack of knowledge of quickest and easiest route to UWA [3]	Bar10: Lack of knowledge of quickest and easiest route	Not included due to statistical reason
Need vehicle for work purposes [3]	Bar3: Need vehicle for other purposes	Not included due to statistical reason

[1] Newly formed by factor analysis and content fit in this article. [2] Own items according to the study "GEDA 2014/2015-EHIS" [44] (p. 119). [3] Barrier items (Shannon et al., 2006) [26]. [4] Krämer & Fuchs (2010) [50] (p. 174). [5] Supplemented due to site-specific hilly conditions of the University of Tübingen.

Table A4. Item's descriptives (frequencies in %; 1 = totally disagree; 2 = more likely to disagree; 3 = more likely to agree; 4 = totally agree), factor loadings, and communalities (h^2) of the explorative factor analysis (EFA) of perceived study environment.

No.	Item Wording	Descriptives							EFA: Factor Number					
		n	1	2	3	4	M	SD	1	2	3	4	5	h^2
G2	There is so much traffic along nearby streets that it makes it difficult or unpleasant to walk in my study environment.	996	17.77	54.02	25.30	2.91	2.13	0.73	**0.76**	−0.18	−0.03	−0.04	0.03	0.61
G3	The traffic speed in most surrounding streets is normally low (30 km/h or less).	992	13.31	36.49	37.50	12.70	2.50	0.88	**0.54**	−0.18	0.05	−0.26	−0.41	0.56
New1	Because of the heavy traffic in my study environment, one feels insecure when walking/cycling.	991	18.97	49.45	24.22	7.37	2.20	0.83	**0.72**	0.16	−0.05	−0.05	0.26	0.61
G8	When walking in my study environment there are a lot of noticeable exhaust fumes (e.g., from cars and buses).	996	7.93	36.95	39.36	15.76	2.63	0.84	**0.72**	0.03	−0.14	0.05	0.17	0.57
E1	There are sidewalks on most of the streets in my study environment.	994	0.70	4.73	31.09	63.48	3.57	0.62	0.04	**0.83**	0.00	0.08	−0.13	0.71
E3	There are bicycle or pedestrian trails in or near my study environment that are easy to get to.	995	1.21	9.85	43.52	45.43	3.33	0.70	−0.17	**0.73**	0.10	0.28	−0.05	0.66
G6	There are crosswalks and pedestrian signals to help walkers cross busy streets in my study environment.	996	1.31	7.83	46.39	44.48	3.34	0.68	−0.25	**0.57**	0.04	0.01	0.02	0.39
F1	There are trees along the streets in my study environment.	993	3.02	22.96	51.96	22.05	2.93	0.75	−0.01	0.21	**0.70**	−0.32	0.02	0.63
F3	There are many interesting things to look at while walking in my study environment.	997	7.12	36.61	40.52	15.75	2.65	0.83	−0.14	0.04	**0.62**	0.48	0.04	0.64
F5	There is a lot of nature in my study environment that is beautiful to look at (such as landscapes, viewpoints).	996	6.73	32.33	44.78	16.16	2.70	0.82	−0.08	−0.06	**0.83**	0.14	−0.05	0.73
C7	There are many canyons/hillsides in my study environment that limit the number of routes for getting from place to place.	994	15.59	33.10	30.68	20.62	2.56	0.99	0.05	−0.21	0.18	**−0.67**	0.05	0.53
D5	There are many alternatives (walking/biking) routes for getting from place to place in my study environment. You do not always have to take the same route.	996	5.22	28.71	46.79	19.28	2.80	0.81	−0.01	0.08	0.21	**0.67**	0.01	0.51
New2	I feel unsafe in my study environment during the day due to crime.	997	79.34	17.35	2.71	0.60	1.25	0.53	0.10	−0.15	0.01	0.00	**0.71**	0.54
New3	It is unsafe to leave even a locked bicycle in my study environment.	990	17.88	52.83	21.62	7.68	2.19	0.82	0.18	0.00	−0.01	−0.07	**0.75**	0.60

The backgrounds highlight the largest part of the frequency distribution of the scale in each case. The bolds highlight the largest rotated factor loading in each case.

Table A5. Item's descriptives (frequencies in %; 1 = totally disagree; 2 = more likely to disagree; 3 = more likely to agree; 4 = totally agree), factor loadings, and communalities (h^2) of the explorative factor analysis (EFA) of motivator items.

No.	Item Wording	Descriptives							EFA: Factor Number		
		n	1	2	3	4	M	SD	1	2	h^2
Mot8	Being more efficient for study and work.	977	15.05	34.60	28.05	22.31	2.58	1.00	**0.79**	0.11	0.63
Mot7	Enjoyment in transportation	987	6.48	29.08	33.13	31.31	2.89	0.92	**0.79**	−0.04	0.62
Mot5	Active balance between and after courses.	989	7.08	23.05	34.48	35.39	2.98	0.93	**0.79**	0.10	0.63
Mot3	Improvement to health/fitness	989	3.24	22.04	36.10	38.62	3.10	0.85	**0.71**	0.33	0.61
Mot1	Potential to save money	986	24.04	31.95	24.85	19.17	2.39	1.10	0.06	**0.81**	0.66
Mot4	Personal contribution to reducing air pollution levels	983	12.31	31.03	32.25	24.42	2.69	0.95	0.48	**0.48**	0.46
Mot2	Avoiding the search for a parking space	893	22.06	16.46	28.78	32.70	2.72	1.14	0.07	**0.81**	0.66

The backgrounds highlight the largest part of the frequency distribution of the scale in each case. The bolds highlight the largest rotated factor loading in each case.

Table A6. Item's descriptives (frequencies in %; 1 = totally disagree; 2 = more likely to disagree; 3 = more likely to agree; 4 = totally agree), factor loadings and communalities (h^2) of the explorative factor analysis (EFA) of barrier items.

No.	Item Wording	Descriptives							EFA: Factor Number			
		n	1	2	3	4	M	SD	1	2	3	h^2
Bar4	Physical effort involved	992	49.29	39.62	8.57	2.52	1.64	0.74	**0.69**	0.33	0.01	0.58
Bar11	Time involved.	985	41.32	31.68	17.36	9.64	1.95	0.99	**0.68**	0.09	0.31	0.57
Bar12	I lack motivation, I'm not in the mood.	990	51.21	32.42	11.72	4.65	1.70	0.85	**0.82**	0.11	0.08	0.69
Bar10	Lack of knowledge of quickest and easiest route.	932	61.48	20.39	12.12	6.01	1.63	0.92	**0.51**	0.16	0.27	0.35
Bar5	I feel uncomfortable participating in university courses after physical exertion.	982	37.17	33.20	18.84	10.79	2.03	1.00	0.31	**0.75**	0.10	0.68
Bar6	Necessity of bringing a change of clothes	934	37.37	27.30	20.24	15.10	2.13	1.08	0.18	**0.82**	0.20	0.74
Bar7	Lack of or poor changing/shower facilities	861	36.82	24.16	20.56	18.47	2.21	1.13	0.09	**0.80**	0.15	0.68
Bar1	Inappropriate weather	995	12.56	43.12	25.73	18.59	2.50	0.94	0.22	0.23	**0.67**	0.55
Bar2	Inappropriate time of day.	991	38.14	32.90	19.07	9.89	2.01	0.98	0.34	0.06	**0.71**	0.62
Bar3	Need vehicle for other purposes	875	58.63	22.06	14.17	5.14	1.66	0.90	−0.01	0.12	**0.72**	0.53

The backgrounds highlight the largest part of the frequency distribution of the scale in each case. The bolds highlight the largest rotated factor loading in each case.

Table A7. Results (inter-item-correlation-coefficients r, β-coefficients and significant *p*-value) for the bivariate correlation and multivariate regression models A1 (sociodemographics and perceived study environment) and A2 (A1 plus Motivators & Barriers) for the transportation mode "walk".

Walk	Bivariate Correlation with Walking (MET/Week)		Model A1		Model A2 (A1 Plus Motivators & Barriers)	
Predictors	r	p	β	p	β	p
Sociodemographic						
Sex	0.03	0.39	0.03	0.33	0.02	0.56
Age	0.01	0.74	0.00	0.92	−0.01	0.88
Resident in university town	−0.06	0.06	−0.06	0.07	−0.07	0.03 *
Perceived study environment						
Active transportation: uphill	−0.03	0.39	−0.01	0.68	0.01	0.87
Active transportation: connectivity	−0.06	0.07	0.03	0.31	0.03	0.41
Active transportation: walking/cycling facilities	−0.05	0.13	0.03	0.40	0.03	0.45
Aesthetics	−0.08	0.02 *	0.07	0.04 *	0.05	0.16
High automobile traffic	−0.00	0.94	0.01	0.84	0.00	0.96
General crime	0.00	0.99	−0.02	0.59	−0.02	0.61
Bicycle-related crime	0.05	0.12	0.06	0.09	0.07	0.04 *

Table A7. Cont.

Walk	Bivariate Correlation with Walking (MET/Week)		Model A1		Model A2 (A1 Plus Motivators & Barriers)	
Predictors	r	p	β	p	β	p
Psychological determinants-Motivators						
Study-related motivator	0.08	0.02 *			0.02	0.71
Personal benefits	0.10	0.00 **			0.07	0.12
Instrumental extrinsic	−0.02	0.59			−0.06	0.08
Avoid air pollution	0.07	0.03 *			0.05	0.22
Psychological determinants-Barriers						
Personal	−0.05	0.12			0.02	0.69
Discomfort with study life	−0.09	0.01 *			−0.08	0.04 *
External	−0.03	0.40			0.01	0.79
R²			0.01		0.03	
ΔR²			0.01		0.02	
RMSEA			0.03		0.04	
CFI			0.95		0.95	
CMIN/DF			1.772		2.396	

* The probability of error is less than 5%. ** The probability of error is less than or equal to 1%.

Table A8. Results (inter-item-correlation-coefficients r, β-coefficients and significant p-value) for the bivariate correlation and multivariate regression models B1 (sociodemographics and perceived study environment) and B2 (B1 plus Motivators & Barriers) for the transportation mode "cycle".

Cycle	Bivariate Correlation with Cycling (MET/Week)		Model B1		Model B2 (B1 Plus Motivators & Barriers)	
Predictors	r	p	β	p	β	p
Sociodemographic:						
Sex	−0.05	0.16	−0.06	0.07	−0.04	0.22
Age	0.02	0.50	0.02	0.52	0.01	0.80
Resident in university town	0.21	<0.01 ***	0.20	<0.01 ***	0.14	<0.01 ***
Perceived study environment:						
Active transportation: uphill	−0.06	0.045 *	−0.08	0.02 *	0.01	0.70
Active transportation: connectivity	0.01	0.83	−0.00	0.96	−0.03	0.26
Active transportation: walking/cycling facilities	0.03	0.32	−0.04	0.22	−0.07	0.02 *
Aesthetics	0.00	0.998	0.02	0.56	−0.05	0.12
High automobile traffic	0.06	0.05 *	0.12	<0.01 ***	0.08	0.01 **
General crime	−0.10	0.00 **	−0.07	0.04 *	−0.02	0.52
Bicycle-related crime	−0.14	<0.01 ***	−0.14	<0.01 ***	−0.13	<0.01 ***
Psychological determinants-Motivators:						
Study-related motivator	0.17	<0.01 ***			−0.01	0.71
Personal benefits	0.25	<0.01 ***			0.13	0.00 **
Instrumental extrinsic	0.08	0.015 *			0.06	0.08
Avoid air pollution	0.18	<0.01 ***			0.05	0.11
Psychological determinants-Barriers:						
Personal	−0.38	<0.01 ***			−0.24	<0.01 ***
Discomfort with study life	−0.16	<0.01 ***			0.04	0.23
External	−0.35	<0.01 ***			−0.23	<0.01 ***
R²					0.08	0.24
ΔR²					0.03	0.16
RMSEA					0.03	0.04
CFI					0.955	0.957
CMIN/DF					1.767	2.401

* The probability of error is less than 5%. ** The probability of error is less than or equal to 1%. *** The probability of error is less than or equal to 0.1%.

Table A9. Results (inter-item-correlation-coefficients r, and significant p-value) for the bivariate correlation between all variables of the regression models.

		1	2	3	4	5	6	7	8	9	10	11	12	13	14	15	16	17
1	Sex	r p n	1 950															
2	Age	r p n	−0.04 0.19 947	1 994														
3	Resident in university town	r p n	0.050 0.13 950	−0.02 0.50 994	1 997													
4	Active transportation: uphill	r p n	−0.00 0.98 948	−0.07 * 0.03 991	0.05 0.12 994	1 994												
5	Active transportation: connectivity	r p n	0.00 1.00 949	−0.04 0.23 993	0.02 0.48 996	0.18 ** 0.00 993	1 996											
6	Active transportation: walking/Cycling facilities	r p n	0.03 0.43 946	0.05 0.14 990	0.04 0.22 993	0.25 ** 0.00 990	0.21 ** 0.00 992	1 993										
7	Aesthetics	r p n	0.00 0.89 945	−0.05 0.14 989	0.02 0.63 992	0.03 0.37 989	0.21 ** 0.00 991	0.17 ** 0.00 988	1 992									
8	High automobile traffic	r p n	0.08 * 0.02 942	0.02 0.45 986	−0.01 0.69 989	0.09 ** 0.00 986	0.09 ** 0.00 988	0.25 ** 0.00 985	0.18 ** 0.00 984	1 989								
9	General crime	r p n	0.07 * 0.03 950	−0.01 0.74 994	−0.10 ** 0.00 997	0.03 0.43 994	−0.01 0.78 996	0.16 ** 0.00 993	0.03 0.29 992	0.19 ** 0.00 989	1 997							
10	Bicycle-related crime	r p n	0.03 0.41 943	0.06 0.09 988	−0.06 0.07 990	0.09 ** 0.01 987	−0.01 0.86 989	0.09 ** 0.00 987	0.05 0.13 985	0.24 ** 0.00 983	0.26 ** 0.00 990	1 990						
11	Study-related motivator	r p n	0.12 ** 0.00 924	−0.01 0.55 968	0.03 0.41 971	−0.03 0.33 968	−0.04 0.19 970	−0.06 0.08 967	−0.14 ** 0.00 966	0.13 ** 0.00 963	0.04 0.19 971	0.01 0.73 965	1 971					
12	Personal benefits	r p n	0.11 ** 0.00 936	0.09 ** 0.01 980	0.06 * 0.05 983	−0.08 * 0.01 980	−0.10 ** 0.00 982	−0.05 0.16 979	−0.17 ** 0.00 979	0.09 ** 0.00 975	−0.01 0.80 983	−0.02 0.58 976	0.66 ** 0.00 962	1 983				
13	Instrumental extrinsic benefits	r p n	0.04 0.31 846	−0.01 0.73 885	−0.05 0.14 888	−0.04 0.270 885	−0.10 ** 0.00 887	−0.03 0.32 884	−0.07 * 0.04 883	0.10 ** 0.01 881	0.09 ** 0.01 888	−0.01 0.89 883	0.22 ** 0.00 868	0.21 ** 0.00 877	1 888			

Table A9. Cont.

		1	2	3	4	5	6	7	8	9	10	11	12	13	14	15	16	17
14	Avoid air pollution	r p n	0.08 * 0.02 936	−0.01 0.86 980	0.00 0.92 983	−0.06 * 0.05 980	−0.10 ** 0.00 982	−0.06 0.06 979	−0.13 ** 0.00 978	0.12 ** 0.00 976	−0.01 0.83 983	−0.06 0.06 977	0.36 ** 0.00 961	0.44 ** 0.00 971	0.33 ** 0.00 881	1 983			
15	Personal barrier	r p n	0.04 0.22 929	−0.04 0.27 972	−0.16 ** 0.00 975	0.23 ** 0.00 972	0.11 ** 0.00 974	0.15 ** 0.00 971	0.12 ** 0.00 970	0.05 0.10 967	0.12 ** 0.00 975	0.07 * 0.03 969	−0.26 ** 0.00 952	−0.33 ** 0.00 962	−0.02 0.60 870	−0.162 ** 0.000 964	1 975		
16	Discomfort with study life	r p n	−0.00 0.98 798	−0.03 0.42 834	−0.08 * 0.02 837	0.26 ** 0.00 834	0.12 ** 0.00 836	0.11 ** 0.00 833	0.12 ** 0.00 832	0.18 ** 0.00 830	0.05 0.18 837	0.17 ** 0.00 832	−0.06 0.12 823	−0.08 * 0.03 826	0.01 0.77 756	−0.076 * 0.029 828	0.46 ** 0.00 825	1 837	
17	External barrier	r p n	0.13 ** 0.00 943	−0.02 0.48 987	−0.09 ** 0.00 990	0.18 ** 0.00 987	0.08 ** 0.01 989	0.13 ** 0.00 986	0.09 ** 0.00 985	0.11 ** 0.00 982	0.16 ** 0.00 990	0.08 * 0.02 983	−0.09 ** 0.01 965	−0.14 ** 0.00 976	0.02 0.59 882	−0.118 ** 0.000 977	0.44 ** 0.00 969	0.38 ** 0.000 832	1 990

* The probability of error is less than 5%. ** The probability of error is less than or equal to 1%.

References

1. Grützmacher, J.; Guysy, B.; Lesener, T.; Sudheimer, S.; Willige, J. *Gesundheit Studierender in Deutschland 2017: Ein Kooperationsprojekt zwischen dem Deutschen Zentrum für Hochschul-und Wissenschaftsforschung, der Freien Universität Berlin und der Technike Krankenkasse*; Fischer Druck GMbH Peine: Hannover, Germany, 2018.
2. Brandl-Bredenbeck, H.P.; Kämpfe, A.; Köster, C. *Studium Heute—Gesundheitsfördernd Oder Gesundheitsgefährdend?: Eine Lebensstilanalyse*; Meyer & Meyer Verlag: Aachen, Germany, 2013.
3. Meier, S.; Mikolajczyk, R.T.; Helmer, S.; Akmatov, M.K.; Steinke, B.; Krämer, A. Prävalenz von Erkrankungen und Beschwerden bei Studierenden in NRW. *Prävention Und Gesundh.* **2010**, *5*, 257–264. [CrossRef]
4. Möllenbeck, D.; Göring, A. Sportliche Aktivität, Gesundheitsressourcen und Befinden von Studierenden: Eine Frage des Geschlechts? In *Aktiv und Gesund?* Becker, S., Ed.; Springer: Wiesbaden, Germany, 2014; pp. 449–474. [CrossRef]
5. TK-CampusKompass: Umfrage zur Gesundheit von Studierenden; TK-Hausdruckerei: Hamburg, Germany, 2015.
6. Möllenbeck, D. Gesundheitliche Ressourcen und Belastungen von Studierenden. In *Bewegungsorientierte Gesundheitsförderung an Hochschulen*, 3rd ed.; Göring, A., Möllenbeck, D., Eds.; Universitätsverlag Göttingen: Göttingen, Germany, 2014; pp. 167–182. [CrossRef]
7. García-Hermoso, A.; Quintero, A.P.; Hernández, E.; Correa-Bautista, J.E.; Izquierdo, M.; Tordecilla-Sanders, A.; Prieto-Benavides, D.; Sandoval-Cuellar, C.; González-Ruíz, K.; Villa-González, E. Active commuting to and from university, obesity and metabolic syndrome among Colombian university students. *BMC Public Health* **2018**, *18*, 523. [CrossRef] [PubMed]
8. Bopp, M.; Bopp, C.; Schuchert, M. Active transportation to and on campus is associated with objectively measured fitness outcomes among college students. *J. Phys. Act. Health* **2015**, *12*, 418–423. [CrossRef] [PubMed]
9. Gropper, H.; John, J.M.; Sudeck, G.; Thiel, A. The impact of life events and transitions on physical activity: A scoping review. *PLoS ONE* **2020**, *15*, e0234794. [CrossRef]
10. Irwin, J.D. Prevalence of university students' sufficient physical activity: A systematic review. *Percept. Mot. Ski.* **2004**, *98*, 927–943. [CrossRef] [PubMed]
11. Parra-Saldías, M.; Castro-Piñero, J.; Castillo Paredes, A.; Palma Leal, X.; Díaz Martínez, X.; Rodríguez-Rodríguez, F. Active commuting behaviours from high school to university in Chile: A retrospective study. *Int. J. Environ. Res. Public Health* **2019**, *16*, 53. [CrossRef]
12. Bauman, A.E.; Reis, R.S.; Sallis, J.F.; Wells, J.C.; Loos, R.J.F.; Martin, B.W.; Lancet Physical Activity Series Working Group. Correlates of physical activity: Why are some people physically active and others not? *Lancet* **2012**, *380*, 258–271. [CrossRef]
13. Bucksch, J.; Claßen, T.; Schneider, S. Förderung körperlicher Aktivität im Alltag auf kommunaler Ebene. In *Handbuch Bewegungsförderung und Gesundheit*; Geuter, G., Hollederer, A., Eds.; Verlag Hands Huber: Bern, Switzerland, 2012.
14. Stokols, D. Establishing and maintaining healthy environments: Toward a social ecology of health promotion. *Am. Psychol.* **1992**, *47*, 6. [CrossRef]
15. Sallis, J.F.; Owen, N.; Fisher, E.B. Ecological models of health behavior. In *Health Behavior and Health Education: Theory, Research, and Practice*, 4th ed.; Glanz, K., Rimer, B.K., Viswanath, K., Eds.; Jossey-Bass: San Francisco, CA, USA, 2008; pp. 456–486.
16. Sallis, J.F.; Cervero, R.B.; Ascher, W.; Henderson, K.A.; Kraft, M.K.; Kerr, J. An ecological approach to creating active living communities. *Annu. Rev. Public Health* **2006**, *27*. [CrossRef]
17. Van Dyck, D.; Cardon, G.; Deforche, B.; Sallis, J.F.; Owen, N.; De Bourdeaudhuij, I. Neighborhood SES and walkability are related to physical activity behavior in Belgian adults. *Prev. Med.* **2010**, *50*, S74–S79. [CrossRef]
18. Giles-Corti, B.; King, A.C. Creating active environments across the life course:"thinking outside the square". *Br. J. Sports Med.* **2009**, *43*, 109–113. [CrossRef] [PubMed]
19. Agarwal, A.; North, A. Encouraging bicycling among university students: Lessons from queen's university, Kingston, Ontario. *Can. J. Urban Res.* **2012**, *2*, 151–168.
20. Balsas, C.J. Sustainable transportation planning on college campuses. *Transp. Policy* **2003**, *10*, 35–49. [CrossRef]
21. Cole, R.; Leslie, E.; Donald, M.; Cerin, E.; Neller, A.; Owen, N. Motivational readiness for active commuting by university students: Incentives and barriers. *Health Promot. J. Aust.* **2008**, *19*, 210–215. [CrossRef] [PubMed]
22. Horacek, T.M.; Dede Yildirim, E.; Kattelmann, K.; Brown, O.; Byrd-Bredbenner, C.; Colby, S.; Greene, G.; Hoerr, S.; Kidd, T.; Koenings, M. Path analysis of campus walkability/bikeability and college students' physical activity attitudes, behaviors, and body mass index. *Am. J. Health Promot.* **2018**, *32*, 578–586. [CrossRef]
23. Molina-García, J.; Castillo, I.; Sallis, J.F. Psychosocial and environmental correlates of active commuting for university students. *Prev. Med.* **2010**, *51*, 136–138. [CrossRef]
24. Molina-García, J.; Menescardi, C.; Estevan, I.; Martínez-Bello, V.; Queralt, A. Neighborhood built environment and socioeconomic status are associated with active commuting and sedentary behavior, but not with leisure-time physical activity, in university students. *Int. J. Environ. Res. Public Health* **2019**, *16*, 3176. [CrossRef]
25. Rybarczyk, G.; Gallagher, L. Measuring the potential for bicycling and walking at a metropolitan commuter university. *J. Transp. Geogr.* **2014**, *39*, 1–10. [CrossRef]
26. Shannon, T.; Giles-Corti, B.; Pikora, T.; Bulsara, M.; Shilton, T.; Bull, F. Active commuting in a university setting: Assessing commuting habits and potential for modal change. *Transp. Policy* **2006**, *13*, 240–253. [CrossRef]
27. Titze, S.; Stronegger, W.J.; Janschitz, S.; Oja, P. Environmental, social, and personal correlates of cycling for transportation in a student population. *J. Phys. Act. Health* **2007**, 66–79. [CrossRef]

28. Wang, C.-H.; Akar, G.; Guldmann, J.-M. Do your neighbors affect your bicycling choice? A spatial probit model for bicycling to The Ohio State University. *J. Transp. Geogr.* **2015**, *42*, 122–130. [CrossRef]
29. Wang, X.; Khattak, A.J.; Son, S. What can be learned from analyzing university student travel demand? *Transp. Res. Rec.* **2012**, *2322*, 129–137. [CrossRef]
30. Wuerzer, T.; Mason, S.G. Cycling Willingness: Investigating Distance as a Dependent Variable in Cycling Behavior Among College Students. *Appl. Geogr.* **2015**, *60*, 95–106. [CrossRef]
31. Cerin, E.; Conway, T.L.; Cain, K.L.; Kerr, J.; De Bourdeaudhuij, I.; Owen, N.; Reis, R.S.; Sarmiento, O.L.; Hinckson, E.A.; Salvo, D.; et al. Sharing good NEWS across the world: Developing comparable scores across 12 countries for the neighborhood environment walkability scale (NEWS). *BMC Public Health* **2013**, *13*, 309. [CrossRef] [PubMed]
32. De Bourdeaudhuij, I.; Sallis, J.F.; Saelens, B.E. Environmental correlates of physical activity in a sample of Belgian adults. *Am. J. Health Promot.* **2003**, *18*, 83–92. [CrossRef]
33. Duncan, M.J.; Spence, J.C.; Mummery, W.K. Perceived environment and physical activity: A meta-analysis of selected environmental characteristics. *Int. J. Behav. Nutr. Phys. Act.* **2005**, *2*, 11. [CrossRef]
34. Frank, L.; Kavage, S. A national plan for physical activity: The enabling role of the built environment. *J. Phys. Act. Health* **2009**, *6* (Suppl. 2), 186–195. [CrossRef]
35. Giles-Corti, B.; Timperio, A.; Bull, F.; Pikora, T. Understanding physical activity environmental correlates: Increased specificity for ecological models. *Exerc. Sport Sci. Rev.* **2005**, *33*, 175–181. [CrossRef]
36. Humpel, N.; Owen, N.; Leslie, E. Environmental factors associated with adults' participation in physical activity: A review. *Am. J. Prev. Med.* **2002**, *22*, 188–199. [CrossRef]
37. Owen, N.; Humpel, N.; Leslie, E.; Bauman, A.; Sallis, J.F. Understanding Environmental Influences on Walking. *Am. J. Prev. Med.* **2004**, *27*, 67–76. [CrossRef]
38. Saelens, B.E.; Sallis, J.F.; Frank, L.D. Environmental correlates of walking and cycling: Findings from the transportation, urban design, and planning literatures. *Ann. Behav. Med.* **2003**, *25*, 80–91. [CrossRef] [PubMed]
39. Sallis, J.F.; Bowles, H.R.; Bauman, A.; Ainsworth, B.E.; Bull, F.C.; Craig, C.L.; Sjöström, M.; De Bourdeaudhuij, I.; Lefevre, J.; Matsudo, V.; et al. Neighborhood environments and physical activity among adults in 11 countries. *Am. J. Prev. Med.* **2009**, *36*, 484–490. [CrossRef] [PubMed]
40. Wallmann, B.; Bucksch, J.; Froboese, I. The association between physical activity and perceived environment in German adults. *Eur. J. Public Health* **2011**, *22*, 502–508. [CrossRef] [PubMed]
41. Wendel-Vos, W.; Droomers, M.; Kremers, S.; Brug, J.; van Lenthe, F. Potential environmental determinants of physical activity in adults: A systematic review. *Obes. Rev.* **2007**, *8*, 425–440. [CrossRef] [PubMed]
42. Finger, J.D.; Tafforeau, J.; Gisle, L.; Oja, L.; Ziese, T.; Thelen, J.; Mensink, G.B.; Lange, C. Development of the European health interview survey-physical activity questionnaire (EHIS-PAQ) to monitor physical activity in the European Union. *Arch. Public Health* **2015**, *73*, 1–11. [CrossRef]
43. Ainsworth, B.E.; Haskell, W.L.; Herrmann, S.D.; Meckes, N.; Bassett Jr, D.R.; Tudor-Locke, C.; Greer, J.L.; Vezina, J.; Whitt-Glover, M.C.; Leon, A.S. 2011 Compendium of Physical Activities: A second update of codes and MET values. *Med. Sci. Sports Exerc.* **2011**, *43*, 1575–1581. [CrossRef]
44. Bödeker, M.; Bucksch, J.; Fuhrmann, H. Bewegungsfreundlichkeit von Wohnumgebungen messen: Entwicklung und Einführung der deutschsprachigen "Neighborhood Environment Walkability Scale". *Prävention Und Gesundh.* **2012**, *7*, 220–226. [CrossRef]
45. Gauvin, L.; Richard, L.; Craig, C.L.; Spivock, M.; Riva, M.; Forster, M.; Laforest, S.; Laberge, S.; Fournel, M.-C.; Gagnon, H. From walkability to active living potential: An "ecometric" validation study. *Am. J. Prev. Med.* **2005**, *28*, 126–133. [CrossRef]
46. Krosnick, J.A. Survey research. *Annu. Rev. Psychol.* **1999**, *50*, 537–567. [CrossRef]
47. Franzen, A. Antwortskalen in standardisierten Befragungen. In *Handbuch Methoden der Empirischen Sozialforschung*; Springer: Wiesbaden, Germany, 2014; pp. 701–711. [CrossRef]
48. Engel, U.; Schmidt, B.O. Unit-und Item-Nonresponse. In *Handbuch Methoden der Empirischen Sozialforschung*; Springer: Wiesbaden, Germany, 2014; pp. 331–348. [CrossRef]
49. Saß, A.-C.; Lange, C.; Finger, J.D.; Allen, J.; Born, S.; Hoebel, J.; Kuhnert, R.; Müters, S.; Thelen, J.; Schmich, P. Gesundheit in Deutschland aktuell—Neue Daten für Deutschland und Europa: Hintergrund und Studienmethodik von GEDA 2014/2015-EHIS. *J. Health Monit.* **2017**, *2*, 83–89. [CrossRef]
50. Krämer, L.; Fuchs, R. Barrieren und Barrierenmanagement im Prozess der Sportteilnahme: Zwei neue Messinstrumente. *Z. Für Gesundh.* **2010**, 170–182. [CrossRef]
51. Schermelleh-Engel, K.; Moosbrugger, H.; Müller, H. Evaluating the Fit of Structural Equation Models: Tests of Significance and Descriptive Goodness-of-Fit Measures. *Methods Psychol. Res.* **2003**, *8*, 23–74.
52. McDonald, R.P.; Marsh, H.W. Choosing a multivariate model: Noncentrality and goodness of fit. *Psychol. Bull.* **1990**, *107*, 247–255. [CrossRef]
53. Cohen, J. *Statistical Power Analysis for the Behavioral Sciences*, 2nd ed.; Lawrence Erlbaum Associates: New York, NY, USA, 1988.
54. Peachey, A.A.; Baller, S.L. Perceived Built Environment Characteristics of On-Campus and Off-Campus Neighborhoods Associated With Physical Activity of College Students. *J. Am. Coll. Health* **2015**, *63*, 337–342. [CrossRef] [PubMed]
55. Nordfjærn, T.; Egset, K.S.; Mehdizadeh, M. "Winter is coming": Psychological and situational factors affecting transportation mode use among university students. *Transp. Policy* **2019**, *81*, 45–53. [CrossRef]

56. Zannat, E.K.; Adnan, M.S.G.; Dewan, A. A GIS-based approach to evaluating environmental influences on active and public transport accessibility of university students. *J. Urban Manag.* **2020**, *9*, 331–346. [CrossRef]
57. Cruz-Rodríguez, J.; Luque-Sendra, A.; Heras, A.d.l.; Zamora-Polo, F. Analysis of Interurban Mobility in University Students: Motivation and Ecological Impact. *Int. J. Environ. Res. Public Health* **2020**, *17*, 9348. [CrossRef] [PubMed]
58. Grimes, A.; Baker, M. The Effects of a Citywide Bike Share System on Active Transportation Among College Students: A Randomized Controlled Pilot Study. *Health Educ. Behav.* **2020**, *47*, 412–418. [CrossRef] [PubMed]
59. Ly, H.; Irwin, J.D. Skip the wait and take a walk home! The suitability of point-of-choice prompts to promote active transportation among undergraduate students. *J. Am. Coll. Health* **2020**, 1–9. [CrossRef] [PubMed]
60. Chim, H.Q.; Oude Egbrink, M.G.A.; Van Gerven, P.W.M.; de Groot, R.H.M.; Winkens, B.; Savelberg, H.H.C.M. Academic Schedule and Day-to-Day Variations in Sedentary Behavior and Physical Activity of University Students. *Int. J. Environ. Res. Public Health* **2020**, *17*, 2810. [CrossRef]
61. Irwin, J.D. Designing effective point-of-choice prompts to promote active transportation and staircase use at a Canadian University. *J. Am. Coll. Health* **2019**, *67*, 215–223. [CrossRef]
62. Limanond, T.; Butsingkorn, T.; Chermkhunthod, C. Travel behavior of university students who live on campus: A case study of a rural university in Asia. *Transp. Policy* **2011**, *18*, 163–171. [CrossRef]
63. Chillón, P.; Molina-García, J.; Castillo, I.; Queralt, A. What distance do university students walk and bike daily to class in Spain. *J. Transp. Health* **2016**, *3*, 315–320. [CrossRef]

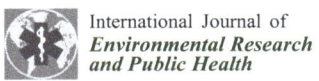

Article

Environmental and Psychosocial Barriers Affect the Active Commuting to University in Chilean Students

Antonio Castillo-Paredes [1,*], Natalia Inostroza Jiménez [2,3], Maribel Parra-Saldías [4], Ximena Palma-Leal [4], José Luis Felipe [5], Itziar Págola Aldazabal [5], Ximena Díaz-Martínez [6] and Fernando Rodríguez-Rodríguez [4]

1. Grupo AFySE, Investigación en Actividad Física y Salud Escolar, Escuela de Pedagogía en Educación Física, Facultad de Educación, Universidad de Las Américas, Santiago 8370035, Chile
2. Área Salud, Universidad Tecnológica de Chile INACAP, La Serena 1700000, Chile; ninostrozajimenez@gmail.com
3. Magíster en Nutrición para la Actividad Física y el Deporte, Escuela de Nutrición y Dietética, Facultad de Ciencias, Universidad Mayor, Santiago 8580745, Chile
4. IRyS Research Group, School of Physical Education, Pontificia Universidad Católica de Valparaíso, Valparaíso 2374631, Chile; maribel.parra@pucv.cl (M.P.-S.); ximena.palmaleal@gmail.com (X.P.-L.); fernando.rodriguez@pucv.cl (F.R.-R.)
5. School of Sport Sciences, Universidad Europea de Madrid, 28670 Madrid, Spain; joseluis.felipe@universidadeuropea.es (J.L.F.); itziar.pagola@universidadeuropea.es (I.P.A.)
6. Quality of Life Research Group in Different Populations, Department of Education Sciences, Universidad del Bíobío, Chillan 3800949, Chile; xdiaz@ubiobio.cl
* Correspondence: acastillop85@gmail.com; Tel.: +56-988388592

Citation: Castillo-Paredes, A.; Inostroza Jiménez, N.; Parra-Saldías, M.; Palma-Leal, X.; Felipe, J.L.; Págola Aldazabal, I.; Díaz-Martínez, X.; Rodríguez-Rodríguez, F. Environmental and Psychosocial Barriers Affect the Active Commuting to University in Chilean Students. *IJERPH* **2021**, *18*, 1818. https://doi.org/10.3390/ijerph18041818

Academic Editors: Gregory Heath and Adilson Marques
Received: 22 December 2020
Accepted: 2 February 2021
Published: 13 February 2021

Publisher's Note: MDPI stays neutral with regard to jurisdictional claims in published maps and institutional affiliations.

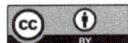

Copyright: © 2021 by the authors. Licensee MDPI, Basel, Switzerland. This article is an open access article distributed under the terms and conditions of the Creative Commons Attribution (CC BY) license (https://creativecommons.org/licenses/by/4.0/).

Abstract: Biking and walking are active commuting, which is considered an opportunity to create healthy habits. Objective: The purpose of this study was to determine the main environmental and psychosocial barriers perceived by students, leading to less Active Commuting (AC) to university and to not reaching the Physical Activity (PA) recommendations. Material and Methods: In this cross-sectional study, 1349 university students (637 men and 712 women) were selected. A self-reported questionnaire was applied to assess the mode of commuting, PA level and barriers to the use of the AC. Results: Women presented higher barriers associated with passive commuting than men. The main barriers for women were "involves too much planning" (OR: 5.25; 95% CI: 3.14–8.78), "It takes too much time" (OR: 4.62; 95% CI: 3.05–6.99) and "It takes too much physical effort" (OR: 3.18; 95% CI: 2.05–4.94). In men, the main barriers were "It takes too much time" (OR: 4.22; 95% CI: 2.97–5.99), "involves too much planning" (OR: 2.49; 95% CI: 1.67–3.70) and "too much traffic along the route" (OR: 2.07; 95% CI: 1.47–2.93). Psychosocial barriers were found in both sexes. Conclusions: Psychosocial and personal barriers were more positively associated with passive commuting than environmental barriers. Interventions at the university are necessary to improve the perception of AC and encourage personal organization to travel more actively.

Keywords: active; commuting; active transport; physical activity; active behavior; college

1. Introduction

Sedentary lifestyle represents an important risk factor for health, since it participates in the development of chronic non-communicable diseases such as cardiovascular diseases, type 2 diabetes and some types of cancer [1,2]. Sedentarism constitutes one of the main causes of mortality worldwide, especially among those who fail to comply with the recommendations of physical activity (PA) for the adult population [3].

This decrease in PA has not only been related to weight gain and worse psychological well-being [4], but also contributes to an increased risk of developing non-communicable diseases and lower life expectancy [5].

Active commuting (walking or cycling from one place to another), is considered an opportunity to create healthy habits, which improve PA levels, decrease cardiovascular risk [6,7] and help achieve a healthier body composition in the young and adult population [8]. Although there is limited evidence in developing countries about the association between active commuting (AC) and health benefits [9,10], Steell et al. [11] showed that, in Chile, 30 min of AC was associated with less adiposity and a healthier metabolic profile that includes a lower risk of obesity, diabetes and metabolic syndrome. Another prospective study, which included a cohort of 263,540 participants from the United Kingdom (Biobank), reported that AC on a bicycle was associated with a lower risk of cardiovascular disease, cancer and all-cause mortality [12].

The university stage is a period of transition from adolescence to adulthood, which is characterized by long days of study, a high sitting time [13], little time for PA [14] and generally bad eating habits [15]. The decrease in PA [16] is mainly due to the fact that the subject of physical education is not mandatory in university, as it is at school [17]. Likewise, sports practice improves physical self-concept, which improves physical appearance, physical ability and weight control behaviors [18]. In Chile, it has been shown that men and women who perform sports activities have a more positive self-concept as compared to men and women who do not perform sports activities [14]. This positive physical self-concept could be associated with lower barriers to PA and AC, but this has not been studied to date.

Studies have shown that the main barriers to PA among university students are related to a lack of time, lack of social support, lack of motivation/enjoyment and economic reasons [19–21]. PA behaviors are influenced by personal (knowledge, skills, attitudes, and self-esteem) and environmental factors (social support, institutional characteristics and built environment [22,23]. However, there is no clarity as t which barriers affect PA in university students, especially considering the different dynamics of different universities [24].

In the same way, the choice of AC, such as walking, can be influenced by several barriers, such as distance and socioeconomic status. It was observed in a study in Spanish university students that those who lived less than 2 km (km) away from the university and those who had a low socioeconomic status used to walk [25]. A short travel distance, high connectivity on the streets, living in an urban area and high density on the roads have been positively associated with higher levels of AC [26,27].

In order to follow the World Health Organization (WHO) recommendation that urban planning in cities promote PA and AC through the design of urban spaces [28], it is important to analyze the previous patterns of population commuting [29,30] to achieve the implementation of promotion programs, improvements in bikeway and walking infrastructure, and road safety [31].

According to the evidence presented and the importance of increasing the level of PA in university students by active commuting, it is necessary to get an idea of the mode of commuting in Chilean university students. The objective of this study was to determine the main environmental and psychosocial barriers perceived by students and associated with less AC to university and not reaching the PA recommendations.

2. Materials and Methods

2.1. Study Design and Participants

This cross-sectional study had a non-probabilistic sample (intentional) and had a descriptive and correlational analysis in university students from three Chilean regions.

A total of 1349 students (637 men and 712 women), with an average age of 22.7 ± 5.8 years, from three public (two in Valparaíso, Viña del Mar and one in Chillán) and one private university (Santiago) were selected. They all agreed to participate voluntarily in the study. They were regular students from the first to fifth academic year studying in fields such as Education (n = 265), Health (n = 308), Engineering (n = 716) and Social Sciences (n = 60). More information and inclusion criteria are shown in Figure 1.

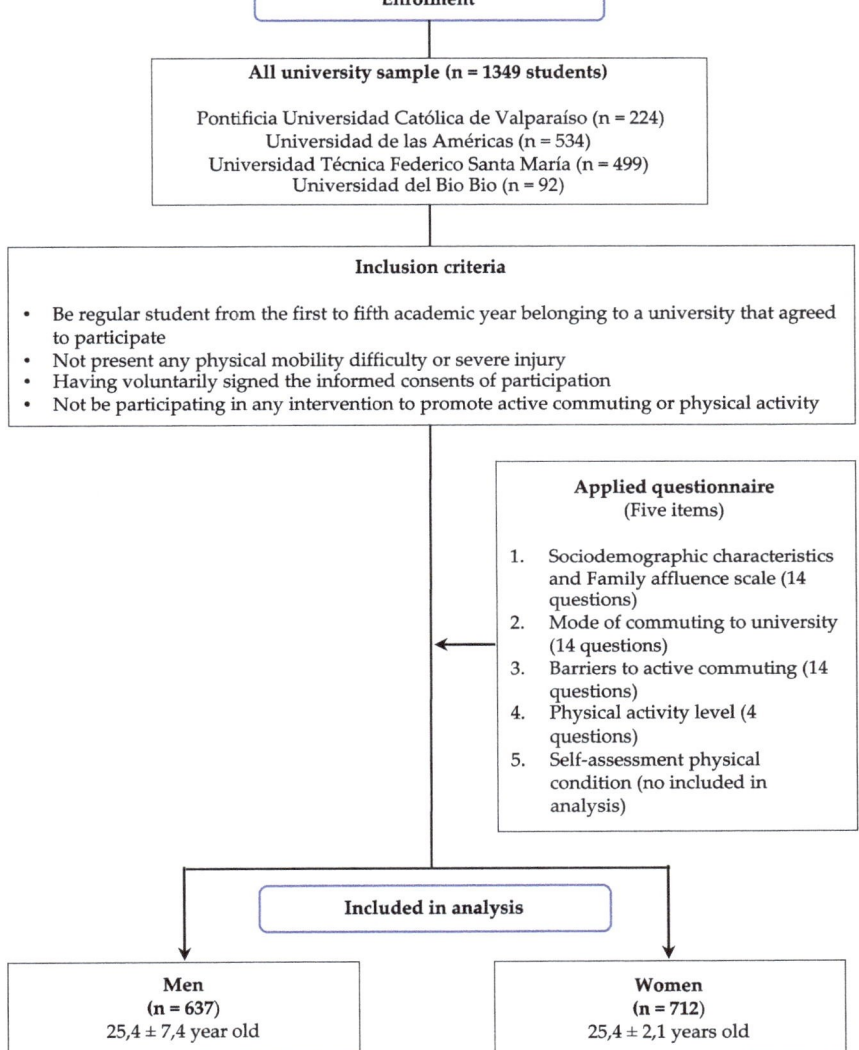

Figure 1. Methodological diagram to explain the sample and instrument.

2.2. Instruments

A self-reported questionnaire was applied to assess the mode of commuting [32], PA level [33] and barriers to the use of the AC in university students [34]. The instrument consisted of five items: sociodemographic characteristics (14 questions); mode of commuting (14 questions); barriers to AC (14 questions); PA level (4 questions) and a self-assessment questionnaire on physical condition—IFIS (International Fitness Scale) (not included in present analysis). This instrument was previously subjected to a specific reliability process for Chilean university students [35] In order to evaluate the reliability of this questionnaire, a test–retest process was performed. Kappa coefficient and Intraclass Correlation Coefficient (ICC) were calculated. Commuting to and from university was found to be in almost perfect agreement, with Kappa coefficient values of 0.882 and 0.822, respectively. ICC scores on distance to and from university and time to and from university showed good reliability in all its items, with high according values.

The sociodemographic characteristics item was sex, age, field of study (*health, education, social science, engineer*), university (*public, private*), residence area (*urban, rural*), live with family and socioeconomic level. To determine socioeconomic level, the Family Affluence Scale (FAS) was used, with the following questions: *(1) "Does your family own a car?"* (No = 0; Yes, one = 1; Yes, two or more = 2), *(2) "How many computers does your family own?"* (None = 0; One = 1; Two = 2; More than two = 3), *(3) "Do you have your own bedroom for yourself?"* (No = 0; Yes = 1) and *(4) "Do you have internet access?"* (No = 0; Yes = 1). Each answer was summed to obtain the total points. A score was assigned, and participants were classified into three categories regarding the FAS: low (0–3 points), medium (4–5 points) and high (6–7 points) [36].

The mode of commuting to university was defined with the questions: *(1) "How do you usually get to university?"* and *(2) "How do you usually get home from university?"*, with a choice of answer options such as walking, bicycle, car, motorcycle, public bus, metro/train and other modes. Walking and bicycle were categorized as "active" modes and other motorized modes as "passive" commuting. The items pertaining to mode of commuting and barriers to the use of AC were used.

The barriers to AC were indicated, such as "There are no sidewalk or bikeways"; "Bikeways occupied by people who walk"; "There is too much traffic along the route"; "Are dangerous crossing along the way"; "Walking or biking is insecure due to crime"; "Are no places to leave the bicycle safely"; "Streets are dangerous because of the cars"; "I get hot and sweat when I'm walking or biking"; "I'm too loaded to go walking or cycling", "It is easier to move with car or motorcycle"; "Walk or biking involves too much planning"; "It takes too much time"; "It takes too much physical effort"; "I need the car or the motorcycle to university". These questions had a categorical like-type response with the alternatives: totally agree = 1; agree = 2; disagree = 3; and strongly disagree = 4 [34].

The International Physical Activity Questionnaire (IPAQ, short version) was used to determine PA levels [33,37]. The PA was classified into sedentary time (min/day), light PA (min/week), moderate PA (min/week), vigorous PA (min/week) and moderate-vigorous (MVPA) as has been reported in a previous study [16]. Regarding the MVPA recommendations for adults ($\geq$150 min/week) [38], students were classified as "Reaching" or "Not reaching" the weekly recommendations.

2.3. Procedure

With the authorization of the academic direction of each university and the knowledge of the career directors, the questionnaire was applied in paper format.

The application of the questionnaire was carried out from Monday to Friday in the day, evening and executive programs, in the same classroom. The application was carried out in 15–20 min and between the months of April and July 2017. Informed consent was obtained from each student before their participation, which requested the authorization to participate in the research project and explained the objectives and that the collected data were anonymous, private, confidential and for exclusive use in the study.

All the participants voluntarily agreed to participate in the study, which was approved by the Ethics Committee of the corresponding university (Code: CCF02052017) and governed by the Declaration of Helsinki 2013 [39].

2.4. Statistical Analysis

The results are presented in frequencies for categorical variables and for continuous variables, in means and standard deviations (M $\pm$ SD). To establish the associations between barriers and mode of commuting and barriers and compliance with MVPA, a binary logistic regression was applied to obtain the Odds Ratio (OR) and Confidence Interval (95% CI). Mode of commuting was included in the model as the dependent variable and barriers were included individually as independent variables. The score was also calculated for the barriers, which were grouped into the categories of Environment and Psychosocial. Significant values of $p < 0.05$ were considered. For the analyses, the statistical software IBM SPSS, version 26, was used.

3. Results

Table 1 present the description and sociodemographic characteristics of the participants. The distribution of the sample by sex was similar (52.8% women and 47.2% men). In both sexes, there was a higher percentage of students in the age range from 18 to 24 years (79.2%), belonging to the engineering study field (53.1%), who reside in urban areas (96.1%), live with their families (73.41%), and have a medium socioeconomic level (52.9%).

Table 1. Sociodemographic characteristics of the participants by sex.

Sociodemographic	All		Women		Men	
	n	(%)	n	(%)	n	(%)
Sex	1349	(100)	712	(52.8)	637	(47.2)
Age (years old)						
18–24	1041	(79.2)	669	(95.0)	372	(61.0)
25–31	159	(12.1)	32	(4.5)	127	(20.8)
32–38	69	(5.3)	3	(0.4)	66	(10.8)
39–46	32	(2.4)	0	(0)	32	(5.2)
47–54	13	(1.0)	0	(0)	13	(2.1)
Study field						
Health	308	(22.8)	216	(30.3)	92	(14.4)
Education	265	(19.6)	206	(28.9)	59	(9.3)
Social sciences	60	(4.4)	37	(5.2)	23	(3.6)
Engineer	716	(53.1)	253	(35.5)	463	(72.7)
Type of university						
Public	815	(60.4)	349	(48.9)	466	(73.1)
Private	534	(39.6)	363	(51.0)	171	(26.8)
Residence area						
Urban	1296	(96.1)	681	(95.6)	615	(96.5)
Rural	53	(3.9)	31	(4.4)	22	(3.5)
Live in family						
Yes	963	(71.4)	565	(79.4)	398	(62.5)
No	386	(28.6)	147	(20.6)	239	(37.5)
Socioeconomic level						
Low	12	(0.9)	9	(1.3)	3	(0.5)
Medium	713	(52.9)	373	(52.4)	340	(53.4)
High	624	(46.3)	330	(46.3)	294	(46.2)

Table 2 shows the mode of commuting of university students according to sex. A total of 82.2% commuters were passive commuters and 17.8% were active commuters, with men (33.8%) forming a higher percentage of those who moved actively. In both sexes, the main mode of commuting was by public bus. The proportion of women and men who reported walking to university was 16.9% and 32%, respectively, while bicycle use was 1% and 1.7%, respectively.

Table 2. Mode of commuting for the university students by sex.

	All		Women		Men	
	n	(%)	n	(%)	n	(%)
Mode of commuting						
Passive	1007	(74.6)	585	(82.2)	422	(66.2)
Active	342	(25.4)	127	(17.8)	215	(33.8)
Commuting to university						
Walking	324	(24.0)	120	(16.9)	204	(32.0)
Bike	18	(1.3)	7	(1.0)	11	(1.7)
Car	179	(13.3)	103	(14.5)	76	(11.9)
Moto	7	(0.5)	1	(0.1)	6	(0.9)
Public bus	681	(50.5)	407	(57.2)	274	(43.0)
Train/metro	140	(10.4)	74	(10.4)	66	(10.4)

Table 3 exhibits the PA of university students according to sex. According to the PA, the mean sitting min/day for the entire sample was 495.7 ± 696.9. Similar data were found in both sexes for minutes/day sitting (women 508.4 ± 751.7 and men 481.6 ± 630.2). Most of the sample (83.5%) did not comply with the recommendation of MVPA for 150 min a week.

Table 3. Physical activity and recommendations of the university students by sex.

	All		Women		Men	
	Mean	±SD	Mean	±SD	Mean	±SD
Physical activity						
Sedentary (min/day)	495.7	±696.9	508.4	±751.7	481.6	±630.2
Light PA (min/week)	262.3	±348.8	224.9	±316.6	304.2	±377.5
Moderate PA (min/week)	113.0	±186.3	100.5	±174.5	126.9	±197.8
Vigorous PA (min/week)	115.6	±160.1	73.6	±118.0	162.5	±185.9
Moderate-vigorous (MVPA)	78.9	±70.6	65.3	±68.0	94.2	±70.3
Recommendation weekly MVPA						
No reach [n (%)]	1127	(83.5)	627	(88.1)	500	(78.5)
Reach [n (%)]	222	(16.5)	85	(11.9)	137	(21.5)

Abbreviations: (mean ± SD) Mean ± Standard Deviation; (PA) Physical Activity (MVPA) Moderate-Vigorous Physical Activity.

Table 4 shows the association between barriers and passive commuting by sex. In women, the barriers *"Walk or biking involves too much planning"* (OR: 5.25; 95% CI: 3.14–8.78; $p < 0.001$), *"It takes too much time"* (OR: 4.62; 95% CI: 3.05–6.99; $p < 0.001$), *"It takes too much physical effort"* (OR: 3.18, 95% CI: 2.05–4.94, $p < 0.001$), were the main barriers. The perception of barriers *"The bikeways are occupied by people who walk"* (OR: 2.54; 95% CI: 1.69–3.84; $p < 0.001$), and *"I'm too loaded to go walking or cycling"* (OR: 2.44; 95% CI: 1.65–3.61; $p < 0.001$), is associated with the probability of passive commuting increasing by two times. In men, *"It takes too much time"* (OR: 4.22; 95% CI: 2.97–5.99; $p < 0.001$) increases the probability of choosing passive commuting four times, while *"Walk or biking involves too much planning"* (OR: 2.49; 95% CI: 1.67–3.70, $p < 0.001$) and *"There is too much traffic along the route"* (OR: 2.07; 95% CI: 1.47–2.93; $p < 0.001$) increases the probability of passive commuting two times. In general, women presented a greater association between barriers and passive commuting than men.

Table 4. Association between barriers and passive commuting by sex.

Barriers	Passive Commuting to University					
	Women			Men		
	OR	(CI 95%)	p Value	OR	(CI 95%)	p Value
Environmental						
There are no sidewalk or bikeways	1.27	(0.84–1.92)	0.264	0.87	(0.60–1.26)	0.446
Bikeways occupied by people who walk	**2.54**	**(1.69–3.84)**	**<0.001**	1.28	(0.91–1.78)	0.152
There is too much traffic along the route	**1.51**	**(1.00–2.27)**	**0.049**	**2.07**	**(1.47–2.93)**	**<0.001**
Are dangerous crossings along the way	**2.12**	**(1.36–3.31)**	**0.001**	**1.55**	**(1.09–2.22)**	**0.016**
Walking or biking is insecure due to crime	1.23	(0.83–1.84)	0.308	0.75	(0.53–1.04)	0.086
Are no places to leave the bicycle safely	1.04	(0.71–1.52)	0.850	1.02	(0.73–1.43)	0.898
Streets are dangerous because of the cars	**2.18**	**(1.39–3.40)**	**0.001**	**1.70**	**(1.17–2.45)**	**0.005**
Psychosocial						
I get hot and sweat when I'm walking or biking	**1.52**	**(1.03–2.24)**	**0.034**	**1.60**	**(1.14–2.23)**	**0.007**
I'm too loaded to go walking or cycling	**2.44**	**(1.65–3.61)**	**<0.001**	1.10	(0.79–1.53)	0.590
It is easier to move with car or motorcycle	1.38	(0.94–2.02)	0.104	**1.75**	**(1.26–2.44)**	**0.001**
Walk or biking involves too much planning	**5.25**	**(3.14–8.78)**	**<0.001**	**2.49**	**(1.67–3.70)**	**<0.001**
It takes too much time	**4.62**	**(3.05–6.99)**	**<0.001**	**4.22**	**(2.97–5.99)**	**<0.001**
It takes too much physical effort	**3.18**	**(2.05–4.94)**	**<0.001**	**1.86**	**(1.30–2.65)**	**0.001**
I need the car or the motorcycle to work	1.09	(0.72–1.66)	0.680	0.96	(0.68–1.37)	0.837

Significant association in bold as $p < 0.05$ and $p < 0.001$.

Table 5 indicates the association between barriers to AC and complying with the MVPA recommendation by sex. The statement "There are no sidewalk or bikeways" (OR: 1.81; 95% CI: 1.02–3.19; $p < 0.05$) was positively associated with non-compliance with the recommendations for MVPA in women. In addition, women who reported being "I get hot and sweat when I'm walking or biking" (OR: 0.56; 95% CI: 0.35–0.89; $p < 0.05$) as a barrier, and men who referred to "It takes too much physical effort" (OR: 0.66; 95% CI: 0.44–0.99; $p < 0.05$) as a barrier, are less likely to comply with the recommendations for MVPA, since the perception of these barriers is negatively associated with compliance with the recommendations.

Table 5. Association between barriers to active commuting and compliance with the MVPA recommendation by sex.

Barriers	Reach MVPA Recomendation					
	Women			Men		
	OR	(CI 95%)	p Value	OR	(CI 95%)	p Value
Environmental						
There are no sidewalk or bikeways	**1.81**	**(1.02–3.19)**	**0.042**	0.90	(0.59–1.36)	0.610
Bikeways occupied by people who walk	0.87	(0.55–1.37)	0.538	0.93	(0.63–1.36)	0.707
There is too much traffic along the route	1.03	(0.62–1.71)	0.918	1.30	(0.85–1.97)	0.225
Are dangerous crossings along the way	1.54	(0.79–3.00)	0.201	1.50	(0.96–2.35)	0.076
Walking or biking is insecure due to crime	0.95	(0.59–1.54)	0.839	0.83	(0.57–1.21)	0.332
Are no places to leave the bicycle safely	0.89	(0.57–1.40)	0.621	0.79	(0.54–1.17)	0.246
Streets are dangerous because of the cars	1.51	(0.78–2.94)	0.224	1.03	(0.67–1.60)	0.889
Psychosocial						
I get hot and sweat when I'm walking or biking	**0.56**	**(0.35–0.89)**	**0.014**	1.05	(0.72–1.54)	0.793
I'm too loaded to go walking or cycling	0.98	(0.60–1.58)	0.917	0.83	(0.57–1.22)	0.345
It is easier to move with car or motorcycle	0.79	(0.50–1.25)	0.311	1.29	(0.83–1.78)	0.312
Walk or biking involves too much planning	1.26	(0.80–1.98)	0.328	0.94	(0.62–1.42)	0.752
It takes too much time	1.15	(0.72–1.84)	0.566	0.76	(0.52–1.11)	0.159
It takes too much physical effort	0.94	(0.59–1.48)	0.780	**0.66**	**(0.44–0.99)**	**0.044**
I need the car or the motorcycle to work	0.74	(0.44–1.23)	0.239	0.85	(0.56–1.28)	0.424

Significant differences in bold were set at $p < 0.05$.

4. Discussion

The main objective was to determine the barriers perceived by students to active commuting to university and the association with physical activity. The main findings were that the passive commuting was the most-used commuting mode to university in Chilean students. The most common barriers associated with passive commuting were "walk or biking involves too much planning" and "it takes too much time" in both sexes.

4.1. Mode of Commuting

The mode of commuting to university in the current study was mainly non-active commuting (82.2%). Similar results were reported in Spain, where a study of 518 students from two universities revealed that 65.1% of participants engaged in non-active commuting [19]. On the other hand, a study conducted at Kansas State University found a prevalence of 34.7% for non-active commuting and 65.3% for active commuting [40], a higher percentage compared to our study. In this regard, a study carried out by the Autonomous University of Barcelona justified the use of the non-active commuting mode for long distances between the university campuses, because the infrastructure was only available for motorized transportation [41]. In the United States, in a study conducted by the University of Kent, students were classified according to their place of residence (on the university campus or outside of it), revealing that only 4% of the students who lived off-campus walked, compared to 42% of students who lived on campus that walked, and 3% who cycled, highlighting the importance of distance in the choice of commuting mode [42]. In another study, also conducted in the United States, 76.1% of students actively moved [43]. These are high figures compared to this Chilean study, because students reside in different districts of the cities, since universities do not have on-campus housing. Thus, in our study, the main passive mode of commuting was public bus, with 50.5%, which was higher in women than in men. A Spanish study done on university students defined the use of the metro/train (31.1%) as the main non-active commuting mode [19], revealing the difference that exists in commuting modes compared with Chilean students. Public transport is more often classified as passive commuting [44]. However, there could be a small benefit associated with its use, since students usually have to walk to public bus stops [45]. In this sense, the choice of the mode of commuting to university is extremely important, not only for the benefits of AC, but also for the increase in daily PA.

4.2. Barriers Perception for Active Commuting

The perception of barriers was divided into "Environmental" and "Psychosocial", and both variables had a significant association with the choice of commuting to university. In both sexes, the most often perceived barriers were "Walk or biking involves too much planning" and "It takes too much time". In an Australian study of AC to and from university, travel time was the most important barrier to AC [46], which is consistent with our study. Another study conducted in university students in Ireland showed that an increase in travel time to university decreased the probability of being classified in a group containing AC and recreational PA at university [47]. This could indicate that students seek to minimize their commuting time, and that it is necessary to provide advice on travel planning and promote walking and cycling, especially for those who live near the university.

In our study, it was possible to appreciate that there were more barriers caused by the personal (psychosocial) compared to environmental barriers. A study carried out on university students from Spain showed that both the psychosocial and environmental variables had a significant correlation with AC to the university [48]. Another study in Spain on AC showed that socioeconomic factors are the most decisive with respect to the use of passive commuting, followed by social behavior variables [41]. A study in Africa on the effect of various motivators and barriers in cycling showed that addressing physical or environmental barriers individually has little impact on promoting cycling, as the perceived motivating variables were more personal [49]. In this sense, and according to the results of our study, it is important to take a comprehensive approach to psychosocial and environmental barriers, since the understanding of psychosocial barriers provides a useful framework to understand the mindset of travelers when designing policies that promote AC.

On the other hand, women showed a greater negative association between AC and the perception of environmental barriers compared to men. In a study on the influence of AC in college students, it was observed that men were more likely to use AC than women, and that, among women, there was a relationship between appearance (e.g., being sweaty) and AC [50]. In addition, this is in agreement with other studies that indicate that women are more concerned about access to services such as showers [51], and that clothing can play an important role in travel decision [52], which coincides with some perceived psychosocial barriers in this study. Another study on the sex gap in choosing to use bicycles showed that women choose bicycles 30% less often than men for their trips to campus and that there are various factors for not commuting by bicycle, such as an unsafe environment [53], which is also consistent with several environmental barriers perceived in this study by women. These findings reinforce the idea that the design of future interventions to promote AC should consider the specific barriers of women and men. Looking at the environmental and social factors that affect the perspective of women and men could directly contribute to increasing rates of AC.

In our study, it was possible to appreciate that there is a perception of both psychosocial and environmental barriers that would affect the use of bicycles as an active means of transport, with the former being the ones that have the greatest influence. Although it has been described that bicycle use not only depends on the individual mobility behaviors of the user but is also associated with the environment, urban cycling interacts with other modes of travelling, such as public buses, cars, motorcycles and pedestrians [54]. The use of a bicycle is associated more with the cyclist, as long as he/she controls the conditions of the trip, such as the distance travelled [55], physical effort and greater exposure to the weather, which conditions the mobility behaviors that stand out as individual, sociodemographic and psychological factors [56].

A study carried out in Argentina showed a lack of road safety when sharing the road with motorized vehicles as a main barrier to bicycle use [57]. In Chile, a study showed that the bicycle is used downtown through the streets, since bikeways are located in certain sectors of the metropolitan region (137 bikeways in 14 districts), which are mainly concentrated in districts of higher socioeconomic status and greater motorization [58]. As safety is an important factor in the choice of the bicycle as a means of AC, it would be important to promote changes in the cycling infrastructure that would make students perceive cycling as safer, such as improvements to local bike routes and the creation of more off-street bikeways. It is fundamental to improve the behaviors of PA practices through programs aimed at people that decrease the personal barriers to the use of this means of AC and to invest in road education.

In relation to the use of vehicles, an investigation showed that postgraduate students have a greater tendency to use passive modes of commuting (bus or car) due to their work or the possibility of acquiring a vehicle [59]. In Chile, the statistics show that the automotive fleet continues to increase [60], which could become a barrier with greater weight for AC. In our study, car use was only a barrier in men. However, in this university stage, students have low purchasing power; young people do not own cars and it is not presented as a significant barrier.

4.3. Barriers Perception for MVPA Recommendation

The barriers associated with non-compliance with MVPA are greater in women than in men. In women, in terms of environmental barriers, we find "There are no sidewalk or bikeways" and in the psychosocial barrier is "I get hot and sweat when I'm walking or biking", compared to men who only have the psychosocial barrier "It takes too much physical effort". It is important, at this point, to emphasize that the perceived barriers associated with MVPA coincide with AC, that is, a lot of effort and sweating are repeated reasons for women for not doing PA in this study.

In the literature, it was found that the barriers to compliance with the MVPA were economic levels, interest in the use of sports facilities, residence, intrapersonal and interpersonal barriers [22], distance [61] and psychosocial factors [47]. In the other study, carried out in university students, it is mentioned that the barriers to compliance with PA are economic levels, health, peer support, self-efficacy and effect related to the practice, which were increased in men compared to women [62]. In comparison with other investigations, women face greater barriers to the practice of PA [63].

On the other hand, Sevil et al. [64] analyzed the relationships between physical activity and the perceived barriers to physical activity, motivation and stages of change in Spanish university students, where they found that the barriers to participation were related negatively to the levels of PA and more self-determined forms of motivation. Recommendations include intervention from a medical area to help to comply with the recommendations of physical activity for optimal health [65], due to the high incidence of sedentary lifestyle in university students [66]. A study of Peruvian medical college students from a private university indicates that of the 312 students, just under a third performed MVPA for $\geq$150 min/week, and slightly more than a third performed MVPA for $\leq$30 min/week [67]. In turn, a study carried out with 244 adults mentions environmental barriers, where they indicate that cold days with little light are a barrier to compliance with the MVPA, because the increase of 10° is associated with an additional increase of 1.5 min/day and every extra hour of light in the day adds 2.23 min to the practice of PA [68]. Moreover, in an investigation in 507 adolescents, they mention internal and external barriers, such as "I am not interested in physical activity" and "I need equipment I don't have", and no significant differences between sex were found [69]. In this sense, a better understanding of the barriers that prevent compliance with the MPVA between both sexes is essential to minimize passive commuting and obtain the variety of benefits associated with AC.

4.4. Limitations and Implications

Despite the numerous significant findings in our study, there were some limitations, including that the student questionnaire was self-reported, and therefore could be subject to bias. On the other hand, the data used were only related to travel between home and university, and cannot be extrapolated to other environments. Our study only recorded the main mode used for commuting, so we did not consider mixed modes. Finally, only four universities were consulted in the research and the geographical characteristics of the three cities where they are located are heterogeneous, and a representative sample per university was not calculated. Therefore, precaution must be taken when generalizing the current results. However, this study makes a significant contribution to the literature on the variety of influences that can affect active commuting. A change in the culture of mobility must begin from within communities and in this sense, university students can be an important target group, especially women, who show a greater negative association between the perception of environmental barriers and AC, as well as with non-compliance with MVPA. Therefore, these findings, in combination with existing research, provide a solid foundation for future studies in this area and the development of policies and programs to improve AC in the university, suggesting that a strong association between the government and university organizations can produce positive results.

5. Conclusions

This study provided important information on perceived barriers to AC and MVPA compliance in Chilean university students. The results of the present study suggest that psychosocial or personal barriers were more positively associated with passive commuting to university than environmental barriers. In other words, aspects based on personal decision to commute actively intervene to a greater extent than the barriers imposed by the environment. Therefore, implementing policies that address the psychosocial factors more, but environmental factors as well, are necessary to increase AC rates, and thus achieve an impact in terms of both health and PA in university students. In addition, our study suggests that it is necessary to target women over men for AC and PA interventions, since women present more barriers and less active commuting. In this way, the measures should not only be applied by the government, but should mainly include universities as the lead actor for the development of educational strategies that promote and increase AC.

Author Contributions: Data collection, conceptualization, methodology, formal analysis, writing,—original draft, visualization, A.C.-P.; conceptualization, formal analysis, writing, N.I.J.; review and editing, M.P.-S., J.L.F. and I.P.A.; data collection—review and editing, X.P.-L. and X.D.-M.; conceptualization, writing—review and editing, supervision and project administration, F.R.-R.; critical review, A.C.-P., N.I.J., F.R.-R., X.P.-L., M.P.-S., X.D.-M., J.L.F. and I.P.A. All authors have read and agreed to the published version of the manuscript.

Funding: This research received no external funding.

Institutional Review Board Statement: The study was conducted according to the guidelines of the Declaration of Helsinki, and approved by the Ethics Committee of Pontificia Universidad Católica de Valparaíso (Code: CCF02052017).

Informed Consent Statement: Informed consent was obtained from all subjects involved in the study.

Acknowledgments: We appreciate the university students who participated in and the academics who supported this project and to Universidad de Las Américas, Universidad Técnica Federico Santa María, Universidad del BioBio and Research Unit of Pontificia Universidad Católica de Valparaíso.

Conflicts of Interest: The authors declare no conflict of interest.

References

1. Dempsey, P.; Matthews, C.; Dashti, S.G.; Doherty, A.; Bergouignan, A.; van Roekel, E.; Dunstan, D.; Wareham, J.; Yates, T.; Wijndaele, K.; et al. Sedentary behavior and chronic disease: Mechanisms and future directions. *J. Phys. Act. Health* **2020**, *17*, 52–61. [CrossRef]
2. OMS. Actividad Física. Available online: https://www.who.int/dietphysicalactivity/pa/es/ (accessed on 27 July 2020).
3. Diaz-Martinez, X.; Petermann, F.; Leiva, A.M.; Garrido-Mendez, A.; Salas-Bravo, C.; Martínez, M.A.; Labraña, A.M.; Duran, E.; Valdivia-Moral, P.; Zagalaz, M.L.; et al. Association of physical inactivity with obesity, diabetes, hypertension and metabolic syndrome in the chilean population. *Rev. Med. Chile* **2018**, *146*, 585–595. [CrossRef]
4. Molina-García, J.; Queralt, A.; Castillo, I.; Sallis, J. Changes in physical activity domains during the transition out of high school: Psychosocial and environmental correlates. *J. Phys. Act. Health* **2015**, *12*, 1414–1420. [CrossRef] [PubMed]
5. Masselli, M.; Ward, P.; Gobbi, E.; Carraro, A. Promoting physical activity among university students: A systematic review of controlled trials. *Am. J. Health Promot.* **2018**, *32*, 1602–1612. [CrossRef]
6. Chillón, P.; Gottrand, F.; Ortega, F.B.; Gonzalez-Gross, M.; Ruiz, J.; Ward, D.; De Bourdeaudhuij, I.; Moreno, L.; Martínez-Gómez, D.; Castillo, M.; et al. Active commuting and physical activity in adolescents from Europe: Results from the HELENA study. *Pediatric Exerc. Sci.* **2011**, *23*, 207–2017. [CrossRef]
7. García-Hermoso, A.; Quintero, A.; Hernández, E.; Correa-Bautista, J.; Izquierdo, M.; Tordecilla-Sanders, A.; Prieto-Benavides, D.; Sandoval-Cuellar, C.; González-Ruíz, K.; Villa-González, E.; et al. Active commuting to and from university, obesity and metabolic syndrome among Colombian university students. *BMC Public Health* **2018**, *18*, 523. [CrossRef] [PubMed]
8. Larouche, R.; Saunders, T.J.; Faulkner, G.E.J.; Colley, R.; Tremblay, M. Associations between active school transport and physical activity, body composition, and cardiovascular fitness: A systematic review of 68 studies. *J. Phys. Act. Health* **2014**, *11*, 206–227. [CrossRef] [PubMed]
9. McKay, A.; Laverty, A.; Shridhar, K.; Alam, D.; Dias, A.; Williams, J.; Millet, C.; Ebrahim, S.; Dhillon, P. Associations between active travel and adiposity in rural India and Bangladesh: A cross-sectional study. *BMC Public Health* **2015**, *15*, 1087. [CrossRef]
10. Sadarangani, K.P.; Von Oetinger, A.; Cristi-Montero, C.; Cortínez-O'Ryan, A.; Aguilar-Farías, N.; Martínez-Gómez, D. Beneficial association between active travel and metabolic syndrome in Latin-America: A cross-sectional analysis from the Chilean National Health Survey 2009–2010. *Prev. Med.* **2018**, *107*, 8–13. [CrossRef]
11. Steell, L.; Garrido-Méndez, A.; Petermann, F.; Díaz-Martínez, X.; Martínez, M.; Leiva, A.; Salas-Bravo, C.; Alvarez, C.; Ramirez-Campillo, R.; Cristi-Montero, C.; et al. Active commuting is associated with a lower risk of obesity, diabetes and metabolic syndrome in Chilean adults. *J. Public Health* **2018**, *40*, 508–516. [CrossRef]
12. Celis-Morales, C.; Lyall, D.; Welsh, P.; Anderson, J.; Steell, L.; Guo, Y.; Maldonado, R.; Mackay, D.; Pell, J.; Sattar, N.; et al. Association between active commuting and incident cardiovascular disease, cancer, and mortality: Prospective cohort study. *Br. Med. J.* **2017**, *357*, j1456. [CrossRef]

13. Buckworth, J.; Nigg, C. Physical activity, exercise, and sedentary behavior in college students. *J. Am. Coll. Health* **2004**, *53*, 28–34. [CrossRef]
14. Oteíza, L.; Rodríguez-Rodríguez, F.; Carvajal, J.; Vargas, P.; Yañez, R. Valoración del autoconcepto físico en estudiantes universitarios y su relación con la práctica deportiva. *J. Mov. Health* **2011**, *12*. [CrossRef]
15. Mardones, M.; Olivares, S.; Araneda, J.; Gómez, N. Etapas del cambio relacionadas con el consumo de frutas y verduras, actividad física y control del peso en estudiantes universitarios chilenos. *Arch. Lat. Nutr.* **2009**, *59*, 304–309.
16. Barranco-Ruiz, Y.; Cruz, C.; Villa-González, E.; Palma-Leal, X.; Chillón, P.; Rodríguez-Rodríguez, F. Active Commuting to University and its Association with Sociodemographic Factors and Physical Activity Levels in Chilean Students. *Medicina* **2019**, *55*, 152. [CrossRef]
17. Lipošek, S.; Planinšec, J.; Leskošek, B.; Pajtler, A. Physical activity of university students and its relation to physical fitness and academic success. *Ann. Kinesiol.* **2018**, *9*, 89–104. [CrossRef]
18. Navas, L.; Soriano, J. Autoconcepto físico y práctica deportiva en estudiantes del Bíobio (Chile). Revista INFAD de Psicología. *Int. J. Dev. Educ. Psychol.* **2014**, *1*, 399–408. [CrossRef]
19. Aceijas, C.; Waldhausl, S.; Lambert, N.; Cassar, S.; Bello-Corassa, R. Determinants of health-related lifestyles among university students. *Perspect. Public Health* **2017**, *137*, 227–236. [CrossRef]
20. Ashton, L.M.; Hutchesson, M.J.; Rollo, M.E.; Morgan, P.J.; Collins, C.E. Motivators and barriers to engaging in healthy eating and physical activity: A cross-sectional survey in young adult men. *Am. J. Men's Health* **2016**, *11*, 330–343. [CrossRef] [PubMed]
21. Ashton, L.M.; Hutchesson, M.J.; Rollo, M.E.; Morgan, P.J.; Thompson, D.I.; Collins, C.E. Young adult males' motivators and perceived barriers towards eating healthily and being active: A qualitative study. *Int. J. Behav. Nutr. Phys. Act.* **2015**, *12*, 93. [CrossRef] [PubMed]
22. Deliens, T.; Deforche, B.; De Bourdeaudhuij, I.; Clarys, P. Determinants of physical activity and sedentary behaviour in university students: A qualitative study using focus group discussions. *BMC Public Health* **2015**, *15*, 201. [CrossRef]
23. Sallis, J.F.; Owen, N.; Fisher, E.B. Ecological models of health behavior. In *Health Behavior and Health Education: Theory, Research, and Practice*, 4th ed.; Jossey-Bass: San Francisco, CA, USA, 2008.
24. Hilger-Kolb, J.; Loerbroks, A.; Diehl, K. When I have time pressure, sport is the first thing that is cancelled': A mixed-methods study on barriers to physical activity among university students in Germany. *J. Sports Sci.* **2020**, *38*, 2479–2488. [CrossRef] [PubMed]
25. Molina-García, J.; Sallis, J.; Castillo, I. Active commuting and sociodemographic factors among university students in Spain. *J. Phys. Act. Health* **2014**, *11*, 359–363. [CrossRef]
26. Humpel, N.; Owen, N.; Leslie, E. Environmental factors associated with adults' participation in physical activity: A review. *Am. J. Prev. Med.* **2002**, *22*, 188–199. [CrossRef]
27. Saelens, B.; Sallis, J.; Frank, L. Environmental correlates of walking and cycling: Findings from the transportation, urban design, and planning literatures. *Ann. Behav. Med.* **2003**, *25*, 80–91. [CrossRef] [PubMed]
28. Raustorp, J.; Koglin, T. The potential for active commuting by bicycle and its possible effects on public health. *J. Transp. Health* **2019**, *13*, 72–77. [CrossRef]
29. Molina-García, J.; Menescardi, C.; Estevan, I.; Martínez-Bello, V.; Queralt, A. Neighborhood built environment and socioeconomic status are associated with active commuting and sedentary behavior, but not with leisure-time physical activity, in university students. *Int. J. Environ. Res. Public Health* **2019**, *16*, 3176. [CrossRef]
30. Goltermann, C.; Juel, C.; Lykke, M.; Schneller, M.B.; Helms, A.; Aadahl, M. Temporal changes in active commuting from 2007 to 2017 among adults living in the Capital Region of Denmark. *J. Transp. Health* **2019**, *14*, 100608. [CrossRef]
31. Palma-Leal, X.; Chillón, P.; Rodríguez-Rodríguez, F.; Barranco-Ruiz, Y.; Huertas-Delgado, F. Perceived parental barriers towards active commuting to school in Chilean children and adolescents of Valparaíso. *Int. J. Sustain. Transp.* **2020**, *14*, 525–532. [CrossRef]
32. Rodríguez-Rodríguez, F.; Cristi-Montero, C.; Celis-Morales, C.; Escobar-Gómez, D.; Chillón, P. Impact of distance on mode of active commuting in Chilean children and adolescents. *Int. J. Environ. Res. Public Health* **2017**, *14*, 1334. [CrossRef]
33. Roman-Viñas, B.; Serra-Majem, L.; Hagströmer, M.; Ribas-Barba, L.; Sjöström, M.; Segura-Cardona, R. International physical activity questionnaire: Reliability and validity in a Spanish population. *Eur. J. Sport Sci.* **2010**, *10*, 297–304. [CrossRef]
34. Molina-García, J.; Queralt, A.; Estevan, I.; Álvarez, O.; Castillo, I. Barreras percibidas en el desplazamiento activo al centro educativo: Fiabilidad y validez de una escala. *Gac. Sanit.* **2016**, *30*, 426–431. [CrossRef]
35. Palma-Leal, X.; Gómez, D.; Garzón, P.; Rodríguez-Rodríguez, F. Fiabilidad de un cuestionario de modos, tiempo y distancia de desplazamiento en estudiantes universitarios. *Retos Nuevas Tend. Educ. Física Deporte Recreación* **2020**, 210–214. [CrossRef]
36. Boyce, W.; Torsheim, T.; Currie, C.; Zambon, A. The family affluence scale as a measure of national wealth: Validation of an adolescent self-report measure. *Soc. Indic. Res.* **2006**, *78*, 473–487. [CrossRef]
37. Craig, C.; Marshall, A.; Sjöström, M.; Bauman, A.; Booth, M.; Ainsworth, B.; Pratt, M.; Ekelund, U.; Yngve, A.; Sallis, J.F.; et al. International physical activity questionnaire: 12-country reliability and validity. *Med. Sci. Sports Exerc.* **2003**, *35*, 1381–1395. [CrossRef]
38. Bull, F.; Al-Ansari, S.; Biddle, S.; Borodulin, K.; Buman, M.; Cardon, G.; Carty, C.; Chaput, J.; Chastin, S.; Chou, R.; et al. World Health Organization 2020 guidelines on physical activity and sedentary behaviour. *Br. J. Sports Med.* **2020**, *54*, 1451–1462. [CrossRef] [PubMed]

39. World Medical Association. Declaration of Helsinki: Ethical Principles for Medical Research Involving Human Subjects. Available online: https://www.wma.net/policies-post/wma-declaration-of-helsinki-ethical-principles-for-medical-research-involving-human-subjects/ (accessed on 27 July 2020).
40. Bopp, M.; Kaczynski, A.; Wittman, P. Active commuting patterns at a large, midwestern college campus. *J. Am. Coll. Health* **2011**, *59*, 605–611. [CrossRef]
41. Soria-Lara, J.; Marquet, O.; Miralles-Guasch, C. The influence of location, socioeconomics, and behaviour on travel-demand by car in metropolitan university campuses. *Transp. Res. Part D Transp. Environ.* **2017**, *53*, 149–160. [CrossRef]
42. Kaplan, D. Transportation sustainability on a university campus. *Int. J. Sustain. High. Educ.* **2015**, *16*, 173–186. [CrossRef]
43. Bopp, M.; Bopp, C.; Schuchert, M. Active transportation to and on campus is associated with objectively measured fitness outcomes among college students. *J. Phys. Act. Health* **2015**, *12*, 418–423. [CrossRef]
44. Parra-Saldías, M.; Castro-Piñero, J.; Castillo-Paredes, A.; Palma-Leal, X.; Díaz-Martínez, X.; Rodríguez-Rodríguez, F. Active commuting behaviours from high school to university in Chile: A retrospective study. *Int. J. Environ. Res. Public Health* **2019**, *16*, 53. [CrossRef]
45. Rissel, C.; Curac, N.; Greenaway, M.; Bauman, A. Physical activity associated with public transport use—a review and modelling of potential benefits. *Int. J. Environ. Res. Public Health* **2012**, *9*, 2454–2478. [CrossRef] [PubMed]
46. Shannon, T.; Giles-Corti, B.; Pikora, T.; Bulsara, M.; Shilton, T.; Bull, F. Active commuting in a university setting: Assessing commuting habits and potential for modal change. *Transp. Policy* **2006**, *13*, 240–253. [CrossRef]
47. Murphy, J.; MacDonncha, C.; Murphy, M.; Murphy, N.; Nevill, A.; Woods, C. What psychosocial factors determine the physical activity patterns of university students? *J. Phys. Act. Health* **2019**, *16*, 325–332. [CrossRef]
48. Molina-García, J.; Castillo, I.; Sallis, J. Psychosocial and environmental correlates of active commuting for university students. *Prev. Med.* **2010**, *51*, 136–138. [CrossRef] [PubMed]
49. Nkurunziza, A.; Zuidgeest, M.; Brussel, M.; Van Maarseveen, M. Examining the potential for modal change: Motivators and barriers for bicycle commuting in Dar-es-Salaam. *Transp. Policy* **2012**, *24*, 249–259. [CrossRef]
50. Sims, D.; Bopp, M.; Wilson, O. Examining influences on active travel by sex among college students. *J. Transp. Health* **2018**, *9*, 73–82. [CrossRef]
51. Kaczynski, A.T.; Bopp, M.J.; Wittman, P. Peer reviewed: Association of workplace supports with active commuting. *Prev. Chronic Dis.* **2010**, *7*, A127. [PubMed]
52. Broache, A. Perspectives on Seattle Women's Decisions to Bike for Transportation. Master's Thesis, University of Washington, Seattle, WA, USA, 2012.
53. Abasahl, F.; Kelarestaghi, K.B.; Ermagun, A. Gender gap generators for bicycle mode choice in Baltimore college campuses. *Travel Behav. Soc.* **2018**, *11*, 78–85. [CrossRef]
54. Bernasconi, O.; Tham, M. Un enfoque praxiográfico a la bici-movilidad en Santiago de Chile. El ciclismo urbano como un logro colectivo. *Antropol. Exp.* **2016**, *16*, 87–110. [CrossRef]
55. Manaugh, K.; Boisjoly, G.; El-Geneidy, A. Overcoming barriers to cycling: Understanding frequency of cycling in a University setting and the factors preventing commuters from cycling on a regular basis. *Transportation* **2017**, *44*, 871–884. [CrossRef]
56. Caballero, R.; Franco, P.; Mustaca, A.; Jakovcevic, A. Uso de la bicicleta como medio de transporte: Influencia de los factores psicológicos. Una revisión de la literatura. *Psico* **2014**, *45*, 316–327. [CrossRef]
57. Jakovcevic, A.; Franco, P.; Dalla Pozza, M.V.; Ledesma, R. Percepción de los beneficios individuales del uso de la bicicleta compartida como modo de transporte. *Suma Psicol.* **2016**, *23*, 33–41. [CrossRef]
58. Arellano, C.; Saavedra, F. El uso de la bicicleta en Santiago de Chile¿ es una opción? *EchoGéo* **2017**. [CrossRef]
59. Assi, K.; Gazder, U.; Al-Sghan, I.; Reza, I.; Almubarak, A. A Nested Ensemble Approach with ANNs to Investigate the Effect of Socioeconomic Attributes on Active Commuting of University Students. *Int. J. Environ. Res. Public Health* **2020**, *17*, 3549. [CrossRef] [PubMed]
60. INE. Permisos de Circulación. Available online: https://www.ine.cl/estadisticas/economia/transporte-y-comunicaciones/permiso-de-circulacion/parque-de-vehiculos (accessed on 27 July 2020).
61. Audrey, S.; Fisher, H.; Cooper, A.; Gaunt, D.; Garfield, K.; Metcalfe, C.; Hollingworth, W.; Gillison, F.; Gabe-Walters, M.; Rodgers, S.; et al. Evaluation of an intervention to promote walking during the commute to work: A cluster randomised controlled trial. *BMC Public Health* **2019**, *19*, 427. [CrossRef] [PubMed]
62. Seo, Y.J.; Ha, Y. Gender differences in predictors of physical activity among Korean college students based on the Health Promotion Model. *Asian/Pac. Isl. Nurs. J.* **2019**, *4*, 1. [CrossRef]
63. Pengpid, S.; Peltzer, K.; Kassean, H.K.; Tsala, J.; Sychareun, V.; Müller-Riemenschneider, F. Physical inactivity and associated factors among university students in 23 low-, middle-and high-income countries. *Int. J. Public Health* **2015**, *60*, 539–549. [CrossRef] [PubMed]
64. Sevil, J.; Praxedes, A.; Abarca-Sos, A.; Del Villar, F.; Garcia-Gonzalez, L. Levels of physical activity, motivation and barriers to participation in university students. *J. Sports Med. Phys. Fit.* **2015**, *56*, 1239–1248.
65. Downes, L. Physical activity and dietary habits of college students. *J. Nurse Pract.* **2015**, *11*, 192–198. [CrossRef]
66. Arias-Palencia, N.M.; Solera-Martinez, M.; Gracia-Marco, L.; Silva, P.; Martinez-Vizcaino, V.; Canete-Garcia-Prieto, J.; Sanchez-Lopez, M. Levels and patterns of objectively assessed physical activity and compliance with different public health guidelines in university students. *PLoS ONE* **2015**, *10*, e0141977. [CrossRef] [PubMed]

67. Zevallos-Morales, A.; Luna-Porta, L.; Medina-Salazar, H.; Yauri, M.; Taype-Rondan, A. Association between migration and physical activity among medical students from a university located in Lima, Peru. *PLoS ONE* **2019**, *14*, e0212009. [CrossRef] [PubMed]
68. Welch, W.; Spring, B.; Phillips, S.; Siddique, J. Moderating effects of weather-related factors on a physical activity intervention. *Am. J. Prev. Med.* **2018**, *54*, e83–e89. [CrossRef] [PubMed]
69. Gunnell, K.; Brunet, J.; Wing, E.; Bélanger, M. Measuring perceived barriers to physical activity in adolescents. *Pediatric Exerc. Sci.* **2015**, *27*, 252–261. [CrossRef] [PubMed]

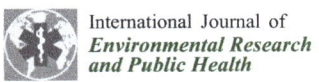

Article

12-Year Trends in Active School Transport across Four European Countries—Findings from the Health Behaviour in School-Aged Children (HBSC) Study

Ellen Haug [1,2,*], Otto Robert Frans Smith [3], Jens Bucksch [4], Catherina Brindley [4], Jan Pavelka [5], Zdenek Hamrik [5], Joanna Inchley [6], Chris Roberts [7], Frida Kathrine Sofie Mathisen [1] and Dagmar Sigmundová [8]

1. Department of Health Promotion and Development, University of Bergen, 5020 Bergen, Norway; frida.mathisen@uib.no
2. Department of Teacher Education, NLA University College, 5012 Bergen, Norway
3. Department of Health Promotion, Norwegian Institute of Public Health, 5015 Bergen, Norway; robert.smith@fhi.no
4. Department of Prevention and Health Promotion, Faculty of Natural and Human Sciences, Heidelberg University of Education, 69120 Heidelberg, Germany; bucksch@ph-heidelberg.de (J.B.); brindley@ph-heidelberg.de (C.B.)
5. Department of Recreation and Leisure Studies, Faculty of Physical Culture, Palacký University Olomouc, 77111 Olomouc, Czech Republic; jan.pavelka@upol.cz (J.P.); zdenek.hamrik@upol.cz (Z.H.)
6. MRC/CSO Social and Public Health Sciences Unit, University of Glasgow, Glasgow G3 7HR, UK; Joanna.Inchley@glasgow.ac.uk
7. Social Research and Information Division, Welsh Government, Cardiff CF10 3NQ, UK; Chris.Roberts@gov.wales
8. Institute of Active Lifestyle, Faculty of Physical Culture, Palacký University Olomouc, 77111 Olomouc, Czech Republic; dagmar.sigmundova@gmail.com
* Correspondence: ellen.haug@uib.no; Tel.: +47-958-095-48

Abstract: Active school transport (AST) is a source of daily physical activity uptake. However, AST seems to have decreased worldwide over recent decades. We aimed to examine recent trends in AST and associations with gender, age, family affluence, and time to school, using data from the Health Behaviour in School-Aged Children (HBSC) study collected in 2006, 2010, 2014, and 2018 in the Czech Republic, Norway, Scotland, and Wales. Data from 88,212 students (11, 13 and 15 years old) revealed stable patterns of AST from 2006 to 2018, apart from a decrease in the Czech Republic between 2006 and 2010. For survey waves combined, walking to and from school was most common in the Czech Republic (55%) and least common in Wales (30%). Cycling was only common in Norway (22%). AST differed by gender (Scotland and Wales), by age (Norway), and by family affluence (everywhere but Norway). In the Czech Republic, family affluence was associated with change over time in AST, and the effect of travel time on AST was stronger. The findings indicate that the decrease in AST could be levelling off in the countries considered here. Differential associations with sociodemographic factors and travel time should be considered in the development of strategies for AST.

Keywords: active school transport; trends; cross-national; HBSC; gender; age; SES

1. Introduction

In recent years, active travel has become an integral part of international initiatives aimed at increasing levels of physical activity within the population [1–4]. Walking and cycling to school have gained considerable attention as sources of young peoples' daily physical activity. More recently, there has also been an increased focus on active commuting as a sustainable form of transport that can reduce problems caused by motorised vehicles, with potentially significant economic benefits and public health impacts [3,5–8].

Reviews of the growing body of literature in the field strongly support a positive relationship between active school transport (AST) and levels of physical activity [9,10].

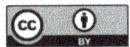

Positive associations have also been found between cycling to and from school and cardiovascular fitness [9–12]. A relationship between AST and body composition indicators is less clear [9,10]. Other potential co-benefits of AST relate to improved navigation and road safety abilities [13,14], better processing of the physical surroundings [15], higher activation (i.e., alertness and activity) during school hours [16], and the development of long-term physical activity and active transportation habits [17,18].

Despite the potential benefits, the number of children and youths that walk or cycle to school seems to have decreased worldwide in recent decades [19–28]. However, large cross-country variations are observed in the prevalence of AST and the magnitude of decline [21]. In the United States, the prevalence of AST among children dropped from 49 to 13% between 1969 and 2009 [25], whereas it declined from 44 to 21% among 10–14 year old children in Australia between 1971 and 2003 [24]. Findings from Europe display a more mixed picture, with generally higher proportions of AST being reported, but decreasing trends have also been observed in European studies [22,26,29,30]. Many of the existing studies on trends in AST span over several decades, covering a period when use of motorised vehicles increased dramatically. Furthermore, the studies are limited to data from individual countries preventing reliable cross-national comparisons. More recently, policy initiatives and national programs to promote active school commuting have been initiated in many countries [3,6,31–33], which may have affected schoolchildren's travel behaviours.

Contemporary studies suggest that AST is associated with a wide range of factors, such as demographic (gender, ethnicity, age), family (parental education, household income, car ownership), social (individual and parental attitudes and concerns, social and cultural norms), environmental (school distance, safety, walkability, traffic calming, infrastructure, recreational facilities, centralization), and policy-related factors [6,25,29,34–36]. It is to be expected that some of the underlying drivers of AST will vary between and within countries [23]. However, a large body of research has identified the distance between home and school and time taken to travel to school as the strongest predictors of AST [6,14,29,36,37], and findings from several countries point towards an increase in the distance to school over time [20,27,29,38].

Gender, age, and socioeconomic status (SES) have been identified as potential moderators of AST [39]. Findings from North America, Australia, New Zealand, and the Czech Republic indicate higher levels of AST for boys more often than girls [14,32,36,40,41], while gender differences have not been observed in studies from Switzerland [26] and Norway [11]. Regarding gender difference trends in recent times, there is no clear pattern, with no differences [41,42], a decline only for girls [43] and a decline in boys and an increase in girls [27] having been observed. The relationship between age and AST is expected to be curvilinear, with an initial age-related increase due to more independent mobility and parental allowances, followed by a decrease because of generally longer distances to secondary schools compared with localised primary schools [14]. Socioeconomic differences in AST have been less well studied. The literature from North America and New Zealand generally shows that low-income households and lower parental education correlate with more AST [14,36]. Nevertheless, the lack of standardised measures and comparable control variables across different studies makes it difficult to compare, aggregate and interpret findings [35,36,44,45].

Cross-national studies of current time trends with a comparable methodological approach are of interest because they can provide unique insights into how recent developments, as well as national and local level policies, may have had an impact on AST. It has been suggested that future research should also consider changes in key AST correlates over time to support the development of new policies, regulations, designs, and programme interventions [36]. To improve the understanding of young peoples' transport to school in different regions in Europe between 2006 and 2018, the current study aimed to examine secular trends in AST and their associations with gender, age, SES, and time to school across Northern Europe (Norway), western Europe (Scotland and Wales) and central Europe (the Czech Republic).

2. Materials and Methods

2.1. Study Population and Procedures

The Health Behaviour in School-Aged Children study (HBSC) is unique in collecting comparable cross-national data on representative samples of young peoples' health behaviours every fourth year. A standardised international protocol ensures the consistency of measures, sampling, and implementation procedures prepared by the HBSC International Coordinating Centre [46].

Data stem from the HBSC studies conducted in 2006, 2010, 2014, and 2018 in the Czech Republic, Norway, Scotland, and Wales. Data on AST were obtained from a total of 88,212 children across the four time points (2006: n = 18,317, 50.3 % girls; 2010: n = 18,902, 51.0% girls; 2014: n = 17,699, 51.3 % girls; 2018: n = 33,294, 50.6 % girls). The age and gender distributions were fairly stable across countries and survey years (Table S1). Students were surveyed to produce representative national estimates for 11, 13, and 15 year old children. Classes within schools were selected with variations in sampling criteria which allowed us to fit country-level circumstances (e.g., national regions, type of school, and size of schools). Ethical approval for the surveys was obtained at the national level. Participation was voluntary and the children were informed about confidentiality and anonymity. Classroom teachers or trained administrators conducted the survey and consent (explicit or implicit) was given from school administrators and/or parents before participation. More details on the HBSC study procedures can be found elsewhere [46].

2.2. Survey Items

2.2.1. Active School Transport

Mode of travel to and from school was assessed with two questions: "On a typical day is the main part of your journey to school made by . . . ?" and "On a typical day is the main part of your journey from school made by . . . ?". Response options were "Walking", "Bicycle", "Bus, train, tram, underground or boat", "Car, motorcycle or moped" or "Other means". A slightly different version of the AST items used earlier in the 1985/86 HBSC study have been examined, with the reliability in terms of Cronbach's alpha found to be 0.83 and a correlation with the total weekday physical activity score—measured by accelerometers—of 0.20 (p < 0.01) [47]. In the present study, only 1–1.5% reported "Other means"; this category was included in non-active transport. For the prevalence and trend analyses, AST was both used as a categorical variable based on 4 categories (walking both ways, cycling both ways, active one-way only, non-active transport), and as a categorical variable based on 2 categories (active transport both ways vs. one-way only or non-active transport). The latter categories in both cases were used as a reference in the analysis that follows.

Time to school was assessed with one question "How long does it usually take you to travel to school from your home?" and was used as a proxy for distance to school. Response options were "Less than 5 min", "5–15 min", "15–30 min", 30 min to 1 h" and "More than 1 h". For the analyses, this variable was recoded into three categories (Less than 5 min, 5–15 min, >15 min). Again, the latter category was used as reference. Travel time to school increased between 2006 and 2018 in Czech Republic and Wales, whereas this remained fairly stable in Norway and Scotland (Supplementary Table S1).

2.2.2. Sociodemographic Variables

Gender (boys vs. girls), age groups (11, 13, and 15 year olds), and individual family affluence (FAS—Family Affluence Scale (FAS-II)) were included in the analysis. The latter is a validated HBSC measure of SES [48]. Family affluence is a composite sum score, which resembles a valid measure of household material affluence derived from participants' responses to 4 items describing the material conditions of their household (respondents' own household bedrooms, family holidays, family vehicle ownership, and PC ownership). FAS has changed through time but this version was used in 2006, and was therefore applied in the current study. Responses to the individual items are summed on a 9-point scale with set cut-points for low (0 to 3), medium (4 to 5), and high (6 to 9) affluence. The individual FAS responses were combined and standardised by using ridit transformation to give a linear SES-score (0–1). The regression coefficient of the FAS score can be directly interpreted as the predicted difference in AST between the least deprived individual and the most deprived individual. When using this procedure, ordered categorical variables are converted to cumulative probabilities, and the individuals are thus ranked on this continuum. Ridit transformation has previously been applied in inequality studies using SES scales with ordinal measurements [49–51] and is recommended for comparisons of the effects of FAS [52]. Family affluence increased between 2006 and 2018 in the Czech Republic, Scotland, and Wales, and remained relatively stable in Norway (Supplementary Table S1).

2.3. Data Analysis

All analyses were conducted using Stata version 15 (StataCorp LLC, College Station, Texas, USA). Stata's survey command (svyset) was used to adjust for sampling weight, clustering, and stratification in the sampling design. The alpha level was set to 0.001 given the large sample size and the number of tests. Joint significance of regression terms containing polytomous categorical variables was determined by means of adjusted F-tests. Secular trends were examined both for AST based on 4 categories and for AST based on 2 categories by means of multinomial and logistic regression, respectively. The initial model included age, gender, and country (Section 3.1). In the next step, the country-by-survey year interaction was added (Section 3.2). Pending statistical significance of this interaction term, age- and gender-adjusted results were presented separately for each country. Results were adjusted for age and gender to make sure that changes in AST could not be attributed to changes in age or gender distributions across survey years. Separate analyses were conducted for each survey year, modelled as a categorical variable and as a continuous variable (linear trend). For categorical time, backward difference coding was used to allow for the comparison between consecutive survey years. To determine whether SES and time to school were related to trends in AST, these two variables were added to the model as main effects (Section 3.2). These factors were considered to be potentially explanatory when the OR associated with survey year was reduced by $\geq 10\%$ [53]. For ease of interpretation, the remaining models were only conducted for AST based on 2 categories and with survey year modelled as a categorical variable (Section 3.3). Country differences were explored further by adding the two-way interactions of country by gender, age, SES, and time to school, respectively. Finally, potential country differences over time were explored by testing a model with three-way interactions of country by survey year by, respectively, gender, age, SES, and time taken to travel to school. For statistically significant interaction terms, country differences were examined across survey years.

3. Results

3.1. AST by Country across Surveys

For AST based on four categories, the adjusted F-test for country was $F_{(9, 2258)} = 204.5$, $p < 0.001$, and for AST based on two categories $F_{(3, 2264)} = 136.1$, $p < 0.001$. This indicated significant variation in AST by country for all survey waves combined (Table 1). Walking to school both ways was most common in the Czech Republic (55%) and least common in Wales (30%), whereas cycling to school was limited, with the exception of Norway (22%). One-way AST was relatively uncommon and there was also only modest variation in its prevalence between countries (6–10%). When considering active travel both ways (Table 1) the prevalence in the Czech Republic (57%) and Norway (59.4%) was significantly higher as compared to Scotland (46%) and Wales (31%).

Table 1. Age/gender-adjusted prevalence of active school transport (AST) by country across survey years.

AST Based on 4 cat.	Country	% (99.9% CI)	OR (99.9% CI)
Walking both ways	Czech Republic	54.6 (51.9, 57.3)	**1.53 (1.21, 1.93)**
	Scotland	44.6 (42.5, 46.7)	0.95 (0.76, 1.19)
	Wales	30.1 (26.5, 33.7)	**0.47 (0.36, 0.62)**
	Norway	36.6 (33.0, 40.3)	Ref.
Cycling both ways	Czech Republic	2.4 (1.7, 3.2)	**0.11 (0.07, 0.16)**
	Scotland	1.3 (.08, 1.7)	**0.04 (0.03, 0.06)**
	Wales	0.8 (.04, 1.2)	**0.02 (0.01, 0.03)**
	Norway	22.2 (19.2, 25.2)	Ref.
One-way AST	Czech Republic	8.7 (7.8, 9.6)	**1.53 (1.21, 1.94)**
	Scotland	9.6 (8.7, 10.4)	**1.29 (1.02, 1.62)**
	Wales	8.6 (7.5, 9.8)	0.85 (0.65, 1.12)
	Norway	5.9 (5.0, 6.7)	Ref.
AST based on 2 cat.			
AST both ways	Czech Republic	57.2 (54.5, 59.8)	0.91 (.74, 1.12)
	Scotland	46.0 (43.9, 48.1)	**0.58 (0.48, 0.70)**
	Wales	31.0 (27.3, 34.6)	**0.30 (0.24, 0.39)**
	Norway	59.4 (55.3, 63.6)	Ref.

Ref. active travel 4 cat. = no AST based on multinominal logistic regression, ref. active travel 2 cat. = no AST/one-way AST. Estimates in bold = $p < 0.001$, logistic regression.

3.2. Secular Trends in AST by Country

The country-by-categorical survey year interaction was statistically significant for both AST based on four categories ($F_{(9, 2258)} = 204.5$, $p < 0.001$) and AST based on two categories ($F_{(9, 2258)} = 204.5$, $p < 0.001$), indicating that the effect of survey year varied across countries. Similar results were obtained for treating time as a continuous variable. As shown in Table 2, AST changed significantly over time in Czech Republic, but remained stable in the other three countries. In the Czech Republic, there was a relatively sharp decrease in walking both ways between 2006 and 2010, followed by a stable pattern between 2010 and 2018. A similar, though less pronounced, pattern was found for cycling both ways. A small linear increase over time was observed for one-way AST in the Czech Republic. For AST based on two categories, this translated into a decrease in AST both ways between 2006 and 2010, followed by a stable pattern between 2010 and 2018. Despite the overall decrease in the Czech Republic between 2006 and 2018, the prevalence of AST both ways remained higher when compared to Scotland and Wales (Figure 1).

Adding family affluence and time to school to the basic country-specific model (gender, survey year) did not change the effect of survey year in Norway, Scotland, Wales. In the Czech Republic, the odds ratio representing the change from 2006 in walking both ways (based on four categories) changed from 0.57 to 0.64 after family affluence, 0.59 after adding time to school, and 0.65 after adding both. This equates to an OR-change of, respectively, 16, 5, and 19%. Family affluence school did not change the significant effect of survey year on cycling both did these variables change the linear effect of survey year on one-way AST on two categories, the odds ratio representing a change from 2006 to ways changed from 0.54 to 0.60 after adding family affluence, 0.56 af school, and 0.62 after adding both variables. This equates to OR-chan respectively. Overall, these results indicated that change over time i associated with a change in walking both ways in the Czech Repu that all the mentioned effects of survey year in the Czech Repub significant after adding family affluence and time to school to the

Gender-adjusted prevalence and secular trends in AST by country and survey year*.

		2010 (%)	2014 (%)	2018 (%)	2010 vs. 2006 OR (99.9%CI)	2014 vs. 2010 OR (99.9%CI)	2018 vs. 2014 OR (99.9%CI)	Adj. F-Test (p-Value)	Linear trend OR (99.9%CI)
AST 4 cat.									
	Czech Republic	67.0	54.9	50.0	51.5	**0.57 (0.37, 0.87)**	0.85 (0.58, 1.27)	1.11 (0.81, 1.51)	**<0.001**	**0.96 (0.94, 0.99)**
	Norway	41.9	32.1	37.5	34.1	0.61 (0.35, 1.07)	1.43 (0.83, 2.45)	0.77 (0.43, 1.37)	0.01	0.98 (0.93, 1.02)
	Scotland	45.7	46.0	43.9	42.1	0.99 (0.77, 1.27)	0.92 (0.70, 1.21)	0.90 (0.66, 1.21)	0.08	0.98 (0.96, 1.01)
	Wales	33.5	31.6	29.9	28.8	0.94 (0.56, 1.58)	0.91 (0.54, 1.54)	0.92 (0.56, 1.49)	0.34	0.98 (0.94, 1.02)
	Czech Republic	3.8	1.8	2.3	2.2	**0.33 (0.13, 0.85)**	1.20 (0.43, 3.30)	1.02 (0.40, 2.61)	**<0.001**	0.94 (0.88, 1.02)
	Norway	20.2	22.0	24.1	23.5	0.81 (0.43, 1.51)	1.38 (0.78, 2.43)	0.85 (0.44, 1.65)	0.30	1.00 (0.95, 1.06)
	Scotland	1.0	1.0	2.0	1.1	0.90 (0.40, 2.04)	1.88 (0.81, 4.40)	0.55 (0.22, 1.35)	0.06	1.02 (0.96, 1.08)
	Wales	0.7	0.7	0.5	0.9	0.92 (0.29, 2.93)	0.73 (0.15, 3.48)	1.68 (0.37, 7.55)	0.70	1.02 (0.93, 1.12)
One-way AST	Czech Republic	4.1	7.3	9.5	10.8	1.25 (0.77, 2.06)	1.23 (0.80, 1.88)	1.21 (0.87, 1.68)	**<0.001**	**1.05 (1.02, 1.08)**
	Norway	5.1	6.1	5.8	6.9	0.94 (0.55, 1.62)	1.22 (0.71, 2.08)	1.02 (0.56, 1.85)	0.48	1.01 (0.97, 1.06)
	Scotland	10.0	9.5	9.2	9.6	0.94 (0.69, 1.27)	0.94 (0.68, 1.30)	0.98 (0.70, 1.36)	0.40	0.99 (0.96, 1.01)
	Wales	8.9	10.8	10.4	7.3	1.20 (0.68, 2.13)	0.93 (0.52, 1.65)	0.67 (0.40, 1.10)	0.005	0.97 (0.93, 1.00)
AST based on 2 cat.									
AST both ways	Czech Republic	71.0	56.9	52.6	53.7	**0.54 (0.36, 0.80)**	0.84 (0.59, 1.20)	1.05 (0.79, 1.40)	**<0.001**	**0.95 (0.93, 0.97)**
	Norway	62.7	54.9	62.0	58.4	0.68 (0.42, 1.10)	1.36 (0.87, 2.12)	0.80 (0.48, 1.31)	0.02	0.98 (0.94, 1.03)
	Scotland	46.8	47.2	46.0	43.3	1.01 (0.80, 1.26)	0.95 (0.75, 1.21)	0.88 (0.67, 1.16)	0.11	0.99 (0.97, 1.01)
	Wales	34.3	32.4	30.4	29.8	0.91 (0.57, 1.45)	0.92 (0.57, 1.46)	0.98 (0.63, 1.52)	0.44	0.98 (0.95, 1.02)

* Ref. AST 4 cat. = no AST, ref. AST 2 cat. = no AST/one-way AST. Estimates in bold = $p < 0.001$. The reported results of the adjusted F-tests and linear trends for the 4-category active travel variable are within country and within the relevant outcome category. The joint significance of survey year across outcome categories was only statistically significant for Czech Republic ($p < 0.001$).

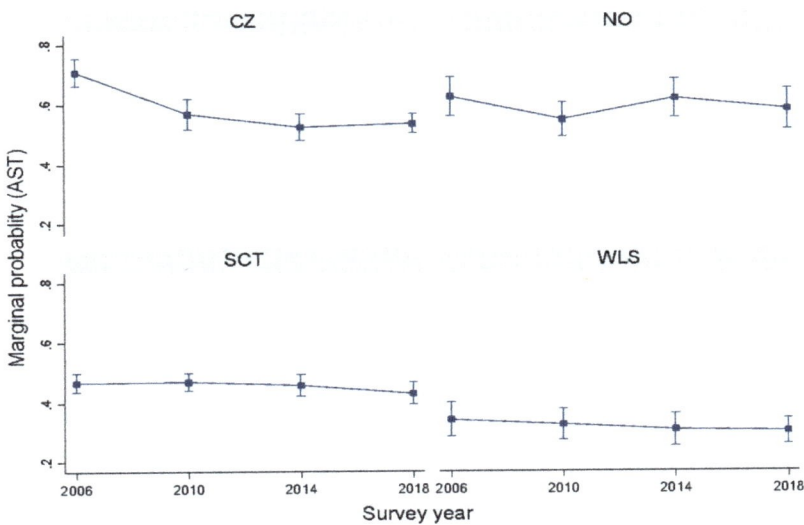

Figure 1. Age and gender adjusted prevalence of AST both ways by country and survey year. (CZ = Czech Republic, NO = Norway, SCT = Scotland, WLS = Wales).

3.3. Country Differences in AST Both Ways by Gender, Age Group, Family Affluence and Time to School

All four two-way interactions of gender, age group, family affluence, and time to school by country were statistically significant ($p < 0.001$), indicating that the effects of these variables varied by country. As shown in both Table 3 and Figure 2, there were significant gender differences in Scotland and Wales, with boys being more likely to exhibit AST both ways as compared to girls in these two countries. There was a particularly strong age group effect in Norway with 11 year olds being much more likely to exhibit AST both ways as compared to 13 and 15 year olds. Family affluence did not impact the probability of AST in Norway, whereas children in the other countries from more affluent families were less likely to have AST both ways as compared to their counterparts from less affluent families. The estimated probability difference of AST between children coming from the least affluent families (0) and children coming from the most affluent families (1) is displayed in Figure 2. Finally, the effect of time to school on AST was much stronger in the Czech Republic when compared with the other three countries. Children from the Czech Republic with a travel time of less than 5 min were more likely to engage in AST (86%), whereas this was much less likely in Scotland (62%) and Wales (50%). This was also true for travel times between 5–15 min, but the country differences were somewhat less pronounced for this category. Across surveys, the prevalence of travel time less than 5 min was 21% for the Czech Republic, 17% for Norway, 22% for Scotland, and 14% for Wales, whereas the prevalence of travel time between 5–15 min was 48% for the Czech Republic, 46% for Norway, 44% for Scotland, and 44% for Wales.

Table 3. Adjusted associations with AST both ways by country *.

Variables	Czech Republic OR (99.9%CI)	Norway OR (99.9%CI)	Scotland OR (99.9%CI)	Wales OR (99.9%CI)	Notable Country Differences
Survey year					
2010 vs. 2006	**0.61 (0.43, 0.89)**	0.67 (0.41, 1.08)	1.11 (0.88, 1.39)	0.96 (0.61, 1.52)	Change in AST in CZ only
2014 vs. 2010	0.99 (0.72, 1.36)	1.35 (0.87, 2.10)	0.96 (0.76, 1.22)	0.99 (0.63, 1.55)	-
2018 vs. 2014	1.01 (.78, 1.31)	0.83 (0.51, 1.34)	0.91 (0.70, 1.19)	1.06 (0.70, 1.60)	-
Female gender	0.97 (0.87, 1.08)	0.93 (0.81, 1.07)	**0.85 (0.76, 0.94)**	**0.79 (0.70, 0.90)**	Gender differences in SCT, WLS only
Age group					
13 year olds	0.97 (0.83, 1.14)	**0.51 (0.37, 0.71)**	**0.80 (0.64, 0.99)**	1.13 (0.97, 1.31)	Age group effect in NO, SCT only
15 year olds	1.18 (1.00, 1.40)	**0.49 (0.36, 0.67)**	0.83 (0.67, 1.03)	1.11 (0.92, 1.35)	Age group effect in NO only
Time to school					
<5 min.	**20.10 (15.81, 25.56)**	**6.88 (5.23, 9.05)**	**3.15 (2.62, 3.79)**	**2.97 (2.20, 4.01)**	Stronger time to school effects in CZ, NO
5–15 min.	**5.58 (4.81, 6.57)**	**2.90 (2.41, 3.50)**	**1.65 (1.43, 1.90)**	**1.36 (1.09, 1.69)**	Stronger time to school effects in CZ, NO
Family affluence	**0.40 (0.32, 0.50)**	0.96 (0.70, 1.31)	**0.46 (0.37, 0.56)**	**0.55 (0.43, 0.70)**	Social gradient absent in NO only

* Estimates by country for model AST = Survey year + gender + Age group + Time to school + Family affluence. Ref. AST 2 cat. = no AST/one-way AST. CZ = Czech Republic, NO = Norway, SCT = Scotland, WLS = Wales. Ref. Age group = 11 year olds, Ref. Time to school = >15 min. Family affluence ridit transformed to a linear score (0–1). Estimates in bold = $p < 0.001$.

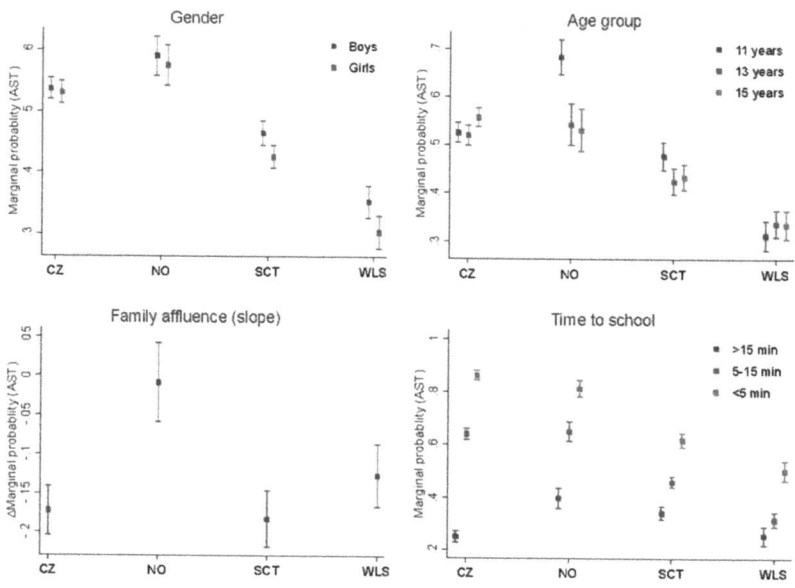

Figure 2. Country differences in AST both ways by gender, age, family affluence, and time to school.

None of the four three-way interactions of country by survey year by, respectively, gender, age, SES, and time to school were statistically significant, indicating that the observed country differences did not change over time.

4. Discussion

The current study provides recent trends in AST and their associations with gender, age, SES, and time to school across four European countries. The findings demonstrate that, apart from the Czech Republic, there were generally stable patterns of partly low levels of AST in the period from 2006 to 2018. However, the prevalence and association with moderating factors varied considerably between countries. For all survey waves combined, walking to school both ways were most common in the Czech Republic (55%), followed by Scotland (45%), Norway (37%), and Wales (30%). Cycling to school was only common in Norway, with the highest prevalence of total AST (59%). One-way AST was relatively uncommon with modest variation between countries. Overall, the results show that active travel both ways was considerably higher in the Czech Republic and Norway when compared to Scotland and Wales. Although, there was a general direction towards a decline across all four countries, this was non-significant. The stable trends in AST observed in the current study contrast with most studies [19–28] but are in line with one study from Australia that assessed trends between 2004–2010 [54] and the findings from 28 studies in Spain between 2010 to 2017 [41]. The findings suggest that a general decline in AST may have levelled out in various regions in Europe.

The prevalence of AST changed significantly over time only in the Czech Republic, with a relatively sharp decrease observed between 2006 and 2010, followed by a stable pattern between 2010 and 2018. This is in line with a previous study [42]. A small linear increase over time was also observed for one-way AST in the Czech Republic. The extent to which the recent initiation of services, such as bike shares, has contributed to this increase is unknown, but a topic worth further investigation. The market demand for micro-mobility is also expected to grow significantly. The availability of these personal vehicles may also influence AST in the future. The negative trend observed in the Czech Republic might be explained by increasing car ownership [55], insufficient cycling infrastructure at a municipal and school level [56], and barriers dealing with safety concerns [57]. The Czech Republic was also the only country where family affluence was associated with change over time in walking both ways. It may, therefore, be the case that the change in family affluence contributed to some of the change in AST, for example, through increased availability of family cars. In all countries, except Norway, children from more affluent families were less likely to engage in AST both ways when compared to their counterparts from less affluent families. This finding is in line with studies from North America and New-Zealand [14,36]. In addition to the possibility of reduced access to a private car in lower-income families, constraints on the time available for single-parents to drive has been identified as a potential reason for family affluence differences [36].

The travel time to school increased between 2006 and 2018 in the Czech Republic and Wales, whereas this remained relatively stable in Norway and Scotland. School distance and time to school have been identified as strong correlates of AST [6,14,29,36,58]. It has been suggested that the development of bigger school units and the closing of neighbourhood schools and school choice policies are contributors to the increased distance and time to school [29,36]. Nevertheless, the literature suggests that many children live within a reasonable walking distance from school [59–61]. In the current study, the prevalence of a travel time less than 15 min was relatively similar across countries. An interesting finding was that the effect of time to school on AST was strongest in the Czech Republic, as Czech children with a travel time of less than 5 min were much more likely to engage in AST, as compared to children in Scotland and Wales. This was also observed for travel times between 5–15 min, but the country differences were less pronounced. Thus, there seems to be potential, especially for countries such as Scotland and Wales, to increase their levels of AST by targeting families who live within a "threshold" distance. This is reported to be less than 1.5–2.0 km for walking and 3.0 km for biking [62–64]. However, environmental factors (e.g., how many busy roads to cross, presence of staff to help crossing roads) could also be influential in short distances. The findings highlight the need for comprehensive local approaches, which should also include some form of risk assessment and environmental modifications.

The relatively high and stable levels of AST observed in Norway may partly be a result of a substantial proportion of schoolchildren cycling to school. Cycling to school allows students to move faster and they can cover greater distances [65]. Unlike studies from many other European countries, schoolchildren from Scotland, Wales and the Czech Republic did not use cycling as a mode of travel. However, the findings are in line with studies from Ireland [66]. Higher rates of cycling versus walking to school among adolescents have been found in other Nordic countries, such as Denmark and Finland [29]. In contrast to Denmark, known for its longstanding cycling traditions, cycling-friendly infrastructure, and flat landscape, the climate, topography, and physical environmental conditions in Norway are diverse. The relatively high prevalence of cycling could be related to social and cultural norms. Nordic countries have a culture where outdoor activities, in general, play an important role in the "way of life" [67] and Norway has a long tradition for outdoor education in primary schools [68]. This could have a positive impact on attitudes towards independent mobility, which has been associated with cycling to school [69]. Another, but perhaps related issue is expectations around school dress codes. In New Zealand, school uniform requirements have been found to influence adolescents' motivation for cycling to school [70]. This could also be the case in Scotland and Wales, where school uniforms can be quite formal, whereas in Norway students do not use school uniforms. In a study from Scotland, wearing helmets were also a barrier for cycling to school, especially among older children [71]. Other essential factors that could explain why school children do not cycle to school, include lack of cycling infrastructure (e.g., dedicated cycle paths), limited facilities at school and children's lack of competence in terms of cycling [66]. The reality is most likely a combination of all the factors noted.

In the current study, an age effect was observed, with lower odds for AST for the 13 and 15 year olds in Norway and the 13 year olds in Scotland. In Wales 11 year olds are already at secondary school which would explain the lack of age effect. In terms of the secular trends in AST, we did not observe any age interactions. The effect of age was considerable in Norway. This is in line with previous studies that have found substantially higher levels of AST among primary as compared to secondary school children [11,47]. Secondary schools are typically bigger school units with increased travel distances for most students [14], which might explain this finding.

Combining the data from all study waves, it appears that gender was a significant factor influencing AST in Wales and Scotland. Gender differences have been confirmed in several previous studies [14,32,36,39,40]. In terms of secular trends in AST, we did not observe any gender interactions, suggesting that the gender differences in Wales and Scotland remained constant throughout the years. Findings from other trend studies have shown comparable results [25,34,41,72]. In two studies from Spain and Brazil, no gender differences were observed [27,43]. However, over time there was a decline for Spanish girls [43], and a decline for boys and an increase for girls among Brazilian youth [27]. Suggested explanations for girls showing lower AST levels relate mainly to safety concerns (e.g., traffic and crime) and independent mobility, with boys more likely to be allowed to explore their neighbourhood environment to a greater extent without supervision [10]. It has also been suggested that the current generation of parents have more concerns about safety that might be responsible for some of the differences in AST levels [31]. Nevertheless, the differential gender differences observed across countries, suggests cultural variations that future studies should seek to understand more in depth.

Strengths and Limitations

The key strengths of this study include the large sample size and ability to compare across four European countries, with representative samples of adolescents, using a shared research protocol. Furthermore, the use of standard methodology for data collection and measurement of AST, with consistent wording throughout the waves, ensured internationally comparable data and robust trend analyses. The analyses were conducted with rigour, by adjusting for sampling weight, clustering and stratification in the sampling design, and the alpha level was set to 0.001, given the large sample size and the number of tests. The possibility of differentiating between cycling and walking in this study was also important, as it gave a more detailed picture of students' travel behaviours to school.

However, there are also limitations. The analysis is based on a repeated cross-sectional design conducted every fourth year. Interpretation of trends should be made carefully because there is no information available between the different survey waves. Data collection was conducted by self-report, and therefore, may be susceptible to recall bias. However, it is a challenge to objectively assess AST because of its versatile nature [73]. The AST measure does not detect day-to-day variations in transport behaviour and the students were categorised based on their main method of travel, which could misrepresent the amount of activity. For example, respondents who used passive transport may have accumulated some amount of physical activity for a segment of the journeys, that could add to their daily physical activity uptake. Furthermore, distance to school was approximated by the included time to school variable, which was a suboptimal solution as time to school partly dependents on transportation mode and could also be influenced by time spent stopping somewhere during the journey and other environmental factors. Nevertheless, a strength of HBSC lies in its breadth, which as a consequence, unfortunately means that not all issues can be explored in great depth.

5. Conclusions

The study found stable patterns of AST in the period from 2006 to 2018, except for a reduction in the Czech Republic from the first to the second wave. These findings could indicate that the previously observed decrease in AST has been flattening off in the countries studied here. Still, the findings suggest that there is a great potential to increase the level of active commuting to school, especially in Scotland and Wales where the levels were low despite government action. This indicates that tackling active travel alone (e.g., with a focus on infrastructure) is not enough and points to the fact that action really does need to be cross-cutting and comprehensive. The variation in the prevalence of AST and the observed associations with gender, age, family affluence and time to school, suggest there are most likely country-specific factors influencing students' choice of travel mode to school.

Supplementary Materials: The following are available online at https://www.mdpi.com/1660-4601/18/4/2118/s1, Table S1: Sample size and descriptive statistics of independent variables.

Author Contributions: Conceptualization, E.H., J.I., C.R., J.B.; methodology, E.H., O.R.F.S., D.S.; software, E.H., O.R.F.S., D.S.; validation, E.H., O.R.F.S., D.S.; formal analysis, O.R.F.S.; investigation, E.H., O.R.F.S., J.B., C.B., J.P., Z.H., D.S., J.B., C.B., J.P., Z.H., D.S.; data curation, D.S., O.R.F.S.; writing—original draft preparation, E.H.; writing—review and editing, J.B., C.B., J.P., Z.H., D.S., F.K.S.M., J.I., C.R.; visualization, O.R.F.S.; supervision, E.H., J.B.; project administration, J.I. All authors have read and agreed to the published version of the manuscript.

Funding: This research is based on data from the HBSC study. In Scotland, the HBSC study is funded by NHS Health Scotland. J.I. is supported by the UK Medical Research Council (MC_UU_12017/14) and Chief Scientist Office (SPHSU14). For further details on HBSC, see http://www.hbsc.org (accessed on 19 February 2021). The HBSC study in Norwegian partly funded by the Norwegian Directorate of Health. The HBSC study in the Czech Republic is supported by the European Regional Development Fund-Project "Effective Use of Social Research Studies for Practice (No. C.02.1.01/0.0/16_025/0007294), by the Technology Agency of the Czech Republic (ÉTA TL01000335) and by the Ministry of Education, Youth and Sports, Inter-Excellence, LTT18020. The HBSC study in Wales is funded by Welsh Government.

Institutional Review Board Statement: All participating countries within the HBSC network adhere to ethical guidelines and principles as described in the HBSC study protocols. The HBSC study is conducted according to the guidelines of the Declaration of Helsinki. Ethical approval for the surveys was obtained at the national level, and adherence to protocol requirements was managed by the HBSC International Data Management Centre in Bergen, Norway (see http://www.hbsc.org/methods/ (accessed on 19 February 2021)).

Informed Consent Statement: Informed consent (explicit or implicit) was given from school administrators and or parents before participation. Participation was voluntary and the children were informed about confidentiality and anonymity. More details on the HBSC study procedures can be found elsewhere [46].

Data Availability Statement: The University of Bergen is the data-bank manager for the HBSC study. Please contact the corresponding author for data requests.

Acknowledgments: HBSC is an international study carried out in collaboration with WHO/EURO. The HBSC International Coordinator was Candace Currie (2006, 2010, 2014 surveys) and Jo Inchley (2018 survey). The Data Bank Manager was Oddrun Samdal. We are grateful to the Principal Investigators in the participating countries. We also wish to thank all the participating students, staff and schools that took part in the study.

Conflicts of Interest: The authors declare no conflict of interest.

References

1. Giles-Corti, B.; Kerr, J.; Pratt, M. Contributing to helping to achieve the UN Sustainable Development Goals: Truly shifting from niche to norm. *Prev. Med.* **2017**, *103S*, S1–S2. [CrossRef]
2. Khreis, H.; Sudmant, A.; Gouldson, A.; Nieuwenhuijsen, M. Transport policy measures for climate change as drivers for health in cities. In *Integrating Human Health into Urban and Transport Planning*; Springer: Cham, Switzerland, 2019; pp. 583–608.
3. World Health Organization. *Physical Activity Strategy for the WHO European Region 2016–2025*; WHO Regional Office for Europe: Copenhagen, Denmark, 2016.
4. Winters, M.; Buehler, R.; Götschi, T. Policies to promote active travel: Evidence from reviews of the literature. *Curr. Env. Health Rep.* **2017**, *4*, 278–285. [CrossRef]
5. Doorley, R.; Pakrashi, V.; Ghosh, B. Quantifying the health impacts of active travel: Assessment of methodologies. *Transp. Rev.* **2015**, *35*, 559–582. [CrossRef]
6. Mehdizadeh, M.; Mamdoohi, A.; Nordfjaern, T. Walking time to school, children's active school travel and their related factors. *J. Transp. Health.* **2017**, *6*, 313–326. [CrossRef]
7. Xia, T.; Zhang, Y.; Crabb, S.; Shah, P. Cobenefits of replacing car trips with alternative transportation: A review of evidence and methodological issues. *J. Env. Public Health* **2013**, *2013*, 797312. [CrossRef] [PubMed]
8. Dinu, M.; Pagliai, G.; Macchi, C.; Sofi, F. Active commuting and multiple health outcomes: A systematic review and meta-analysis. *Sports Med.* **2019**, *49*, 437–452. [CrossRef] [PubMed]
9. Larouche, R.; Saunders, T.J.; Faulkner, G.E.J.; Colley, R.; Tremblay, M. Associations between active school transport and physical activity, body composition, and cardiovascular fitness: A systematic review of 68 studies. *J. Phys. Act. Health.* **2014**, *11*, 206–227. [CrossRef] [PubMed]
10. Schoeppe, S.; Duncan, M.J.; Badland, H.; Oliver, M.; Curtis, C. Associations of children's independent mobility and active travel with physical activity, sedentary behaviour and weight status: A systematic review. *J. Sci. Med. Sport* **2013**, *16*, 312–319. [CrossRef]
11. Østergaard, L.; Kolle, E.; Steene-Johannessen, J.; Anderssen, S.A.; Andersen, L.B. Cross sectional analysis of the association between mode of school transportation and physical fitness in children and adolescents. *Int. J. Behav. Nutr. Phys Act.* **2013**, *10*, 91. [CrossRef]
12. Henriques-Neto, D.; Peralta, M.; Garradas, S.; Pelegrini, A.; Pinto, A.A.; Sánchez-Miguel, P.A.; Marques, A. Active commuting and physical fitness: A systematic review. *Int. J. Env. Res. Public Health* **2020**, *17*, 2721. [CrossRef]
13. Brown, B.; Mackett, R.; Gong, Y.; Kitazawa, K.; Paskins, J. Gender differences in children's pathways to independent mobility. *Child Geogr.* **2008**, *6*, 385–401. [CrossRef]
14. Ikeda, E.; Stewart, T.; Garrett, N.; Egli, V.; Mandic, S.; Hosking, J.; Witten, K.; Hawley, G.; Tautolo, E.S.; Rodda, J. Built environment associates of active school travel in New Zealand children and youth: A systematic meta-analysis using individual participant data. *J. Transp. Health.* **2018**, *9*, 117–131. [CrossRef]
15. Rissotto, A.; Tonucci, F. Freedom of movement and environmental knowledge in elementary school children. *J. Environ. Psychol.* **2002**, *22*, 65–77. [CrossRef]

16. Westman, J.; Johansson, M.; Olsson, L.E.; Mårtensson, F.; Friman, M. Children's affective experience of every-day travel. *J. Transp. Geogr.* **2013**, *29*, 95–102. [CrossRef]
17. Roberts, I. Children and sport. Walking to school has future benefits. *Br. Med. J.* **1996**, *312*, 1229. [CrossRef]
18. Telama, R.; Yang, X.; Leskinen, E.; Kankaanpää, A.; Hirvensalo, M.; Tammelin, T.; Viikari, J.S.; Raitakari, O.T. Tracking of physical activity from early childhood through youth into adulthood. *Med. Sci. Sports Exerc.* **2014**, *46*, 955–962. [CrossRef] [PubMed]
19. Buliung, R.N.; Mitra, R.; Faulkner, G. Active school transportation in the Greater Toronto Area, Canada: An exploration of trends in space and time (1986–2006). *Prev. Med.* **2009**, *48*, 507–512. [CrossRef] [PubMed]
20. Cui, Z.; Bauman, A.; Dibley, M.J. Temporal trends and correlates of passive commuting to and from school in children from 9 provinces in China. *Prev. Med.* **2011**, *52*, 423–427. [CrossRef]
21. Larouche, R. Last Child Walking?—Prevalence and Trends in Active Transportation. In *Children's Active Transportation*; Elsevier: Amsterdam, The Netherlands, 2018; pp. 53–75.
22. Pavelka, J.; Sigmundová, D.; Hamřík, Z.; Kalman, M.; Sigmund, E.; Mathisen, F. Trends in Active Commuting to School among Czech Schoolchildren from 2006 to 2014. *Cent. Eur. J. Public Health* **2017**, *25* (Suppl. 1), S21–S25. [CrossRef] [PubMed]
23. Yang, Y.; Xue, H.; Liu, S.; Wang, Y. Is the decline of active travel to school unavoidable by-products of economic growth and urbanization in developing countries? *Sustain. Cities Soc.* **2019**, *47*, 101446. [CrossRef] [PubMed]
24. Van der Ploeg, H.P.; Merom, D.; Corpuz, G.; Bauman, A.E. Trends in Australian children traveling to school 1971–2003: Burning petrol or carbohydrates? *Prev. Med.* **2008**, *46*, 60–62. [CrossRef]
25. McDonald, N.C.; Brown, A.L.; Marchetti, L.M.; Pedroso, M.S. US school travel, 2009: An assessment of trends. *Am. J. Prev. Med.* **2011**, *41*, 146–151. [CrossRef]
26. Grize, L.; Bringolf-Isler, B.; Martin, E.; Braun-Fahrländer, C. Trend in active transportation to school among Swiss school children and its associated factors: Three cross-sectional surveys 1994, 2000 and 2005. *Int. J. Behav. Nutr. Phys. Act.* **2010**, *7*, 28. [CrossRef] [PubMed]
27. Costa, F.F.; Silva, K.S.; Schmoelz, C.P.; Campos, V.C.; de Assis, M.A.A. Longitudinal and cross-sectional changes in active commuting to school among Brazilian schoolchildren. *Prev. Med.* **2012**, *55*, 212–214. [CrossRef] [PubMed]
28. Trang, N.H.; Hong, T.K.; Dibley, M.J. Active commuting to school among adolescents in Ho Chi Minh City, Vietnam: Change and predictors in a longitudinal study, 2004 to 2009. *Am. J. Prev. Med.* **2012**, *42*, 120–128. [CrossRef]
29. Fyhri, A.; Hjorthol, R.; Mackett, R.L.; Fotel, T.N.; Kyttä, M. Children's active travel and independent mobility in four countries: Development, social contributing trends and measures. *Transp. Policy* **2011**, *18*, 703–710. [CrossRef]
30. Reimers, A.K.; Marzi, I.; Schmidt, S.C.; Niessner, C.; Oriwol, D.; Worth, A.; Woll, A. Trends in active commuting to school from 2003 to 2017 among children and adolescents from Germany: The MoMo Study. *Eur. J. Public Health* **2020**. [CrossRef] [PubMed]
31. Chillón, P.; Evenson, K.R.; Vaughn, A.; Ward, D.S. A systematic review of interventions for promoting active transportation to school. *Int. J. Behav. Nutr. Phys. Act.* **2011**, *8*, 10. [CrossRef] [PubMed]
32. Hollein, T.; Vašíčková, J.; Bucksch, J.; Kalman, M.; Sigmundová, D.; van Dijk, J.P. School physical activity policies and active transport to school among pupils in the Czech Republic. *J. Transp. Health* **2017**, *6*, 306–312. [CrossRef]
33. *Welsh Government An Active Travel Action Plan for Wales*; Welsh Government: Cardiff, UK, 2016.
34. Ikeda, E.; Hinckson, E.; Witten, K.; Smith, M. Associations of children's active school travel with perceptions of the physical environment and characteristics of the social environment: A systematic review. *Health Place* **2018**, *54*, 118–131. [CrossRef]
35. Lu, W.; McKyer, E.L.J.; Lee, C.; Goodson, P.; Ory, M.G.; Wang, S. Perceived barriers to children's active commuting to school: A systematic review of empirical, methodological and theoretical evidence. *Int. J. Behav. Nutr. Phys. Act.* **2014**, *11*, 140. [CrossRef] [PubMed]
36. Rothman, L.; Macpherson, A.K.; Ross, T.; Buliung, R.N. The decline in active school transportation (AST): A systematic review of the factors related to AST and changes in school transport over time in North America. *Prev. Med.* **2018**, *111*, 314–322. [CrossRef]
37. Rahman, M.L.; Pocock, T.; Moore, A.; Mandic, S. Active transport to school and school neighbourhood built environment across urbanisation settings in Otago, New Zealand. *Int. J. Env. Res. Public Health* **2020**, *17*, 9013. [CrossRef]
38. Ham, S.A.; Martin, S.; Kohl, H.W. Changes in the percentage of students who walk or bike to school—United States, 1969 and 2001. *J. Phys. Act. Health.* **2008**, *5*, 205–215. [CrossRef] [PubMed]
39. McMillan, T.E. Urban form and a child's trip to school: The current literature and a framework for future research. *J. Plan. Lit.* **2005**, *19*, 440–456. [CrossRef]
40. Larsen, K.; Buliung, R.N.; Faulkner, G. School travel route measurement and built environment effects in models of children's school travel behavior. *J. Transp. Land Use* **2016**, *9*, 5–23. [CrossRef]
41. Gálvez-Fernández, P.; Herrador-Colmenero, M.; Esteban-Cornejo, I.; Castro-Piñero, J.; Molina-García, J.; Queralt, A.; Aznar, S.; Abarca-Sos, A.; González-Cutre, D.; Vidal-Conti, J. Active commuting to school among 36,781 Spanish children and adolescents: A temporal trend study. *Scand. J. Med. Sci. Sports* **2020**. [CrossRef]
42. Dygrýn, J.; Mitáš, J.; Gába, A.; Rubín, L.; Frömel, K. Changes in active commuting to school in Czech adolescents in different types of built environment across a 10-year period. *Int. J. Env. Res. Public Health* **2015**, *12*, 12988–12998. [CrossRef] [PubMed]
43. Chillón, P.; Martínez-Gómez, D.; Ortega, F.B.; Pérez-López, I.J.; Díaz, L.E.; Veses, A.M.; Veiga, O.L.; Marcos, A.; Delgado-Fernández, M. Six-year trend in active commuting to school in Spanish adolescents. *Int. J. Behav. Med.* **2013**, *20*, 529–537. [CrossRef]

44. Pang, B.; Kubacki, K.; Rundle-Thiele, S. Promoting active travel to school: A systematic review (2010–2016). *BMC Public Health* **2017**, *17*, 638. [CrossRef]
45. Villa-González, E.; Barranco-Ruiz, Y.; Evenson, K.R.; Chillón, P. Systematic review of interventions for promoting active school transport. *Prev. Med.* **2018**, *111*, 115–134. [CrossRef]
46. Inchley, J.; Currie, D.; Cosma, A.; Samdal, O. *Health Behaviour in School-Aged Children (HBSC) Study Protocol: Background, Methodology and Mandatory Items for the 2017/18 Survey*; CAHRU: St Andrews, UK, 2018.
47. Ommundsen, Y.; Klasson-Heggebø, L.; Anderssen, S.A. Psycho-social and environmental correlates of location-specific physical activity among 9-and 15-year-old Norwegian boys and girls: The European Youth Heart Study. *Int. J. Behav. Nutr. Phys. Act.* **2006**, *3*, 32. [CrossRef] [PubMed]
48. Boyce, W.; Torsheim, T.; Currie, C.; Zambon, A. The family affluence scale as a measure of national wealth: Validation of an adolescent self-report measure. *Soc. Indic. Res.* **2006**, *78*, 473–487. [CrossRef]
49. Leversen, I.; Torsheim, T.; Samdal, O. Gendered leisure activity behavior among Norwegian adolescents across different socio-economic status groups. *Int. J. Child Youth Fam. Stud.* **2012**, *3*, 355–375. [CrossRef]
50. Levin, K.A.; Torsheim, T.; Vollebergh, W.; Richter, M.; Davies, C.A.; Schnohr, C.W.; Due, P.; Currie, C. National income and income inequality, family affluence and life satisfaction among 13 year old boys and girls: A multilevel study in 35 countries. *Soc. Indic. Res.* **2011**, *104*, 179–194. [CrossRef]
51. Mackenbach, J.P.; Kunst, A.E. Measuring the magnitude of socio-economic inequalities in health: An overview of available measures illustrated with two examples from Europe. *Soc. Sci. Med.* **1997**, *44*, 757–771. [CrossRef]
52. Schnohr, C.W.; Kreiner, S.; Due, E.; Currie, C.; Boyce, W.; Diderichsen, F. Differential item functioning of a family affluence scale: Validation study on data from HBSC 2001/02. *Soc. Indic. Res.* **2008**, *89*, 79–95. [CrossRef]
53. Jeuring, H.W.; Comijs, H.C.; Deeg, D.J.; Stek, M.L.; Huisman, M.; Beekman, A.T. Secular trends in the prevalence of major and subthreshold depression among 55–64-year olds over 20 years. *Psychol. Med.* **2018**, *48*, 1824–1834. [CrossRef]
54. Meron, D.; Rissel, C.; Reinten-Reynolds, T.; Hardy, L.L. Changes in active travel of school children from 2004 to 2010 in New South Wales, Australia. *Prev. Med.* **2011**, *53*, 408–410. [CrossRef] [PubMed]
55. Kastlova, O.; Houšť, R. *Transport Yearbook Czech Republic 2018*; Ministry of Transport of Czech Republic: Prague, Czech Republic, 2018.
56. Ministry of Transport of the Czech Republic. *Czech National Cycling Development Strategy 2013—2020*; Ministry of Transport of the Czech Republic: Praha, Czech Republic, 2013.
57. Pavelka, J.; Sigmundová, D.; Hamřík, Z.; Kalman, M. Active transport among Czech school-aged children. *Acta Gymnica* **2012**, *42*, 17–26. [CrossRef]
58. Wong, B.Y.-M.; Faulkner, G.; Buliung, R. GIS measured environmental correlates of active school transport: A systematic review of 14 studies. *Int. J. Behav. Nutr. Phys. Act.* **2011**, *8*, 39. [CrossRef] [PubMed]
59. Nelson, N.M.; Foley, E.; O'gorman, D.J.; Moyna, N.M.; Woods, C.B. Active commuting to school: How far is too far? *Int. J. Behav. Nutr. Phys. Act.* **2008**, *5*, 1. [CrossRef]
60. .Sleap, M.; Warburton, P. Are primary school children gaining heart health benefits from their journeys to school? *Child Care Health Dev.* **1993**, *19*, 99–108. [CrossRef] [PubMed]
61. Zaccari, V.; Dirkis, H. Walking to school in inner Sydney. *Health Promot. J. Austr.* **2003**, *14*, 137–140. [CrossRef]
62. D'Haese, S.; De Meester, F.; De Bourdeaudhuij, I.; Deforche, B.; Cardon, G. Criterion distances and environmental correlates of active commuting to school in children. *Int. J. Behav. Nutr. Phys. Act.* **2011**, *8*, 88. [CrossRef]
63. McDonald, N.C. Travel and the social environment: Evidence from Alameda County, California. *Transp. Res. D* **2007**, *12*, 53–63. [CrossRef]
64. Campos-Sánchez, F.S.; Abarca-Álvarez, F.J.; Molina-García, J.; Chillón, P. A Gis-based method for analysing the association between school-built environment and home-school route measures with active commuting to school in urban children and adolescents. *Int. J. Env. Res. Public Health* **2020**, *17*, 2295. [CrossRef]
65. Krizek, K.; Forsyth, A.; Baum, L. *Walking and Cycling International Literature Review*. Victoria Department of Transport, Melbourne, Australia. 2009. Available online: https://www.pedbikeinfo.org/cms/downloads/Krizek%20Walking%20and%20Cycling%20Literature%20Review%202009-1.pdf (accessed on 18 February 2021).
66. Costa, J.; Adamakis, M.; O'Brien, W.; Martins, J. A Scoping Review of Children and Adolescents' Active Travel in Ireland. *Int. J. Env. Res. Public Health* **2020**, *17*, 2016. [CrossRef]
67. Bergsgard, N.A.; Bratland-Sanda, S.; Giulianotti, R.; Tangen, J.O. Sport, outdoor life and the Nordic world: An introduction. *Sport Soc.* **2019**, *22*, 515–524. [CrossRef]
68. Skaugen, R.; Fiskum, T.A. How schools with good academic results justify their use of outdoor education. *Int. Educ. Res.* **2015**, *3*, 16–31. [CrossRef]
69. Ducheyne, F.; De Bourdeaudhuij, I.; Spittaels, H.; Cardon, G. Individual, social and physical environmental correlates of 'never'and 'always' cycling to school among 10 to 12 year old children living within a 3.0 km distance from school. *Int. J. Behav. Nutr. Phys. Act.* **2012**, *9*, 142. [CrossRef]
70. Mandic, S.; Hopkins, D.; Bengoechea, E.G.; Flaherty, C.; Williams, J.; Sloane, L.; Moore, A.; Spence, J.C. Adolescents' perceptions of cycling versus walking to school: Understanding the New Zealand context. *J. Transp. Health* **2017**, *4*, 294–304. [CrossRef]

71. Kirby, J.; Inchley, J. Active travel to school: Views of 10-13 year old schoolchildren in Scotland. *Health Educ.* **2009**, *109*, 169–183. [CrossRef]
72. Ferreira, R.W.; Varela, A.R.; Monteiro, L.Z.; Häfele, C.A.; Santos, S.J.D.; Wendt, A.; Silva, I.C.M. Sociodemographic inequalities in leisure-time physical activity and active commuting to school in Brazilian adolescents: National School Health Survey (PeNSE 2009, 2012, and 2015). *Cad. Saude Publica* **2018**, *34*, e00037917. [PubMed]
73. Larouche, R.; Eryuzlu, S.; Livock, H.; Leduc, G.; Faulkner, G.; Trudeau, F.; Tremblay, M.S. Test-Retest reliability and convergent validity of measures of children's travel behaviours and independent mobility. *J. Transp. Health* **2017**, *6*, 105–118. [CrossRef]

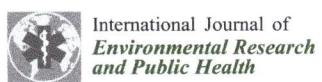

Article
Health Impacts of Urban Bicycling in Mexico

David Rojas-Rueda

Department of Environmental and Radiological Health Sciences, Colorado State University, Fort Collins, CO 80523, USA; David.Rojas@colostate.edu; Tel.: +1-(970)-491-7038; Fax: +1-(970)-491-2940

Abstract: Background: Bicycling has been associated with health benefits. Local and national authorities have been promoting bicycling as a tool to improve public health and the environment. Mexico is one of the largest Latin American countries, with high levels of sedentarism and non-communicable diseases. No previous studies have estimated the health impacts of Mexico's national bicycling scenarios. **Aim:** Quantify the health impacts of Mexico urban bicycling scenarios. **Methodology:** Quantitative Health Impact Assessment, estimating health risks and benefits of bicycling scenarios in 51,718,756 adult urban inhabitants in Mexico (between 20 and 64 years old). Five bike scenarios were created based on current bike trends in Mexico. The number of premature deaths (increased or reduced) was estimated in relation to physical activity, road traffic fatalities, and air pollution. Input data were collected from national publicly available data sources from transport, environment, health and population reports, and surveys, in addition to scientific literature. **Results:** We estimated that nine premature deaths are prevented each year among urban populations in Mexico on the current car-bike substitution and trip levels (1% of bike trips), with an annual health economic benefit of US $1,897,920. If Mexico achieves similar trip levels to those reported in The Netherlands (27% of bike trips), 217 premature deaths could be saved annually, with an economic impact of US $45,760,960. In all bicycling scenarios assessed in Mexico, physical activity's health benefits outweighed the health risks related to traffic fatalities and air pollution exposure. **Conclusion:** The study found that bicycling promotion in Mexico would provide important health benefits. The benefits of physical activity outweigh the risk from traffic fatalities and air pollution exposure in bicyclists. At the national level, Mexico could consider using sustainable transport policies as a tool to promote public health. Specifically, the support of active transportation through bicycling and urban design improvements could encourage physical activity and its health co-benefits.

Keywords: bicycling; transport; Mexico; health impact assessment; environmental health

Citation: Rojas-Rueda, D. Health Impacts of Urban Bicycling in Mexico. *IJERPH* **2021**, *18*, 2300. https://doi.org/10.3390/ijerph18052300

Academic Editors: Adilson Marques and Paul B. Tchounwou

Received: 1 January 2021
Accepted: 23 February 2021
Published: 26 February 2021

Publisher's Note: MDPI stays neutral with regard to jurisdictional claims in published maps and institutional affiliations.

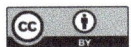

Copyright: © 2021 by the author. Licensee MDPI, Basel, Switzerland. This article is an open access article distributed under the terms and conditions of the Creative Commons Attribution (CC BY) license (https:// creativecommons.org/licenses/by/ 4.0/).

1. Introduction

The United Nations has reported that more than 50% of the global population lived in urban settings in 2018, and the urbanization trend is expected to increase in the coming years [1]. Urban and transport planning has been suggested as a critical health determinant, impacting physical activity, air and noise quality, traffic safety, blue and green spaces, among others [2,3]. Specifically, bicycling has been suggested as a tool to promote physical activity [4–6].

Sedentarism is one of the leading risk factors for mortality worldwide [7]. The global prevalence of insufficient physical activity in 2016 was 23%, and the Latin American region had the highest prevalence of insufficient physical activity (39%) [8]. Mexico is the second most populated country in the Latin American region, with 127 million inhabitants [9], with more than 80% of its population living in urban areas [1]. Mexico has reported 29% of the population has insufficient physical activity [8].

Active transport policies have been promoted extensively in Latin America, being the open street programs (where main streets in cities are closed for walking and cycling), one of the most known active transport policy originated in Latin America [10–12]. Although bicycling has played an essential role in personal mobility around the world, current trends show that motorized traffic is gaining more relevance [13]. Compared to other modes of transportation, bicycles offer a convenient and affordable transport option that could capture a higher proportion of urban transport passengers than is currently the case [13].

Previous studies have estimated the health impacts of local bicycling transport scenarios, but most of them have been focused on developed countries [14–16]. To our knowledge, no study has assessed the health impact of bicycling scenarios in Mexico. This study aims to estimate the health impacts, risks, and benefits of Mexico bicycling scenarios at the national level.

2. Methodology

2.1. Study Design and Data Collection

This study follows a quantitative health impact assessment (HIA) approach, assessing bicycling scenarios in the urban population in Mexico. Transport data were collected from the "Global High Shift Cycling" study [13]. The "Global High Shift Cycling" study provides bicycling data at a national level, describing transport patterns such as trips per person per day, trip length, kilometers traveled by a person, and mode of transport (Table 1). Methods and descriptions of the "Global High Shift Cycling" study have been reported elsewhere [13]. National population data were obtained from the United Nations population forecast [1]. Mortality rates by age and country were collected from the year 2017, which was reported by the Global Burden of Disease (GBD) project [17]. Air pollution data of particulate matter less than 2.5 micrometers of diameter (PM2.5) annual average national concentration was collected from the World Health Organization (WHO) Global Ambient Air Quality Database [18]. National annual traffic fatalities by mode of transport were collected from the Road Safety Annual Reports [19] and the global observatory data from the World Health Organization from years 2009 to 2018 [20]. National physical activity data in metabolic equivalent of task (MET) were collected from scientific publications [21,22]. Dose–response functions used in this quantitative Health Impact Assessment (HIA) for physical activity and air pollution on all-cause mortality were collected from the published meta-analysis [23,24].

Table 1. Input data used in the analysis.

Basal Level of Physical Activity (METs)						
Group 1		Group 2		Group 3		
%	METs	%	METs	%	METs	
19.4	8.95	28.8	26.85	51.8	35.8	

Urban population (20 to 64 years old, in 2010)	Mortality rate (per 100,000 people, 2017)	Air pollution (PM2.5 annual concentration µg/m3)	Car Speed (km/h)	Bike Speed (km/h)	Average trips per person per day (trips/day)	Average trip length by mode of transport (km/trip)
51,718,756	369.36	23.38	30	11.6	3.75	2

Traffic fatalities by car per year	Traffic fatalities per billion kilometers traveled by car			Traffic fatalities by bike per year	Traffic fatalities per billion kilometers traveled by bike		
	Mean	Lower uncertainty interval	Upper uncertainty interval		Mean	Lower uncertainty interval	Upper uncertainty interval
4704	19.77	9.15	63.09	301	41.21	22.6	133.29

MET: Metabolic Equivalent of Task; PM2.5: Particulate Matter with a dimeter <2.5 µm.

2.2. Scenarios

Five scenarios were included in this study (Figure 1): (a) current bike levels in Mexico (based on the bike trips reported at the national level for adults in urban population, 1.07%) [13]; (b) double the national bike-share (assuming as transport goal doubling the current levels of bike trips, 2.13%); (c) arriving at bike levels reported in Brazil (Brazil was the Latin America country with the largest bike mode share reported, 3%) [13]; (d) achieving the Danish bike levels (Denmark is reference country for bicycling, 16%) [25]; and (e) achieving the Dutch bike levels (The Netherlands is the country with the largest bike share in the world, 27%) [26]. All the scenarios assumed an 8% car-bike substitution based on the average reported substitution among 26 cities worldwide [14,27–30]. All scenarios assumed a conservative average bike trip distance in Mexico of 2 km.

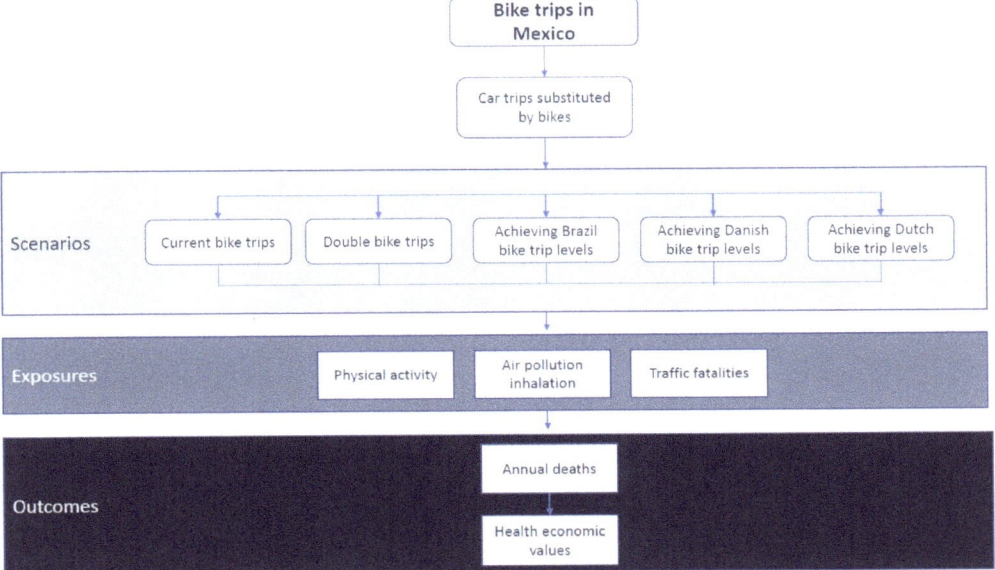

Figure 1. Conceptual framework of the study.

2.3. Quantitative Model

A quantitative health impact assessment approach was followed to estimate the number of annual premature deaths related to each scenario and health determinant (Figure 1). All-cause mortality was estimated considering three different health determinants (physical activity, road traffic fatalities, and air pollution (PM2.5)). The "TAPAS (transportation, air pollution, and physical activities) tool" developed and used in previous quantitative HIA was used to estimate the health impacts in this study [6,14]. A detailed description of the TAPAS tool methods has been reported in the supplemental material and elsewhere [6,14,31,32]. TAPAS tool is a quantitative HIA run on Microsoft Excel for Office 365, version 2008 (Microsoft, Redmond, USA, 2020). The dose–response functions used in the TAPAS tool, between physical activity, PM2.5, and all-cause mortality, were selected from meta-analyses of cohort studies from adult populations. The risk estimated from traffic fatalities by kilometer traveled was obtained from national transport and health data. Levels of each determinant were estimated for each country and scenario. An all-cause mortality relative risk (RR) was estimated for each health determinant and scenario and transformed into a population attributable fraction (PAF). Using the Mexico mortality rate for adults (20–64 years old) and the national urban adult population (20–64 years old) in each scenario, the number of expected premature deaths was estimated for each scenario. Finally, the PAF from each scenario was multiplied with the corresponding expected number of premature deaths in the population to obtain the number of attributable premature deaths. For the economic assessment, the value of statistical life was used to estimate the economic impacts of preventing deaths in each scenario, using the value of statistical life reported for Mexico (US $210,880) [33].

2.3.1. Physical Activity

The physical activity level was estimated based on the trip duration, trip frequency, and physical activity intensity, using the metabolic equivalent of task (MET) (Table 1). The physical activity was defined as 6.8 METs for bikes and 2 METs for car travelers. The relative risk of all-cause mortality was based on the dose–response function (DRF) provided by a meta-analysis of cohort studies (RR = 0.81 (0.76–0.84) for each increment of 8.6 METs, with a power transformation of 0.25)) [24], assuming a non-linear DRF. The physical activity assessment considers the basal levels of physical activity in the Mexican population [21,22] to estimate the relative risk for each scenario before being translated into a population attributable fraction and then to the estimated attributable premature deaths (see Supplemental Material Figures S1 and S2).

2.3.2. Air Pollution

The air pollution assessment focused only on the exposure to particulate matter with a diameter < 2.5 µm (PM2.5), which has shown a strong association with all-cause mortality [34–36]. We obtained the annual average PM2.5 concentrations in Mexico, using the World Health Organization database of air quality [18] (Table 1). We estimated the concentration of PM2.5 in each microenvironment (bike and car), using background/car or bike ratios provided by a previous meta-analysis [37], following a similar approach as reported in previous studies [14,16,31] (see Supplemental Material Figure S3 and Tables S1–S3). The inhaled dose was estimated using the minute ventilation according to the intensity of physical activity (in METs) in each mode of transport (bike and car), PM2.5 concentration in the mode of transport, and trip duration [14,16,31] (see Supplemental Material Tables S2 and S3). The DRF for PM2.5 and all-cause mortality from a meta-analysis were used (RR = 1.06 (1.04, 1.08)) for each increment of 10 µg/m3 of PM2.5) [23]. Finally, using the comparative risk assessment approach, we estimated the relative risk, population attributable fraction, and the expected number of premature deaths for each scenario, as reported before (see Supplemental Material Figure S3).

2.3.3. Road Traffic Fatalities

The road traffic fatalities in Mexico were obtained from the annual traffic fatalities reported at the national level through transport mode from years 2009 to 2018 (Table 1). For each scenario, we estimated the number of kilometers traveled by car and bike. The expected traffic fatalities by mode of transport were estimated using the traffic fatalities per billion kilometers traveled and the distance traveled in each mode of transport [31,34]. Then a relative risk of traffic fatalities for cyclists compared with car drivers was estimated. The relative risk was translated to an attributable fraction and a final number of prevented premature deaths in each scenario (see Supplemental Material Table S1 and Figure S4).

3. Results

The national bike share in Mexico was 1.07% of all trips. We estimated an average of 2,068,750 daily bike trips among adults in urban settings in Mexico (Table 1). The number of bike trips per day (<2 km) was estimated to substitute car trips in Mexico where 165,500. In all the scenarios, the health benefits (in preventable deaths) of physical activity related to bicycling outweighed the health risks associated with traffic fatalities and air pollution inhalation (Table 2).

Table 2. Results of current and hypothetical bicycling scenarios in Mexico.

Variable	Current Situation	Double Bike Share	Achieving Brazil Levels	Achieving Danish Levels	Achieving Dutch Levels
Bike modal share (%)	1.07	2.13	3	16	27
Total bike trips Mexico (trips/day)	2,068,750	4,137,501	5,818,515	31,032,081	52,366,637
Expected bike trips coming from cars in Mexico (trips/day)	165,500	331,000	465,481	2,482,567	4,189,331
Annual prevented deaths (deaths/year)	9	17	24	129	217
Low uncertanty interval	6	11	16	84	142
Upper uncertainty interval	25	49	69	370	625
Annual economic benefit on mortality (US $/year)	1,897,920	3,584,960	5,061,120	27,203,520	45,760,960

3.1. Impacts of Current Bicycling Levels in Mexico

It was estimated that the current levels of bike trips in Mexico (that are expected to substitute car trips, 165,500 trips per day) resulted in 9 (95% UI: 6–25) premature deaths avoided each year among the urban adult population. In terms of economic values, it was estimated that the current bike trips could result in US $1,897,920 annual health economic benefits related to mortality (Table 2). In terms of risks and benefits, traffic fatalities were estimated to increase 2 annual deaths and air pollution exposure 1 annual death. Physical activity resulted in the prevention of 12 annual deaths (Figure 2 and Supplemental Material Table S4)

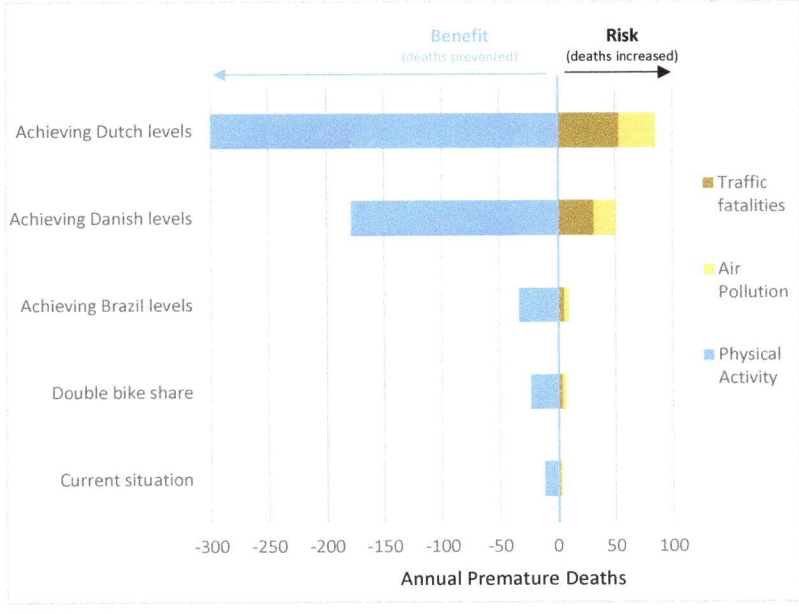

Figure 2. Risks and benefits of bicycling scenarios in Mexico, in annual premature deaths by scenario and risk factor.

3.2. Impacts of Future Bicycling Scenarios in Mexico

If Mexico doubles the current levels of bike trips to 2.13% (assuming similar trips substitution from cart to bike, that current levels), the annual premature deaths prevented could arrive at 17 (95% UI: 11–49), with an economical translation of US $3,584,960. If Mexico achieves the bike trip levels reported in Brazil (3%), the annual benefits could arrive at 24 (95% UI: 16–69), with an economic impact of US $5,061,120. If Mexico arrives at bike trip levels reported in Denmark (16% of bike trips), the health impacts will be translated into 129 (95% UI: 84–370) annual prevented deaths and US $27,203,520. Finally, suppose Mexico achieves bike trip levels similar to those reported by The Netherlands. In that case, the health impacts will be an annual reduction of 217 (95% UI: 142–625) prevented deaths, with an annual health economic benefit of US $45,760,960.

4. Discussion

This study found that bikes in Mexico have the potential to prevent up to 217 annual premature deaths if bike trip levels, similar to those reported in the Netherlands, are achieved with an annual economic benefit of more than 45 million US dollars (Table 1). In the current situation, bike trip levels in Mexico are expected to prevent 9 premature deaths each year (Table 1). In the five scenarios assessed, the health benefits (due to physical activity) outweighed the health risks (air pollution inhalation and traffic incidents) (Figure 2).

This is the first study assessing the health impacts of national bicycling scenarios in Mexico. This study included the 51,718,756 adult urban inhabitants in Mexico. This study includes five different bicycling scenarios comparing the current bike levels in Mexico with reference counties in Latin America (Brazil) and worldwide (Denmark and the Netherlands, the global reference countries for bicycling trends). This study provides a conservative estimation of the bicycle health impacts in Mexico. The analysis only includes a small portion of bike trips (those assumed to came from cars (8% of all bike trips)), assuming short trip distances 2 km, including only adult population (20–64 years old) and urban settings. The overall health impacts of bicycling in Mexico are expected to be larger if all bicycle trips and populations are counted.

These results are in accordance with previous quantitative health impact assessment studies on bicycling scenarios using similar exposures (physical activity, air pollution, and traffic fatalities) [14,31,38–40]. A previous study in seven European cities found that achieving 10% of bike trips will prevent between 0 to 31 deaths in Antwerp and Vienna [38]. In this study was assumed that 28% of bicycling increments came from cars [38]. Another study on the health impacts of bike-sharing systems in Barcelona, Spain, was found that if 90% of the bike-sharing trips came from cars (around 38,000 trips per day), 12 deaths could be avoided each year [31]. Another study with more ambitious scenarios from six European cities estimated the health impacts of bicycling scenarios in Paris, Prague, Warsaw, Basel, and Barcelona [2]. In this study, the aim was to assess "what if" those cities achieve the bike share from Copenhagen (35%) [2]. In this case, the study estimated among 5 to 113 premature deaths prevented each year between the six European cities [2]. Unlike previous studies that have been focused on single cities [2,6,14,31], our study focused on the national urban populations, providing a broader perspective of policy scenarios in Lat America. Like previous studies, this analysis focused on car trip substitution, considering that sifting car trips to active transportation will have larger health benefits and important climate co-benefits [2].

This study found that the current bicycling levels in Mexico will benefit public health at a national scale, preventing nine premature deaths annually among adult urban populations (that are expected to shift from car to bike). Those results were also translated into economic impacts related to mortality, using the value of statistical life, a standard metric used by transport planners and engineers to measure traffic safety impacts. We estimated that Mexico's current car-bike substitution levels have an economic benefit of up to 1.8 million US dollars annually. This study also included different hypothetical policy scenarios related to bike share. We selected four extra bike scenarios to compare "what if" Mexico increases their bike levels to double the current bike share (2.13%); or to those reported by Brazil (3%) that was the Latin American country with the highest bicycling levels; or to those reported in Denmark (16%) or the Netherlands (27%), the reference countries for bicycling around the globe. In those scenarios, the health benefits ranged between 17 to 217 annual premature deaths that could be prevented each year, with an economic benefit between 3.5 to 45 million US dollars annually (Table 1). These results highlight the importance of active transportation policies in Mexico and the potential of transport policies to support public health.

Among the exposures included in this quantitative health impact assessment, physical activity produced the most considerable health impacts (Figure 2). Physical activity is well known as a health-protective factor for multiple diseases and causes of death, such as cardiovascular, metabolic, and mental diseases, among others [16]. Our analyses focused on all-cause mortality as a health outcome because it has been proposed as the best indicator of health impacts on active transport assessments compared to morbidity [6,16]. This analysis utilized the "TAPAS tool," a quantitative health impact assessment tool for bicycling, walking, and public transport, reported in previous transport health impact assessments [2,6,14,31]. The "TAPAS tool" for bicycling estimated the health impacts of physical activity using a non-linear dose–response function (DRF) from a meta-analysis of cohort studies [24], and it was calibrated with the corresponded physical activity levels reported by the adult population in Mexico and applied to the exposure levels by each scenario. The non-linear function considers that those who already were physically active would gain fewer health benefits than those who are more sedentary. This non-linear approach results in a conservative result estimating fewer health benefits than using a linear DRF [2].

In this study, air pollution analysis only considers the exposure to PM2.5 inhalation during the trip. Although air quality improvements can be expected from changes in modal share, these health-related impacts were not in the scope of this study, and the study only focused on the PM2.5 exposure of bicyclists during the trip. PM2.5 was selected because it was expected to produce the largest health burden compared to other air pollutants such as NO2 or black carbon [6].

Traffic safety analysis was based on traffic fatalities. This study quantified fatal traffic incidents per billion kilometers traveled, using the reported national road safety estimates provided by the World Health Organization (WHO) [20]. This study only considered the traffic fatality risk by mode of transport (bike vs. car). It did not assess the impacts of other traffic risk factors such as the type of route or traveler demographics due to the lack of data available in these aspects.

Our study was limited by data availability and the necessity to make assumptions to model likely scenarios. In terms of the scenarios modeled, we select national bicycling goals similar to those that already exist in other nations in Latin America and globally. However, one limitation is the transferability of the policy scenarios to the Mexican context. In Denmark and the Netherlands, geographical and social characteristics differ from the Mexican context (i.e., population density, transport infrastructure, or land use and cartography). Another limitation was the lack of specific modal shift (car to bike) data from Mexico. Thus, the data available from 26 cities from China, Europe, and the US was summarized to estimate the average percentage of bike trips that can shift from car trips [14,27,29,30]. Our estimates' uncertainty was also assessed, providing uncertainty intervals composed of the input data's variability (maximum and minimum) and the confidence intervals from the DRF from air pollution and physical activity. Another limitation in this study was the need to assume an average trip distance in Mexico. In this study, we selected 2 km as a conservative scenario. But a sensitivity analysis was conducted to estimate the health impacts in the five scenarios if a similar bike trip length (5 km) was used as reported in a previous study in Europe [38]. In this sensitivity analysis, we found that the health benefits of urban bike trips in Mexico could be estimated between

15 to 384 preventable annual deaths among the five scenarios (see Supplemental Material Tables S5 and S6).

Furthermore, if national and local authorities improve traffic safety and air quality, in addition, to increase bike levels, more health benefits could be expected in Mexico. In all our scenarios, we assume only an 8% of car–bike trip substitution. This is of particular relevance because if authorities achieve attracting more car drivers and passengers to bicycles, the health benefits could increase largely in addition to the overall levels of bike trips. This study only considers a population between 20 and 64 years old. If policymakers and transport planners achieve the goal of attracting younger and older age groups to bicycles, the health benefits from bicycling in Mexico could be more extensive. As in many other countries, the aging process is also affecting the Mexican population [1]. Healthy aging starts with integrating a healthy lifestyle since the early stages of life, and bicycling could be used as a tool to promote healthy aging. Some general recommendations for policymakers and stakeholders to promote bicycling in Mexico are (a) the support of active transport policies, specifically on interventions to promote bicycling and reduce car driving; (b) support traffic safety and air quality improvements in urban settings in Mexico; and (c) improve data collection and quality improvement in terms of physical activity, traffic safety, air quality, and transport characteristics. For health practitioners, this study can help to dimension the relevance of transport policies to improve public health. Researchers should support local and national data collection on transport and health with a vision of harmonization and comparability. A summary of the policies needed to increase bicycling in Mexico is listed in Table 3.

Table 3. Policy recommendations to support bicycling in Mexico.

Bicycling
• Rapidly implement bicycling infrastructure on a large scale
• Implement bike share programs in medium and large-size cities, prioritizing connections to public transport
• Prioritize bicycling infrastructure design based on safety, accessibility, connectivity, and aesthetics
• Implement and enforce laws and regulations to prioritize bicycling safety
• Support bicycling through fiscal and economic incentives and information campaigns
• Support open streets in large and medium-sized cities

Motorize transport
• Eliminate policies that subsidize additional motor vehicle use, such as minimum parking requirements, free on-street parking, and fuel subsidies
• Implement motorize transport policies that consider their negative externalities, such as congestion pricing or vehicle kilometers traveled fees
• Invest fuel taxes, driving fees, and other transport-system revenues in sustainable transport.
• Reduce speed limits to support traffic safety

Table 3. *Cont.*

Urban planning

- Coordinate metropolitan transport and land-use plans, aiming that all new investments result in more bicycling and fewer trips by motorized vehicles
- Support transit-oriented and mixed-use developments
- Implement car-free streets and neighborhoods
- Support a network of green and blue spaces that help to connect bicycling infrastructure
- Prioritize a universal design aiming for more inclusive and equitable use of public space and transport networks

Environment

- Develop laws and regulations that protect the population from harmful air pollution and traffic noise levels
- Increase awareness of air pollution sources, especially from motorized vehicles in urban settings
- Implement stricter air pollution and noise emission limits from motorized vehicles
- Reduce bicyclist air pollution exposure by prioritizing bike infrastructure away from emission sources, such as motorized vehicles

Public health

- Consider bicycling as a health promotion and prevention tool
- Support active transport policies to improve traffic safety
- Support active transport policies to improve air quality and reduce noise pollution
- Increase collaboration with urban and transport planners
- Design public health campaigns to support a healthy lifestyle through active transportation

5. Conclusions

The study found that bicycling promotion in Mexico would provide important health benefits. At the national level, Mexico could consider using sustainable transport policies as a tool to promote public health. Specifically, the support of active transportation through bicycling interventions could promote physical activity, reduce mortality and increase health economic benefits. The attraction of bike users could be supported by bike investments and interventions (e.g., bike lanes, bike parking, and bike-sharing systems), combined with interventions to reduce car use (e.g., parking pricing and reduction, and congestion pricing). To meet ambitious bicycling scenarios in Mexico, strong transport, urban planning, energy, environmental, and health policies should be adopted at national and local levels.

Supplementary Materials: The following are available online at https://www.mdpi.com/1660-4601/18/5/2300/s1, Figure S1. Physical activity model; Figure S2. Dose response functions (DRF) for physical activity and all cause mortality; Figure S3 Air pollution model; Figure S4. Traffic fatality model; Table S1. Relative risk formulas for each model; Table S2. General formulas; Table S3. Air pollution variables; Table S4. Results in annual premature deaths in each scenario by risk factor; Table S5. Sensitivity results in premature deaths prevented each year in each scenario, assuming a 5km bike trip length; Table S6. Sensitivity results in premature deaths prevented each year in each scenario, using the HEAT for walking and cycling V.3* (5 km trip distance).

Funding: None.

Institutional Review Board Statement: Not applicable.

Informed Consent Statement: Not applicable.

Data Availability Statement: Publicly available datasets were analyzed in this study. This data can be found in the references, supplemental material and here: [https://itdpdotorg.wpengine.com/wp-content/uploads/2015/11/A-Global-High-Shift-Cycling-Scenario_Nov-2015.pdf accessed on 1 March 2021] [https://www.who.int/airpollution/data/cities/en/ accessed on 1 March 2021] [https://population.un.org/wup/Publications/Files/WUP2018-Report.pdf accessed on 1 March 2021] [https://www.itf-oecd.org/sites/default/files/docs/irtad-road-safety-annual-report-2019.pdf accessed on 1 March 2021]

Conflicts of Interest: The author declares they have no actual or potential competing financial interests.

References

1. United Nations. *World Urbanization Prospects: The 2018 Revision*; UN: New York, NY, USA, 2018.
2. Rojas-Rueda, D.; de Nazelle, A.; Andersen, Z.J.; Braun-Fahrländer, C.; Bruha, J.; Bruhova-Foltynova, H.; Desqueyroux, H.; Praznoczy, C.; Ragettli, M.S.; Tainio, M.; et al. Health Impacts of Active Transportation in Europe. *PLoS ONE* **2016**, *11*, e0149990. [CrossRef]
3. Mueller, N.; Rojas-Rueda, D.; Basagaña, X.; Cirach, M.; Cole-Hunter, T.; Dadvand, P.; Donaire-Gonzalez, D.; Foraster, M.; Gascon, M.; Martinez, D.; et al. Health impacts related to urban and transport planning: A burden of disease assessment. *Environ. Int.* **2017**, *107*, 243–257. [CrossRef]
4. Mulley, C.; Tyson, R.; McCue, P.; Rissel, C.; Munro, C. Valuing active travel: Including the health benefits of sustainable transport in transportation appraisal frameworks. *Res. Transp. Bus. Manag.* **2013**, *7*, 27–34. [CrossRef]
5. Sahlqvist, S.; Song, Y.; Ogilvie, D. Is active travel associated with greater physical activity? The contribution of commuting and non-commuting active travel to total physical activity in adults. *Prev. Med.* **2012**, *55*, 206–211. [CrossRef]
6. Rojas-Rueda, D.; de Nazelle, A.; Teixidó, O.; Nieuwenhuijsen, M.J.; De Nazelle, A.; Teixidó, O.; Nieuwenhuijsen, M.J.; de Nazelle, A. Replacing car trips by increasing bike and public transport in the greater Barcelona metropolitan area: A health impact assessment study. *Environ. Int.* **2012**, *49*, 100–109. [CrossRef]
7. Stanaway, J.D.; Afshin, A.; Gakidou, E.; Lim, S.S.; Abate, D.; Abate, K.H.; Abbafati, C.; Abbasi, N.; Abbastabar, H.; Abd-Allah, F.; et al. Global, regional, and national comparative risk assessment of 84 behavioural, environmental and occupational, and metabolic risks or clusters of risks for 195 countries and territories, 1990–2017: A systematic analysis for the Global Burden of Disease Stu. *Lancet* **2018**, *392*, 1923–1994. [CrossRef]
8. Guthold, R.; Stevens, G.A.; Riley, L.M.; Bull, F.C. Articles Worldwide trends in insufficient physical activity from 2001 to 2016: A pooled analysis of 358 population-based surveys with 1.9 million participants. *Lancet Global Health* **2016**, *6*, e1077–e1086. [CrossRef]
9. United Nations. *World Population Prospects 2019: Data Booklet*; UN: New York, NY, USA, 2019.
10. O'Donovan, G.; Lee, I.-M.; Hamer, M.; Stamatakis, E. Association of "weekend warrior" and other leisure time physical activity patterns with risks for all-cause, cardiovascular disease, and cancer mortality. *JAMA Intern. Med.* **2017**, *177*, 335–342. [CrossRef]
11. Lydon, M.; Garcia, A. *Tactical Urbanism: Short-Term Action for Long-Term Change*; Island Press-Center for Resource Economics: Washington, DC, USA, 2015; ISBN 9781610915670.
12. Sarmiento, O.L.; Schmid, T.L.; Parra, D.C.; Díaz-Del-Castillo, A.; Gómez, L.F.; Pratt, M.; Jacoby, E.; Pinzón, J.D.; Duperly, J. Quality of life, physical activity, and built environment characteristics among colombian adults. *J. Phys. Act. Health* **2010**, *7*, 181–195. [CrossRef]
13. Mason, J.; Fulton, L.; Mcdonald, Z.; Mayne, C.; Pardo, C.; Cherry, B.; Margevicius, M.; Replogle, R.; Neufeld, A.; Leal, G.; et al. *A Global High Shift Cycling Scenario: The Potential for Dramatically Increasing Bicycle and E-Bike Use in Cities Around the World, with Estimated Energy, CO_2, and Cost Impacts*; Institute for Transportation & Development Policy: New York, NY, USA; The University of California: Davis, CA, USA, 2015.
14. Otero, I.; Nieuwenhuijsen, M.J.; Rojas-Rueda, D. Health impacts of bike sharing systems in Europe. *Environ. Int.* **2018**, *115*, 387–394. [CrossRef]
15. Wanner, M.; Götschi, T.; Martin-Diener, E.; Kahlmeier, S.; Martin, B.W. Active transport, physical activity, and body weight in adults: A systematic review. *Am. J. Prev. Med.* **2012**, *42*, 493–502. [CrossRef] [PubMed]
16. Mueller, N.; Rojas-Rueda, D.; Cole-hunter, T.; De Nazelle, A.; Dons, E.; Gerike, R.; Götschi, T.; Int, L.; Kahlmeier, S.; Nieuwenhuijsen, M. Health impact assessment of active transportation: A systematic review. *Prev. Med.* **2015**, *76*, 103–114. [CrossRef] [PubMed]
17. Roth, G.A.; Abate, D.; Abate, K.H.; Abay, S.M.; Abbafati, C.; Abbasi, N.; Abbastabar, H.; Abd-Allah, F.; Abdela, J.; Abdelalim, A.; et al. Global, regional, and national age-sex-specific mortality for 282 causes of death in 195 countries and territories, 1980–2017: A systematic analysis for the Global Burden of Disease Study 2017. *Lancet* **2018**, *392*, 1736–1788. [CrossRef]

18. WHO. WHO Global Ambient Air Quality Database. Available online: https://www.who.int/airpollution/data/cities/en/ (accessed on 28 May 2020).
19. OECD; ITF. *Road Safety Annual Report 2019*; ITF: Paris, France, 2019; Volume 8.
20. WHO. *Global Status Report on Road Safety 2018*; World Health Organization: Geneva, Switzerland, 2018; ISBN 9788566800197.
21. Ding, D.; Lawson, K.D.; Kolbe-Alexander, T.L.; Finkelstein, E.A.; Katzmarzyk, P.T.; van Mechelen, W.; Pratt, M. The economic burden of physical inactivity: A global analysis of major non-communicable diseases. *Lancet* 2016, *388*, 1311–1324. [CrossRef]
22. Medina, C.; Janssen, I.; Campos, I.; Barquera, S. Physical inactivity prevalence and trends among Mexican adults: Results from the National Health and Nutrition Survey (ENSANUT) 2006 and 2012. *BMC Public Health* 2013, *13*, 43. [CrossRef]
23. Hoek, G.; Krishnan, R.M.; Beelen, R.; Peters, A.; Ostro, B.; Brunekreef, B.; Kaufman, J.D. Long-term air pollution exposure and cardio-respiratory mortality: A review. *Environ. Health* 2013, *12*, 43. [CrossRef] [PubMed]
24. Woodcock, J.; Franco, O.H.; Orsini, N.; Roberts, I. Non-vigorous physical activity and all-cause mortality: Systematic review and meta-analysis of cohort studies. *Int. J. Epidemiol.* 2011, *40*, 121–138. [CrossRef] [PubMed]
25. ECF Cycling Data Denmark. Available online: https://ecf.com/cycling-data/denmark?field_cd_country_region_tid=1549 (accessed on 31 December 2020).
26. ECF Cycling Data The Netherlands. Available online: https://ecf.com/cycling-data/netherlands?field_cd_country_region_tid=1700 (accessed on 31 December 2020).
27. Ma, X.; Cao, R.; Wang, J. Effects of psychological factors on modal shift from car to dockless bike sharing: A case study of Nanjing, China. *Int. J. Environ. Res. Public Health* 2019, *16*, 3420. [CrossRef]
28. Oakil, A.T.; Ettema, D.; Arentze, T.; Timmermans, H.; Oakil, T.; Ettema, D.; Arentze, T.; Timmermans, H. Bicycle commuting in the Netherlands: An analysis of modal shift and its dependence on life cycle and mobility events. *Int. J. Sustain. Transp.* 2016, *10*, 376–384. [CrossRef]
29. Bjørnarå, H.B.; Berntsen, S.; te Velde, S.J.; Fyhri, A.; Deforche, B.; Andersen, L.B.; Bere, E. From cars to bikes—The effect of an intervention providing access to different bike types: A randomized controlled trial. *PLoS ONE* 2019, *14*, e0219304. [CrossRef] [PubMed]
30. Scheepers, C.E.; Wendel-Vos, G.C.W.; den Broeder, J.M.; van Kempen, E.E.M.M.; van Wesemael, P.J.V.; Schuit, A.J. Shifting from car to active transport: A systematic review of the effectiveness of interventions. *Transp. Res. Part A Policy Pract.* 2014, *70*, 264–280. [CrossRef]
31. Rojas-Rueda, D.; de Nazelle, A.; Tainio, M.; Nieuwenhuijsen, M.J.; David, R.; Audrey, D.N.; Marko, T.; Nieuwenhuijsen, M.J. The health risks and benefits of cycling in urban environments compared with car use: Health impact assessment study. *Br. Med. J.* 2011, *343*, d4521. [CrossRef]
32. Rojas-Rueda, D.; de Nazelle, A.; Teixidó, O.; Nieuwenhuijsen, M.J. Health impact assessment of increasing public transport and cycling use in Barcelona: A morbidity and burden of disease approach. *Prev. Med.* 2013, *57*, 573–579. [CrossRef] [PubMed]
33. De Lima, M. The value of a statistical life in Mexico. *J. Environ. Econ. Policy* 2019, *9*, 140–166. [CrossRef]
34. Johan de Hartog, J.; Boogaard, H.; Nijland, H.; Hoek, G.; Hartog, J.J. De Do the health benefits of cycling outweigh the risks? *Environ. Health Perspect.* 2010, *118*, 1109–1116. [CrossRef] [PubMed]
35. Beelen, R.; Raaschou-Nielsen, O.; Stafoggia, M.; Andersen, Z.J.; Weinmayr, G.; Hoffmann, B.; Wolf, K.; Samoli, E.; Fischer, P.; Nieuwenhuijsen, M.; et al. Effects of long-term exposure to air pollution on natural-cause mortality: An analysis of 22 European cohorts within the multicentre ESCAPE project. *Lancet* 2014, *383*, 785–795. [CrossRef]
36. Cohen, A.J.; Brauer, M.; Burnett, R.; Anderson, H.R.; Frostad, J.; Estep, K.; Balakrishnan, K.; Brunekreef, B.; Dandona, L.; Dandona, R.; et al. Estimates and 25-year trends of the global burden of disease attributable to ambient air pollution: An analysis of data from the Global Burden of Diseases Study 2015. *Lancet* 2017, *389*, 1907–1918. [CrossRef]
37. De Nazelle, A.; Bode, O.; Orjuela, J.P. Comparison of air pollution exposures in active vs. passive travel modes in European cities: A quantitative review. *Environ. Int.* 2017, *99*, 151–160. [CrossRef] [PubMed]
38. Mueller, N.; Rojas-Rueda, D.; Salmon, M.; Martinez, D.; Ambros, A.; Brand, C.; de Nazelle, A.; Dons, E.; Gaupp-Berghausen, M.; Gerike, R.; et al. Health impact assessment of cycling network expansions in European cities. *Prev. Med.* 2018, *109*, 62–70. [CrossRef]
39. Jarrett, J.; Woodcock, J.; Griffiths, U.K.; Chalabi, Z.; Edwards, P.; Roberts, I.; Haines, A. Effect of increasing active travel in urban England and Wales on costs to the National Health Service. *Lancet* 2012, *379*, 2198–2205. [CrossRef]
40. Thondoo, M.; Mueller, N.; Rojas-Rueda, D.; de Vries, D.; Gupta, J.; Nieuwenhuijsen, M.J. Participatory quantitative health impact assessment of urban transport planning: A case study from Eastern Africa. *Environ. Int.* 2020, *144*, 106027. [CrossRef] [PubMed]

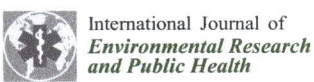

Article

Psychosocial and Social Environmental Factors as Moderators in the Relation between the Objective Environment and Older Adults' Active Transport

Linda M. Nguyen [1] and Lieze Mertens [2,3,*]

[1] Faculty of Health, Medicine & Life Sciences, Maastricht University, Universiteitssingel 40, 6229 ER Maastricht, The Netherlands; lindanguyen395@gmail.com
[2] Department of Movement and Sport Sciences, Faculty of Medicine and Health Sciences, Ghent University, Watersportlaan 2, B-9000 Ghent, Belgium
[3] Research Foundation—Flanders (FWO), Egmontstraat 5, B-1000 Brussels, Belgium
* Correspondence: lieze.mertens@ugent.be

Abstract: In order to develop tailored interventions aiming to encourage active transport among older adults, it is important to gain insights into the modifiable moderators affecting active transport behavior considering the neighborhood in which one lives. Therefore, this study aimed to determine which objective physical environmental factors have an impact on the active transport behavior of Belgian older adults (≥65 years old) and which psychosocial and social environmental moderators influence those relationships. Data from 503 independent living older adults who participated the Belgian Environmental Physical Activity Study in Seniors were included. Multilevel negative binomial regression models (participants nested in neighborhoods) with log link function were fitted for the analyses. Our resulted indicated that older adults living in an environment with higher residential density, higher park density, lower public transport density, and more entropy index had higher active transport levels. Furthermore, different types of neighborhood in which older adults live can lead to different moderators that are decisive for increasing older adults' active transport behavior. Therefore, based on our results some recommendations towards tailored interventions could be given to increase older adults' active transport behavior depending on the environment in which one lives.

Keywords: walking; cycling; elderly; neighborhood; interaction effects; socio-ecological model

1. Introduction

Despite the well-known physical, mental and social health benefits of regular physical activity (PA), 62% of the older adults living in Flanders (Belgium) aged from 65- to 74-year-olds and 87% of those aged 75 years [1] do not meet the recommended 150 min of moderate-to-vigorous physical intensity activity (MVPA) per week [1–3]. Walking and cycling are considered as accessible and inexpensive forms of MVPA [4,5] and are well-liked by Flemish older adults [6]. It was shown that regular walking and cycling (equivalent to 150 min of MVPA/week) were related to a decreased risk of all-mortality of 11% and 10% respectively, after adjustment for other PA [7]. As older adults eventually have to stop driving their car due to physiological restrictions (e.g., hearing, reaction time, muscle strength, vision), acceptable transportation alternatives to driving must be sought, of which active transport (AT) might be one [8,9]. AT or walking and cycling to a destination (e.g., to do groceries, to visit a friend) can be considered as an activity that is easy to integrate into older adults' daily routines [10,11], benefit one's health condition, and it is also beneficial for the economics and environment in terms of reduction in noise, traffic jams, and CO_2-emissions [5]. However, in Belgium, respectively hardly 17% and 9% of the older adults (≥65 years) indicated walking or cycling as their main means of transport. Knowing that

22%, 47% or 63% of the trips older adults make are shorter than respectively 1, 3 and 5 km [12] AT is still not sufficiently embodied yet into their daily life routines.

AT can be influenced by both individual and environmental factors [13]. Individual factors include influences within the individual, such as demographics, biological, or psychological factors (i.e., self-efficacy, perceived benefits or barriers) and/or that are close to the individual, such as the social climate at home or in a neighborhood (i.e., social environmental factors) [13,14]. Environmental factors include influences that are beyond the individual, such as the presence of pedestrian/cycling facilities, parking, and traffic (i.e., physical environmental factors) [13,14]. AT can thus be explained by an interplay between several types of factors at multiple levels: individual (i.e., socio-demographic and psychosocial factors), social environmental, and physical environmental factors [13].

In a recent review and meta-analysis, strong evidence was found between the neighborhood physical environment and older adults' walking for transport [15]. Whilst, limited evidence was available on the combination of walking and cycling for transport or cycling for transport solely [15]. Moreover, neighborhood environmental factors were more frequently assessed using self-reports instead of objective measures [15–17]. However, it is important to gain insights into determinants affecting AT behavior considering the neighborhood in which one lives. As the objective physical environment is often difficult to alter in short term, it is important to determine which individual and social environmental factors can be modified that may increase older adults' AT behavior. In that way tailored interventions can be developed depending on the environment in which one lives. Unfortunately, knowledge about modifiable moderators between environment-AT associations is still lacking [15]. We hypothesized that older adults living in a less encouraging objective determined neighborhood will engage more in AT if they have a positive psychosocial view towards PA (i.e., more self-efficacy, perceiving more benefits/less barriers towards PA) [18], or live in a supportive social physical environment (i.e., a trustworthy and socially cohesive neighborhood) [19,20]. It is known from previous studies that self-efficacy, perceptions about benefits and barriers towards PA were observed as the major determinants of PA among older adults [21,22]. Furthermore, research on the social environmental factors of PA, especially among older adults, is still limited. Hence, more studies about determinants and moderators concerning environment-AT associations are needed to gain complete insights.

Therefore, the aim of this study was to determine which objective physical environmental factors have an impact on the AT behavior of older adults ($\geq$65 years old) and which psychosocial and social environmental moderators influence those relationships.

2. Materials and Methods

2.1. Study Design

The cross-sectional data derived from the Belgian Environmental Physical Activity Study in Seniors (BEPAS Seniors) [23] were used for the current study. The BEPAS Seniors was a cross-sectional study which focused on independent living older adults aged 65 and over, living across twenty different neighborhoods in Ghent and its suburbs (Flanders, Belgium). This study aimed to examine the relationship between the neighborhood in which older adults live and their PA levels. The study protocol was approved by the Ghent University Hospital Ethics Committee. The BEPAS Seniors is detailed described in the original study conducted by Van Holle and colleagues [23].

2.2. Sampling

In short, data collection was performed between October 2010 and September 2012. Neighborhoods were stratified on Geographical Information System (GIS) -based data in Ghent (Flanders, Belgium) to determine neighborhood walkability (high vs. low) and matched on neighborhood annual household income level (high vs. low) [23]. Four types of neighborhood strata resulted: high walkability-high income, high walkability-low income, low walkability-high income, and low walkability-low income. In total twenty different neighborhood samples in Ghent and its suburbs were selected; five neighborhoods were allocated under each type of neighborhood.

Subsequently, older adults were randomly recruited in each type of neighborhood stratified based on gender and age (<75 versus ≥75 years old). Selected older adults were approached by sending an information letter by postal mail in which the aim of the study was indicated including the announcement of the home visit by a trained interviewer during the next two weeks. During the home visits, and after signing the informed consent, a face-to-face interview collected information about socio-demographic, self-reported physical functioning, residential self-selection, PA levels in the last week, psychosocial factors, and perceived social environmental factors. The following inclusion criteria were applied: aged ≥65 years old, able to understand and speak Dutch/Flemish, able to walk a few hundred meters without heavy difficulties in physical functioning and lived independently.

2.3. Measures

2.3.1. Socio-Demographic Factors and Residential Self-Selection

During the face-to-face interview, the following participants' information was retrieved: age, gender, origin (yes: Belgium as country of birth vs. no), education (tertiary vs. no tertiary level), occupation (household, blue-, or white collar), living situation (with vs. without partner) and owning motorized vehicles (at least one vehicle vs. no). Participants' self-reported physical functioning was derived from the Short Form 36 item Survey (SF-36) [24]. Participants had to denote on a 3-point scale (severely limited; somewhat limited; not limited) to what extent they were physically limited while performing ten general activities, such as lifting or carrying groceries, climbing stairs, and walking short distances. Subsequently, activities in which participants reported to be severely or somewhat limited were summed. Participants' physical functioning, ranging from zero to ten, was obtained by reversing this latter variable. Residential self-selection was assessed based on an eight-item scale derived from a study [25]. Respondents were asked to rate how important eight possible reasons (e.g., proximity of open spaces, sense of community) were for selecting their neighborhood. Internal consistency of the scale in the current sample was good (Cronbach's alpha = 0.83).

2.3.2. Self-Reported Active Transport Behavior

The dependent variable, AT, was measured using the long version of the International Physical Activity Questionnaire (IPAQ) [26,27]. The frequency (i.e., number of days) and duration (i.e., average time/day) of walking and cycling for transport in the last seven days was assessed. The IPAQ was proven reliable and valid specific among older adults [27], whereby its test-retest reliability was overall moderate to good [28].

2.3.3. Psychosocial Factors towards PA

In total six psychosocial factors towards PA were included in the current study. A more detailed description of the content of the items and scoring of the factors can be found in the original study of Van Holle and colleagues [29]. In short, self-efficacy, consisted of five items, referred to one's confidence to be physically active in difficult circumstances. Perceived benefits, likewise, consisted of five items, reflected on benefits, such as health benefits and meeting new people. Perceived barriers, consisted of seven items, reflected on barriers, such as feeling for 'not being good enough' and bad weather conditions. Furthermore, social support indicated the partner's/friends' supportive attitude towards PA. Social norm indicated what the partner/friends think(s) about one should perform PA. Lastly, modeling referred to what extent the partner/friend(s) is/are being physically active. Therefore, these last three factors consisted of each two items. The items were based on existing validated questionnaires used among Belgian adults [30,31]. Those psychosocial factors were assessed on a 3-, 5- or 7-point scale, see Table 1 for a detailed overview. Each factor variable was calculated by averaging the scores on the items and considered as continuous variable.

Table 1. Descriptive statistics of the participants ($n = 503$).

Characteristics	Values
Age in years (M ± SD)	74.4 ± 6.2
Women (%)	53.4
Living with a partner (%)	65.3
Tertiary education (%)	38.0
Physical functioning (M ± SD)	7.05 ± 2.37
No motorized vehicles in the household (%)	20.8
Active transport (min/week) (M ± SD)	121.8 ± 163.6
No active transport (%)	31.4
Psychosocial factors towards physical activity (M ± SD)	
Self-efficacy [a]	2.1 ± 0.5
Perceived benefits [b]	3.4 ± 0.8
Perceived barriers [b]	1.9 ± 0.7
Social norm [b]	2.9 ± 1.4
Social support [b]	2.8 ± 1.5
Modeling [c]	2.8 ± 1.9
Social neighborhood environmental factors (M ± SD)	
Talking to neighbors [c]	5.5 ± 1.4
Social interactions with neighbors [c]	2.2 ± 1.1
Neighborhood social trust and cohesion [d]	3.7 ± 0.8
Neighborhood social diversity [b]	4.2 ± 0.7
Objective neighborhood environmental factors, buffer 500 m (M ± SD)	
Residential density [e]	4871.1 ± 3261.1
Park density [f]	10.9 ± 8.6
Public transport density [g]	33.3 ± 19.7
Intersection density [h]	162.7 ± 70.0
Entropy [i]	0.5 ± 0.2

M = mean; SD = standard deviation; [a] = assessed on a 3-point scale; [b] = assessed on a 5-point scale; [c] = assessed on a 7-point scale; [d] = assessed on a 4-point scale; [e] = number of dwellings per surface buffer 500 m; [f] = number of public parks of all sizes per surface buffer 500 m; [g] = number of public transportation stops of any kind per surface buffer 500 m; [h] = number of intersections per surface buffer 500 m; [i] = range from 0 (= perfect homogeneous land use) to 1 (= perfect heterogeneous land use).

2.3.4. The Perceived Social Neighborhood Environment

In total four perceived social environmental factors were included in the current study: talking to neighbors, social interactions with neighbors, neighborhood social trust and cohesion, and neighborhood social diversity. 'Talking to neighbors' referred to informal social interactions with neighbors and consisted of two items, while 'social interaction with neighbors' referred to formal social interactions and consisted of three items. These two factors measured the extent of social interactions between older adults and their neighbors [32,33]. 'Neighborhood social trust and cohesion' was derived from a questionnaire by Sampson [34] and consisted of four items assessed participants' agreement about their local neighborhood (e.g., 'people in this neighborhood can be trusted'). 'Neighborhood social diversity' gives an indication of the social composition of the neighborhood (e.g., proportion of immigrants, youngsters, older people in the neighborhood), consisted of three items and was assessed analogous to previous research in older adults [35]. Each factor variable was calculated by averaging the scores on the items and considered as continuous variable. See Table 1 for a detailed overview concerning the scoring of the factors. A more detailed description of the content of the items can be found once again in the original study of Van Holle and colleagues [36].

2.3.5. The Objective Physical Neighborhood Environment

The BEPAS Seniors included objective GIS-data for all participants using a sausage buffer of 500 m around their home address [23]. The near and direct neighborhood environment may be important for older adults, as they are more likely to walk/cycle in streets they are familiar with and they are overall less commutable to other locations compared to other age groups [15,21,37,38]. The density of the following five physical environmental factors were objectively calculated in a 500 m buffer zone surrounding each participant's home address: residential density, park density, public transport density, intersection density and entropy. First, residential density was described as the ratio between the number of single- and multifamily domiciles and the area of all parcels within or partial within the buffer zone. Second, park density was defined as the ratio between the number of parks that are full or partial in the buffer zone and the total land area in the buffer zone. Third, public transport density was described as the ratio between the number of transport stops (i.e., bus, tram, train) and the total buffer zone. Additionally, intersection density was the ratio between the number of three- or more-way crossings and the total buffer zone. Lastly, entropy referred to the index of land use mix diversity within the buffer zone [39]. The entropy index was calculated by using Dobesova's and Krivka's formula [39]:

$$H(S) = \frac{-\sum_{i=1}^{k}[(\rho_i)\cdot(\ln\rho_i)]}{\ln k}$$

where $H(S)$ indicates the entropy index (also called Shannon index), ρ_i is the area of a category of land use over the total area of all categories (within one neighborhood), and k is the number of land use categories in the particular neighborhood. Five land use categories were included in the formula: residential, commercial, civic, entertainment, food and private/public recreational.

2.4. Data Analyses

Descriptive statistics of the total study sample were obtained using SPSS 26.0 software (IBM Corp, Armonk, New York, United States). Generalized estimating equations (GEE) in the SPSS software was used to examine the main associations between objective physical environmental factors and AT, and to determine the moderating effects of psychosocial and social environmental factors. Multilevel negative binominal regression models (participants nested in neighborhoods) with log link function were fitted for the analyses as the dependent variable, AT (combined minutes walking and cycling for transport per week), was positively skewed and contained a considerable number of null values (31.4%).

First, single predictor models (i.e., two-level negative binominal regression models) for each potential covariate (i.e., age, gender, living status, education, vehicles, physical functioning and residential self-selection) were fitted. Only the significant covariates (i.e., living status and physical functioning), see Table A1 in Appendix A, were added as covariates in the further analyses, given the complexity of the models. Second, single predictor models for each objective environmental factor, for each psychosocial and social environmental factor were separately fitted and added in Appendix A (see Table A1) for completeness. Third, 50 single interactions models were separately estimated between the objective physical environmental factors and each potential moderator (i.e., psychosocial and social environmental factors), and can be found in Appendix A Table A2. Fourth, all single interaction effects from the third step surpassing the statistical threshold of $p < 0.10$ were simultaneously added in the final model. The final model is presented in Table 2. Only the significant interaction effects observed in the final model are further described in the text and visualized with graphs. To facilitate model convergence and interpretation, all objective environmental factors were standardized. Level of significance was defined at $\alpha = 0.10$ (trend) and $\alpha = 0.05$.

Table 2. Final model.

Factors	ExpB (95% CI)
Living status (ref: living with a partner)	0.97 (0.70–1.33)
Physical functioning	1.18 (1.14–1.23)
Residential density	2.63 (1.09–6.35) *
Park density	1.35 (1.02–1.77) *
Public transport density	0.31 (0.15–0.64) **
Intersection density	0.99 (0.72–1.36)
Entropy	3.89 (0.80–18.86) ^
Self-efficacy	1.40 (1.06–1.84) *
Perceived benefits	0.93 (0.84–1.04)
Perceived barriers	0.92 (0.76–1.11)
Social support	1.09 (1.00–1.19) *
Modeling	0.96 (0.90–1.03)
Neighborhood social trust and cohesion	1.15 (0.96–1.36)
Talking to neighbors	1.20 (1.04–1.38) *
Social interaction to neighbors	0.90 (0.81–1.00) *
Residential density * self-efficacy	0.78 (0.60–1.02) ^
Residential density * social support	1.02 (0.90–1.16)
Residential density * modeling	0.97 (0.91–1.03)
Residential density * social trust and cohesion	1.02 (0.81–1.02)
Park density * perceived barriers	0.90 (0.81–1.02) ^
Public transport density * perceived benefits	1.22 (1.07–1.38) **
Public transport density * talking to neighbors	1.08 (0.99–1.18) ^
Intersection density * social support	0.96 (0.87–1.06)
Entropy * perceived benefits	0.83 (0.71–0.96) *
Entropy * perceived barriers	1.25 (1.00–1.56) *
Entropy * neighborhood social trust and cohesion	0.80 (0.56–1.10)
Entropy * social interactions to neighbors	0.95 (0.87–1.03)

^ $p < 0.10$; * $p < 0.05$; ** $p < 0.01$; ref = reference category.

3. Results

3.1. Descriptive Statistics

In total, 503 older adults ranged in age from 65 to 97 years old participated the BEPAS Seniors study. The socio-demographics, the self-reported AT behavior and the psychosocial, social environmental, and objective physical environmental factors of the total study sample are presented in Table 1. Just over half of the sample (53.4%) were women, 38.0% of the participants performed tertiary education, and 65.3% lived with a partner. On average, the sample performed 121.8 ± 163.6 min per week AT, and 31.4% of the total study sample did not engage in AT.

3.2. Final Model

Main Effects Objective Environmental Factors

The final model is presented in Table 2. Older adults living in an environment with higher residential density, higher park density, lower public transport density, and more entropy (trend) had significantly higher AT levels. Living in a neighborhood that is one standard deviation higher in residential density was associated with 263% more minutes AT per week. Older adults living in a neighborhood that is one standard deviation higher in park density were associated with 35% more AT per week. Older adults living in a neighborhood that is one standard deviation lower in public transport stops were associated with 69% more AT. Living in an environment with one standard deviation higher in entropy was marginally associated with 389% more AT.

3.3. Interactions with Psychosocial, and Social Environmental Factors

The association between objective residential density and AT was marginally significantly moderated by self-efficacy ($p = 0.067$). Older adults living in low residential density neighborhoods with high self-efficacy towards PA performed more AT in comparison to older adults perceiving low self-efficacy towards PA. In high residential neighborhoods, older adults with low self-efficacy performed more AT in comparison to older adults perceiving high self-efficacy (see Figure 1).

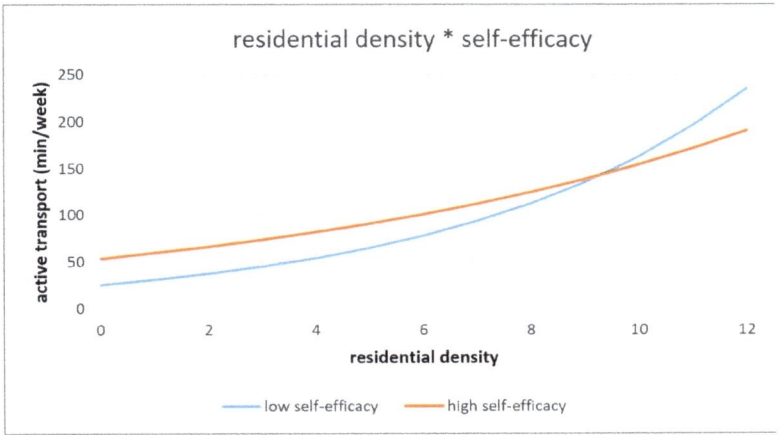

Figure 1. Interaction effect of residential density and self-efficacy on active transport.

The association between objective park density and AT was marginally significantly moderated by perceived barriers towards PA ($p = 0.088$). The positive effect of park density on AT was greater for older adults who perceived low barriers towards PA in comparison to older adults perceiving high barriers towards PA (see Figure 2).

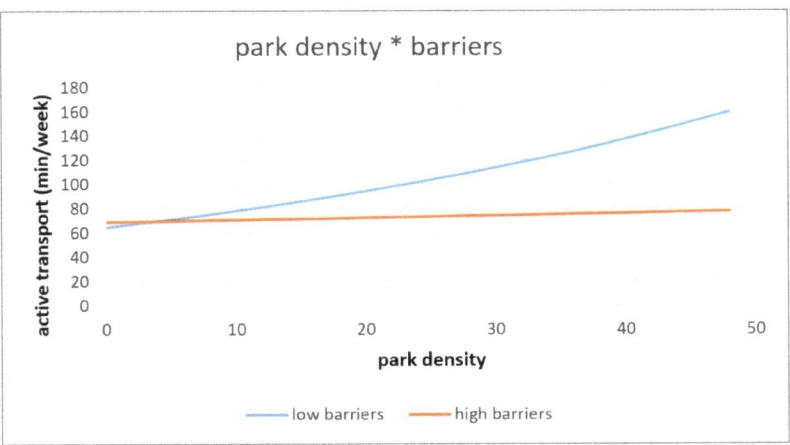

Figure 2. Interaction effect of park density and barriers towards PA on active transport.

The association between objective public transport density and AT was significantly moderated by perceived benefits towards PA ($p = 0.002$). Older adults living in low transport dense environments with low benefits towards PA performed more AT in comparison to older adults with high benefits towards PA. While, in high dense environments, older adults with high benefits towards PA performed more AT in comparison to older adults with low benefits towards PA (see Figure 3).

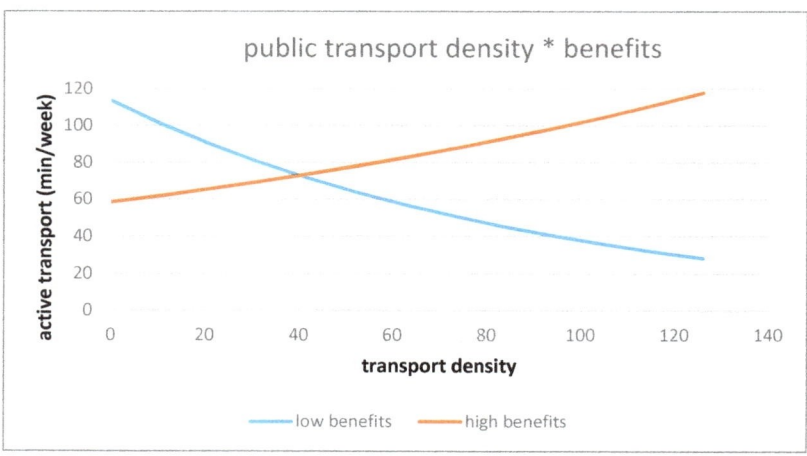

Figure 3. Interaction effect of public transport density and benefits towards PA on active transport.

The association between objective public transport density and AT was marginally significantly moderated by talking to neighbors ($p = 0.080$). The negative effect of transport dense environments on AT is greater for people who talked less with their neighbors in comparison to older adults who talked more with their neighbors (see Figure 4).

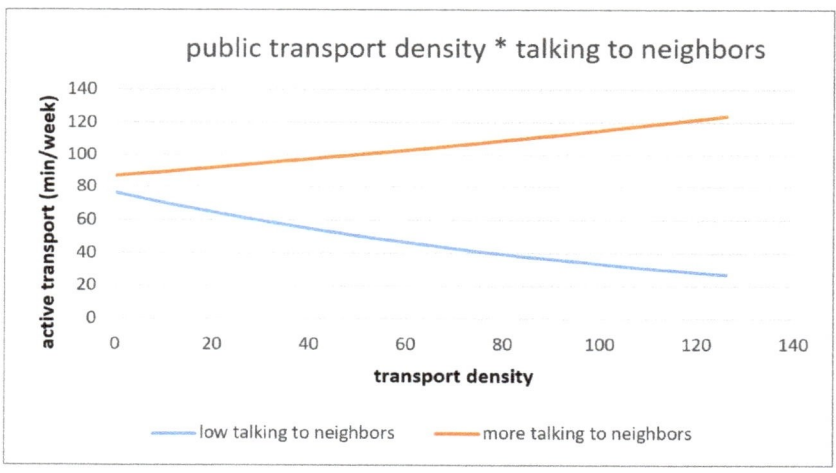

Figure 4. Interaction effect of public transport density and talking to neighbors on active transport.

The association between objective entropy and AT was significantly moderated by barriers towards PA ($p = 0.046$). Only for older adults with high barriers there was a difference depending on the entropy index of the neighborhood on AT. Older adults living in low entropy index neighborhoods with high barriers towards PA performed less AT in comparison to older adults with low barriers towards PA. While older adults living in high entropy index neighborhoods with high barriers towards PA performed more AT in comparison to older adults with low barriers towards PA (see Figure 5).

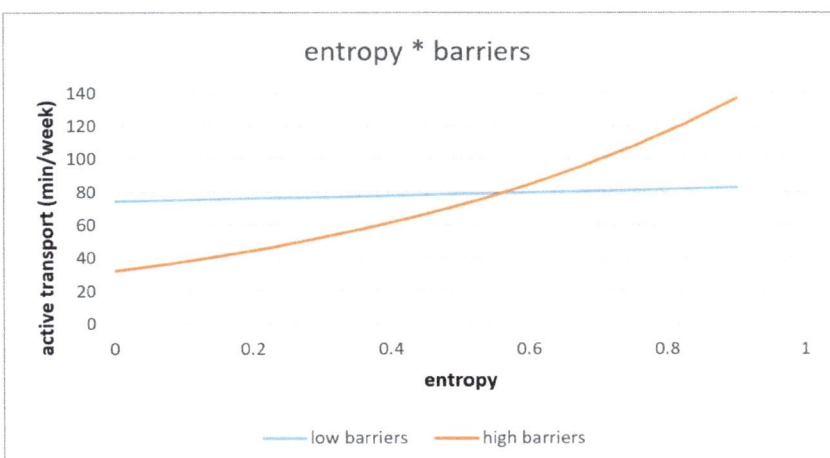

Figure 5. Interaction effect of entropy and barriers towards PA on active transport.

The association between objective entropy and AT was significantly moderated by benefits towards PA ($p = 0.015$). Only for older adults with low benefits towards PA there was a difference depending on the entropy index of the neighborhood on AT. Older adults living in low entropy index neighborhood with low benefits towards PA performed less AT in comparison to older adults with high benefits towards PA. While older adults living in high entropy index neighborhood with low benefits towards PA did more AT in comparison to older adults with high benefits towards PA (see Figure 6).

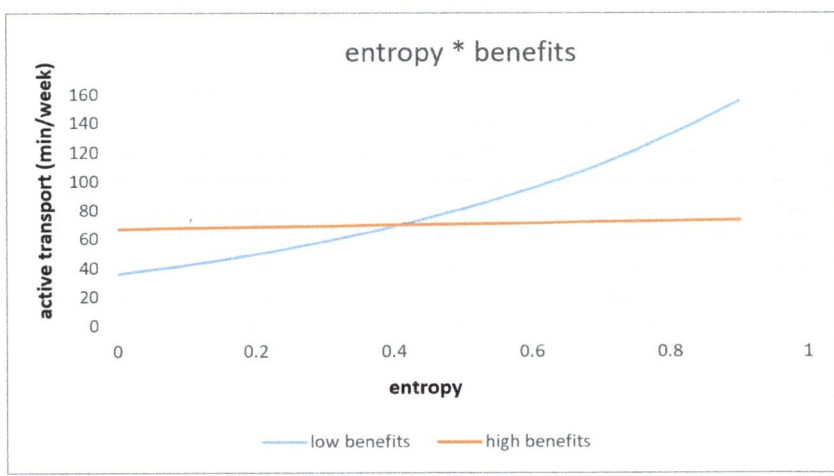

Figure 6. Interaction effect of entropy and benefits towards PA on active transport.

4. Discussion

The aim of this study was to determine which objective physical environmental factors have an impact on the AT behavior of older adults (≥ 65 years old) and which psychosocial and social environmental moderators have an impact on those relationships. Our results indicated that older adults living in an environment with higher residential density, higher park density, lower public transport density, and more entropy had higher AT levels. Similar results among older adults were found in a recent meta-analysis but for the perceived measure of residential density, park availability and land use mix diversity [15].

Residential density and land use mix diversity are two components of walkability, which reflects the ease of walking to destinations in a neighborhood [40]. Among Belgian older adults, high neighborhood walkability was found to be related to higher levels of transportation walking experiences [23]. However, for the third component of walkability, intersection density or street connectivity, we did not find a significant association with AT, while in the literature objective [15] or perceived [22] street connectivity was often correlated to more AT. Van Cauwenberg [22] indicated that a higher street connectivity could make AT more attractive as older adults are supported to choose more alternative routes (e.g., avoid busy streets or steep slopes) [22]. A possible explanation why we did not find this association in our study might be the small buffer size (i.e., 500 m). Even though using a small buffer size for older adults is recommended [15,37,38], it might be interesting to look at different or larger buffer sizes. Furthermore, contrary to our expectations and previous results, a contradictory result was found for public transport accessibility. Our results indicated that low public transport dense neighborhoods were associated with more AT, while a positive association was found previously [15]. A possible explanation for this finding might be that older adults have to walk further distances to access destinations because they do not have access to public transport. This might be a sign that those neighborhoods need more investment in public transport accessibility. Given the conflicting results with the literature, these findings need further exploration.

In order to better respond to such relationships with the purpose of interventions, it is good to have insight into the possible moderators between environment-AT associations. We hypothesized that older adults living in a less encouraging objective determined neighborhood will do more AT if they have a positive psychosocial view towards PA [18], or live in a supportive social physical environment [19,20]. A first interesting result is that the negative effect found on AT according to high public transport dense neighborhoods could be reduced if older adults perceiving high benefits towards PA or when they often talk to their neighbors. According to the Health Belief Model [41], older adults' AT behavior change is influenced by both perceived benefits and barriers of change. Therefore, for older adults living in high public transport dense neighborhoods the benefits towards PA should be more emphasized. Additional, if older adults talk more to their neighbors, they get more familiar with their neighborhood and nearby surroundings, which might increase their willingness to do more AT. A recent longitudinal study of Josey and Moore [42] among adults indicated that a more favorable personal social network may be essential for bringing change into physical inactivity behavior. Research on the social environmental factors of PA among older adults is still limited, therefore, further exploration on these findings are certainly needed.

Second, as stated in our results, park density increases AT, and also from previous research we know that good accessibility of parks (e.g., low traffic on route, slope of terrain <5%) increases the likelihood that older adults will visit a park [43,44]. Furthermore, our results indicated that the positive effect of park density on AT among older adults could be strengthened if they perceived low barriers towards PA (e.g., lack of time, bad weather conditions, fear of falling) in comparison to older adults perceiving high barriers towards PA. From a recent longitudinal study among older adults, we learn that by decreasing the perceived barriers towards PA the engagement in cycling for transport over time can be increased [17]. Moreover, previous cross-sectional research showed that perceived barriers and benefits were the most important correlates in relation to overall MVPA [29,45]. In other words, when older adults perceiving high barriers and these are not reduced, it might discourage them even more their intention to be physically active, despite living in higher park dense neighborhoods.

Third, we found that older adults living in low residential dense neighborhoods perceiving a higher self-efficacy will do more AT than older adults perceiving less self-efficacy. Previous studies confirmed the association between higher self-efficacy towards

PA (e.g., confidence to be physically active when the weather is bad, or when you have little time) and higher levels of PA [46], or specifically higher levels of walking for transport [17]. Hereby, self-efficacy, the expectation older adults have about their own ability to do more AT [47], may be important to increase PA levels among older adults. More specifically, according to our results, we can conclude that improving the self-efficacy towards PA may be more essential among older adults living in low residential dense neighborhoods.

Fourth, an unexpected result was found according to the moderating effect of perceived barriers and benefits towards PA for the association between entropy and AT. The entropy index represents how homogenous or heterogeneous the usage of a particular area is [39]; the higher is the diversity of the land use, the higher is the entropy index. Previous longitudinal [17], cross-sectional qualitative [21,48] and quantitative [49–51] research reported similar findings among older adults concerning the positive main association between entropy or land use mix diversity and walking for transport. We found that older adults living in an environment with more entropy will marginally have higher levels of AT which corresponds to the literature. However, for older adults perceiving low barriers towards PA or perceiving high benefits towards PA, no difference will be found according to the entropy index of the neighborhood in which older adults live. Nevertheless, for older adults perceiving high barriers towards PA or perceiving low benefits towards PA, there will be a difference in AT depending on the entropy index of the neighborhood in which one lives. Older adults living in low entropy index neighborhood with high barriers or low benefits towards PA will do less AT in comparison to older adults perceiving low barriers or high benefits towards PA. While older adults living in high entropy index neighborhood with high barriers or low benefits towards PA do more AT in comparison to older adults with low barriers or high benefits towards PA. In other words, older adults who consider AT as more beneficial to them and have lower barriers towards PA will do it regardless of where they live, while older adults who think AT is less beneficial and have more barriers, would not do it in an environment that is not conducive to it. Consequently, a more entropy dense neighborhood enables walking and makes it easy, even for older adults who would not normally walk or cycle. Therefore, older adults living in neighborhoods where the diversity of land use mix is low, it is important to encourage benefits towards PA and decrease the barriers towards PA.

In summary, interventions aiming to promote AT are necessary, since a small number of older adults perform AT. It is important to be aware that different types of neighborhood in which older adults live can lead to different moderators that are decisive for increasing older adults' AT behavior. Based on our results, the following suggestions could be made for future intervention. Interventions focusing on increasing the benefits towards PA as well as talking to neighbors might help to increase AT behavior of older adults living in high public transport dense neighborhoods which is negative correlated to older adults' AT. For older adults living in high park dense neighborhoods, decreasing barriers towards PA could increase older adults' AT. Furthermore, interventions focusing on providing self-efficacy training to older adults to boost their confidence and ability to do more physical activities might rise older adults' AT living in low residential dense neighborhoods. Lastly, declining barriers and increasing benefits towards PA will enhance older adults' AT behavior if they live in an environment with a low entropy index. Although, this study gives a first indication of possible changeable psychosocial and social environmental moderators in the relation between the objective physical environment and older adults' AT, longitudinal studies are crucial to gain better insights into which moderators could predict the relationship over time.

The current study has several strengths and limitations. A first strength is the investigated moderating effects of psychosocial and social environmental factors which are modifiable factors that can be embedded in interventions aiming to encourage AT taking into account the environment in which one lives. This has hardly been studied before among older adults. Another strength is that the physical environmental factors were objectively assessed, while previous research often used subjectively assessed data which might be more sensitive for biases. Furthermore, older adults' characteristics and factors were largely assessed through a face-to-face interview by trained health professionals. Responses can be more accurately obtained during a guided survey instead of a self-administered survey, especially among older adults as they may experiences more cognitive difficulties when filling in a questionnaire by themselves [52]. A validity study showed that less over-reporting bias occurred when an interview-administered version was used for IPAQ instead of a self-administered version [53]. Lastly, the large sample size enabled to investigate both main and moderating effects.

Limitations of the current study mainly include its cross-sectional design, so no causal inferences of the findings could be made [54]. It is recommended to perform longitudinal and/or experimental studies, which enables to investigate changes in AT behavior over time and to identify causality. Furthermore, psychosocial factors were questioned in relation to PA in general and not AT in specific, which might have led to inaccurate findings [55]. Nevertheless, these psychosocial factors were based on existing validated questionnaires used among Belgian adults [30,31]. Another limitation was the self-report of older adults' AT behavior. GPS devices gives us the opportunity to objectively assess the transport behavior, however there are also concerns such as losing GPS contact or misclassify the travel mode [56,57]. Therefore, it is recommended to combine these GPS devices with activity diaries or accelerometer in order to fulfill the missing information [58,59]. Furthermore, we are aware that we have not included all possible variables that have an impact on active transport, such as vehicle traffic or pleasantness of routes for walking and cycling. Therefore, we have to be careful when drawing policy conclusions. Lastly, as this research is conducted in Belgium, the generalization of these results to Western Europe may be possible due to the similar cycling culture should be approached with caution.

5. Conclusions

Interventions aiming to promote AT are necessary, since a small number of older adults perform AT. It is important to be aware that different types of neighborhood in which older adults live can lead to different moderators that are decisive for increasing older adults' AT behavior. Our results indicated that older adults living in an environment with higher residential density, higher park density, lower public transport density, and more entropy had higher levels of AT. Furthermore, we can give a few recommendations towards interventions based on the results found for the modifiable moderators which will give the opportunity to develop tailored interventions depending on the environment in which the older adult lives. First, increasing the benefits towards PA as well as talking to neighbors might help to increase AT behavior of older adults living in a high public transport dense neighborhood which is negative correlated to older adults' AT. Second, decreasing barriers towards PA, could increase AT for older adults living in high park dense neighborhoods. Third, interventions focusing on providing self-efficacy training to older adults to boost their confidence and ability to do more physical activities might rise older adults' AT living in low residential dense neighborhoods. Lastly, interventions focusing on declining barriers and increasing benefits towards PA will enhance older adults' AT behavior if they live in an environment with a low entropy index.

Author Contributions: Conceptualization, L.M.; methodology, L.M.; software, L.M. and L.M.N.; validation, L.M. and L.M.N.; formal analysis, L.M. and L.M.N.; investigation, L.M.; resources, L.M.; data curation, L.M. and L.M.N.; writing—original draft preparation, L.M. and L.M.N.; writing—review and editing, L.M. and L.M.N.; visualization, L.M.; supervision, L.M.; project administration, L.M.; funding acquisition, L.M. All authors have read and agreed to the published version of the manuscript.

Funding: This work was funded by the Research Foundation Flanders (FWO) [grant number B/13018/01]. Lieze Mertens is supported by a postdoctoral fellowship of the Research Foundation Flanders [grant number FWO17/PDO/140].

Institutional Review Board Statement: The study was conducted according to the guidelines of the Declaration of Helsinki and approved by the Ethics Committee of the Ghent University Hospital (registration number B670201423000).

Informed Consent Statement: Informed consent was obtained from all subjects involved in the study.

Data Availability Statement: The data presented in this study are available on request from the corresponding author.

Acknowledgments: The authors would like to thank Veerle Van Holle for her contribution in data collection.

Conflicts of Interest: The authors declare no conflict of interest.

Appendix A

Table A1. Single-predictor models related to active transport.

Demographics	ExpB (95% CI)
Age	1.00 (0.83–1.21)
Gender (ref: women)	1.00 (0.97–1.01)
Living status (ref: living with a partner)	0.74 (0.62–0.89) **
Education (ref: tertiary)	0.82 (0.64–1.05)
Vehicles (ref: motorized vehicle)	1.04 (0.82–1.33)
Physical functioning	1.20 (1.14–1.26) ***
Residential self-selection	1.12 (0.91–1.39)
Objective environmental factors, buffer 500 m [a]	
Residential density 500 m	1.56 (1.39–1.74) ***
Park density 500 m	1.09 (0.97–1.24)
Public transport density 500 m	1.16 (1.04–1.30)
Intersection density 500 m	1.29 (1.13–1.47) ***
Entropy 500 m	1.31 (1.12–1.55) **
Psychosocial factors towards physical activity [a]	
Self-efficacy	1.28 (0.93–1.77)
Perceived benefits	1.12 (0.99–1.27) ^
Perceived barriers	0.88 (0.74–1.04)
Social support	1.04 (0.96–1.12)
Social norm	0.96 (0.89–1.04)
Modelling	0.96 (0.89–1.04)
Social environmental factors [a]	
Talking to neighbors	1.19 (1.08–1.32) **
Social interaction to neighbors	0.97 (0.90–1.05)
Social trust and cohesion	1.05 (0.88–1.26)
Social diversity	1.00 (0.77–1.31)

^ $p < 0.10$; * $p < 0.05$; ** $p < 0.01$; *** $p < 0.001$; ref = reference category; [a] = adjusted for living status and physical functioning, participants nested in neighbourhoods.

Table A2. Single interactions models related to active transport.

Residential Density	ExpB (95% CI)
Residential density * self-efficacy	0.68 (0.52–0.87) **
Residential density * perceived benefits	0.98 (0.88–1.08)
Residential density * perceived barriers	1.12 (0.92–1.37)
Residential density * social support	0.92 (0.88–0.97) **
Residential density * social norm	1.04 (0.96–1.14)
Residential density * modeling	0.93 (0.89–0.97) *
Residential density * social diversity	0.89 (0.63–1.24)

Table A2. Cont.

Residential Density	ExpB (95% CI)
Residential density * social trust and cohesion	0.87 (0.77–0.99) *
Residential density * talking to neighbors	1.04 (0.97–1.11)
Residential density * social interaction to neighbors	0.97 (0.90–1.05)
Park Density	
Park density * self-efficacy	1.09 (0.84–1.41)
Park density * perceived benefits	1.05 (0.96–1.15)
Park density * perceived barriers	0.83 (0.73–0.94) **
Park density * social support	0.97 (0.89–1.07)
Park density * social norm	0.99 (0.94–1.04)
Park density * modeling	0.97 (0.92–1.02)
Park density * social diversity	0.97 (0.75–1.26)
Park density * social trust and cohesion	1.05 (0.91–1.22)
Park density * talking to neighbors	0.94 (0.85–1.04)
Park density * social interaction to neighbors	1.04 (0.94–1.15)
Public Transport Density	
Public transport density * self-efficacy	1.03 (0.80–1.31)
Public transport density * perceived benefits	1.13 (1.02–1.24) *
Public transport density * perceived barriers	0.98 (0.82–1.16)
Public transport density * social support	1.03 (0.99–1.08)
Public transport density * social norm	1.04 (0.98–1.10)
Public transport density * modeling	1.04 (0.98–1.10)
Public transport density * social diversity	0.94 (0.78–1.12)
Public transport density * social trust and cohesion	1.10 (0.94–1.28)
Public transport density * talking to neighbors	1.07 (0.99–1.16) ^
Public transport density * social interaction to neighbors	1.02 (0.94–1.11)
Intersection Density	
Intersection density * self-efficacy	0.92 (0.69–1.21)
Intersection density * perceived benefits	1.00 (0.91–1.10)
Intersection density * perceived barriers	1.04 (0.87–1.24)
Intersection density * social support	0.94 (0.89–0.99) *
Intersection density * social norm	1.05 (0.96–1.14)
Intersection density * modeling	0.97 (0.93–1.02)
Intersection density * social diversity	0.91 (0.66–1.26)
Intersection density * social trust and cohesion	0.93 (0.78–1.11)
Intersection density * talking to neighbors	1.00 (0.91–1.10)
Intersection density * social interaction to neighbors	0.99 (0.91–1.09)
Entropy	
Entropy * self-efficacy	0.86 (0.61–1.22)
Entropy * perceived benefits	0.87 (0.76–1.00) *
Entropy * perceived barriers	1.25 (1.00–1.54) *
Entropy * social support	0.97 (0.87–1.08)
Entropy * social norm	1.05 (0.92–1.19)
Entropy * modeling	1.01 (0.92–1.10)
Entropy * social diversity	1.04 (0.73–1.47)
Entropy * social trust and cohesion	0.81 (0.69–0.95) *
Entropy * talking to neighbors	0.95 (0.74–1.07)
Entropy * social interaction to neighbors	0.93 (0.88–1.00) *

^ $p < 0.10$; * $p < 0.05$; ** $p < 0.01$; ref = reference category; all single interactions models were adjusted for living status and physical functioning.

References

1. Van Acker Ragnar, V.O. *Samen Sterk Voor Ouderen in Beweging: In de Vrije Tijd Inclusief Sport, Thuis, TIJDENS verplaatsingen en op Het (Vrijwillers) werk. Basisvisie, Werkkader en Inspiratie Voor Vlaamse Middenveldorganisaties Uit Verschillende Sectoren*; Vlaams Instituut Gezond Leven en Vlaamse Ouderenraad: Brussel, Belgium, 2018.

2. World Health Organization. *Physical Activity Strategy for the WHO European Region 2016–2025*; World Health Organization (WHO) Regional Office for Europe: Copenhagen, Denmark, 2015.
3. US Department of Health and Human Services. *2008 Physical Activity Guidelines for Americans*; US Department of Health and Human Services: Hyattsville, MD, USA, 2008.
4. Ison, S.; Shaw, J. *Cycling and Sustainability*; Emerald Group Publishing: Bingley, West Yorkshire, UK, 2012.
5. Rabl, A.; De Nazelle, A. Benefits of shift from car to active transport. *Transp. Policy* **2012**, *19*, 121–131. [CrossRef]
6. De Fré, B.; De Martelaer, K.; Philippaerts, R.; Scheerder, J.; Lefevre, J. Sportparticipatie en fysieke (in) activiteit van de Vlaamse bevolking: Huidige situatie en seculaire trend (2003–2009). In *Participatie in Vlaanderen 2 Eerste Analyse van de Participatiesurvey*; Leuven, J.L.W., Ed.; Acco: The Hague, The Netherlands, 2009.
7. Kelly, P.; Kahlmeier, S.; Götschi, T.; Orsini, N.; Richards, J.; Roberts, N.; Scarborough, P.; Foster, C. Systematic review and meta-analysis of reduction in all-cause mortality from walking and cycling and shape of dose response relationship. *Int. J. Behav. Nutr. Phys. Act.* **2014**, *11*, 1–15. [CrossRef]
8. Coughlin, J.F. Beyond Health and Retirement: Placing Transportation on the Aging Policy Agenda. *Public Policy Aging Rep.* **2001**, *11*, 1–23. [CrossRef]
9. Adler, G.; Rottunda, S. Older adults' perspectives on driving cessation. *J. Aging Stud.* **2006**, *20*, 227–235. [CrossRef]
10. Heesch, K.C.; Giles-Corti, B.; Turrell, G. Cycling for transport and recreation: Associations with socio-economic position, environmental perceptions, and psychological disposition. *Prev. Med.* **2014**, *63*, 29–35. [CrossRef]
11. Van den Berg, P.; Arentze, T.; Timmermans, H. Estimating social travel demand of senior citizens in the Netherlands. *J. Transp. Geogr.* **2011**, *19*, 323–331. [CrossRef]
12. Vlaamse overheid Departement Mobiliteit en Openbare Werken. *Onderzoek Verplaatsingsgedrag Vlaanderen 4*; Vlaamse Overheid, Departement Mobilitieit en Openbare Werken: Brussel, Belgium, 2014.
13. Sallis, J.F.; Cervero, R.B.; Ascher, W.L.; Henderson, K.A.; Kraft, M.K.; Kerr, J. An ecological approach to creating active living communities. *Annu. Rev. Public Health* **2006**, *27*, 297–322. [CrossRef]
14. Spence, J.C.; Lee, R.E. Toward a comprehensive model of physical activity. *Psychol. Sport Exerc.* **2003**, *4*, 7–24. [CrossRef]
15. Cerin, E.; Nathan, A.; Van Cauwenberg, J.; Barnett, D.W.; Barnett, A. The neighbourhood physical environment and active travel in older adults: A systematic review and meta-analysis. *Int. J. Behav. Nutr. Phys. Act.* **2017**, *14*, 1–23. [CrossRef] [PubMed]
16. Hoehner, C.M.; Ramirez, L.K.B.; Elliott, M.B.; Handy, S.L.; Brownson, R.C. Perceived and objective environmental measures and physical activity among urban adults. *Am. J. Prev. Med.* **2005**, *28*, 105–116. [CrossRef] [PubMed]
17. Mertens, L.; Van Dyck, D.; Deforche, B.; De Bourdeaudhuij, I.; Brondeel, R.; Van Cauwenberg, J. Individual, social, and physical environmental factors related to changes in walking and cycling for transport among older adults: A longitudinal study. *Health Place* **2019**, *55*, 120–127. [CrossRef]
18. Kosteli, M.-C.; Williams, S.E.; Cumming, J. Investigating the psychosocial determinants of physical activity in older adults: A qualitative approach. *Psychol. Health* **2016**, *31*, 730–749. [CrossRef] [PubMed]
19. Van Cauwenberg, J.; Cerin, E.; Timperio, A.; Salmon, J.; Deforche, B.; Veitch, J. Park proximity, quality and recreational physical activity among mid-older aged adults: Moderating effects of individual factors and area of residence. *Int. J. Behav. Nutr. Phys. Act.* **2015**, *12*, 46. [CrossRef]
20. Van Cauwenberg, J. Insights into the Complex Interplay between the Environment and Physical Activity Behaviours among Community-Dwelling Older Adults. Ph.D. Thesis, Ghent University, Ghent, Belgium, 2015.
21. Van Cauwenberg, J.; Van Holle, V.; Simons, D.; DeRidder, R.; Clarys, P.; Goubert, L.; Nasar, J.; Salmon, J.; De Bourdeaudhuij, I.; Deforche, B. Environmental factors influencing older adults' walking for transportation: A study using walk-along interviews. *Int. J. Behav. Nutr. Phys. Act.* **2012**, *9*, 85. [CrossRef]
22. Van Cauwenberg, J.; Clarys, P.; De Bourdeaudhuij, I.; Ghekiere, A.; De Geus, B.; Owen, N.; Deforche, B. Environmental influences on older adults' transportation cycling experiences: A study using bike-along interviews. *Landsc. Urban Plan.* **2018**, *169*, 37–46. [CrossRef]
23. Van Holle, V.; Van Cauwenberg, J.; Van Dyck, D.; Deforche, B.; Van De Weghe, N.; De Bourdeaudhuij, I. Relationship between neighborhood walkability and older adults' physical activity: Results from the Belgian Environmental Physical Activity Study in Seniors (BEPAS Seniors). *Int. J. Behav. Nutr. Phys. Act.* **2014**, *11*, 1–9. [CrossRef] [PubMed]
24. Ware, J.; Sherbourne, C. A 36-item short form health survey (SF-36): Results from the Medical Outcomes Study. *Med. Care* **1992**, *30*, 473–483. [CrossRef] [PubMed]
25. Frank, L.D.; Saelens, B.E.; Powell, K.E.; Chapman, J.E. Stepping towards causation: Do built environments or neighborhood and travel preferences explain physical activity, driving, and obesity? *Soc. Sci. Med.* **2007**, *65*, 1898–1914. [CrossRef]
26. IPAQ. International Physical Activity Questionnaire. Long. last 7 days self-Adm. Format 71. 2002. Available online: www.ipaq.ki.se (accessed on 15 September 2010).
27. Rzewnicki, R.; Auweele, Y.V.; De Bourdeaudhuij, I. Addressing overreporting on the International Physical Activity Questionnaire (IPAQ) telephone survey with a population sample. *Public Health Nutr.* **2003**, *6*, 299–305. [CrossRef]
28. Van Holle, V.; De Bourdeaudhuij, I.; Deforche, B.; Van Cauwenberg, J.; Van Dyck, D. Assessment of physical activity in older Belgian adults: Validity and reliability of an adapted interview version of the long International Physical Activity Questionnaire (IPAQ-L). *BMC Public Health* **2015**, *15*, 1–14. [CrossRef]

29. Van Holle, V.; Van Cauwenberg, J.; Deforche, B.; Van De Weghe, N.; De Bourdeaudhuij, I.; Van Dyck, D. Do psychosocial factors moderate the association between objective neighborhood walkability and older adults' physical activity? *Health Place* **2015**, *34*, 118–125. [CrossRef]
30. Van Dyck, D.; Cardon, G.; Deforche, B.; Giles-Corti, B.; Sallis, J.F.; Owen, N.; De Bourdeaudhuij, I. Environmental and Psychosocial Correlates of Accelerometer-Assessed and Self-Reported Physical Activity in Belgian Adults. *Int. J. Behav. Med.* **2011**, *18*, 235–245. [CrossRef] [PubMed]
31. De Bourdeaudhuij, I.; Sallis, J. Relative Contribution of Psychosocial Variables to the Explanation of Physical Activity in Three Population-Based Adult Samples. *Prev. Med.* **2002**, *34*, 279–288. [CrossRef]
32. Lochner, K.; Kawachi, I.; Kennedy, B.P. Social capital: A guide to its measurement. *Health Place* **1999**, *5*, 259–270. [CrossRef]
33. Unger, D.G.; Wandersman, A. The importance of neighbors: The social, cognitive, and affective components of neighboring. *Am. J. Community Psychol.* **1985**, *13*, 139–169. [CrossRef]
34. Sampson, R.J.; Raudenbush, S.W.; Earls, F. Neighborhoods and Violent Crime: A Multilevel Study of Collective Efficacy. *Science* **1997**, *277*, 918–924. [CrossRef]
35. Van Cauwenberg, J.; De Donder, L.; Clarys, P.; De Bourdeaudhuij, I.; Buffel, T.; De Witte, N.; Dury, S.; Verté, D.; Deforche, B. Relationships between the perceived neighborhood social environment and walking for transportation among older adults. *Soc. Sci. Med.* **2014**, *104*, 23–30. [CrossRef]
36. Van Holle, V.; Van Cauwenberg, J.; De Bourdeaudhuij, I.; Deforche, B.; Van De Weghe, N.; Van Dyck, D. Interactions between Neighborhood Social Environment and Walkability to Explain Belgian Older Adults' Physical Activity and Sedentary Time. *Int. J. Environ. Res. Public Health* **2016**, *13*, 569. [CrossRef]
37. Carlson, J.A.; Sallis, J.F.; Conway, T.L.; Saelens, B.E.; Frank, L.D.; Kerr, J.; Cain, K.L.; King, A.C. Interactions between psychosocial and built environment factors in explaining older adults' physical activity. *Prev. Med.* **2012**, *54*, 68–73. [CrossRef]
38. Gómez, L.F.; Parra, D.C.; Buchner, D.; Brownson, R.C.; Sarmiento, O.L.; Pinzón, J.D.; Ardila, M.; Moreno, J.; Serrato, M.; Lobelo, F. Built Environment Attributes and Walking Patterns Among the Elderly Population in Bogotá. *Am. J. Prev. Med.* **2010**, *38*, 592–599. [CrossRef] [PubMed]
39. Dobesova, Z.; Krivka, T. Walkability Index in the Urban Planning: A Case Study in Olomouc City. In *Advances in Spatial Planning*; Burian, J., Ed.; IntechOpen: Rijeka, Croatia, 2012; pp. 179–197. [CrossRef]
40. Frank, L.D.; Sallis, J.F.; Saelens, B.E.; Leary, L.; Cain, K.; Conway, T.L.; Hess, P.M. The development of a walkability index: Application to the Neighborhood Quality of Life Study. *Br. J. Sports Med.* **2010**, *44*, 924–933. [CrossRef]
41. Rosenstock, I.M. Historical Origins of the Health Belief Model. *Health Educ. Monogr.* **1974**, *2*, 328–335. [CrossRef]
42. Josey, M.J.; Moore, S. The influence of social networks and the built environment on physical inactivity: A longitudinal study of urban-dwelling adults. *Health Place* **2018**, *54*, 62–68. [CrossRef]
43. Alves, S.; Aspinall, P.A.; Thompson, C.W.; Sugiyama, T.; Brice, R.; Vickers, A. Preferences of older people for environmental attributes of local parks. *Facilities* **2008**, *26*, 433–453. [CrossRef]
44. Parra, D.C.; Gomez, L.F.; Fleischer, N.L.; Pinzon, J.D. Built environment characteristics and perceived active park use among older adults: Results from a multilevel study in Bogotá. *Health Place* **2010**, *16*, 1174–1181. [CrossRef] [PubMed]
45. Van Holle, V.; McNaughton, S.A.; Teychenne, M.; Timperio, A.; Van Dyck, D.; De Bourdeaudhuij, I.; Salmon, J. Social and Physical Environmental Correlates of Adults' Weekend Sitting Time and Moderating Effects of Retirement Status and Physical Health. *Int. J. Environ. Res. Public Health* **2014**, *11*, 9790–9810. [CrossRef]
46. Baert, V.; Gorus, E.; Mets, T.; Geerts, C.; Bautmans, I. Motivators and barriers for physical activity in the oldest old: A systematic review. *Ageing Res. Rev.* **2011**, *10*, 464–474. [CrossRef]
47. Bandura, A. *Self-Efficacy: The Exercise of Control*; W.H. Freeman: New York, NY, USA, 1997. [CrossRef]
48. Michael, Y.L.; Green, M.K.; Farquhar, S.A. Neighborhood design and active aging. *Health Place* **2006**, *12*, 734–740. [CrossRef]
49. Van Cauwenberg, J.; Clarys, P.; De Bourdeaudhuij, I.; Van Holle, V.; Verté, D.; De Witte, N.; De Donder, L.; Buffel, T.; Dury, S.; Deforche, B. Physical environmental factors related to walking and cycling in older adults: The Belgian aging studies. *BMC Public Health* **2012**, *12*, 142. [CrossRef] [PubMed]
50. Nathan, A.; Pereira, G.; Foster, S.; Hooper, P.; Saarloos, D.; Giles-Corti, B. Access to commercial destinations within the neighbourhood and walking among Australian older adults. *Int. J. Behav. Nutr. Phys. Act.* **2012**, *9*, 133. [CrossRef]
51. Cerin, E.; Lee, K.-Y.; Barnett, A.; Sit, C.H.P.; Cheung, M.-C.; Chan, W.-M.; Johnston, J.M. Walking for transportation in Hong Kong Chinese urban elders: A cross-sectional study on what destinations matter and when. *Int. J. Behav. Nutr. Phys. Act.* **2013**, *10*, 78. [CrossRef]
52. Matthews, C.; Welk, G. Use of self-report instruments to assess physical activity. *Phys. Act. Assess. Health Relat. Res.* **2002**, *107*, 123.
53. Van Dyck, D.; Cardon, G.; Deforche, B.; De Bourdeaudhuij, I. IPAQ interview version: Convergent validity with accelerome-ters and comparison of physical activity and sedentary time levels with the self-administered version. *J. Sports Med. Phys. Fit.* **2015**, *55*, 776–786.
54. Bouter, L.M.; Zielhuis, G.; Zeegers, M.P. *Textbook of Epidemiology*, 1st ed.; Bohn Stafleu van Loghum: Houten, The Netherlands, 2018.
55. Giles-Corti, B.; Timperio, A.; Bull, F.; Pikora, T. Understanding physical activity environmental correlates: Increased specific-ity for ecological models. *Exerc. Sport Sci. Rev.* **2005**, *33*, 175–181. [CrossRef]

56. Dill, J.; Gliebe, J. Understanding and Measuring Bicycling Behavior: A Focus on Travel Time and Route Choice. Oregon Transportation Research and Education Consortium. 2008. Available online: https://pdxscholar.library.pdx.edu/usp_fac/28/ (accessed on 10 January 2021).
57. Carlson, J.A.; Jankowska, M.M.; Meseck, K.; Godbole, S.; Natarajan, L.; Raab, F.; Demchak, B.; Patrick, K.; Kerr, J. Validity of PALMS GPS Scoring of Active and Passive Travel Compared with SenseCam. *Med. Sci. Sports Exerc.* **2015**, *47*, 662–667. [CrossRef]
58. Huss, A.; Beekhuizen, J.; Kromhout, H.; Vermeulen, R. Using GPS-derived speed patterns for recognition of transport modes in adults. *Int. J. Health Geogr.* **2014**, *13*, 40. [CrossRef]
59. Eellis, K.; Egodbole, S.; Emarshall, S.; Elanckriet, G.; Estaudenmayer, J.; Ekerr, J. Identifying Active Travel Behaviors in Challenging Environments Using GPS, Accelerometers, and Machine Learning Algorithms. *Front. Public Health* **2014**, *2*, 36. [CrossRef]

MDPI
St. Alban-Anlage 66
4052 Basel
Switzerland
Tel. +41 61 683 77 34
Fax +41 61 302 89 18
www.mdpi.com

International Journal of Environmental Research and Public Health Editorial Office
E-mail: ijerph@mdpi.com
www.mdpi.com/journal/ijerph

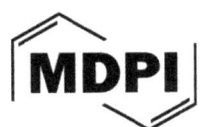

www.ingramcontent.com/pod-product-compliance
Lightning Source LLC
LaVergne TN
LVHW070251100526
838202LV00015B/2206